Psychiatry

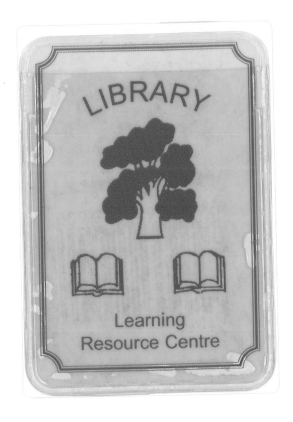

LIBRARY

Learning
Resource Centre

PSYCHIATRY

THIRD EDITION

Janis L. Cutler, MD

Professor of Psychiatry at Columbia University Medical Center
Director of Medical Student Education, College of Physicians
and Surgeons of Columbia University and New York State
Psychiatric Institute
Faculty, Columbia University Center
for Psychoanalytic Training and Research

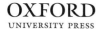
OXFORD
UNIVERSITY PRESS

OXFORD
UNIVERSITY PRESS

Oxford University Press is a department of the University of
Oxford. It furthers the University's objective of excellence in research,
scholarship, and education by publishing worldwide.

Oxford   New York
Auckland   Cape Town   Dar es Salaam   Hong Kong   Karachi
Kuala Lumpur   Madrid   Melbourne   Mexico City   Nairobi
New Delhi   Shanghai   Taipei   Toronto

With offices in
Argentina   Austria   Brazil   Chile   Czech Republic   France   Greece
Guatemala   Hungary   Italy   Japan   Poland   Portugal   Singapore
South Korea   Switzerland   Thailand   Turkey   Ukraine   Vietnam

Oxford is a registered trademark of Oxford University Press
in the UK and certain other countries.

Published in the United States of America by
Oxford University Press
198 Madison Avenue, New York, NY 10016

Library of Congress Cataloging-in-Publication Data
Psychiatry (Cutler)
Psychiatry / [edited by] Janis L. Cutler.—Third edition.
     p. ; cm.
Includes bibliographical references and index.
ISBN 978–0–19–932607–5 (alk. paper)
I. Cutler, Janis L., editor of compilation.   II. Title.
[DNLM: 1. Mental Disorders. WM 140]
RC454
616.89—dc23
2013042497

The science of medicine is a rapidly changing field. As new research and clinical experience broaden
our knowledge, changes in treatment and drug therapy occur. The author and publisher of this
work have checked with sources believed to be reliable in their efforts to provide information that
is accurate and complete, and in accordance with the standards accepted at the time of publication.
However, in light of the possibility of human error or changes in the practice of medicine, neither
the author, nor the publisher, nor any other party who has been involved in the preparation or
publication of this work warrants that the information contained herein is in every respect accurate
or complete. Readers are encouraged to confirm the information contained herein with other
reliable sources, and are strongly advised to check the product information sheet provided by the
pharmaceutical company for each drug they plan to administer.

9 8 7 6 5 4 3 2 1
Printed in the United States of America
on acid-free paper

To RCP, with love

CONTENTS

Acknowledgments	ix
Contributors	xi
Introduction	xv

1. **Psychiatric Assessment and Treatment Planning** — 1
   Janis L. Cutler

2. **The Psychiatric Interview** — 22
   Anand Desai and Lyle Rosnick

3. **Mood Disorders** — 46
   Licínia Ganança, David A. Kahn, and Maria A. Oquendo

4. **Schizophrenia and Other Psychotic Disorders** — 97
   Matthew D. Erlich, Thomas E. Smith, Ewald Horwath, and Francine Cournos

5. **Neurocognitive Disorders and Mental Disorders Due to Another Medical Condition** — 129
   Jennifer M. Rucci and Robert E. Feinstein

6. **Anxiety, Obsessive-Compulsive, and Stress Disorders** — 168
   Franklin R. Schneier, Hilary B. Vidair, Leslie R. Vogel, and Philip R. Muskin

7. **Substance-Related and Addictive Disorders** — 204
   Benjamin R. Bryan and Frances R. Levin

8. **Personality Disorders** — 257
   Eve Caligor, Frank Yeomans, and Ze'ev Levin

9. **Feeding and Eating Disorders** — 291
   Michael J. Devlin and Joanna E. Steinglass

10. **Somatic Symptom and Related Disorders** — 323
    Kelli Jane K. Harding and Brian A. Fallon

11. **Psychological Factors Affecting Medical Conditions**   351
    Sara Siris Nash, Lucy Hutner, and Eve Caligor

12. **Suicide**   387
    Brian Rothberg and Robert E. Feinstein

13. **Violence**   403
    Robert E. Feinstein and Brian Rothberg

14. **Child, Adolescent, and Adult Development**   418
    Jonathan A. Slater, Katharine A. Stratigos, and Janis L. Cutler

15. **Child and Adolescent Psychiatry**   456
    *Daniel T. Chrzanowski, Elisabeth B. Guthrie, Matthew B. Perkins,
    and Moira A. Rynn*

16. **Pharmacotherapy, ECT, and TMS**   513
    Jessica Ann Stewart, L. Mark Russakoff, and Jonathan W. Stewart

17. **Psychotherapy**   557
    David D. Olds and Fredric N. Busch

Index   611

ACKNOWLEDGMENTS

I am fortunate to have spent my entire psychiatric career in the Department of Psychiatry at the College of Physicians and Surgeons of Columbia University and New York State Psychiatric Institute. I am grateful to the medical school and departmental leadership, my faculty colleagues, and the bright, idealistic, intellectually curious medical students with whom I have had the privilege of working. In particular, I would like to thank Dr. Jeffrey Lieberman, Department Chair, and Dr. Maria Oquendo, Vice-chair for Education, for their support of medical student education, as well as Dr. Ronald Rieder, previous Vice-chair for Education, for his support and mentorship. Dr. Eric Marcus, Director of the Columbia University Psychoanalytic Center for Training and Research, inspired and co-edited the previous two editions of *Psychiatry*. He is an exemplary role model of a great teacher who has devoted his career to psychiatric education.

I have also had the good fortune to learn about psychiatry and psychiatric education from my colleagues nationwide in the Association for Directors of Medical Student Education in Psychiatry. I am grateful for their enthusiasm and creativity. In particular I would like to thank Dr. John Spollen for his suggestions with regard to the reorganization of the Suicide and Violence chapters.

Edith White deserves special recognition and gratitude for her long-standing role as administrator for the Division of Medical Student Education. It has been a pleasure to work with Christopher Reid and Craig Panner of Oxford University Press. Finally, the continued support of my family makes the work worthwhile. Special thanks and appreciation go to Dr. Reed Perron and Alexander and Joshua Weiss.

CONTRIBUTORS

Benjamin R. Bryan, MD
Instructor in Clinical Psychiatry
College of Physicians and Surgeons of
    Columbia University
New York, NY

Fredric N. Busch, MD
Clinical Professor of Psychiatry
Weill Cornell Medical College
Faculty, Columbia University Center for
    Psychoanalytic Training and Research
New York, NY

Eve Caligor, MD
Clinical Professor of Psychiatry
NYU School of Medicine
Director, Psychotherapy Division
Columbia University Center for
    Psychoanalytic Training and Research
New York, NY

Daniel T. Chrzanowski, MD
Assistant Clinical Professor of Psychiatry
College of Physicians and Surgeons of
    Columbia University
New York, NY

Francine Cournos, MD
Professor of Clinical Psychiatry (in
    Epidemiology)
Mailman School of Public Health,
    Columbia University
New York, NY

Janis L. Cutler, MD
Professor of Psychiatry at Columbia
    University Medical Center
Director of Medical Student Education in
    Psychiatry
College of Physicians and Surgeons of
    Columbia University and New York
    State Psychiatric Institute
Faculty, Columbia University Psychoanalytic
    Center for Training and Research
New York, NY

Anand Desai, MD
Assistant Clinical Professor of Psychiatry
College of Physicians and Surgeons of
    Columbia University and New York
    State Psychiatric Institute
New York, NY

Michael J. Devlin, MD
Professor of Clinical Psychiatry
College of Physicians and Surgeons of
    Columbia University
Associate Director, Eating Disorders
    Research Unit
New York State Psychiatric Institute
Attending Psychiatrist, New York
    Presbyterian Hospital, Columbia
    University Medical Center
New York, NY

Matthew D. Erlich, MD
Assistant Professor of Clinical Psychiatry
College of Physicians and Surgeons of
    Columbia University
Director, OMH Consultation Service
New York State Office of Mental Health
New York, NY

Brian A. Fallon, MD
Professor of Psychiatry at Columbia
    University Medical Center
Director, Center for Neuroinflammatory
    Disorders and Biobehavioral Medicine
New York State Psychiatric Institute
Director, Lyme & Tick-Borne Diseases
    Research Center
Columbia University Medical Center
New York, NY

Robert E. Feinstein, MD
Professor of Psychiatry
Vice Chair of Clinical Education Quality
    & Safety
Practice Director Psychiatry
University of Colorado Hospital
Aurora, CO

Licínia Ganança, MD
Columbia University
Division of Molecular Imaging and
    Neuropathology
New York State Psychiatric Institute
New York, NY

Elisabeth B. Guthrie, MD
Associate Professor of Psychiatry and
    Pediatrics at Columbia University
    Medical Center
Associate Director, New York Presbyterian
    Child and Adolescent Psychiatry
    Residency Training Program of
    Columbia and Cornell Universities
New York, NY

Kelli Jane K. Harding, MD
Assistant Professor of Psychiatry at
    Columbia University Medical Center
Emergency Psychiatry Attending
NY-Presbyterian Hospital/
    Columbia Campus
New York, NY

Ewald Horwath, MD, MS
Professor and Chair, Department of
    Psychiatry
Case Western Reserve University
The Metro Health System
Cleveland, OH

Lucy Hutner, MD
Assistant Professor of Psychiatry
Associate Director of Residency Training
NYU School of Medicine
Adjunct Assistant Clinical Professor of
    Psychiatry
College of Physicians and Surgeons of
    Columbia University
New York, NY

David A. Kahn, MD
Diane Goldman Kemper Family Professor
    of Psychiatry Emeritus
Columbia University Medical Center
New York, NY

Frances R. Levin, MD
Kennedy-Leavy Professor of Psychiatry at
    Columbia University Medical Center
New York State Psychiatric Institute
New York, NY

Ze'ev Levin, MD
Clinical Professor of Psychiatry
NYU School of Medicine
New York, NY

Philip R. Muskin, MD
Professor of Psychiatry
Columbia University Medical Center
Chief, Consultation-Liaison Psychiatry
NY-Presbyterian Hospital/
    Columbia Campus
Faculty, Columbia University
    Psychoanalytic Center
Research Psychiatrist, New York State
    Psychiatric Institute
New York, NY

Sara Siris Nash, MD
Assistant Professor of Psychiatry
Consultation Liaison Division
Columbia University Medical Center
New York, NY

David D. Olds, MD
Clinical Professor of Psychiatry
College of Physicians and Surgeons of
Columbia University
New York, NY

Maria A. Oquendo, MD
Professor of Psychiatry and Vice-Chair for
Education
Columbia University Medical Center
Research Psychiatrist, New York State
Psychiatric Institute
Residency Training Director, Department
of Psychiatry
College of Physicians and Surgeons of
Columbia University
New York, NY

Matthew B. Perkins, MD, MBA, MPH
Medical Director, Division of Children and
Family Services
New York State Office of Mental Health
New York, NY

Lyle Rosnick, MD
Assistant Professor of Clinical Psychiatry
College of Physicians and Surgeons of
Columbia University
Assistant Attending Psychiatrist, New York
Presbyterian Hospital, Columbia
University Medical Center
Faculty, Columbia University
Psychoanalytic Center for Training and
Research
New York, NY

Brian Rothberg, MD
Assistant Professor
University of Colorado School of Medicine
Aurora, CO

Jennifer M. Rucci, MD
OnsiteCare
Director of Mental Health
Charlotte, NC
Davis Regional Medical Center
Attending psychiatrist
Statesville, NC

L. Mark Russakoff, MD
Director of Psychiatry
Phelps Memorial Hospital Center
Sleepy Hollow, NY

Moira A. Rynn, MD
Chief, Division of Child and Adolescent
Psychiatry
Associate Professor of Clinical Psychiatry
College of Physicians and Surgeons of
Columbia University and New York
State Psychiatric Institute
New York, NY

Franklin R. Schneier, MD
Professor of Psychiatry
Columbia University Medical Center
Research Scientist, New York State
Psychiatric Institute
New York, NY

Jonathan A. Slater, MD
Clinical Professor of Psychiatry
College of Physicians and Surgeons of
Columbia University
Director, Consultation and Emergency
Service
Morgan Stanley Children's Hospital of
New York
New York, NY

Thomas E. Smith, MD
Associate Professor of Psychiatry
Columbia University Medical Center
New York, NY

Joanna E. Steinglass, MD
Assistant Professor
Columbia University Medical Center
New York State Psychiatric Institute
New York, NY

Jessica Ann Stewart, MD
Clinical Fellow in Child and Adolescent
Psychiatry
New York Presbyterian Hospital
New York, NY

Jonathan W. Stewart, MD
Professor of Clinical Psychiatry
College of Physicians and Surgeons of
Columbia University
Research Psychiatrist, New York State
Psychiatric Institute
New York, NY

Katharine A. Stratigos, MD
Assistant Clinical Professor of Psychiatry
College of Physicians and Surgeons of
  Columbia University
New York, NY

Hilary B. Vidair, PhD
Co-Director of Clinical Training
Assistant Professor, Clinical Psychology
  Doctoral Program
Long Island University
Brookville, NY

Leslie R. Vogel, MD
Private Practice
New York, NY

Frank Yeomans, MD
Clinical Associate Professor of Psychiatry
Director of Training
Personality Disorders Institute
Weill Medical College of Cornell
  University
Adjunct Associate Professor
Columbia University Psychoanalytic
  Center for Training and Research
New York, NY

INTRODUCTION

Psychiatry is the field of medicine that concerns itself with those illnesses that have emotional or behavioral manifestations. Psychiatric illnesses are extremely common and exact a great personal and social cost in disability, suffering, and even death. This book is intended as an introductory text that prepares medical students, physicians, and other health professionals for the clinical task of working with psychiatric patients. As such, it emphasizes recognition and assessment of psychiatric illness. The text's clinical orientation is equally well suited for medical students during their preclinical introduction to psychiatry course and core psychiatry clerkship, as well as nonpsychiatric physicians, psychiatric residents, and other health professionals who work with patients with psychiatric disorders, including psychologists, social workers, nurses, and occupational therapists.

Patients with emotional and behavioral difficulties are often discouraged from seeking help by the stigma that they, their families, and even physicians tend to attach to psychiatric illnesses. All health care providers should be sensitive to the shame that patients with psychiatric problems may have. Being well informed about the signs and symptoms of the most common psychiatric disorders improves the physician's chances of recognizing these disorders in patients. Familiarity with the course and prognosis of these conditions enhances the ability to refer patients for appropriate treatment and to complete the first step in the referral process, which is frequently education and reassurance.

The first two chapters in the book provide a framework for the evaluation of psychiatric patients, focusing on clinical assessment and the psychiatric interview. These chapters demonstrate how to obtain and synthesize clinical data and generate an appropriate differential diagnosis and treatment plan. Subsequent chapters cover the major psychiatric disorders; the special topics of suicide, violence, and the medically ill patient; and an overview of the stages of child, adolescent, and adult development. An additional chapter is devoted to the assessment and treatment of children and adolescents. The book concludes with chapters covering pharmacotherapy and psychotherapy.

DIAGNOSTIC AND CLINICAL FEATURES

The use of diagnostic categories has a particular history in psychiatry, and over the past several decades, the field has been concerned with improving diagnostic reliability and consistency. Throughout this book, reference is made to the *Diagnostic and Statistical Manual of Mental Disorders*, 5th edition (DSM-5), which is published by the American Psychiatric Association, the professional organization of psychiatrists in the United States. The publication of the DSM-5 in 2013 incorporates a more dimensional approach to psychiatric diagnosis. Previous editions of the DSM had used a polythetic approach (i.e., more than one combination of symptoms will qualify for a particular diagnosis). The aim of the DSM system is descriptive. It is the best and most widely referenced psychiatric diagnostic system currently available. It is not, however, a perfect system but rather an evolving one. Ultimately, the criteria are intended only as guidelines for physicians who must use their own best judgment in making an appropriate diagnosis.

THE INTERVIEW

In all of medicine the clinical interview is the basis by which diagnoses are made and therapeutic alliances between patients and physicians are forged. Even in this age of advanced medical technology, no sophisticated test can take the place of a careful, complete history that is empathically obtained. Clinical interviewing as a sophisticated art is perhaps nowhere more apparent than in psychiatry. The central importance of the clinical psychiatric interview is reflected in the central positioning of a section devoted to the interview, accompanied by Interviewing Guideline summaries, in each disorder chapter.

ETIOLOGY

As in the rest of medicine, the description of psychiatric syndromes and their effective treatments has generally preceded an understanding of their pathophysiology and etiology. The past several decades has witnessed an explosion in the understanding of some of the neurobiological mechanisms that underlie many psychiatric disorders. Advances in neuroimaging, molecular genetics, and other basic science techniques hold the promise for even more knowledge in the not too distant future. But enthusiasm must be tempered by the sobering realization that the mind and the ways in which it can become disturbed are exceedingly complex—so much so that, for example, researchers struggling to understand the etiology of schizophrenia have compiled many probably significant but currently isolated observations and thus do not seem to be much closer to solving the mystery of how and why 1% of the world's population is afflicted with this devastating illness.

Some in the field have worried that the emphasis on neurobiology has replaced the previous tradition of the biopsychosocial model, which attempts to consider the whole patient, encompassing a biologically endowed human being with a particular psychology and social context. Psychiatrists continue to struggle with the issue of how much of an effect external factors such as family, environment, and psychic trauma have on the onset and course of psychiatric disorders. A fundamental assumption of this book is that, in the "nature versus nurture" debate, both sides have validity: Genetic loading and intrauterine exposure may play important roles in the etiology of many psychiatric disorders, but interpersonal, developmental, and other "nurture" issues seem to be crucial as well.

TREATMENT

Patients come to physicians and other health professionals to receive help. Treatment planning requires a collaborative effort between patient and clinician. While detailed treatment guidelines are beyond the scope of this book, a summary of specific treatment options available for each of the major psychiatric illnesses, including psychotherapeutic and pharmacotherapeutic modalities, is provided. Psychiatry's strong clinical tradition should serve its patients and the entire field of medicine well. It is the intent of this book to provide the practicing clinician with a foundation that is biopsychosocially based and psychiatrically well informed.

USE OF THE BOOK

We have strived to maintain an appropriate balance between thoroughness and ease of use. Clinical illustrations, included to bring the material to life, are set off from the main text. Essential information is highlighted in tables and with key words to allow *Psychiatry*'s use as a resource for successful exam preparation.

/// 1 /// Psychiatric Assessment and Treatment Planning

JANIS L. CUTLER

When patients come to physicians with complaints and concerns, they hope to receive help, comfort, and information. They do not necessarily think in terms of diseases or syndromes, and they frequently do not know what information about themselves and their problems physicians need to have. Patients initially describe and organize their complaints and concerns in a way that makes sense to themselves. The presentation varies from patient to patient and is affected by many factors, including their medical knowledge, level of anxiety, coping and defense mechanisms, and attitude toward physicians. Physicians should listen to the complaints from the patient's perspective and add their own questions and observations to develop a complete picture of the patient's problems, resources, and strengths, which will facilitate treatment planning. In psychiatric assessment, both the diagnosis (which categorizes conditions according to signs and symptoms) and the description of patients' strengths and vulnerabilities (i.e., what makes them unique) play important roles in determining the best treatment approach.

The psychiatric case write-up is an essential means of communication among health care professionals who may be involved in the patient's treatment. It also serves as documentation of the physician's evaluation (patients and other parties, such as insurance companies and the courts, may be able to gain access to the written psychiatric case formulation, which is a legal and official part of patients' medical records).

The case write-up should reflect the process of case formulation and involves a number of steps, which also serve to organize the write-up (see Figure 1.1). The focus varies, depending on the **setting** in which the patient is being evaluated and the **goals** of the interview (which relate to the chief complaint). The quantity and depth of information in the case write-up also vary. The write-up may be based on a brief emergency room interview, a one-hour outpatient visit, an extensive outpatient evaluation consisting of several sessions, or days to weeks of inpatient sessions. In general, the less time spent with the patient, the less information available for the assessment and the more questions that will be left unanswered in the formulation. The written record may be an admission note to an inpatient unit or day program, an off-service note (summarizing treatment by the previous staff when psychiatrists change), an outpatient evaluation summary, or a discharge

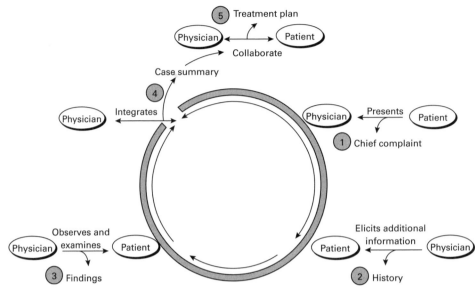

FIGURE 1.1 Steps in creating the case write-up. (1) The patient presents the chief complaint to the physician. (2) As the interview proceeds, the physician elicits additional information from the patient in order to obtain the history of the present illness and the past psychiatric history, medical history, psychosocial history, and family history. The physician also conducts a review of systems. (3) Findings from the physical examination, mental status examination (including how the patient relates to the physician), and laboratory and other test results are collected. (4) The physician then integrates all of the information and generates a descriptive and diagnostic impression. (5) Together, the patient and physician create a theoretically sound and feasible treatment plan.

summary (a review of completed treatment course, usually of an inpatient). Every institution has its own requirements and vocabularies for case formulations, but the objectives are always the same: the case write-up communicates the physician's understanding of a patient and his or her needs to other clinical staff persons and helps the physician and staff crystallize this information and integrate it into a treatment plan.

A psychiatric case write-up is recorded in the same format as a medical case write-up, with some modifications (see Table 1.1). If a patient is seen more than once, additional sections may be added to indicate the course of the patient throughout the evaluation process or hospital admission, including all changes in symptoms and functioning.

The case material is rarely organized in the way the patient presents it in the interview. In fact, beyond the basic headings, almost invariably it is not. The written record more closely reflects the organization and thought processes of the physician as he or she comes to understand and integrate the patient's problems. The interview and the written formulation do, however, begin at the same place: the chief complaint.

CHIEF COMPLAINT

The chief complaint is the reason the patient gives for seeking help. It does not necessarily reflect the problem that the patient needs help with most—in fact, the chief complaint may be misleading (see Box 1.1). Patients with the same disorder may nonetheless

TABLE 1.1 Components of the Case Write-up

Identifying information (ID)
    Age
    Relationship/marital status
    Occupation/source of support
Chief complaint (CC)
History
    History of the present illness (HPI)
    Past psychiatric history
    Past medical history (PMH)
    Current medications
    Review of systems (ROS)
    Psychosocial history
    Family history (FH)
Findings
    Physical examination (PE)
    Mental status examination (MSE)
    Laboratory and other tests
Impression
    Case summary
    Differential diagnosis
    Predisposing and precipitating factors
Treatment plan
Prognosis

BOX 1.1
MISLEADING CHIEF COMPLAINTS

A patient who complains of feeling "nervous," a seemingly innocuous symptom, may be suffering from a number of psychiatric disorders, ranging from depression to psychosis. A man whose chief complaint is that he is "losing his mind" is just as likely, if not more so, to be suffering from panic attacks as from psychosis. One elderly man who had little formal education, no history of mental illness, and a tendency to be unaware of his emotional state gave this initial description of what turned out to be a clear-cut case of depression: "I'm not long for this world—I'm very weak, I have a funny feeling in my stomach, my head is full, I can't eat or sleep."

BOX 1.2

DIFFERENT CHIEF COMPLAINTS FOR IDENTICAL PROBLEMS

Two middle-aged women noticed breast lumps and made appointments with their internists. One woman's chief complaint was fatigue. She "forgot" the lump until her physician began to examine her. At that time, she mentioned the lump, which was of much more concern to her, and to her physician, than the fatigue, which may have been related to her worry about the lump and may not have had a more specific basis. The second woman's "chief complaint" was the lump, which she talked about in a straightforward manner, complete with her own assessment of the diagnostic possibilities.

Arriving at an overall formulation for these two patients involves different processes, although the "differential diagnosis" is the same: cyst, benign tumor, or malignant tumor. For one patient, the true chief complaint is easily identified; for the other, it nearly slips by without mention. Each woman's unique response to her anxiety-provoking symptom is reflected in her presenting complaint and should be included in the case summary and overall formulation: one woman tends to use denial as a coping mechanism when she is under stress; the other, intellectualization (see Box 17.3, Chapter 17, Psychotherapy). Their different responses will also be reflected in their treatment plans. The denial of the first patient could impede a prompt workup and should be regarded as part of the problem, not necessarily to be changed but certainly to be kept in mind. The intellectualization of the second patient can be regarded as a strength to be used by her and her physician as the evaluation proceeds. If both of these women are eventually diagnosed with invasive cancer with widespread metastases, a defensive personality style that had been detrimental could become a strength, and vice versa (denial may be helpful when a patient is facing a terminal illness, whereas intellectualization, although it contributes to the patient's understanding of the illness, may block an associated emotional reaction and make the patient more vulnerable to depression).

---

give entirely different chief complaints (see Box 1.2). The chief complaint is generally recorded in the patient's own words.

HISTORY

History of the Present Illness

The physician begins the interview by eliciting the history of the present illness, starting with the chief complaint (keeping in mind that it may be misleading) and working backward. The physician allows the interview to follow any number of different paths, depending on the patient's leads and the physician's intuition, in order to develop a **chronological, systematic outline** of the **signs and symptoms** of the current episode, which culminated in the patient's decision to come for help. Explanations as to why the patient has come for help at this time (i.e., **why *now***) and why the need for help is presented in the way that it is are crucial to the history. Only when this history-taking process is complete do the "present illness" and its chronology become apparent. The history of the present illness is best composed after the differential diagnosis has been generated because the history should support the differential diagnosis. Attempting to complete the written assessment while interviewing the patient usually results in a confused record that lacks the integration and synthesis required, by definition, for a formulation, because the physician has not had sufficient time to process the information before recording it.

If the patient's current episode of illness exists within the context of a chronic psychiatric syndrome, the history of the present illness can begin with the symptoms of the first episode of illness ever experienced, *or* with the current exacerbation, leaving the early symptoms and previous episodes to be summarized in the past history. If the diagnosis is unclear or should be modified, it may be most useful for the history of the present illness to cover the entire illness course of the illness. If the diagnosis has been clearly established, previous episodes can be summarized in the past psychiatric history section. In addition, if the current episode is complex, it may be simplest to include previous episodes in the past history.

Eliciting a history from patients with **personality disorders** is often challenging because the maladaptive patterns of behavior and emotional responses characteristic of personality disorders tend to be **egosyntonic** (i.e., understood by the individual as part of her or his personality and not the result of a disease process), in contrast to the egodystonic symptoms characteristic of most other psychiatric disorders, which patients regard as foreign and separate from themselves. Patients with personality disorders may have great difficulty in articulating their problems (see Chapter 8, Personality Disorders). When a personality disorder is suspected, the physician should conduct the interview in a way that allows the patient's **interpersonal relationships,** as well as certain aspects of his or her inner life, to be assessed (see Box 1.3).

The history of the present illness should include **brief specific examples** to illustrate particular problems. **Pertinent negatives** should be included as well. The list of symptoms and conditions that have not been present should not be all-inclusive. In fact, not all of the information obtained in the interview should be recorded. Instead, positive and negative findings should be of sufficient detail to provide someone reading it with the information necessary to generate a case formulation but should not contain extraneous information. It can be a challenge to know what is important and what is not, what fits a particular clinical pattern and should be highlighted, what fits but is of secondary importance, what does not fit but should be included because it is so significant that it calls the working diagnosis into question, and what does not fit but can be minimized because it is probably a spurious finding. Informed focusing can be difficult, but it is the goal. A clearly formulated, well-presented history should lead all readers to generate the same differential diagnosis.

Past Psychiatric History

The past psychiatric history should include descriptions of **previous episodes of psychiatric illnesses,** the **treatment** received, the **outcome** of that treatment, and pertinent negatives. The presence or absence of prior hospitalizations, instances of impaired impulse control, and suicidal and homicidal ideation should *always* be included. Historical information particularly relevant to the current clinical questions should be addressed (see Box 1.4).

BOX 1.3

HISTORY OF A PATIENT WITH A PERSONALITY DISORDER

BACKGROUND

A 25-year-old graduate student complaining of "depression" described a confusing mixture of vague symptoms, which she subsequently dismissed. She presented long, overly detailed complaints about people in her life who were not clearly differentiated from one another. During the interview, the physician focused on the patient's distorted perceptions of others, her inability to describe herself in a coherent fashion, her self-destructive behavior, and her chronic feelings of emptiness. A clinical picture of borderline personality disorder gradually emerged. Although the written history of the present illness and the past history will not reflect the confusion of the first half of the interview, the physician may comment on the patient's circumstantiality and tangentiality in the mental status examination portion of the case formulation.

HISTORY

The patient reports chronic feelings of emptiness. She avoids being alone at all costs and experiences intense anxiety when she is alone. She has repeatedly engaged in self-destructive behavior, including superficially cutting her arm with a razor blade. The patient denies substance abuse and suicide attempts. Her patterns of relationships have been stormy. She rapidly becomes involved in intense relationships and then, just as quickly, becomes disillusioned with and enraged by the same person she had been idealizing. In one instance, she began meeting several times a week with one of her male professors, initially talking about course work and issues relevant to her field of interest but soon confiding in him about her personal concerns. She saw him as warm and supportive, "a treasure." After one occasion when he had to cut an appointment short, she became furious and reported, "I thought he was special, but he's just like everyone else—selfish and self-centered."

COMMENT

This history of the present illness summarizes the patient's narrative in a succinct manner that facilitates arriving at the appropriate diagnosis. Without directly referring to the diagnostic criteria, the history of the present illness points the reader in the general direction of a personality disorder, and specifically to the diagnosis of borderline personality disorder. This focus is a conscious editorial decision on the part of the interviewer. In other situations, it would not be necessary or appropriate to include such detailed information about the patient's relationships.

Past Medical History

The past medical history is an essential part of all psychiatric case formulations. Many medical conditions have direct psychiatric manifestations (see Chapter 5, Neurocognitive Disorders and Mental Disorders Due to Another Medical Condition). Chronic illnesses such as diabetes, asthma, and arthritis, as well as acute and short-lived but stressful

---

BOX 1.4

PAST PSYCHIATRIC HISTORY

A patient who had had schizophrenia for 10 years suffered a psychotic exacerbation after the sudden death of her mother. She presented to the emergency room with this chief complaint: "I'm hearing voices telling me to kill myself." The woman had been followed since the onset of her illness by a psychiatrist who was on the staff at the same hospital. Her past history was clearly documented in previous chart entries and could be briefly summarized in the current case formulation, highlighting the information that was most relevant for the decisions to be made: Has the patient been suicidal before? Has she ever had command auditory hallucinations? Has she acted on them or done anything to hurt herself? Has she had to deal with other losses, and, if so, how did she do so? Is she usually adherent to treatment? This information should be the focus of the past psychiatric history. In other words, this patient's history of difficulty dealing with loss and impulse control is more essential than is a complete review of her previous psychotic symptoms. It is important to remember that the purpose of the written record is to communicate needed information.

---

medical events such as an emergency appendectomy or severe pneumonia requiring hospitalization, may be significant stressors with which patients must cope (see Chapter 11, Psychological Factors Affecting Medical Conditions). The patient's approach to health and illness and to physicians, including issues such as adherence to prescribed treatments and avoidance of prohibited risk-taking behaviors such as smoking, can be elicited in the context of the past medical history.

Review of Systems

The review of systems, as the name implies, records the **presence or absence of current symptoms** in each **major organ system**, including the central nervous system. Psychiatric and medical symptoms that appear to be *unrelated* to the patient's present illness should be recorded in this section of the case formulation (see Chapter 2, The Psychiatric Interview, for suggestions on eliciting a comprehensive psychiatric review of systems, and *DeGowin's Diagnostic Evaluation* [LeBlond and Brown 2009] for suggestions on conducting a medical review of systems).

Psychosocial History

The psychosocial history encompasses the patient's **childhood, adolescence, and adulthood**. The childhood history should address any unusual findings with regard to childbirth, infancy, and the attainment of **developmental milestones**. Profiles of significant people present in the family during childhood should be obtained, as well as the family atmosphere, including conflicts, **losses**, and changes in the status of significant adults. Inquiries must always be made about the possibility of **physical and sexual abuse**.

An **educational history**, including performance at school, and a description of **peer relationships** should be obtained. **Childhood illnesses** and symptoms should be noted. **Earliest memories** can sometimes be useful.

A picture of school and occupational functioning, friendships, and intimate relationships should be provided for adolescence and adulthood. The **sexual history** and **alcohol and drug history** are generally included in this section. Whereas the other sections of the case formulation tend to focus on disease and disability, the psychosocial history should include **areas of health** and **strength** (see sample in Box 1.5).

Assessment of the patient's **cultural identity** is an important aspect of the psychosocial history. This will include the culture in which the patient was raised (i.e., **ethnic** and **religious** background), current **cultural reference groups, language** abilities, and cultural conceptualizations of **distress** and **coping**.

BOX 1.5
SAMPLE PSYCHOSOCIAL HISTORY

BACKGROUND

The patient is a 19-year-old woman who was admitted to an inpatient unit with the diagnosis of an eating disorder. While the following psychosocial history is not all-inclusive, the information provided is important for understanding the patient as an individual and will contribute to an initial treatment plan, part of which may be to obtain further information to fill in some of the gaps.

The patient is the youngest of three children born to middle-class parents living in an affluent suburb. Her father, who teaches college biology, is a nervous, suspicious man, who gets drunk every night in front of the television set. Her attractive mother dominates the family and participates in an active social life. The patient's two sisters have been successful academically, athletically, and socially and are currently at various stages of completing graduate work at Ivy League schools. Her family is superficially warm and supportive, but the emphasis is apparently on remaining pleasant to the exclusion, as much as possible, of any problems or bad feelings.

The patient describes herself as having been a withdrawn and shy child. She felt excluded from, and inferior to, her peers and frequently stayed home, complaining of "stomach aches." She was a good student, nonetheless, earning grades of B+ and A. During adolescence, with her mother's coaching, she became popular, participating in extracurricular activities with a circle of superficial friends whom she would go out of her way to please. She spent weekends "partying," abusing alcohol, amphetamines, cocaine, and marijuana. She was "never without a boyfriend," molding herself to her latest boyfriend's specifications in order to be the "perfect girlfriend," and she became sexually active. After graduation from high school, she attended a prestigious college several hundred miles away, where she immediately felt lonely and out of place. She left after her first semester and spent the rest of the year isolated at home.

> ## BOX 1.6
> ## PARALLEL PSYCHOSOCIAL HISTORY
>
> A woman in her thirties reported that her depression occurred in March of 2012 and then later stated that her mother died in December of 2012. When the physician double-checked this sequence, the patient corrected the physician, and her own dates, with surprise, saying, "The depression must have been in March of 2013, because it was definitely after my mother's death." Patients are not necessarily aware of these connections and sequences, but they may be of great importance. For example, a man in his fifties presented with a depression. While obtaining a parallel psychosocial history, the physician learned that the patient's father was dying of cancer. When the physician raised the possibility that the patient might be "upset" about his father's impending death (but did not suggest that the depression might be causally related), the patient completely denied any such reaction, insisting that he was prepared for his father's death because his father had been ill for several years and was in his eighties. Later in his treatment it became apparent that the patient had an ambivalent relationship with his father and that his impending death was, indeed, having a profound impact on him.

It can be extremely helpful to note the **timing of events** in the personal history in **parallel** with the timing of events in the patient's psychiatric history. While obtaining the personal history, the physician should keep in mind the key psychiatric events in the patient's life and make note of when they occur in relation to life circumstances. Important errors can be made if the physician does not specifically inquire about this sequence (see case examples in Box 1.6).

Family History

While some family information will be included in the psychosocial history, the presence or absence of psychiatric disorders in first-degree relatives should be noted in the family history section of the case formulation.

MENTAL STATUS EXAMINATION

The mental status examination is the most essential part of the "findings" section of the case write-up. It is comprised of **observed** data, in contrast to the subjectively reported history. The mental status examination is an **objective description** of an individual's **current mental state**, based on his or her speech and behavior. The format of the mental status examination provides a particular structure for listening, observing, and recording (see summary of major categories in Table 1.2 and definitions of mental status examination findings in Table 1.3). Like the physical examination, the mental status examination **does not include historical information**, nor does it include subjective complaints (with the exception of mood, see definition). The mental status examination is recorded in a systematic fashion following a **standard structure** with specific headings

TABLE 1.2 Mental Status Examination

Category	Definition	Common "Normal" Descriptors	"Abnormal" Descriptors (see definitions of individual items in Table 1.3)
Appearance, behavior, speech, and attitude	A detailed description of the individual as he or she appears during the clinical encounter, including grooming and clothing; motor behavior; the rate, volume, and modulation of speech and interactions with the interviewer	See sample mental status examination in Box 1.7	
Mood	Subjective feeling state of the individual sustained over much of the interview	Euthymic	Depressed (dysthymic), sad, irritable, expansive, euphoric, nervous, angry
Affect	Objective description of the individual's emotional state as observed by the clinician	Full range	Constricted, blunted, flat, inappropriate, labile
Thought process	The organization of the individual's thoughts as reflected in his or her verbal productions	Coherent and goal directed	Tangential, circumstantial, flight of ideas, loosening of associations, word salad, blocking, neologisms
Thought content	Overt signs and symptoms of psychopathology; the themes of the individual's thoughts during the interview should be mentioned only if preoccupations and ruminations are present; presence or absence of delusions, suicidal and homicidal ideation should always be included	No evidence of delusions; denies obsessions and suicidal and homicidal ideation	Presence of delusions (specify type—grandiose, paranoid, somatic, religious, reference), overvalued ideas (including paranoid ideation and ideas of reference), obsessions, ruminations, suicidal and homicidal ideation; paucity of thought—describe and give examples
Perception	Assessment of perceptual symptoms: illusions, depersonalization, derealization, hallucinations	Denies auditory and visual hallucinations	Specify type of hallucination (auditory, visual, olfactory, tactile) and describe
Cognitive	Assessment of the individual's abilities with regard to attention and orientation as well as intellectual functions, including memory, calculations, fund of knowledge, and capacity for abstract thought	Alert, attentive, and oriented × 3. Describe findings of each test administered (see Chapter 5, Neurocognitive Disorders and Mental Disorders Due to Another Medical Condition)	
Insight	The individual's understanding of himself or herself in the context of wanting or needing help; also referred to in psychodynamic terms as "observing ego"	Intact, excellent	Fair, impaired (include explanation)
Judgment	Closely related to insight but refers specifically to actions the individual will take based on insight; usually reflects impulse control	Intact, excellent	Fair, impaired (include explanation)

TABLE 1.3 Definitions of Mental Status Examination Findings

Descriptor	Definition
Behavior	
Psychomotor agitation	Noticeable and marked increase in body movements, e.g., hand wringing, pacing
Psychomotor retardation	Significant slowing of speech and body movements, lack of usual fidgetiness
Mood	
Expansive	Enthusiastic
Euphoric	Feeling great, as if one just won the lottery
Affect	
Blunted	Decrease in amplitude of emotional expression
Constricted	Normal amplitude but restricted range
Flat	Virtually complete absence of affective expression
Inappropriate	Emotions expressed are not congruent with content of patient's thoughts (occasional nervous smiling or laughter is not sufficient)
Labile	Unpredictable shifts in emotional state
Thought Process	
Circumstantial	Organized but overly inclusive, eventually gets to the point in a painstakingly slow manner
Tangential	Occasional lapses in organization such that the patient suddenly changes the subject and never returns to it; if a question is asked, it isn't answered
Flight of ideas	Flow of thoughts is extremely rapid but connections remain intact
Loosening of associations	Frequent lapses in connection between thoughts, disorganized
Word salad	Incomprehensible speech due to lapses in connections even within a single sentence; incoherent, a "tossed salad" of ideas
Blocking	Patient loses his or her train of thought; by definition, the patient should confirm the subjective experience of being blocked; the term should not be based on the interviewer's observation alone
Neologism	A created word with an idiosyncratic meaning
Thought Content	
Delusion	A firmly held, false belief not shared by members of the patient's culture (by definition, reality testing is not intact, i.e., the patient is unable to consider the possibility that the belief is incorrect)
Obsession	An idea that is intrusive and egodystonic (by definition, reality testing is preserved, i.e., the patient will readily acknowledge that the obsession makes no sense); should not be confused with ruminations, which are egosyntonic, or delusions
Overvalued idea	A false belief not shared by members of the patient's culture that is not fixed, i.e. it is held to more firmly than one would expect but reality testing is maintained
Paranoid ideation	Specific type of overvalued idea characterized by suspiciousness about others' motives
Ideas of reference	Specific type of overvalued idea characterized by misinterpretation of external events as having particular meaning for the individual
Phobia	A specific fear that results in avoidance of a situation despite the individual's realization that the fear is irrational

(continued)

TABLE 1.3 Continued

Descriptor	Definition
Perception	
Illusion	Misinterpretation of a sensory stimulus that can occur in any sensory modality (e.g., misperceiving billowing curtains in a darkened room to be an intruder)
Hallucination	Perceiving a sound, sight, taste, smell, or touch in the absence of external sensory stimulation that seems indistinguishable from such an experience in reality
Depersonalization	The sense that one is outside of oneself
Derealization	A vague sense of unreality in one's perception of the external world

(see guidelines in Table 1.4). **Detailed descriptions** should be included, interspersed with carefully chosen examples and brief patient quotes. **Pertinent negative findings** should be included, as they are in the history section. Common physical examination descriptors such as "within normal limits" or "well developed, well nourished" do not belong in the recorded mental status examination, as they do not adequately convey how a particular individual appeared, behaved, and sounded, even if the mental status examination is "normal." On the other hand, an overly inclusive written report is not useful in providing a clear description of an individual's unique mental status. A wealth of information can be efficiently conveyed by a well-organized, descriptive, and concise mental status examination (see sample mental status examination within the Sample Case Write-up in Box 1.7).

OTHER FINDINGS

Physical Examination

A thorough physical examination should be performed and documented in the case formulation for all psychiatric patients. The physical examination should be thorough because, even if there are no neurological findings, a systemic illness may be present that is producing psychiatric symptoms. Patients with clear-cut psychiatric disorders can also have other medical conditions that can be missed if a thorough physical examination is not performed. Vital signs and a detailed neurological examination are of particular importance.

TABLE 1.4 Guidelines for Recording the Mental Status Examination

- Objectively describe the patient's current mental state.
- Convey a clear description of the patient's unique mental status examination.
- Provide detailed descriptions, including examples and brief patient quotes.
- Record information systematically, following a standard structure with specific headings.
- Identify positive findings and psychopathology.
- Mention pertinent negatives.
- Include assessment of suicidal and homicidal ideation and psychotic symptoms, whether or not they are present.
- Be concise.

BOX 1.7

SAMPLE CASE WRITE-UP

IDENTIFYING DATA

A 24-year-old single unemployed man supported by Social Security Disability Insurance and living with his grandmother

CHIEF COMPLAINT

"I tried to commit suicide."

HISTORY OF THE PRESENT ILLNESS

The patient is currently being transferred to a psychiatric inpatient unit from the medical service following a suicide attempt requiring admission to the intensive care unit 1 week ago. For approximately 1 month prior to admission he had been feeling "depressed" and "paranoid," convinced that people on the street as well as his family wanted to hurt him. He also believed that people were moving their eyes in a particular way as they tried to look at him surreptitiously because they were afraid that he had hostile intentions toward them. The experience was "really, really scary" and he felt "alone," as he spent hours in his room "praying that the feeling would go away."

Over the course of the month he became increasingly frustrated with being ill and unable to work, and he began to have thoughts of wanting to be dead. He did not lose his appetite, but he had trouble sleeping, was fatigued, and didn't enjoy anything. He heard a voice outside of his head repeating his name and saying "hi." His psychiatrist increased the dose of his risperidone (an antipsychotic). The increased dose made him feel sedated, but otherwise didn't seem to help. On the day of his suicide attempt he began to hear a "satanic" voice telling him repeatedly "kill yourself." He took about 30 risperidone pills as well as a handful of lithium. His grandmother came home earlier than expected and called 911 when she watched him faint as he tried to stand up. He told the emergency medical technicians that he had only taken health food supplements, hoping to avoid being taken to the hospital so that he would be left at home to die. After checking his blood pressure and pulse they insisted that he be taken to the hospital. In the emergency room he suffered a cardiac arrest and was in a coma for 3 days.

The patient reports that he had been thinking about his mother in the days leading up to his suicide attempt, as it was recently the 10-year anniversary of her apparently accidental death by heroin overdose. He also reports that he had tried to return to work about 6 weeks ago as a part-time outdoor messenger. He had been hoping that he was ready to go back to work, but felt extremely "stressed" within a couple of days and quit within 2 weeks, becoming preoccupied with the many losses that he has suffered, "jobs, the army reserve, my mind."

(continued)

PAST PSYCHIATRIC HISTORY

The patient first developed psychiatric problems 5 years ago. At that time he began regular attendance at a church and believed that the pastor "was God. I had thoughts that I was Jesus Christ. When the pastor preached, I felt like I was supposed to go tell others." He also became convinced that a well-known national political figure was "the anti-Christ." He dressed up in army fatigues and camouflaged his face in order to "go on a mission. I was supposed to kill him." He was picked up by the police and admitted to a psychiatric facility. He did not hear voices at that time. He was treated with risperidone and discharged after about 2 weeks. Since then he has had two additional psychiatric admissions. His previous admissions have been associated with medication nonadherence, as he has tended to discontinue his medications after a period of feeling better. The patient reports experiencing several "high" periods characterized by "super energy" and racing thoughts. He has also been "depressed" at times but he denies previous suicide attempts or significant suicidal ideation. He is somewhat unclear about the details and the precise time course of his mood symptoms. He has been taking lithium for the past year.

PAST MEDICAL HISTORY

The patient denies any significant medical problems or prior hospitalizations. He denies a history of head trauma.

CURRENT MEDICATIONS

Risperidone 6 mg/d, lithium carbonate 1200 mg/d

REVIEW OF SYSTEMS

The patient denies other psychiatric symptoms.

PSYCHOSOCIAL HISTORY

The patient was raised by his grandmother, who immigrated to the United States from the Dominican Republic as a young adult. He describes her as a warm, supportive, and noncritical person. His mother stayed with them, off and on, until her death. His parents were not married and he met his father only once, when he was 16 years old. He does not know where his father is. He has two younger half-brothers, 12 and 18 years old, who each have a different father. He denied a history of sexual or physical abuse.

The patient joined the army at age 17 years and completed 2 years of service. He did not see active duty. He earned his GED while in the army. He worked as a waiter and remained in the army reserve when he returned home. He was discharged from the army reserve at the time of his first psychiatric hospitalization. Since that time he has had a series of short-term jobs (cashier, messenger) but has been unable to work for more than a week or two. He reports some experimentation with marijuana, cocaine, and alcohol during early adolescence and while in the army, but denies recreational drug or alcohol use in the past few years. He has never had a

(continued)

romantic relationship, and he has become increasingly socially isolated over the past few years, aware that many previous friends from his neighborhood avoid him since he's had a mental illness. He has made some friends in his church, which he attends regularly and finds a comfort.

FAMILY HISTORY

The patient reports that his mother had "the same illness," which began after she started using drugs, and she had a long-standing addiction to heroin. His maternal grandfather had the "same illness" as well, and was an alcoholic. The patient is not aware of a history of psychiatric illness in other family members. His younger brothers are currently in school and apparently doing well.

PHYSICAL EXAMINATION

Within normal limits

MENTAL STATUS EXAMINATION

Appearance, Behavior, Speech, and Attitude

The patient is a young man with neatly styled, curly hair, who makes good eye contact and is cooperative with the interviewer. He has a somewhat wide-eyed, blank, unchanging expression on his face and blinks infrequently. His casual shirt is clean and neat. The patient sits quietly in his seat, rarely shifting position. He occasionally uses his hands to emphasize a point. His speech is clear, at times slightly fast, but remains in a monotone throughout the interview.

Mood

"Good, happy to be alive."

Affect

Blunted

Thought Process

Coherent and goal-directed, without loosening of associations

Thought Content

Denies paranoid delusions; "happy to be alive" after suicide attempt; denies[1] current suicidal ideation; no evidence of[2] homicidal ideation but not specifically asked[3]

Perception

Denies hallucinations

Cognitive

Oriented × 3; short-term memory good (3/3 objects in 2 minutes); long-term memory appears good, though dates need to be corroborated; fund of knowledge good (knows current president and recent news events); simple calculations with money correct; difficulty with serial sevens; serial threes slow, with mistakes that the patient immediately caught and corrected

(continued)

Insight

Patient appears to have an excellent understanding of having a "mental illness" that has profoundly affected his life: "I've lost so much." Spontaneously explains that beliefs about people wanting to hurt him and the conviction that he was Jesus Christ were "crazy."

Judgment

Patient appears to be cooperative with his treatment. He feels that his "attitude" is better now in that he understands the need to take his medication. He realizes that he came very close to dying and is relieved that he did not die.

LABORATORY RESULTS

Most recent labs, including creatinine, blood urea nitrogen (BUN), and electrolytes, were within normal limits. Urine toxicology screen at the time of admission was negative for recreational drugs including marijuana, cocaine, and opiates. Brain MRI shows moderate cortical atrophy, including enlarged ventricles; no focal findings.

CASE SUMMARY

The patient is a 24-year-old man with a 5-year history of intermittent psychotic and mood symptoms who was admitted 1 week ago after making a serious suicide attempt in response to command auditory hallucinations. His medical condition is now stable. His mental status examination is notable for blunted affect. The patient no longer appears to be psychotic, and he denies current suicidal ideation.

DIFFERENTIAL DIAGNOSIS

The patient's psychotic symptoms (auditory hallucinations, paranoid and grandiose delusions), blunted affect, and functional deterioration are most suggestive of chronic schizophrenia. His mood symptoms (both depression and mania) suggest the possibility of schizoaffective disorder, most recent episode depressed, although overall it is not clear how predominant those symptoms are in relation to his psychotic symptoms (see Chapter 4, Schizophrenia and Other Psychotic Disorders). A mood disorder with psychotic features seems unlikely as he has been psychotic without mood symptoms (e.g., at the time of his first hospitalization). A substance-related psychotic disorder seems unlikely given his recent abstinence (confirmed by his negative toxicology screen on admission). There is no evidence of another medical cause for his symptoms, and his MRI scan is consistent with chronic schizophrenia (see Chapter 4, Schizophrenia and Other Psychotic Disorders).

Diagnosis: Chronic schizophrenia versus schizoaffective disorder; status post suicide attempt, medical sequelae resolved

PREDISPOSING AND PRECIPITATING FACTORS

Biological Factors

A genetic predisposition seems likely, given his family history. Drug use may have played a role in precipitating his first psychotic episode. Medication nonadherence may be contributing to his recurring symptoms.

(continued)

Psychological Factors

The patient was raised by a loving caregiver, but his childhood was nonetheless marked by deprivation and trauma, as his father was absent and his mother was probably emotionally unavailable to him given her own psychiatric and substance abuse problems, culminating in her unexpected and traumatic death during his adolescence. Recent stressors include the anniversary of his mother's death, and his growing realization that he may never be able to work.

Social Factors

The patient has been struggling with acceptance of his chronic mental illness, which has isolated him to some extent from his family and friends, in part as a direct result of the illness, but also probably due to social stigma.

TREATMENT PLAN

It will be useful to obtain additional information from his treating psychiatrist and his grandmother, as well as records from his previous psychiatric admissions, in order to define better the extent and timing of his mood symptoms in relation to his psychotic symptoms and overall illness course. He may not require a long hospitalization if he remains asymptomatic, and the psychosocial aspects of the treatment plan outlined below may be conducted on an outpatient basis. The role of the hospital staff would be to locate appropriate programs and facilitate the patient's initial referral and connection to them.

Biological Treatment

It may be time to consider a change to new antipsychotic and/or mood-stabilizing medications, given his recent exacerbation. The decision may be informed by further clarifying his degree of medication nonadherence, since his psychotic symptoms are now resolved on the same medications that he was taking prior to admission. A long-acting injectable antipsychotic may help address the nonadherence issue.

Psychological Treatment

Group psychotherapy with other patients with chronic mental illness may be helpful, if he can feel comfortable in a group setting, in order to provide ongoing psychoeducation and support in his struggle to accept the realistic limitations of his likely chronic psychiatric disorder (see Psychosocial Treatment in Chapter 4, Schizophrenia and Other Psychotic Disorders). Supportive psychotherapy on an individual basis may help him to develop better coping skills and, in a carefully modulated manner, better awareness of and control over the continued impact of his childhood marked by deprivation and loss.

Social Treatment

Given his growing demoralization in the face of his apparent inability to work, participation in a day program may be useful to provide a more structured and

(continued)

supportive setting in which to try to be productive. A day program would also help to mitigate his social isolation.

PROGNOSIS

Fair. The patient currently appears to have good insight and judgment, but his repeated episodes of medication nonadherence are of concern, as are his strong family history and recurrent psychotic episodes. The fact that he acted in response to command auditory hallucinations to make a nearly fatal suicide attempt is extremely concerning.

The presence of mood symptoms and the possibility of a diagnosis of schizoaffective disorder are better prognostic indicators, as is the consistent presence in his life of his supportive grandmother (her age and health should be inquired about, as he will be at high risk for decompensation when her health deteriorates).

---

[1]*"denies" implies that the patient has been specifically and directly asked about the symptom.*
[2]*"no evidence of" implies that the interviewer did not observe the symptom, but did not specifically inquire about it.*
[3]*"not specifically asked" should be stated explicitly if the presence or absence of a symptom is of particular importance, as it is in this case.*

Laboratory Tests

Blood and urine tests are frequently crucial adjunctive data to a thorough history in ruling out other medical conditions as possible causes of psychiatric symptoms as well as in identifying unrelated medical illnesses requiring treatment. In addition to the standard chemistry and hematological panels, toxicology screening should always be considered to rule out substance-induced disorders (see Chapter 7, Substance-Related and Addictive Disorders). Specialized blood tests and other modalities such as computerized tomography (CT) scanning, magnetic resonance imaging (MRI), and electroencephalography (EEG) can be used to screen for possible causes of delirium (e.g., fever, metabolic abnormalities) or neurological conditions with behavioral manifestations that could be mistaken for a psychiatric disorder (e.g., a patient with a brain tumor located in the frontal lobes might present with symptoms of a mood disorder). A neuropsychological battery of tests can sometimes be useful. All testing should be done with an eye toward balancing costs (both economic costs and health risks to the patient) with possible benefits. This judgment is based on a realistic estimate of the probability of a particular condition given its prevalence and the patient's presentation (see chapters on individual disorders, particularly Chapter 5, Neurocognitive Disorders and Mental Disorders Due to Another Medical Condition, for specific indications).

IMPRESSIONS

Once the physician has obtained the history and made his or her observations, further integration and planning remains. The physician's impressions of the patient and the patient's symptoms can be organized into three discrete sections that build on one another: (1) the case summary, (2) the differential diagnosis, and (3) predisposing and precipitating factors.

Case Summary

While the history presents the facts in such a way that readers can make their own judgments as to the validity of the interviewer's conclusions, the case summary begins the process of integration. The case summary remains descriptive, but it is more tightly focused and analytical than the patient-focused perspective of the history and the purely observational tone of the mental status examination. As the example in Box 1.7 illustrates, the case summary is mercilessly brief and succinct. Yet it is an important step toward identifying those findings in a particular patient that are similar to those found in other patients (i.e., toward making a diagnosis).

It is also a step toward completing other aspects of the overall assessment that can be at least as important as the diagnosis: Is the patient a danger to himself or herself, or to others? Will the patient be adherent to medication and other treatment recommendations? Thus, the case summary may include statements about the patient's **current level of functioning** and **behavior patterns,** as well as assessments of particular **symptom patterns** and **risks**. For example, the physician might conclude that a patient is **psychotic** (i.e., reality testing is impaired, as indicated by the presence of delusions, hallucinations, or a thought disorder, as described in Chapter 4, Schizophrenia and Other Psychotic Disorders). The term *psychotic* is at a level of overall assessment that does not belong in the mental status examination itself but should be included in the case summary as the physician begins to reach conclusions. Similarly, while the patient's thoughts, fantasies, and plans regarding suicide are recorded in the mental status examination, the physician's impression of the patient's impulse control and **suicide risk** should be included, when relevant, in the case summary.

Differential Diagnosis

The diagnosis summarizes patterns of data, predicts the course of an illness and the recovery from it, and suggests treatment options. In the systematic process of case formulation, the diagnosis is a separate step that is reached only after the patient's psychopathology has been summarized descriptively. Following this sequence keeps physicians disciplined and helps them consider all appropriate diagnoses systematically. This sequence does not mean that physicians are not thinking about diagnoses until this point. On the contrary, diagnostic possibilities are being entertained, patterns are being sought, and hypotheses considered and discarded all the while the physician is gathering data and making observations. By the time the physician begins to create the written record, the most likely diagnoses should have been identified. The entire case write-up is organized with those diagnoses in mind. However, following the formal sequence of steps (i.e., first, the history and observations; next, the summary of the psychopathology and other findings; and, finally, the diagnostic impressions) ensures that each section does indeed follow logically from the previous one.

Identifying specific diagnoses should be relatively simple after the psychopathology has been carefully described. The first question to answer is which **general category of psychopathology** does the patient's symptoms fit into, based on the history of the present illness and the mental status examination. These categories include the mood, psychotic, cognitive, anxiety, and personality disorders. Once the general category is determined, more specific details must be considered. This is where knowledge of characteristic diagnostic and prevalence patterns, including **gender and age differences**, is most crucial.

For example, a 19-year-old with no prior psychiatric history presented with auditory hallucinations and grandiose delusions, which had been occurring for six months. Because of the frequent onset of schizophrenia during adolescence, this disorder quickly became the most likely diagnosis, based on this brief piece of history. Substance-induced psychotic episode and bipolar disorder would be two other possibilities in the differential diagnosis. A 35-year-old woman with the same presentation is much more likely to be suffering from a mood disorder with a manic episode or mixed features, while a 65-year-old woman would be given a diagnosis of psychiatric disorder due to a another medical condition until this was proved otherwise. A closer look at more details about the patient's condition will either confirm the initial diagnosis or suggest other, less obvious diagnoses.

The degree of certainty regarding the diagnosis depends in part on the amount of detailed historical information available. A brief initial evaluation interview will probably generate a long list of possible differential diagnoses, whereas a formulation composed at the end of a lengthy hospital stay should present a fairly definite diagnostic impression.

Predisposing and Precipitating Factors

The formulation is not complete even after a diagnosis has been reached. The diagnosis reflects only those signs and symptoms that the patient shares with other patients who have the same disorder. Assigning a diagnostic label identifies common features but tends to blur the more subtle, and not so subtle, distinctions among individual patients with the same diagnosis. While this diagnostic labeling is crucial for purposes of communicating with others involved with the patient's care and for beginning to establish a prognosis and develop a treatment plan, it is not sufficient for describing an individual person who is suffering from an illness. The **biopsychosocial approach** describes the **patient's strengths and vulnerabilities** and helps to convey the patient's uniqueness. Vulnerabilities can also be labeled as possible predisposing or precipitating factors. In recent years, the biopsychosocial approach has been expanded to include a **cultural formulation**, which considers the patient's symptoms, stressors, supports, vulnerability, and resilience in relation to his or her cultural reference group. The case formulation in Box 1.7 illustrates the three parts of the clinical impressions, based on the history and findings.

TREATMENT PLAN

Having completed a careful description of the patient's problems, their possible origins, and the patient's capacity to deal with those problems, the physician is finally ready to formulate a treatment plan. Immediate and long-term goals and concomitant recommendations for treatment should be delineated. The **patient's goals** must be given prime importance as the treatment plan is being developed. The recommendations should include not only the ideal treatments but also those that are feasible given the patient's resources. Frequently, an initial step in the treatment plan will be obtaining additional information, such as history from family members and records of prior treatment.

The **biopsychosocial perspective** is useful in treatment planning because it focuses on all aspects of the patient's problems and their solutions. **Biological factors** might be treated with medication, electroconvulsive therapy, hypnosis, or bright-light phototherapy; **psychological factors** with various forms of psychotherapy; and **social factors** with hospitalization or other environmental changes, such as mobilizing a wider friendship network, joining a self-help group such as Alcoholics Anonymous, or obtaining additional work skills (see sample treatment plan in Box 1.7).

PROGNOSIS

The prognosis is a prediction of the course an illness will take (i.e., it is the physician's educated guess as to how a particular illness will play itself out in a particular patient). This prediction is based on the physician's specific knowledge of the individual patient and general knowledge of diseases (e.g., a depressive episode tends to resolve with adequate psychopharmacological and psychotherapeutic treatment, whereas schizophrenia tends to be characterized by years of waxing and waning symptoms and progressive impairment). In other words, given the diagnosis, as well as the patient's strengths and vulnerabilities, to what extent will he or she recover and perhaps even achieve better personal adjustment? The sample case formulation in Box 1.7 concludes with the patient's prognosis.

REFERENCE CITED

LeBlond, R., and D. Brown. *DeGowin's Diagnostic Examination*, 9th ed. New York: McGraw-Hill, 2009.

SELECTED READINGS

American Psychiatric Association. Work Group on Psychiatric Evaluation (Vergare M. J., chair). *Practice Guideline for Psychiatric Evaluation of Adults*, 2nd ed., June 2006. DOI: 10.1176/appi.books. 9780890423363.137162. http://psychiatryonline.org/content.aspx?bookid=28&sectionid=2021669

MacKinnon, R. A., and S. C. Yudofsky. *Principles of the Psychiatric Evaluation*. Philadelphia: J.B. Lippincott, 1991.

Perry, S., A. M. Cooper, and R. Michels. The psychodynamic formulation: its purpose, structure, and clinical application. *American Journal of Psychiatry* 144:543–550, 1987.

Shea, S. C. *Psychiatric Interviewing: The Art of Understanding. A Practical Guide for Psychiatrists, Psychologists, Counselors, Social Workers, Nurses, and Other Mental Health Professionals*. Philadelphia: W. B. Saunders, 1998.

ANAND DESAI AND LYLE ROSNICK

The psychiatric interview is the physician's most important tool for arriving at a diagnostic and prognostic assessment as well as formulating a treatment plan. It can be thought of as a clinical procedure, deployed for both diagnostic and therapeutic purposes. When the interview is conducted in a supportive and empathic manner, the very act of the physician's seeking information from the patient should alleviate the patient's suffering. Just as mastery of a procedure for the surgeon requires years of study, repetition, supervised practice, and thoughtful review, it can take years to acquire proficiency and a sense of confidence as a psychiatric interviewer. Nonetheless, even a novice can learn to conduct competent, thorough, and therapeutic evaluations.

GENERAL PRINCIPLES

Psychiatric and other types of medical interviews share certain similarities. Both types of interviews include the patient's subjective account of symptoms and the physician's more objective assessment of the patient's thoughts, feelings, appearance, and behavior. The physician begins both types of interviews by considering the patient's chief complaint, that is, what caused the patient to seek help at that point in time. In both types the patient is asked about the present illness and the past history. The psychiatric interview includes a survey of the major realms of psychopathology, which is analogous to the review of systems in other medical evaluations. In addition, the psychiatric interviewer is interested not only in the patient's illness and the ways that the patient experiences and copes with it but also with his or her social, academic, and vocational functioning in general, past and present.

Within the conceptual framework of the medical model, psychiatric symptoms are seen as direct manifestations of an illness, just as chest pain is seen as a possible symptom of coronary artery disease. The interviewer notes the presence or absence of symptoms of pertinent illnesses or syndromes, tracks the course of symptoms, and looks for factors that exacerbate or alleviate them, including previous treatment. Panic disorder, obsessive-compulsive disorder, and major depression lend themselves particularly well to the medical model.

While adhering to the basic medical model, the psychiatric interview has four additional essential and distinguishing features: a psychological perspective, empathic

> **BOX 2.1**
> ## GENERAL INTERVIEWING GUIDELINES
>
> - Maintain a professional stance that is empathic, respectful, and curious.
> - Begin with open-ended questions.
> - Follow up with focused questions.
> - Avoid technical terms.
> - Make use of silence.
> - Provide periodic summaries.
> - Ask for clarification.
> - Attend to emotional responses.
> - Empathize without offering false reassurance.

listening, particular attention to the physician's emotional responses, and a focus on the interview process (see Box 2.1 for general interviewing guidelines).

Psychological Perspective

To do justice to the complexity of psychiatric illnesses and patients, the physician must employ working models of the mind, in addition to neurobiological models of brain dysfunction. The psychodynamic model is a psychological perspective that views unconscious thoughts and feelings as powerful motivators and inhibitors of behavior. Symptoms are understood not simply as manifestations of brain chemistry but also as reflections of underlying psychological processes, including psychologically determined solutions to problems and conflicts that the patient may not be consciously aware of. From the standpoint of this perspective, the patient's recurring patterns of behavior in significant interpersonal relationships, past and present, are especially relevant. They represent potential clues to how the patient will experience and relate to the interviewer and to subsequent caretakers. The patient's internal psychological conflicts, management of strong affect, and capacity for gratification in love and work are also of primary interest (see sample interview in Box 2.2).

Other psychological, behavioral, and social scientific theories are widely employed by contemporary psychiatrists as well. In addition to the psychodynamic perspective, cognitive, behavioral, and interpersonal theory can be relevant for the assessment and treatment of patients with specific psychiatric disorders. Each theoretical perspective opens up ways of listening to patients, making sense of clinical encounters, and structuring treatments. Theoretical perspectives, or models of the mind, are not mutually exclusive; the psychiatric interviewer views them as complementary and variably useful, depending on the patient, the psychopathology, and the situation.

Empathic Listening

Because psychiatric problems are primarily experienced in the mind, the patient's subjective experience is of paramount importance. Empathic listening involves actively trying to see the world through the patient's eyes. Empathy requires imagination. Imagining a paranoid patient's sense of danger and isolation, for example, or an anxious patient's sense of imminent catastrophe, helps the physician capture the inner world of the patient.

BOX 2.2

INTERVIEW EXAMPLE DEMONSTRATING USEFULNESS OF A PSYCHOLOGICAL PERSPECTIVE

A 31-year-old female bisexual Hispanic graduate student was admitted to the hospital for treatment of a major depressive episode following the death of her mother. She has been in the hospital for 5 days. The female physician interviewer just rotated onto the service and is meeting the patient for the first time.

Interviewer: Can you tell me about the circumstances that led to your hospitalization?

Patient: I'm really not in the mood. They told me this morning that you would be my doctor. I could tell I wasn't going to feel comfortable talking to you. You look younger than I am! [The physician was indeed 3 years younger than the patient. The interviewer did not know quite how to respond. The patient got a bit angrier and looked the physician up and down. The interviewer was tense but remained composed.] You don't look like you can handle me. And I get this feeling that you're too confident, cold and clinical. Very straight. Too straight and middle class. You look perfect, with your outfit and your hair.

I: I see. Well, where do we go from here? You've given up before you've even started.

P: Oh, I have started. Listen, I'm sorry, but I really just can't see you treating me. How do I get assigned another doctor?

I: I don't know, I think you'd have to talk to the director of the unit.

P: Maybe I can be assigned to the other doctor. She looks like she speaks Spanish.

I: Would you be more comfortable speaking Spanish?

P: [The patient snapped angrily.] What the hell do you think?

I: OK, I'm sorry. Let me talk to my director, and I'll get back to you.

In this vignette, the interviewer is faced with a difficult and serious challenge. The patient is overtly hostile and contemptuous, making hurtful and personal attacks, rejecting wholesale the physician as a person as well as anything that she might have to offer. Such situations can be decentering and demoralizing; they can stir up strong feelings toward the patient that impact the present moment as well as the course of ensuing treatment. Conceptualizing what has gone wrong can inform an attempt to salvage the interview and the treatment.

Because the patient has refused to engage in the interview, the physician has correctly chosen to focus on the impasse, although the intervention might have gotten more traction if she had referred specifically to their relationship (changes italicized): "You've given up *on me* before *we've* even started." When the patient redoubled her rejection, the physician remained composed and professional, assessing whether the patient was concerned about a language barrier. The patient snapped back in a dramatically disrespectful manner. Understandably, the interviewer felt taken aback by the attack, and helpless to connect with the patient.

The physician's sense of defeat is in part realistic: there can be no productive interview until the patient's anger is addressed. The patient's behavior and affect may

(continued)

in part constitute rage and irritability due to a mood episode, personality disorder, substance-related disorder, medication side effect, or other underlying process. The evaluation that is necessary to make that determination cannot proceed because the patient's response to the physician has ground the interview to a halt. How can the physician understand and manage this stalemate?

First, the physician must register that the patient has very concretely transferred onto the physician a whole set of assumptions, beliefs, and motivations that belong to the patient's internal world. The patient is displaying an intense emotional and psychological response to the physician, despite not knowing her. Keeping in mind that this response reflects the patient's psychology, and is virtually unrelated to the physician, can help the interviewer to feel less personally affected, rejected, offended, or emotionally reactive. Separating the patient's fantasies from reality will help the interviewer to gain some distance from and perspective on the patient's distortions so that they can be named, thought about, discussed, and understood. The interviewer may then be able to call to mind what little she knows about the patient—for example, that her mother has died and her most recent physician has rotated off service. This information could lead the interviewer to hypothesize that the patient might be feeling abandoned, helpless, and angry, as well as terrified about getting close to and losing another caretaking figure, with all the pain that can entail. This understanding can help the interviewer begin to find seeds of empathy for the patient. Maintaining an attitude of unwavering respect and engaged curiosity, and taking a nondefensive and nonjudgmental approach, the interviewer could then make any one of the interventions listed below that felt most comfortable. Interventions such as these will elaborate more of the patient's inner world and put into words impulses, feelings, and fantasies that the patient is otherwise enacting, thus paving the way for the beginning of a collaborative interview and doctor–patient relationship.

"I can assure you I'm not perfect, but tell me more about why you're so sure I can't help you based only on my appearance."

"You obviously doubt that someone like me can help you."

"You're having a very strong reaction to me, and I'd like to understand it more. What else have you noticed about me to convince you I'm of no use?"

"It sounds like I really seem quite young and incompetent to you right now. And very straight. What kinds of experiences have you had with people who are similar to the way you see me?"

"How do you see me as straight?"

"How do you see yourself as a lot to handle?"

"What were the first things you noticed, when you knew you weren't going to feel comfortable talking to me? It sounds like an awful feeling for you to have."

"It's as if, in your mind, there's an image of me as a detached and uppity doctor, very different from you, almost too different to understand and relate to you in a helpful way."

Patients who feel that the interviewer wants to and can understand their perspective are far more likely to cooperate meaningfully with the interview. The physician's communication of understanding often helps the patient feel less confused, helpless, or alone. This, in turn, may help patients feel better about themselves, crucially mitigating feelings of guilt, humiliation, or shame. The patient's experience of feeling understood, together with the physician's emotional experience of coming to empathic understanding and making empathic contact, constitutes the bedrock of the **therapeutic alliance**. In the process of sharing their suffering with the physician, patients may experience a measure of relief. The interviewer who encounters the patient once only can still effect a truly therapeutic interaction.

Listening to the patient's **verbal communication** involves hearing more than the explicit meaning of the words. The physician tries to register the music of the language. All elements of language, including figures of speech and tonal modulation, convey emotions and contribute to the depth and meaning of verbal communication. Likewise, the interviewer should be attuned to other implicit aspects of the patient's speech—such as the ease or difficulty of following the story; the order in which it is told; omissions, hesitations, contradictions; as well as the congruence or lack thereof between what is being said and how the patient says it. The physician also listens to the patient's **nonverbal communication**, or body language, which includes facial expressions, gestures, and posture.

Physician Emotional Responses

In addition to verbal and nonverbal communication, the psychiatric interviewer tunes in to a third channel of communication: his or her own emotional responses to the patient. The physician who is authentically involved in the interview—listening, imagining, trying to empathize—is bound to have emotional responses in the process. Indeed, the absence of any emotional response in the physician, or a general emotional blandness coming through on this channel, is itself a significant deviation from the expectable and, as such, should prompt reflection and further investigation. There are numerous potential barriers to the physician's ability to make an emotional connection with a patient. Barriers may stem from the patient, the interviewer, or their mutual interaction. Before arriving at any conclusions, the interviewer needs to subject his or her own emotional responses to critical inquiry: Am I having a personal, idiosyncratic response to this patient? Am I feeling something that the patient is having trouble acknowledging? Is it possible that the patient is inducing these feelings in me, and if so, how and why might the patient communicate with me in this way? The physician's awareness of his or her emotional responses to the patient can inform interventions even at the outset of the interview, as the example in Box 2.3 illustrates. The importance of formulating answers to these questions will vary according to the patient's psychopathology, the clinical setting, and the purpose of the interview. The interviewer sometimes integrates this channel of information into the clinical picture only *after* completing the interview. As one eminent psychiatric interviewer framed the charge: "To see into the mind of another we must repeatedly immerse ourselves in the flood of his associations and feelings; we must be ourselves the instrument that sounds him" (Nemiah 1961). Thus, in the psychiatric interview, the physician makes use of his or her whole self as an instrument of healing, a complex and rewarding challenge.

Attention to Process

The psychiatric interview differs from other medical interviews in its emphasis on observing, and then examining, both the content and **process** of the interview as interrelated

BOX 2.3

INTERVIEW EXAMPLE DEMONSTRATING USEFULNESS OF ATTENTION TO THE PHYSICIAN'S EMOTIONAL RESPONSE

Interviewer: What brought you to the hospital today?

Patient (32-year-old woman): Well, my daughter died last winter, and she would have been 6 years old next week, and I began having flashbacks to an incident that occurred at my neighbor's during my childhood. This morning I was having that flashback. I felt as if I were almost reliving the experience and becoming a little girl! [The patient is visibly distraught and on the verge of tears.]

    I: Did the memory come after that?

    P: I can't remember when I first remembered it.

    I: Did your daughter's upcoming birthday stir up these thoughts?

    P: I don't know.

The interviewer began with a classic open-ended question. In response, the patient provided an emotion-laden answer, a confusing hodgepodge about two subjects (i.e., thoughts of her daughter and flashbacks of traumatic memories from her own childhood). Her manner of speaking was difficult to follow, disorganized, impressionistic, and bereft of details. It is logical that the interviewer would have been puzzled and would have wanted to make sense of her initial reply. However, he prematurely adopted a line of questioning that closed off the discussion. The physician tried to fill in the gaps himself by asking a number of unrelated, closed-ended questions, rather than by requesting her to clarify and elaborate on her own on what she already had said. If she had been unable or unwilling to do so, the interviewer might speculate that the nature and intensity of her feelings (and perhaps her fear of being overwhelmed by them) were preventing her from thinking and expressing herself clearly. It would have been more empathic and productive for the physician to show an interest in what the patient was feeling, for example, by saying, "What a terrible loss. You must be feeling overwhelmed." In fact, the interviewer himself was feeling horrified and threatened by the patient's tragic story. He thus was afraid to invite her to share her feelings with him. Because of his inability to contain his own anxiety and to process his other emotions, he was unable to tolerate a deeper exploration of her emotional state. Instead, he chose to sidestep her feelings by reverting to who, what, when, where, and why questions, as a journalist would.

manifestations of the patient's pathology. The process of the interview refers to how the patient communicates and engages with the interviewer, as well as to the type of interaction and rapport that emerges. The physician must create an environment in which a meaningful and informative process can develop. To do this, the physician needs to assume and maintain an attitude of unconditional respect for and interest in the patient. As the interview gets underway, the physician is prepared to listen actively without judgment, neither relinquishing nor seizing control. He or she strives to maintain a state of mind that allows for emotional receptivity and emotional contact with the patient, following the story as it is told. Not every moment of confusion needs to be addressed, as it may be a transient issue that the patient will soon clarify. Remaining curious, engaged, and connected, the clinician can contain the patient's emotions and distress simply by listening. The physician's skill in transiently tolerating confusion and discomfort allows the patient some freedom to think, feel, and speak in his or her own way. The interviewer can promptly intervene if the patient proceeds in a grossly disorganized manner, whether due to psychosis or another underlying deficit in thought, language, or memory. In most situations, however, the psychiatric interviewer is prepared to listen actively, completely focused on the patient and the interview process. The interview will be most informative and, therefore, helpful to both participants if the process is not initially dominated by the physician but rather allowed to emerge from the patient, telling his or her story in his or her own way.

The psychiatric interviewer is often silent, listening attentively. For the psychiatric interview to be most productive, the patient requires time to respond to the interviewer's questions spontaneously and at length. To facilitate this process, the physician can use brief, nondirective interventions. These are relatively neutral phrases or questions. For example, the interviewer may repeat or restate the last thing the patient said before falling silent. At other times, the physician might simply make an observation about the process itself: "You are tearful" or "You stopped yourself." With a hesitant or disengaged patient, the interviewer might ask whether something is making it difficult to talk. Simple, intuitive responses and questions similarly maintain a connection with the patient and his or her story without undue impingement. For example, an "Uh huh," "What happened then?" or "Tell me more about that" can facilitate the flow of the interview in a nondirective manner. The example in Box 2.4 illustrates two basic principles related to interview process: (1) when experiencing strong feelings during an interview, the patient will stonewall the physician unless he or she is given an opportunity to express these emotions, and (2) when a significant impediment to the progress of the interview manifests itself, it must be addressed if the interview is to proceed productively.

CONDUCTING THE INTERVIEW

Preparatory Phase

Setting the Frame
The interviewer greeting a new patient should provide straightforward introductions, aiming for a relatively natural and professionally warm demeanor. Adult patients should be addressed formally by their last names, and the interviewer can follow the patient's lead with regard to shaking hands. The physician then provides a clear statement about the capacity in which he or she will be relating to the patient, as well as expectations of the patient and goals for the interview. If the physician knows something about the patient, this should be addressed by saying something such as, "I understand that you were brought to the emergency room in an ambulance, and I've had a chance to speak with your outpatient doctor briefly. But I am most interested to hear from you directly what has been going, what led to your coming in today, and where you are with all of this now."

From the very beginning of every psychiatric interview, it is crucial to treat the patient as an active collaborator rather than as a passive subject. It is often helpful to explain to the patient how he or she can function to make the interview most useful. The informed

BOX 2.4

INTERVIEW EXAMPLE DEMONSTRATING THE IMPORTANCE OF EARLY PROCESS OBSERVATIONS

Interviewer: What brought you in today? [Silence.] Could you tell me a little bit about yourself? How old are you?

    Female Patient: Nineteen years old. [Silence.]

I: And you live where?

P: Connecticut. [Silence.]

I: Whom do you live with?

P: My mom and my sister. And my three cats.

I: And your father?

P: He lives in Alabama.

I: Oh, I see. Your parents...are...divorced then?

P: Yes.

I: I see. How long have they been divorced?

P: About 4 years.

I: And what do you do?

P: I just finished my freshman year of college.

I: How was that?

P: Fine.

I: So you are home for the summer and go back in the fall?

P: Yes.

The physician began with an **open-ended question**: "What brought you in today?" In response to the patient's silence, the interviewer changed the subject and asked two questions in rapid sequence. When the patient chose to respond with her age, the interview took the form of a series of **closed-ended questions** that required brief, factual answers. The physician sought exclusively demographic information about the patient and her relatives. It is understandable that the physician wanted to know something about the details of the patient's life. Perhaps this interviewer initially felt more comfortable asking questions with predictable, unemotional answers. The early interview process deteriorated into one in which the patient compliantly provided brief answers to numerous "survey" questions. The interview had taken on a ping-pong quality. Too many closed-ended initial questions, not altogether uninformative, miss the mark in terms of establishing an effective psychiatric interview. They inhibit patients from sharing or even learning about their inner, subjective experience as well as what is most important to *them* at the moment.

(continued)

Eventually realizing what had happened, the physician switched gears by returning to an open-ended question about the chief complaint:

I: So how can I be of help to you?

P: I'm not sure right now. [Silence.] You know, I've been on the waiting list for 6 months.

I: You want to tell me about that?

P: I don't know, maybe you can tell me! Six months is a mighty long time.

I: It certainly is! And you clearly have a lot of feelings about it. Please tell me about them.

In actuality the patient did not even answer the question about what initially led her to call for an appointment. Nevertheless, the question and the reply represented a turning point in the interview. At that juncture the interview and the patient came to life. The patient accepted the invitation to open up by sharing her most pressing feelings. It was as if the patient (accurately) interpreted the open-ended question as a signal that the interviewer was now willing and able to let her talk and have some control over the topics discussed. The physician immediately realized that the patient had let him in on her feelings toward the clinic (and, by extension, toward the interviewer himself). The interviewer responded empathically, and wisely asked the patient to elaborate. With this intervention the physician took another giant step toward establishing a therapeutic alliance by explicitly manifesting interest in the patient's emotions. After expressing her frustration, the patient naturally segued into a discussion of her situation.

patient will feel more secure and confident about how to proceed. To develop and maintain a therapeutic alliance, the interviewer should strive to be thoughtful and empathic during every interaction with the patient. Respect and consideration of the patient's needs and concerns should be shown even before the interview begins. Informing the patient in advance of the interview's purpose and duration, and whether it will be the only meeting or the first of many, will begin to establish a **frame**, which is the mutually agreed upon basic structure of the treatment. The frame also includes the location, frequency, and cost of sessions, if applicable.

The process of establishing the frame will vary depending on the setting. *In the emergency room*, for example, the physician may explain as follows: "You and I will talk for 30 minutes now, and I will be here through the night. My primary goal at the moment is to understand in as much detail as possible what led to your coming to the ER and how you are feeling now. From time to time I may interrupt you, because there is a lot I'd like to learn about you and your situation in the limited time we have. After we speak, I'll be reviewing your records, including the blood work and imaging; I'll discuss the situation with the team and come back to figure out with you what's next. Let's begin with what brought you to the ER today." *In the outpatient setting*, the interviewer might say: "Today's evaluation will last for an hour. I will review your records in the coming days and give you a call next week to discuss my impressions with you." *On an inpatient unit*, the physician can let the patient know that they will meet daily for half-hour sessions.

The Interview Setting

Physicians in clinics, emergency rooms, and inpatient units often have little control over the setting of the psychiatric interview. The place available for an interview is likely to be a sparsely furnished, windowless room or even a hallway. Regardless of the locale, the interviewer should arrange the environment as much as possible so that there is privacy and freedom from intrusion, as well as a reasonably comfortable place for both interviewer and patient to sit. Unneeded distractions, or the potential for intrusions, impair the interviewer's ability to be fully present, actively and empathically listening, emotionally available, and receptive. If the setting permits, the interviewer may even ask if the patient is satisfied with the room temperature, inviting input into whether a window should be opened or the air conditioner turned off.

Safety

Both interviewer and patient need to feel emotionally and physically secure. A frightened, preoccupied interviewer cannot conduct a successful interview, and a fearful, distracted patient cannot do his or her part. Certain measures can be taken if either person is frightened. For example, the presence of a security guard in the room might make a paranoid patient feel more comfortable. The interviewer of a potentially assaultive patient might choose to conduct the interview in a patient lounge or waiting room: participants can sit farther apart so as not to feel cornered, and guards or other staff members can be present at close range. The interviewer's fears should never be ignored, even if they seem irrational or exaggerated. Instead, the interviewer should seek advice and direction from someone with more knowledge and experience. Patients should be interviewed only under conditions in which everyone involved feels safe (see Chapter 13, Violence).

Language

Evaluation of the patient's verbal proficiency, when indicated, should be conducted at the beginning of the interview. The interviewer can ask: "What languages do you speak other than English? Which language are you most comfortable speaking?" Using an **experienced translator** with patients whose first language is not English is crucial for psychiatric interviews, which rely on observations of patients' thought patterns and on open discussion about the intimate details of their personal lives. Family members and friends are extremely unreliable as translators. In addition to the obvious fact that patients may feel inhibited about fully disclosing their symptoms and behaviors in the presence of a family member, other pitfalls abound. The family member may be reluctant to translate the interviewer's questions or the patient's responses accurately, particularly when they concern self-destructive thoughts or psychotic symptoms. The family member may also try to present the patient's responses as more organized and coherent than they actually are. These distortions may be conscious or unconscious. An inexperienced translator may make the same errors, but there is generally less motivation to do so.

It is possible to perform an empathic interview that is diagnostically and therapeutically useful despite the use of a translator. The following guidelines are helpful. The interviewer should make eye contact with the patient, not the translator, and the translator should sit off to the side. This arrangement will encourage the patient to focus on the physician. The physician should encourage the translator to maintain the give-and-take flow of the interview but to interrupt if necessary in order to explain areas of confusion or difficulties in fully conveying the patient's meaning. Interviewers should use their usual body language, including hand gestures, facial expressions, and vocal inflections.

History-Taking Phase

In most clinical situations, this phase should begin with an open-ended question, such as "How can I be of help to you?" "What brought you in today?" or "How did you come to be hospitalized?" Some patients require little further prompting to answer such questions in a coherent and detailed manner. When this happens, the interviewer should allow the patient to speak at some length and resist the temptation to interrupt. While listening actively and empathically, the physician can begin to observe such things as the patient's capacity for goal-directed thinking, as reflected in the coherence of the patient's story.

For patients who are able to give their recent history in a spontaneous and comprehensible fashion, the interviewer during this phase needs to employ techniques that encourage the patient to continue speaking. Eye contact, an occasional head-nod, and a succinct restatement of what has been said will let patients know that the physician is following their story. At times, the interviewer can respond with a relatively neutral, nondirective intervention, such as "What happened next?" or "How did you understand that?" or "How did you feel at that point?" The interviewer's goals during this relatively unstructured phase of the interview are to maintain a connection with the patient and to encourage elaboration of the story.

The more open-ended this initial phase of the interview remains, the greater the interviewer's chances of discerning potential clues, the further exploration of which may clarify whether the patient has a psychiatric disorder and, if so, in what broad realm(s) of psychopathology. Of particular relevance in this regard are the patient's report of any symptoms of distress; troubling feelings or ideas; changes in functioning; problems in interpersonal relationships; parts of the story which are particularly difficult to understand or imagine, potentially suggesting an area of psychological conflict; and potential stress due to life events or the patient's environment, taking into account the social and cultural context.

After listening at length, the interviewer follows up on the patient's chief complaint and present illness in a more systematic and structured manner, using specific, closed-ended questions to establish such details as the presence or absence of symptoms; the duration, course, and severity of symptoms; exacerbating or ameliorative factors; associated illnesses; and the patient's understanding of and responses to the symptoms. In effect, the physician begins by surveying the landscape, and then hones in on all areas of potential interest to investigate them in finer detail.

Challenges to History-Taking

Two relatively common scenarios require immediate intervention: the disorganized patient and the difficult-to-engage patient.

The Disorganized Patient

Patients who are in acute distress or actively disorganized are generally not able to communicate their problems effectively to the interviewer. Their difficulty will usually emerge soon after the interviewer's opening question. In these cases, the interviewer will need to impose structured questions earlier, both to contain the patient and to investigate the disorganization. The physician must attempt to clarify the cause of the patient's confusion. Is the patient cognitively impaired, for example, or psychotic, or intoxicated? The interview of the disorganized patient will more closely resemble a detailed mental status examination and a focused medical history. The physician might first establish whether there are cognitive deficits. Formal testing can be introduced by stating, "I have the impression that you may be having difficulty with things like concentration and memory. I'd like to ask you some questions to clarify whether you're having difficulties in these areas" (see Chapter 5, Neurocognitive Disorders and Mental Disorders Due to Another Medical Condition). The next focus should be on the patient's thought process and content, assessing for deficits in reality testing that are indicative of psychosis (see Chapter 4, Schizophrenia and Other Psychotic Disorders).

The Difficult-to-Engage Patient

Some patients may give excessively brief responses, speak repetitively, become vague, or talk about matters that are not immediately relevant. When the difficulty is not related to cognitive impairment or psychosis, the interviewer may attempt to engage the patient through open-ended follow-up questions and nondirective encouragement. If these techniques are unsuccessful, the interviewer must turn his or her attention to the process of the interview.

As a guiding principle, the psychiatric interviewer should focus on process before content whenever there seems to be a barrier to the free flow of information. The physician's role extends beyond simply gathering information to addressing the impediments to communication. In many situations, the very problems the patient is having with the interview may be related to the problems that led to presentation in the first place. As the case example in Box 2.5 illustrates, the most useful interventions in stalled initial interviews are often observations about the process. Once the impediment to the patient's talking freely has been expressed and understood, the flow of information can resume. At the same time, the patient's inner experience will be understood in greater depth, illustrating how the diagnostic and therapeutic dimensions of the psychiatric interview are interwoven.

BOX 2.5

INTERVIEW EXAMPLE DEMONSTRATING USEFULNESS OF ADDRESSING PROCESS BEFORE CONTENT

A 23-year-old man presented to an outpatient clinic for treatment. In the initial evaluation, he began by saying that he had been feeling depressed over the past few weeks. He was unemployed and living with his mother, who supported him financially. The patient explained that he couldn't find a job "because of the depression." At this point, the patient looked at the doctor expectantly. After a pause, the interviewer attempted to draw the patient out.

Interviewer: Tell me more about that.

Patient: That's basically it. I've just been depressed, and I wanted to know what medications were available.

I: It sounds like it's been a difficult time for you. Can you tell me more about what you think happened and what you are experiencing now?

P: Not really. Like I said, I just got depressed a few weeks ago and it's getting in the way of finding a job. And I really need to find a job—to get my mother off my case!

(continued)

I: So your mother has been on your case recently.

P: Yeah.

I: I'd like to understand all this in greater detail so that I can be of help to you. You began by saying you've been depressed for a few weeks. How did that come about and how you do understand it?

P: I don't know. I don't really think it's that important.

A few more attempts at engaging the patient were unsuccessful, with the patient continuing to give terse responses. At this point, very early in the interview, the interviewer might be tempted to resort to the list of symptoms of a major depressive episode, asking yes-no questions about them. This approach would not be altogether misguided, as the interviewer will need to establish answers to these questions before the evaluation is complete. However, the interviewer will have missed a crucial opportunity to understand and address the patient's resistance, which may be conscious or unconscious (see Chapter 17, Psychotherapy). Turning to process before content, the physician can further her understanding of the patient as well as the patient's understanding of himself.

In the vignette, the interviewer observed that the patient grew relatively passive in the interaction, while the interviewer herself became the active member of the team, attempting to engage the patient by repeated questions. It is as if something of what the patient described with his mother was recreated in the interview: the patient is not working, and the interviewer is on his case! The physician could comment on the process by saying, "I wonder whether something is making it difficult to talk freely right now" or, "I have the impression this isn't easy to talk about with me." If the physician speculates that the resistance is due to a displacement of the patient's feelings about his mother onto the physician, she could say: "I can see that it's difficult for you to tell me about the problems for which you're seeking help. Talking at more length feels useless to you. I've noticed that a version of what is happening at home is also happening right now, almost as if I'm getting on your case, asking you to do something you're not doing. And if I were like your mother, whom you've told me is angering you recently, I can understand a bit more about why you might not want to talk or get too invested by sharing more of yourself with me."

These types of interventions can help patients feel understood and reveal more about their inner state. The patient in the example is difficult to engage, but the psychological sources of his resistance are not yet clear. For example, the patient could be feeling hopeless about the treatment already, or paranoid about the doctor's intentions. He might be feeling a sense of shame or even humiliation in revealing that he has been depressed, or he might feel particularly anxious or exposed, or even angry, consciously or unconsciously, toward the doctor for some reason. These would all be important aspects of the patient's experience and clinical presentation to know about and understand in greater depth, as each of these possible sources

(continued)

of difficulty engaging will have implications not only for the remaining conduct of the interview but also for diagnosis and treatment planning. Addressing the process of the interview allows the patient to clarify his experience.

When the physician asked whether something was making it difficult to talk freely, the patient explained that he didn't believe the interviewer could really help him. In fact, he didn't really believe in psychiatry at all; he just wanted to try the medication to appease his mother. Here the interviewer made an empathic comment: "I can see then why it would be difficult for you to tell me about your problems. You feel hopeless that it could lead to anything productive." In response to the physician's intervention, the patient did feel understood and said more about his skepticism of psychiatry. The physician followed the affect: "I wonder whether feelings of hopelessness or a sense of having to appease your mother—whether these things come up in other situations, with other people in your life." The patient then went on to elaborate how futile it seemed that anyone could help him, which led him to elaborate spontaneously on his life situation, significant early losses, and his problematic relationship with his mother. The patient was speaking freely.

Over the course of the initial interview, the patient grew increasingly animated and connected with the physician, who recommended they meet again to continue the evaluation. The patient agreed, and a potential treatment was underway.

Past Psychiatric and Medical History

The interviewer should fill in the details of the patient's past psychiatric and medical problems as well as treatment, inquiring in a systematic and detailed manner. In general, the interviewer will prioritize information according to the clinical situation; in a busy emergency room, for example, the physician will focus this section of the interview on that information which is essential.

Crucial past psychiatric history includes psychiatric hospitalizations, symptoms of psychosis and mood disorders, suicide attempts, self-injury, violence, dangerously impulsive behavior, arrests, incarcerations, and previous outpatient treatment. The task is not simply to compile a disconnected list of facts but instead to make narrative sense of them. For example, if a patient reports two past suicide attempts, the interviewer should address them one by one, inquiring about all details leading up to and surrounding each attempt as well as the subsequent treatment. With regard to past hospitalizations, the psychiatric interviewer wants to know what led to a hospitalization, why it was necessary, what the precipitating factors might have been at the time, what the inpatient course entailed, and what the discharge plan and follow-up treatment involved. For example, if a patient reports that she saw a psychiatrist for 6 months after leaving the hospital, the interviewer will want to know how and why the treatment ended. The more time available for the interview, the more the physician should explore the past history, oscillating between open-ended listening and focused questioning. Even when the time is limited, the facts should be placed in a context. Throughout this section of the history-taking, the principles of empathic listening apply. In gathering past psychiatric and medical history— major events and stories that inevitably entail emotional experiences—the physician will deepen his or her knowledge of the patient, thus enhancing the physician's capacity for empathic understanding of and emotional contact with the patient.

Review of Systems

A psychiatric interview should include a **review of systems**, in which the patient's past and present mental health is surveyed to identify signs and symptoms in the major realms of psychopathology. Here the interviewer uses as a guide the leads noted during the more open-ended phase of history-taking: anything the patient has said—or notably not said—that suggests psychiatric illness, disturbances, or difficulty in functioning. Sometimes, a patient may report one problem but not another—because it occurred in the past, is happening in the present with minor symptoms, or is manifest in the present and the patient does not realize it. Almost always, however, hints of any major illnesses are revealed by the present complaints. The interviewer should pursue the possible presence of certain ailments even when they are not spontaneously elaborated. For example, a patient who has presented for evaluation of panic attacks mentions that he was depressed in college and at another point makes reference to recent weight gain. During the closed-ended questioning, the interviewer should follow up on this lead, working backward from the present by asking how the patient's mood has been recently, given all that has been going on. This opens an exploration of whether the patient is currently depressed. It is neither desirable nor possible to question every patient about every category of symptoms. The physician's judgment will modify how detailed and exhaustive the review of systems should be. Box 2.6 includes examples of the types of questions that can be used in surveying the realms of psychopathology.

BOX 2.6

SCREENING QUESTIONS FOR A PSYCHIATRIC REVIEW OF SYSTEMS

MOOD DISORDERS (SEE CHAPTER 3)

Depression

Have you ever had a period when you were feeling depressed or down most of the day nearly every day? What about a time when you lost interest or pleasure in things you usually enjoyed?

Mania

Have you ever had a period of time when you were feeling so good, "high," excited, or hyper that other people thought you were not your normal self or you were so hyper that you got into trouble? What about a time when you were feeling irritable or angry every day for at least several days?

SCHIZOPHRENIA AND OTHER PSYCHOTIC DISORDERS (SEE CHAPTER 4)

Now I'd like to ask you about unusual experiences that people sometimes have.

Delusions

Has it ever seemed like people were talking about you or taking special notice of you? *If yes:* Were you convinced they were talking about you or did you think it might have been your imagination?

(continued)

What about receiving special messages from the TV, radio, or newspaper, or from the way things were arranged around you? What about anyone going out of their way to give you a hard time, or trying to hurt you? Have you ever felt that you were especially important in some way, or that you had special powers to do things that other people could not do? Have you ever felt that something was very wrong with you physically even though your doctor said nothing was wrong…like you had cancer or some other terrible disease? Have you ever been convinced that something was very wrong with the way a part or parts of your body looked? Have you ever felt that something strange was happening to parts of your body? Have you ever had any unusual religious experiences? Have you ever felt that you had committed a crime or done something terrible for which you should be punished? Were you ever convinced that your spouse or partner was being unfaithful to you? *If yes:* How did you know they were being unfaithful? Did you ever feel you had a special, secret relationship with someone famous, or someone you didn't know very well?

Hallucinations

Did you ever hear things that other people couldn't, such as noises, or the voices of people whispering or talking?

NEUROCOGNITIVE DISORDERS (SEE CHAPTER 5)

Have you or has anyone close to you ever felt that you had a problem with your memory or with remaining alert, knowing where you were, why you were there, or whom you were with?

ANXIETY DISORDERS (SEE CHAPTER 6)

Panic Disorder

Have you ever had a panic attack, when you suddenly felt frightened or anxious or suddenly developed a lot of physical symptoms?

Agoraphobia

Were you ever afraid of going out of the house alone, being in crowds, standing in a line, or traveling on buses or trains?

Social Phobia

Was there anything that you have been afraid to do or felt uncomfortable doing in front of other people, like speaking, eating, or writing?

Generalized Anxiety

In the last 6 months, have you been particularly nervous or anxious? Do you also worry a lot about bad things that might happen?

OBSESSIVE-COMPULSIVE DISORDER (SEE CHAPTER 6)

Have you ever been bothered by thoughts that didn't make any sense and kept coming back to you even when you tried not to have them? Was there ever anything that you had to do over and over again and couldn't resist doing, like washing your

(continued)

hands again and again, counting up to a certain number, or checking something several times to make sure that you'd done it right?

STRESS DISORDERS (SEE CHAPTER 6)

Sometimes things happen to people that are extremely upsetting—things like being in a life-threatening situation like a major disaster, very serious accident, or fire; being physically assaulted or raped; seeing another person killed or dead, or badly hurt; or hearing about something horrible that has happened to someone you are close to. At any time during your life, have any of these kinds of things happened to you? *If yes:*

Sometimes traumatic experiences keep coming back in nightmares, flashbacks, or thoughts that you can't get rid of. Has that ever happened to you? What about being very upset when you were in a situation that reminded you of one of these terrible things?

ALCOHOL AND SUBSTANCE USE DISORDERS (SEE CHAPTER 7)

Has there been any time in your life when you had five or more drinks on one occasion? Have you ever gotten "hooked" on a prescribed medicine or taken a lot more of it than you were supposed to?

Have you or anybody important to you ever thought that you have a problem with alcohol or other drugs?

EATING DISORDERS (SEE CHAPTER 9)

Anorexia Nervosa

Has there ever been a time when you weighed much less than other people thought you ought to weigh? *If yes:* Why was that? How much did you weigh?

At that time, were you very afraid that you could become fat?

At your lowest weight, did you still feel too fat or that part of your body was too fat?

Bulimia Nervosa

Have you often had times when your eating was out of control? *If yes:* Tell me about those times. *If unclear:* During these times, do you often eat within any 2-hour period what most people would regard as an unusual amount of food? Tell me about that.

Did you do anything to counteract the effects of eating that much? Like making yourself vomit; taking laxatives, enemas, or water pills; strict dieting or fasting; or exercising a lot?

Were your body shape and weight among the most important things that affected how you felt about yourself?

SUICIDE (SEE CHAPTER 12)

No psychiatric evaluation is complete without an assessment of suicidal thoughts and attempts.

Have you ever wished you were dead or wished you could go to sleep and not wake up?

(continued)

Have you had any thoughts about killing yourself?

Have you ever done anything, started to do anything, or prepared to do anything to end your life?

_____

From First, M. B., R. L. Spitzer, M. Gibbon, and J. B. W. Williams. Structured Clinical Interview for DSM-IV-TR Axis I Disorders–Patient Edition *(SCID-I/P) revised January 2007.*

Psychosocial History

The prospect of eliciting and organizing a detailed narrative of the patient's life can seem overwhelming. The length of time spent in the interview specifically asking questions about the patient's psychosocial history, and the level of detail elicited, will vary. But the interviewer should appreciate that many contextualized facts about and events in the patient's life may already have emerged in the course of the interview. These include details such as whether the patient is religious; where and with whom the patient lives; his or her education and occupation, activities, and passions. More closed-ended questions will add to the existing sketch (see Box 2.7). Questions about a patient's legal history, drug use, and physical or sexual abuse may not flow naturally in the course of the interview. The interviewer should ask the patient directly about these matters in a straightforward and open fashion, consistent with the rest of the inquiry.

If necessary, the physician can expand this phase of the interview to gather more information about the patient's psychological, social, sexual, and academic development and functioning. A more elaborated psychosocial history may explore in greater depth the patient's family of origin: the personalities and significant events in the lives of parents

---

BOX 2.7

QUESTIONS TO ELICIT THE MINIMUM ESSENTIAL PSYCHOSOCIAL HISTORY

- Where were you born and reared?
- What were your family's financial circumstances?
- Were your parents married?
- Do you have siblings?
- How far did you go in school?
- Do you work and support yourself?
- Are you in a relationship?
- Are you married?
- Do you have children?
- Where and with whom do you live?
- On whom do you rely for support?
- Have you ever been physically or sexually abused?
- Have you ever been arrested or done things that would have gotten you arrested if you had been caught?

and siblings; significant aspects of the family's history and worldview; the relationships among members of the family, and significant events or losses in the life of the family as a whole. The patient's prenatal and perinatal history can be relevant from a biological and a psychological perspective. Was the pregnancy planned? Were there any notable complications during gestation or following delivery? Next, the interviewer will survey the patient's early, middle, and late childhood, inquiring about developmental milestones, important relationships, and significant life events. As the interviewer reviews the years before, during, and after adolescence, the following information will be of interest: school performance; friendships; life outside of family; areas of pleasure and strength; and evidence of identity consolidation, as manifested in coherent, nuanced, consistent, and three-dimensional descriptions of himself or herself and others—that is, their values, priorities, and salient characteristics. The physician should also inquire about the patient's sexual history, including the patient's first sexual experiences, sexual orientation, and current sexual fantasies and behaviors. The interviewer will also want to learn about the patient's significant adult friendships, experiences in love and intimate relationships, as well as the capacity for commitment to these relationships. Finally, the patient should be asked about finances. Do you have financial concerns? Have current difficulties caused problems at work or reduced your income? Are you able to pay your bills? The patient's history of legal problems and substance use should be covered in detail during this phase of the interview if they were not reviewed earlier.

This more elaborate and extensive psychosocial history is generally not covered in a single interview, but emerges in multiple interviews over the course of an evaluation or treatment. Here again, whether in contracted or expanded fashion, the goal is the same: the interviewer is aiming not just for sequential, isolated facts but for the story, the plot, that connects those facts. A series of questions should not be asked in a rote, checklist, impersonal fashion. The interviewer needs to follow the patient's story naturally, being interested in the significant events, who the main characters are, what has motivated the patient, and what conflicts, crises, or tragedies have been encountered. The physician is trying to understand the patient's **emotional history**, which focuses on emotional reaction patterns, typical responses to stress, coping strategies, and the dominant themes and repetitions that occur in relationships. Information about basic relationship patterns and tendencies with significant others will enable the physician to anticipate the characteristic ways in which the patient is likely to respond both to physicians and to treatment. Finally, the patient's **cultural identity** must be taken into account (see Box 2.8).

The most useful interviewing technique for eliciting the psychosocial history is the same technique employed in the opening phase of the interview. The interviewer may begin with a statement as simple as "Tell me about your life." Then the interviewer listens actively, albeit quietly, initially speaking only to encourage the patient to continue talking or to address resistances that the patient cannot overcome alone. Box 2.9 includes additional examples of questions relevant to the psychosocial history.

Family History

The family history of psychiatric and medical illnesses is obtained in the course of any complete psychiatric interview. Psychiatric illnesses result from a combination of biological and environmental factors, and the family history of illness gives information about both. Psychiatric and medical illnesses in parents, siblings, grandparents, aunts, uncles, and cousins should be investigated. The physician should ask specifically about any known history of attempted or completed suicide; mental illnesses including depression,

BOX 2.8
CULTURE AND THE PSYCHIATRIC INTERVIEW

Culture refers to the systems of knowledge, ideas, beliefs, and practices that are inherited, recreated, and molded from generation to generation, within families and other social institutions. The components of a person's culture that are relevant to the psychiatric interview include language, family structure, social and community structure, concepts of health and illness, religion and spirituality, ways of seeing and understanding the world, as well as general beliefs about the stages of the life cycle.

A person's cultural background, beliefs, and ideals shape to varying degrees how he or she characteristically thinks and behaves. The interpretive framework provided by his or her culture determines a person's experience and expression of psychiatric signs and symptoms. It can also influence the patient's encounter with the psychiatric interviewer. In contemporary life, we are exposed to multiple cultures, and we draw from these cultures as we shape our identities and make meaning out of experience. Because culture at large is a dynamic, changing system—individually experienced but collectively maintained—the cultural factors influencing a person's life should not be generalized or stereotyped.

The cultural factors that influence a patient cannot really be separated from who he or she is as a person. The physician should attempt to uncover and define the cultural context within which the patient lives and suffers as they emerge from the patient's individual story and point of view. Cultural considerations apply to everyone, not just underserved or unfamiliar racial or ethnic minorities within a given society. The interviewer should not inquire generically about the views of the groups with which patients self-identify or to which the physician has ascribed them. The intracultural heterogeneity of beliefs should be allowed to emerge. Since individuals create personal beliefs out of diverse cultural influences in their lives, the cultural dimension of a patient's illness must be considered on an individual, personalized basis (Lewis-Fernandez and Aggarwal, 2013).

Culture frames the experience of mental health and illness for both patient and physician in three primary ways. First, what is normal, expected, and acceptable with regard to thoughts, feelings, and behavior may differ across cultures, families, and social institutions. Therefore, the level at which a patient's experience is considered problematic or pathological varies; it is shaped by cultural norms that have been internalized by the physician, the patient, and those around them. When cultural factors are taken into account, the physician can identify the ways in which a patient has culturally interpreted psychopathology that would result in delaying care and prolonging distress. For example, a religious 60-year-old Russian Orthodox woman believes her major depression is punishment for her sins; and an 18-year-old woman's intensely shy, socially reticent behavior, signifying social anxiety disorder, is

(continued)

normalized by her family and experienced by the patient and others as respectful and appropriate for a young, unmarried woman. Culture may also influence the patient's sense of vulnerability and the intensity of his distress. For example, a 50-year-old Dominican man's local family culture, using rich somatic idioms to express emotional states, amplifies his somatization, contributing to fears that maintain panic disorder and frequent emergency room visits.

Second, cultural factors contribute directly both to the degree of stigma associated with mental illness and to the social and familial response. A patient's culture may offer useful coping strategies that enhance resilience. Cultural norms may also determine the types of interventions and treatments the patient seeks out, including alternative and complementary systems of health care. Cultural factors can influence the patient's acceptance or rejection of a psychiatric diagnosis, adherence to treatments, and the patient's concept of mind both biologically and psychologically. All of these have implications for the course of illness and recovery.

Third, cultural similarities or differences between physician and patient can contribute to the accuracy of diagnosis as well as to the patient's acceptance of a diagnosis and engagement in treatment (see case example in Box 2.2). Patients and physicians who appear to share the same cultural background may nevertheless differ in important ways. They may implicitly assume an understanding of each other, and this can lead to overidentification, erroneous or incomplete assumptions, and shorthand manners of speaking that obscure communication, as well as to conscious or unconscious avoidance of certain questions, topics, or realms of psychopathology.

THE INTERVIEW

A detailed inquiry into cultural factors is indicated when significant differences in cultural, religious, or socioeconomic backgrounds between physician and patient cause difficulty in conducting the evaluation, or when the interviewer is uncertain about the fit between the patient's culturally distinctive symptoms and the DSM diagnostic criteria. At other times, the interviewer might have difficulty judging how severe or how impaired the patient is as a result of his or her illness. If the physician and patient disagree about the course of treatment, or if the patient has a history of limited engagement in treatment or nonadherence altogether, specific attention to cultural factors is warranted.

The following are examples of questions that should be asked during a cultural interview. They can be incorporated into the interview at appropriate and natural moments.

- We all understand our problems in our own way, and these may be different from how doctors describe them. Would you describe things differently if you were talking to your family or friends?
- What bothers *you* the most about your situation?

(continued)

- How do you understand what is going on?
- What do you think is causing it?
- How do your family and friends make sense of what's happening with you?
- Is there some kind of specific support that only your family or friends, or your activities, provide? What are they? How do they help?
- What are the most important aspects to you of your background or identity? By that I mean things like communities you belong to, your religion or faith, gender or sexual orientation, languages you speak, your race or ethnic background, your family's history and traditions?
- Does your background or identity affect your illness? How?
- It's natural for people to look for help from people they trust. What kinds of advice or treatment have you sought for your difficulties—from other doctors or other types of healers? How were they? Which ones seemed to help?
- Has anything prevented you from getting help or from coming in sooner?"
- What kind of help do you think you need right now; what would be most helpful from your perspective, for your situation?
- Have family or friends, or others important to you, suggested things they think might be helpful to you?
- It's always possible that doctors and patients don't understand each other— for all kinds of reasons. Are you concerned, today with me, that I've missed something important?
- Have you been worried, today with me, that we've misunderstood each other?

bipolar disorder, schizophrenia and other psychotic disorders; and neurocognitive disorders. The interviewer should also inquire about a family history of alcohol and substance abuse. Throughout this phase, the physician needs to listen empathically, trying to discern the impact on and relevance to the patient of any positive family history of mental illness.

Mental Status Examination

Most of the information needed for the mental status examination is obtained simply through observation and active listening (see Chapter 1, Psychiatric Assessment and Treatment Planning). Establishing the presence of psychotic symptoms can be among the most challenging aspects of the psychiatric interview. Psychotic fears or beliefs may be unrecognized by the patient or actively withheld from the interviewer. The physician's sense that something is off may stem from the content or from the process of the interview. In the course of telling his or her history, the patient may reveal unusual ideas, irrational beliefs, or intense distrust. In the process, the patient may appear vague, rigid, guarded, or evasive. In such cases, or when aspects of a patient's story seem strange, illogical, contradictory, or incomprehensible, the physician should focus on the patient's reasoning and use of evidence to support his or her beliefs. When there is a question of psychosis

---

BOX 2.9

QUESTIONS TO ELICIT AN ELABORATED PSYCHOSOCIAL HISTORY

- What is your earliest memory?
- Tell me about your childhood.
- Where were your parents born?
- When did you (they) come to this country? From where? Under what circumstances?
- Where did you grow up?
- In how many places have you lived?
- Who lived at home? Parents? Siblings? Grandparents?
- Were you ever separated from a parent for any length of time?
- Did you have any operations or serious illnesses or accidents as a child?
- How much schooling have you and your other family members had?
- How did you do in school (elementary school, junior high or middle school, high school, college)?
- Tell me about your friendships (in grade school, adolescence, college, in recent years).
- Does religion play an important role in your life? Do you consider yourself a spiritual person?

---

and the patient is guarded in the interview, the physician could say: "I can see that you'd like to keep that private or are having difficulty talking openly about it with me. Is there something you're worried about?" This can be followed by addressing the doctor–patient relationship, asking: "Are you feeling suspicious of me—my intentions or motivations?" When possible delusions have been identified, the physician should explore the patient's reality testing directly: "I can see how convincing it seems. But I'd like to clarify: is it at all possible that there is another explanation?" or "It makes sense that you're scared, since you believe you have a brain tumor the doctors can't detect. But do you think it's possible that the imaging is correct, and that there is no tumor?"

Formal cognitive testing usually does not flow with the rest of the interview and will need to be introduced specifically with a neutral statement such as, "Now I'm going to ask you some questions to assess your memory and concentration" (see Chapter 5, Neurocognitive Disorders and Mental Disorders Due to Another Medical Condition).

Concluding Phase

The conclusion of a psychiatric interview will depend on the nature and purpose of the interview, as well as on such factors as whether there will be further interviews and whether the situation is an emergency. In all cases, the physician should allow time for the closing phase of the interview. In this phase, the interviewer asks whether any important history was omitted. An introductory statement might be, "We have some time left. I'm wondering whether I've missed anything you think is important. For example, something you had wanted to tell me but didn't." Or: "Is there anything you think I should have asked you but haven't yet?" Even after a lengthy interview, a patient may make surprising revelations.

The physician then shares the impressions and treatment recommendations with the patient in a sensitive, culturally informed manner, employing language and concepts that the patient and other laypersons can comprehend. It is important to allow time for the patient to respond and react to what has transpired. When necessary, patients should be given time to regain their composure and leave with dignity.

REFERENCES CITED

Lewis-Fernandez, R., and N. K. Aggarwal. Culture and psychiatric diagnosis. *Advances in Psychosomatic Medicine* 33:15–30, 2013.

Nemiah, J. C. *Foundations of Psychopathology*. New York: Oxford University Press, 1961.

SELECTED READINGS

Gaw, A. C. *Concise Guide to Cross-Cultural Psychiatry*. Washington, DC: American Psychiatric Publishing, 2001.

Halleck, S. L. *Evaluation of the Psychiatric Patient: A Primer*. New York: Plenum Medical, 1991.

Hays, P. A. *Addressing Cultural Complexities in Practice: Assessment, Diagnosis and Therapy*, 2nd ed. Washington, DC: American Psychological Association, 2008.

Laria, A. J., and R. Lewis-Fernandez. Latino patients. In *Clinical Manual of Cultural Psychiatry*, ed. R. F. Lim. Arlington, VA: American Psychiatric Publishing, 2006.

MacKinnon, R. A., R. Michels, and P. J. Buckley. *The Psychiatric Interview in Clinical Practice*, 2nd ed. Arlington, VA: American Psychiatric Publishing, 2006.

MacKinnon, R. A., and S. C. Yudofsky. *Principles of the Psychiatric Evaluation*. Philadelphia: J.B. Lippincott, 1991.

Mohl, P. Listening to the patient. In *Psychiatry*, 3rd ed., A. Tasman, J. Kay, J. A. Lieberman, M. B. First, and M. Maj, eds. Hoboken, NJ: Wiley-Blackwell, 2008.

Shea, S. C. *Psychiatric Interviewing: The Art of Understanding*, 2nd ed. Philadelphia: W.B. Saunders, 1998.

Trzepacz, P. T., and R. W. Baker. *The Psychiatric Mental Status*. New York: Oxford University Press, 1993.

Wallace, E. R. *Dynamic Psychiatry in Theory and Practice*. Philadelphia: Lea and Febiger, 1983.

/// 3 /// Mood Disorders

LICÍNIA GANANÇA, DAVID A. KAHN, AND MARIA A. OQUENDO

Mood disorders are a significant public health problem. They are relatively common, and their recurrent nature profoundly disrupts patients' lives. Depression afflicts one in eight Americans during his or her lifetime and costs the U.S. economy more than $43 billion annually in medical treatment and lost productivity.

Despite the seriousness of mood disorders, only one-third of individuals with these disorders are properly diagnosed or treated. Studies have found that although 20% of patients in primary care clinics were clinically depressed (Olfson et al. 2000), only one-half were diagnosed as such by a physician (Rost et al. 1998; Wells et al. 1989). Several factors might account for this underrecognition. First, in general medical settings, many patients with mood disorders present with unexplained somatic complaints, especially pain and insomnia, rather than a clearly stated emotional complaint, the so-called masked depression. Second, it can be difficult to distinguish mild mood disorders from the normal emotional ups and downs of life. Third, **stigma** remains a barrier to seeking help for mental illness. Most people—and, sometimes, even physicians—tend to fear, look down upon, or ignore mental illness. In order to avoid the risk of being seen as weak in their own eyes or the eyes of others, many individuals with mood disorders choose not to get professional help, preferring to "tough it out." This attitude sometimes results in dire consequences for ill persons and their families, as 10% to 15% of patients with severe mood disorders die from suicide.

Mood disorders are neither normal variations in mood nor appropriate reactions to severe stress. These disorders are distinguished from normal moods and reactions by the duration and intensity of patients' suffering and the degree of their functional impairment. Mood disorders do not represent a failure of "will power" or some other form of moral weakness. Fortunately, there is a growing recognition that mood disorders are medical illnesses that require aggressive diagnosis and treatment by physicians.

DIAGNOSTIC AND CLINICAL FEATURES

Mood can be understood as the amalgam of emotions that a person feels over time, the general emotional state that "colors" the person's perception of the world. Mood is characterized by features such as intensity, duration, fluctuations, and the adjectival description of type (depressed, expansive, irritable, euthymic). **Emotions** are more ephemeral affective states caused by physiological changes in response to an event and are usually accompanied by somatic symptoms. Examples of emotions are happiness, fear, anger, and disgust. **Affect** is the way in which emotions are displayed as observable behaviors such as through body language, including facial expression. The effects of mood on a person's behavior are complex and widespread. Mood shapes conscious attention, interest, and motivation, and it alters unconscious autonomic functions, such as those related to vagal tone and sleep physiology. Many physical sensations, such as energy, pain, muscle tension, hunger, satiety, and sexual pleasure, have strong emotional components that influence the production and intensity of these sensations; thus, changes in a person's mood state can effect changes in energy and behavior.

Constricted emotional range, a decrease in the usual repertoire of emotional responses the individual displays, can occur in mood disorders and stands in contrast to normal emotional experience. Patients with mood disorders are emotionally stuck. Because one or more emotions persist more intensely and for a much longer time than circumstances warrant, these patients lose much of their emotional flexibility and, therefore, their ability to adapt to changing circumstances; they have trouble "shifting gears" within a normal repertoire of complex emotions. Normally, after a loss or victory, a person has intense feelings of sadness or elation for a time, which gradually give way to new responses to life's events. After the loss of a romantic attachment, for example, some depressed individuals repeatedly experience symptoms so severe that they are unable to get out of bed for weeks. In contrast, some persons experience a manic "high" and become so euphorically obsessed with a speculative investment strategy that they are unable to experience warning signs, such as self-doubt, and eventually suffer financial harm.

Mood is also closely linked to **cognition**. For example, research into memory physiology suggests that perceptions and thoughts (i.e., "what happened") are best retained when they are linked with strong emotional memories (i.e., "how it felt"). In persons with mood disorders, a filter is introduced that distorts normal perceptions and memories or subjects them to selective recall. This distorting process can dramatically affect a central aspect of mood, self-worth. **Self-worth** is one component of a person's permanent self-image that stretches over time and includes perceptions of past experiences, current abilities, and future plans. In patients with mood disorders, the perception of self-worth goes through unstable gyrations. Typically, a depressed patient views past events with undue criticism and guilt, feels worthless, and finds the world an unpromising place. In contrast, manic patients glorify their abilities and find the world a stimulating place.

The mood disorders consist of the **depressive** and **bipolar disorders**. These disorders are recognized as distinct groups because they share both specific symptoms and features of a longitudinal course. The predominant symptom of any mood disorder is **a distinct period of abnormally and persistently altered mood**. Bipolar disorder, also known as **manic-depressive illness**, is distinguished from depressive disorders by the presence of manic or hypomanic (i.e., mildly manic) episodes that can occur in addition to depressive episodes. Of note, a diagnosis of bipolar I disorder can be made in the absence of depressive episodes. Figure 3.1 schematizes these categories. Most depressed patients feel sad or "low," and most manic patients feel irritable, euphoric, or "high." Patients with mood disorders also experience behavioral, cognitive, and psychomotor changes, which may constitute their presenting complaints.

The key feature of the longitudinal course of mood disorders is a tendency toward **cycles of recurrence**. Although some patients have only a single episode during their lives, most have multiple episodes, or recurrences, interspersed with periods of remission,

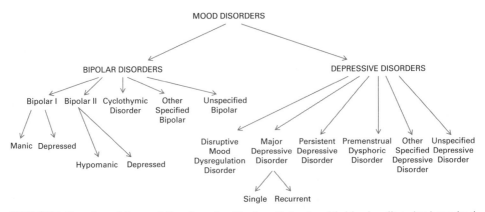

FIGURE 3.1 **Overview of the mood disorders classification.** Patients with bipolar disorder have had at least one episode of mania or hypomania. Bipolar I disorder consists of recurrences of mania and major depression. Bipolar II disorder consists of recurrences of major depression and hypomania (mild mania). Cyclothymic disorder consists of recurrent brief periods of mild depressive symptoms and hypomanic symptoms that do not meet criteria for a hypomanic episode. Other specified bipolar and related disorder is for partial syndromes, such as recurrent hypomania without depression. In unspecified bipolar and related disorder the patient does not meet the full criteria for any of the disorders in the bipolar and other disorders class; this diagnosis is best suited for situations where information is limited, such as in emergency room settings. Depressive disorders include major depressive disorder, which is often recurrent but sometimes occurs as a single lifetime episode, as well as persistent depressive disorder (dysthymia), disruptive mood dysregulation disorder, and premenstrual dysphoric disorder. Other specified depressive disorder is the diagnostic term for partial syndromes, such as patients who are depressed but have too few criteria for major depression and whose depression has been too brief for persistent depressive disorder. Unspecified depressive disorder represent cases where full criteria for any of the depressive disorders are not met and, as for unspecified bipolar disorder, can be used when there is insufficient information to make a more specific diagnosis.

known as **euthymia**, or normal mood. Some patients have chronic symptoms and never achieve full recovery. As with many other major medical illnesses, the prevention of relapse and the recognition of persistent low-grade symptoms between episodes are critical elements in the long-term treatment of patients with mood disorders.

Major Depression

Psychological Symptoms and Signs

Patients with major depression have a persistent, distinct feeling of depression or loss of pleasure or interest in usual activities that lasts for at least 2 weeks, as well as at least four associated symptoms (see Table 3.1). When describing a **depressed mood**, patients often say they feel sad or "blue," are "down in the dumps," have an ache or an empty feeling in their heart or in the pit of their stomachs, or feel the need to cry. In addition, other emotional states such as anxiety, irritability, or even hostility can also appear. **Sad feelings** are often accompanied by persistently lowered self-esteem or self-criticism. These are two features generally not observed in persons who are responding to external losses. In his classic paper "Mourning and Melancholia," Sigmund Freud noted that mourners

TABLE 3.1 DSM-5 Diagnostic Criteria for Major Depressive Disorder

A. Five (or more) of the following symptoms have been present during the same 2-week period and represent a change from previous functioning; at least one of the symptoms is either (1) depressed mood or (2) loss of interest or pleasure:

Note: Do not include symptoms that are clearly attributable to another medical condition.

(1) Depressed mood most of the day, nearly every day, as indicated by either subjective report (e.g., feels sad, empty, or hopeless) or observation made by others (e.g., appears tearful). (**Note:** In children and adolescents, can be irritable mood.)

(2) Markedly diminished interest or pleasure in all, or almost all, activities most of the day, nearly every day (as indicated by either subjective account or observation).

(3) Significant weight loss when not dieting or weight gain (e.g., a change of more than 5% of body weight in a month), or decrease or increase in appetite nearly every day. (**Note:** In children, consider failure to make expected weight gain.)

(4) Insomnia or hypersomnia nearly every day.

(5) Psychomotor agitation or retardation nearly every day (observable by others, not merely subjective feelings of restlessness or being slowed down).

(6) Fatigue or loss of energy nearly every day.

(7) Feelings of worthlessness or excessive or inappropriate guilt (which may be delusional) nearly every day (not merely self-reproach or guilt about being sick).

(8) Diminished ability to think or concentrate, or indecisiveness, nearly every day (either by subjective account or as observed by others).

(9) Recurrent thoughts of death (not just fear of dying), recurrent suicidal ideation without a specific plan, or a suicide attempt or a specific plan for committing suicide.

B. The symptoms cause clinically significant distress or impairment in social, occupational, or other important areas of functioning.

C. The episode is not attributable to the physiological effects of a substance or another medical condition.

Note: Criteria A–C represent a major depressive episode.

Note: Responses to a significant loss (e.g., bereavement, financial ruin, losses from a natural disaster, a serious medical illness or disability) may include the feelings of intense sadness, rumination about the loss, insomnia, poor appetite, and weight loss noted in Criterion A, which may resemble a depressive episode. Although such symptoms may be understandable or considered appropriate to the loss, the presence of a major depressive episode in addition to the normal response to a significant loss should also be carefully considered. This decision inevitably requires the exercise of clinical judgment based on the individual's history and the cultural norms for the expression of distress in the context of loss.

D. The occurrence of the major depressive episode is not better explained by schizoaffective disorder, schizophrenia, schizophreniform disorder, delusional disorder, or other specified and unspecified schizophrenia spectrum and other psychotic disorders.

E. There has never been a manic episode or a hypomanic episode.

Note: This exclusion does not apply if all of the manic-like or hypomanic-like episodes are substance-induced or attributable to physiological effects of another medical condition.

(continued)

TABLE 3.1 Continued

Specifiers for Major Depressive Disorder

Specify (for current clinical status or features):

    With anxious distress

    With mixed features

    With melancholic features

    With atypical features

    With mood-congruent psychotic features

    With mood-incongruent psychotic features

    With catatonia

    With peripartum onset

    With seasonal pattern

Specify (for current or most recent episode):

    Single episode

    Recurrent episode

Specify (for current severity)

    Mild: Few, if any, symptoms in excess of those required to make the diagnosis
are present, the intensity of the symptoms is distressing but manageable, and the
symptoms result in minor impairment in social or occupational functioning.

    Moderate: The number of symptoms, intensity of symptoms, and/or functional
impairment are between those specified for "mild" and "severe."

    Severe: The number of symptoms is substantially in excess of that required to make the
diagnosis, the intensity of the symptoms is seriously distressing and unmanageable, and the
symptoms markedly interfere with social and occupational functioning.

feel sad over the loss of a loved one, but any feelings of guilt or self-blame generally pass
after several weeks. In contrast, depressed patients often feel sad and experience a personal **sense of guilt or inadequacy.** Feelings of guilt or defectiveness may or may not
be related to a specific external loss and may be so disproportional or irrational that they
develop into a specific delusion. Typical examples are found in persons who believe that
they have committed horrible crimes or are emitting foul odors that offend others. These
feelings of guilt and shame may be quite subtle. Mood disorders occur in some people
near retirement age. For example, someone who is facing the loss of the structure and
social reinforcement provided by the workplace may begin to feel that his or her personal
qualities (e.g., talents, vigor) and opportunities are actually declining.

    Another aspect of depression is intense pessimism and hopelessness. Depressed
patients tend to discount the past, feel that the future has been destroyed, and find it
hard to imagine they will ever feel well again. One graduate student, for example, became
depressed about, and felt ashamed of, the difficulty she was having mastering a new field
of study and withdrew from friends and pleasurable activities. Wondering whether she
had deserved the Phi Beta Kappa award she received in college and feeling that she fraud-
ulently presented herself to the world as a promising scholar, she feared that her inade-
quacies would be exposed, at long last, in graduate school and that she would be unable to

complete her degree. **Anxiety** in the form of worry or outright panic often accompanies pessimistic thoughts. Fears of being alone and unable to cope are common. A triad of helplessness, hopelessness, and worthlessness often summarizes the feelings of sadness.

Depressed patients also lose interest and pleasure in things, people, or activities they normally enjoy. When the loss of the ability to experience pleasure is nearly total, it is referred to as **anhedonia**. Patients with anhedonia cannot be cheered by activities they normally enjoy, such as playing with their children or watching television. They feel apathetic and unenthusiastic; their interest in physical pleasures, such as food or sex, seems dull, flat, or deadened. In severe anhedonia, patients lose interest in their most important emotional ties to other people (see case example in Box 3.1).

The DSM-5 criteria for a major depressive episode include either sadness or loss of interest as mandatory criteria to establish the diagnosis, in part because some patients do not sense or articulate the former and focus more on the latter. In extreme cases, patients are unable to verbally express sadness even though they have all of the other objective symptoms of depression. Patients with this condition, known as **alexithymia** (meaning without words for feelings), typically present with fatigue or other vague medical complaints. They say that they are distressed and have lost interest in their normal activities, which they often attribute to their physical problems, but also say that they do not feel sad or worthless. The presence of at least five other symptoms of depression, such as sleep disturbance, establishes the diagnosis. Patients with **"masked" depression** may present with severe pain (often head, pelvic, abdominal, or low back pain) and deny that they feel sad, although they suffer from loss of interest and other symptoms of depression.

Behavioral Symptoms and Signs

Behavioral, cognitive, and psychomotor symptoms may occur with depression. The **behavioral symptoms** are changes in appetite, sleep patterns, energy levels, and sex drive. They are often referred to as **"vegetative"** symptoms because they reflect dysregulation of the simplest survival activities and are likely tied to endocrine, autonomic, and circadian functions of the hypothalamus.

BOX 3.1

CASE EXAMPLE OF ANHEDONIA

A normally vibrant woman with a family and an active career became extremely withdrawn and unable to function when depressed. She stayed in bed as much as possible in a half-waking, half-sleeping state. Initially, she worried about getting her children to school on time and sharing household chores with her husband. Eventually, she became indifferent to these concerns and even stopped feeling anxious. In other words, she gave up. She left her job and felt that it was hopeless to maintain ties that might enable her to return later. Although she seemed to be emotionally dead, she was anything but indifferent to her inner state. She felt acute pain because of the distance she felt from the people who she knew she loved. Her growing sense of burdening them caused her to think constantly about suicide. Thus, the very relationships that had previously given her pleasure now gave her unbearable pain because she could not maintain them.

Depression can be associated with a number of **sleep abnormalities**, including **sleep-onset insomnia**, also referred to as difficulty falling asleep (DFA); **sleep maintenance insomnia**, also known as middle-of-the-night awakening (MNA); and **terminal insomnia**, also known as early-morning awakening (EMA). While difficulty falling asleep is a nonspecific symptom, middle-of-the-night awakening and early-morning awakening are classic symptoms of depression. A patient with terminal insomnia typically falls asleep at the usual hour and then wakes up at 3:00 or 4:00 a.m. with a feeling of deep sadness, dread, or anxiety. In contrast, about 30% of depressed patients have **"atypical," or "reversed," vegetative signs**, which include **hypersomnia**, as well as increased appetite. Hypersomnia is more common among adolescents and those with either bipolar or seasonal (fall/winter) depression. Sleep disturbance may commence before any mood changes are perceived by the patient. Consistent polysomnographic findings in depression include **decreased rapid eye movement (REM) sleep latency**, lengthened first REM sleep episode, shortened first non-REM sleep episode, decreased slow-wave sleep, and reduced sleep continuity. Physical **fatigue** or loss of energy occur independently of sleep and appetite changes and may occur equally as often with either insomnia or hypersomnia.

A common symptom that patients may be embarrassed to report is a **loss of interest in sex**, which can be a source of frustration to them and their partners. Occasional menstrual changes and gastrointestinal complaints, such as nausea or constipation, are other symptoms of possible endocrine or autonomic dysfunction.

Cognitive dysfunction is another way in which patients are affected by depression. Patients may describe reading the same page over and over again or watching television without comprehending what they have read or seen. For example, a habitual reader of novels may be unable to read anything longer than a light magazine article; a student may find it hard to write a term paper; a homemaker may be unable to organize a shopping list; or a factory worker may continually make assembly-line errors. Such patients may say that their minds are "just not working properly." This cognitive deficiency is usually not a simple matter of having distracting thoughts and, in some cases, is more serious than an inability to concentrate on the immediate task at hand. Patients may forget recent events or become disoriented as to the time of day. Some patients exhibit frank confusion and do not recognize people they know or are unable to find their way around. Severe confusion of this sort is called **pseudodementia**, although there is nothing "pseudo" about it. Rather, it is a transient dementia that resolves when the depression is treated. Elderly patients and patients with baseline central nervous system disease are more likely than others to suffer from transient dementia. In fact, depression is important in the differential diagnosis of any patient presenting with dementia characterized by withdrawal, apathy, or irritability.

Psychomotor activity is usually diminished in depressed patients. Their thoughts, speech, and motor movements are often subjectively experienced and objectively observed to be slowed down. This phenomenon is known as **psychomotor retardation**. When psychomotor retardation is at its most extreme, patients can appear mute and virtually immobile. Patients might describe their minds and bodies feeling "trapped in molasses." Basic social behavior, such as looking up at someone entering the room, may disappear. Patients may experience difficulty getting out of bed, getting dressed, taking medicine, attending to personal hygiene, seeing a doctor, or even making a telephone call to ask for help. Decisions as simple as which foods to buy at the grocery store can be overwhelming. If psychomotor retardation is combined with severe apathy, loss of appetite, and overall self-neglect, a medical emergency can result, secondary to malnutrition, dehydration, electrolyte imbalance, or infections from decubitus ulcers or uncleaned urine and feces. In contrast, some patients exhibit **psychomotor agitation**, in which they have rapid, repetitive thoughts and speech and frenzied movements, such as unstoppable crying, pacing, or hand wringing. These patients often feel very anxious and hopeless, complaining sometimes of nearly constant panic. Agitation and akathisia (a subjective state of restlessness leading to an inability to stay still) can often be seen in depressed patients but also can be side effects of antidepressant medication, especially selective serotonin reuptakes inhibitors (SSRIs). Agitated patients may physically cling to others and unintentionally provoke angry responses in families and caregivers. When severe agitation and insomnia are present, it is important to consider the possibility of a mixed affective state, in which patients present with simultaneous symptoms of mania and depression (see Specifiers for Mood Disorder, later in this chapter).

A patient's behavioral, cognitive, and psychomotor symptoms may vary considerably throughout the course of a day. Two special patterns of this variation are diurnal variation and mood reactivity. The patient who is experiencing **diurnal variation** consistently feels worst at one particular time of the day (often, the morning). For example, a patient wakes up early, feels terribly low, and is unable to concentrate, eat, or talk to anyone. Gradually, he or she begins to feel better and, by evening, may feel almost normal. On the next day, however, the pattern repeats itself. The patient with **mood reactivity** can be cheered up briefly or brought out of the depression by a "good" event, such as being praised by another person, eating a favorite meal, having a visit from a grandchild, or receiving romantic attention. Patients with true anhedonia are, by definition, unable to have a reactive mood. However, relative anhedonia is often seen in a patient with marked diurnal variation; although nothing can cheer the person up during the first part of the day, by evening, some glimmers of old interests and pleasures emerge.

To assess depression severity, researchers use standardized numerical rating scales (e.g., the Hamilton Rating Scale for Depression, Beck Depression Inventory, the Young Mania Ratings Scale). Each symptom of depression and each area of impaired functioning are rated on a scale of severity, and the total is added. Practicing physicians usually make this assessment less formally but use the same approach. Moderately severe depression might be characterized by feelings of sadness that occur off and on throughout the day but not an overwhelming feeling of gloom; some disturbance of sleep but not complete exhaustion; minimal weight change; no serious suicidal ideation; and enough concentration to allow patients to continue working or attending school. Severe depression is often equated with melancholia or psychotic depression. These features are not always present, however (e.g., in severe atypical depression).

Persistent Depressive Disorder (Dysthymia)

The fifth edition of the *Diagnostic and Statistical Manual of Mental Disorders* (DSM-5) proposes a new conceptualization of chronic depression. The new diagnosis, persistent depressive disorder, encompasses the previous DSM-IV dysthymic disorder and major depressive disorder with a chronic specifier.

Persistent depressive disorder is a **milder** form of depression, lasting for at least **2 years**, with little or no remission during that time (see DSM-5). Low mood, lack of energy and interest, low self-esteem, and irritability usually form the clinical picture. Sleep disturbance is usually characterized by initial or intermediate insomnia. Early-morning awakening or worsening of mood in the morning, so typical of more severe depression episodes, is very unusual. Psychotic symptoms, such as delusions or hallucinations, are not present. Traditionally, people with these symptoms have been viewed as having personality conflicts or frustrations leading to dissatisfaction with life. It became clear that dysthymia has many similarities with major depression in terms of family history, biological findings, and probably treatment response, and that it could not be satisfactorily differentiated from chronic depression. The difference seems to be more relevant, however, between the chronic and nonchronic forms of depression. *Chronic depressive disorders*, a term used to refer to depressive episodes lasting more than 2 years, are associated with poorer response to treatment, slower rate of improvement over time, younger age of onset, longer episodes, greater disease burden, higher rates of medical and psychiatric comorbidity, and higher rates of suicidal ideation.

This new conceptualization of chronic depression also deals with the so-called double depression (a combination of dysthymia with superimposed major depression episodes) that now falls under this category.

Patients with mild depression fall roughly into two groups: (1) those who have had depressive symptoms since childhood or late adolescence, and (2) those who appear healthy when young but experience major losses, such as the death of a spouse or child, divorce, financial setback, or medical disability at some point in their adult lives and fall into a chronic state of demoralization. Depressive personality is an informal term for a phenomenon that may be seen in individuals with chronic mild depression. Such patients may have long-standing personality difficulties, such as problems in maintaining consistent relationships or in living up to their full academic or occupational potential. They may be irritable, gloomy, and difficult to get along with, tending to complain to those around them that their "glass is always half empty." Alternatively, they may be hardworking, eager to please, and apparently cheerful but also fearful of making mistakes and never satisfied with themselves.

Premenstrual Dysphoric Disorder

Sufficient evidence was gathered to include premenstrual dysphoric disorder in the DSM-5, elevating it from the research criterion stage to the status of a formal diagnosis. Women can experience markedly depressed mood and anhedonia as part of **premenstrual dysphoric disorder** (see DSM-5). Mood and associated physical symptoms (breast tenderness, headaches, bloating) occur in relation to the woman's menstrual cycle as follows: present during the last week of the luteal phase, remit within a few days of the follicular phase, and are absent in the week following menses. Documentation of a **cyclical pattern** must be made using a **prospective daily symptom ratings log** over at least **2 consecutive months** to confirm the diagnosis.

Bipolar Disorder

Patients with bipolar disorder have episodes of mania or hypomania, as well as episodes of depression. The diagnosis of bipolar disorder is made as soon as a patient has one manic episode, even if that person has never had a depressive episode. Almost all patients who become manic will eventually experience depression; about 10% of patients diagnosed with bipolar disorder seem to have only manic episodes. The diagnostic criteria for major depressive episodes are the same for major depressive disorder (also referred to as unipolar depression) and bipolar disorder. The actual diagnostic term is bipolar disorder, current episode depressed. Two major subtypes of bipolar disorder are bipolar I disorder and bipolar II disorder. Patients with **bipolar I** disorder experience mania and a depressive

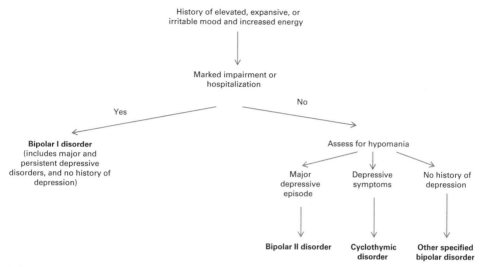

FIGURE 3.2 **Assessing for mania and hypomania**. The decision tree maps the key characteristics differentiating the various bipolar spectrum disorders.

disorder (although only manic episodes are necessary to establish the diagnosis), while those with **bipolar II** disorder experience hypomania and, specifically, major depression (see Figure 3.2). In contrast to the previous editions of the DSM, the DSM-5 permits the diagnosis of bipolar disorder if a full manic or hypomanic episode emerges during antidepressant treatment and persists at a fully syndromal level beyond the immediate effects of the treatment.

Cyclothymia is a milder illness in which patients have hypomania and mild depressive symptoms that are not sufficiently severe to warrant the diagnosis of major depression. If an individual clearly seems to be suffering from some type of bipolar disorder but does not meet the criteria for one of the other subtypes, a diagnosis of Other Specified Bipolar and Related Disorders is assigned. An example would be a patient with hypomania but no history of depressive episodes. A diagnosis of Unspecified Bipolar and Related Disorder can be applied to cases where the patient does not meet full criteria for any of the bipolar disorders, especially in situations where insufficient information is available, such as in emergency room settings.

Mania

The mood of manic patients is characterized by **irritability or abnormal euphoria**, and increased **goal-directed activity** or **energy must be present**. The DSM-5 criteria require 1 week's duration of mania unless the patient requires hospitalization (see DSM-5). Abnormal euphoria is characterized by exaggerated cheerful mood, sense of well-being or happiness, and optimism. Traditionally, euphoric mood has been described as contagious to others, or "infectious gaiety." Patients in manic states have **inflated self-esteem** and heightened interest and pleasure in their surroundings. They often feel they are capable of anything. The world seems to exist for their gratification, and they grandiosely believe that nothing can or should stop them from obtaining what they want. Manic elation quickly blends with irritability if their desires are frustrated. Indeed, **anger** is often the dominant emotion. Along with **grandiosity**, patients frequently deny that anything is wrong. **Impaired insight**, which is ubiquitous in manic patients, is probably caused by the disease itself (not just a "willful" denial of illness) and represents a nearly delusional state. Patients may state that they feel better than ever and not acknowledge that they are ill and in need of treatment. In some patients, it also seems to protect against a feeling of emptiness that underlies the grandiose visions.

The physical, or vegetative, signs in manic patients include insomnia, but unlike in depression, the **need for sleep is decreased**. Patients feel rested after fewer hours of sleep than they usually require. Patients may deny having any trouble sleeping. Only with nearly total insomnia does exhaustion become a problem and, therefore, a cause for complaint. Patients often have **increased energy** for all kinds of activities, such as exercising, working late hours, and socializing. The busy pace may become unpleasant. Patients sometimes say this feeling is similar to a motor that is going too fast. Engagement in multiple projects and tasks is also common. Increased sexual drive and potency and uninhibited social and sexual behavior together with poor judgment may lead to grossly indiscreet behavior, which can become a source of extreme embarrassment later on. Manic patients, unlike depressed patients, have no specific appetite disorder. Some eat robustly and gain weight, whereas others neglect themselves generally, which may lead to weight loss and dehydration.

Manic patients have significant **cognitive change**s, including racing thoughts, a tendency to express thoughts impulsively, distractibility, and difficulty focusing on tasks requiring prolonged attention. Typically, they exhibit a rapid or pressured speech pattern, frequently interrupt others, and have difficulty listening. One of the first indications that a patient is becoming manic may be a family member's observation about pressured speech (e.g., "She just won't shut up! Even when I go out of the room, she keeps blabbering on to herself. No one else can get a word in edgewise."). In order to get other people to listen to them, such patients may make excessive use of the telephone. Although manic patients are often humorous, their humor tends to bore listeners after a while. They can also erupt into anger, especially if people attempt to ignore them or argue with the points they are trying to make.

As the illness becomes severe, the thoughts of manic patients become **disorganized** and skip rapidly among topics that often appear to have little relationship to each other. **Flight of ideas** occurs when tenuously connected thoughts follow each other rapidly, at times giving the impression that there is no logical connection between them (e.g., "Sure, I'm not sleeping. The cars and taxis blew their damn horns all night. You know, I was even late to work because all the cabs were backed up again."). At times the ideas can lose all logical connection and the patient exhibits **loosening of associations**, also seen in schizophrenia. Manic patients sometimes exhibit **clang associations**, which get their name from the German word for "sound" and occur when words are used only for their phonetic sound and not their meaning (e.g., "I got on the bus, I got busted, musted, rusted, like it was Russia!"). When manic patients develop more extreme disorganization of their thought process, exhibiting loosening of associations or word salad, their speech can be indistinguishable from the thought-disordered speech seen in schizophrenia.

Increased motor activity and agitation that are visible to observers are also characteristic of manic patients. Although motor activity may be purposeful at first (e.g., cleaning the house or getting to places in a hurry), it can deteriorate into inappropriate or disorganized actions, such as pacing or fighting. **Manic delirium** occurs when extreme psychomotor agitation is accompanied by disorientation, garbled speech, and chaotic behavior. In this condition, which may be thought of as the counterpart to the

> ### BOX 3.2
> ### CASE EXAMPLE OF MANIC IMPULSIVITY
>
> A divorced woman who was living on her savings planned an affordable vacation within the United States. She became manic shortly before her departure date. When her flight was canceled for mechanical reasons, she exchanged and upgraded her ticket for one to Paris, arrived there with no hotel reservations, spent $5,000 in a few days, and had to call her distraught but wealthy brother to wire money for a return flight. The woman's doctor knew nothing of this until the woman's worried son called after seeing his mother a few weeks later.

pseudodementia found in depression, patients may not be able to care for themselves. Their self-neglect can lead to exhaustion, dehydration, and even death.

Many manic patients behave in impulsive ways: spending sprees, extravagant traveling, sexual affairs, and risky business ventures are the hallmarks of their social dysfunction. Catastrophic ruin may result from the combination of patients' disordered mental attributes (e.g., grandiose plans, rapid thinking, markedly increased sex drive, and denial) and their high level of physical energy that translates ideas into action. Marriages, jobs, lifetime savings, and reputations may be lost. When evaluating manic behavior, it is crucial to obtain a baseline history of the patient's usual patterns of social, sexual, and financial behavior. This information is necessary because patients may deny that they are behaving abnormally. Also, recognition of mania may be delayed in patients who have the resources to compensate for any financial damage. Family and friends often "bail out" manic patients whose indiscretions are mild (see case example in Box 3.2).

Hypomania

Patients who are hypomanic suffer **less functional impairment** than manic patients (see DSM-5). If psychotic symptoms occur, the episode is, by definition, manic and not hypomanic. Hypomanic patients are usually able to carry out their daily tasks at work or home and are generally not ill enough to require hospitalization. People around them notice that they are behaving differently than usual, however. The unusual behavior is sometimes rather likable, especially if their mood is upbeat. Hypomanic people are energetic and can be goal-directed and well organized in their performance at work and at home. Enhanced creativity, sexual capacity, and leadership ability are not unusual. If all activity is pleasurable, the condition does not come to the attention of a doctor. Many bipolar patients view hypomania as a silver lining and resent its being taken away through treatment. Their **heightened cognitive and sensual alertness** combined with the **increased energy** creates a feeling of being superhuman. Phrases like "I've never felt so good before in my life" are characteristic warning signs and should raise the physician's concerns because, as the syndrome escalates, social and occupational catastrophes may occur. The silver lining usually gives way to depression or escalates to a destructive "high." Typically, the patient's expression of grandiosity combined with increasingly unrealistic ideas leads others to begin questioning the judgment of the hypomanic person. Euphoria soon changes to argumentativeness; social or financial failures begin to occur; and the patient either crashes into despair and depression or pushes the level of denial upward into full-blown mania.

Hypomania may last for months, or it may precede by a few days a full-blown manic episode. Patients with repeated cycles often exhibit peculiar changes in behavior, or the so-called **hypomanic alert**, at the start of an episode.

Cyclothymia

Patients with cyclothymia alternate between mild depression, but of short duration, and hypomanic symptoms. The cycles are continuous and last for several weeks to several months. Rarely do these patients complain specifically about the highs and lows they experience. More commonly, patients will complain only of being depressed at times, not realizing that they have been hypomanic at other times. Family members may be aware of the pattern, but they are rarely consulted because the patient's symptoms are generally mild. The physician often makes the diagnosis after observing patients for a period of time and discovering that the "well" periods are, in fact, highs. Individuals with cyclothymia sometimes seek treatment for help with personality or social problems. They often have trouble maintaining relationships, get into arguments when they are hypomanic, and perform inconsistently at school or work. Mild mixed states may also be a part of this illness. In these patients, the predominant complaint is chronic depression with fluctuating sleep patterns, agitation, and irritability. Cyclothymia is sometimes a precursor to the more classic form of bipolar I or bipolar II illness. States resembling cyclothymia can also be seen during incomplete recovery from these more severe disorders.

Specifiers for Mood Disorders

The DSM-5 classifies major depressive disorder and bipolar I disorder on the basis of whether the latest episode (manic or depressive) is single or recurrent, as well as current severity, presence of psychotic features, and remission status. In the specific case of hypomanic episodes in the context of bipolar I disorder, current severity and the presence of psychotic features are not relevant and only different remission statuses are taken into account. Additional features define different specifiers that further portray the clinical picture. As many specifiers as is suitable can be applied to the same episode. On the basis of additional symptoms, specifiers are melancholic features, atypical features, mood-congruent or mood-incongruent psychotic features, catatonic features, mixed features, anxious distress, and level of concern for suicide. Three other specifiers—rapid cycling, seasonal pattern, peripartum onset—are defined by the course of the illness or by particular precipitants.

Melancholic features often occur in patients with severe depression. Historically known as the classic form of the illness, melancholia has sometimes been called endogenous because, more than other forms of depression, it tends to appear spontaneously without psychological precipitants. It is associated with significant neurobiological abnormalities that are thought to reflect a genetic or biological etiology. Antidepressant medications are essential for patients with melancholic features.

Patients with melancholic features experience severe **anhedonia, lack of reactivity** to usually pleasurable stimuli, and at least three of the following features: a **distinct quality** of depressed mood that the patient says is different from feelings of disappointment or loss at other times, **diurnal variation** with a worse state in the morning, **early morning insomnia, marked psychomotor retardation or agitation**, significant decreased appetite with **weight loss**, and excessive guilt.

Up to one-third of depressed patients suffer from depression **with atypical features**, having the atypical symptoms of **increased sleep and appetite** (reversed vegetative signs), extreme fatigue and heaviness in the limbs (**leaden paralysis**), and, sometimes, **mood reactivity**. A lifelong pattern of exaggerated **interpersonal sensitivity** has also been described in these patients. Proper diagnosis of patients with depression with atypical features traditionally was important because of their preferential response to the SSRI and monoamine oxidase inhibitor (MAOI) classes of antidepressant drugs over the tricyclic antidepressants (TCAs), although the latter two classes of medication are now rarely used. Nonetheless, the distinction may still inform the use of current medications that avoid exacerbating the feelings of sedation and urges to overeat. Atypical depression can be every bit as severe and recurrent as melancholic or "typical" depression, and there is no reason to think it has any less association with neurobiological dysfunction than these forms. Reversed vegetative signs are also relatively common in bipolar depression (i.e., major depression that occurs during the course of bipolar disorder).

Psychotic features can occur in **both depressive and manic** episodes. About one-third of manic patients are psychotic, as is the case for about 15% of depressed patients, including 25% of those admitted to hospitals. Patients experience psychotic symptoms such as delusions and (less commonly) hallucinations, in addition to the other symptoms of major depression or mania. These psychotic symptoms occur only during mood episodes and not at other times in their lives.

Psychotic features are classified as mood-congruent or mood-incongruent on the basis of whether or not the delusions focus on themes that are consistent with the current mood episode. In the case of a depressive episode, delusions or hallucinations are considered **mood-congruent** if they focus on a depressive theme such as **guilt, pessimism**, disease, impoverishment, or deserved punishment. The delusions can dramatically reflect guilt, hopelessness, and a sense that one's self or the world has deteriorated beyond repair (see case examples in Box 3.3). Nihilistic delusions are seen in severe depression in which patients deny their existence or even deny the existence of the world around them. In Cotard's syndrome, an extreme form of nihilistic delusion, the patient believes he or she is dead. An example of a mood-incongruent delusion is a depressed woman's belief that her neighbors were talking about her, criticizing her apartment and her clothing. She felt angry and frightened but did not feel that she deserved this criticism or had done anything wrong to provoke it. Persecutory delusions perceived as unjustified or unfair as in this example are usually more characteristic of primary psychotic disorders, whereas in depressed mood-congruent persecutory delusions the patient justifies them as being deserved. Rarely, in some cases of extremely severe psychotic depression, the world is perceived with such pessimism and hopelessness that patients can kill their loved ones, usually followed by suicide, in an "altruistic way," believing that they are saving them from great misfortunes. Patients with mood-incongruent symptoms have a worse prognosis for resuming premorbid functioning. Psychotic symptoms tend to occur repeatedly in some patients, are more common in **bipolar** than in unipolar depression, and may be a major **risk for suicide**.

In mania, psychosis usually develops after earlier manic symptoms have begun to escalate, but it may precede the full syndrome by 1 or 2 weeks, serving as a warning sign. For example, whenever he was about to enter a manic phase, a patient who had a recurrent delusion that he was Jesus Christ would start to grow a beard, which was a sign that he believed he was transforming into the Messiah. The most typical **mood-congruent manic** themes are related to grandiosity, which may take a **euphoric** form (e.g., patients imagining that a celebrity is going to marry them or believing that they possess answers

---

BOX 3.3

CASE EXAMPLES OF DEPRESSED PATIENTS WITH MOOD-CONGRUENT DELUSIONS

One man, an accountant, believed that a minor addition error he had made 10 years earlier was responsible for the demise of his firm. Another man believed that he was "evil incarnate" and that his family would "pay the price for his misdeeds." A woman believed that she was literally burning in hell and had tactile hallucinations of feeling the flames. A man was convinced that he was unable to speak because he thought he had not spoken for a long time while he was depressed, even though he was able to speak loudly and clearly. Another man thought his bowels were obstructed and that no food was able to pass through them. He was also convinced that he was going blind because an examination 2 years earlier had revealed a microembolus. He tried to save his vision by not "using it up," believing that only a finite amount existed. He also believed that his landlord had infused his mind with toxic fumes, which caused his thinking to slow down.

---

to the great problems afflicting humanity), or a hostile, paranoid form in patients who think others envy them or want to kill them because of their greatness. **Grandiose delusions** of being on a special mission or having special abilities or powers are classic in manic patients, and it is important to inquire about these delusions specifically. This grandiosity is in marked contrast to psychotic depression, in which patients fear punishment for being bad. The euphoric and paranoid forms of manic grandiosity are often combined. One man believed he was the "godfather," that he had been hospitalized for his own safety, that the movie *Godfather Part 3* was about him, and that, when the movie was released, the mafia would pick him up at the hospital in a limousine so he could attend the gala benefit premiere.

The behavior of psychotic manic patients can be extremely bizarre and violent toward others, whereas in suicidal psychotic depressive patients, the destructive behavior is directed toward the self. One psychotic manic patient, thinking she was a messenger of God, threw her cat out of a fifth-floor window in order to observe the biblical injunction to "sacrifice one small beast" to the Lord. Mood-incongruent delusions are also seen, as in the case of a woman who believed that the colors of traffic lights had been altered from the usual red, green, and yellow. As with depression, patients with mood-incongruent delusions have poorer outcomes in terms of ability to function socially even after the psychotic and mood disorder symptoms have resolved.

One-tenth to one-third of patients with major depression experience a **seasonal pattern** of recurrence of depressive episodes, in which symptoms emerge predictably in the fall or winter months. The opposite pattern--depression in the summer and nondepressed periods in the winter—has also been described. **Lethargy and fatigue** are common symptoms of **winter** seasonal pattern. Atypical features of **hypersomnia** and **overeating** are frequent but not universal. Seasonal patterns may be seen in bipolar disorder, as well, especially in bipolar II disorder with hypomania in the spring or summer following a depressive episode during the winter. Experiments have shown that the pattern is usually related to **light deprivation** and is more common in northern latitudes. In addition to

BOX 3.4

CASE EXAMPLE OF DEPRESSION WITH SEASONAL PATTERN

A 39-year-old novelist presented in October with fatigue, withdrawal from her friends, and writer's block. She described recent cravings for carbohydrates along with a 7-pound weight gain, and an inability to cope with laundry, cleaning, and other household chores. Her history revealed a pattern of such difficulties occurring since college. Her symptoms had usually been evaluated as physical ailments, although tests for viral or endocrine disorders had been negative. She responded quickly to treatment with a bright bedside lamp set on a timer to go on early in the morning.

the standard treatments for depression, light therapy using **bright lights** that mimic the wavelengths of natural light or trips to southerly locales are uniquely effective in patients with depression with seasonal pattern (see case example in Box 3.4). In the case of bipolar disorder, this pattern needs to exist for at least one type of episode (manic, hypomanic, or depressive). Seasonal pattern is thought to be caused by specific abnormalities of melatonin secretion and other biochemical aspects of the sleep–wake cycle and not by seasonal psychosocial stresses, such as the holiday "blues."

In the weeks after they deliver a child, 10% of women experience mood disorders, and the specifier of major depression with **peripartum onset** should be used. **Psychotic features** rarely occur but are of grave concern. This condition is distinct from the transient "baby blues" that 50% of women experience for a few days immediately after giving birth. The enormous psychological and physical changes, including massive new responsibilities for both the mother and father, sleep deprivation, and hormonal fluctuation, have all been considered as possible causes of depression with peripartum onset, but none has been definitively linked to it. Women with a personal or family history of affective disorders are at greater risk, which suggests an underlying vulnerability. The symptoms and treatment of depression with peripartum onset (or mania) are basically the same as for other mood disorders, although special support may be needed for the mother and the family. Mothers with depression with peripartum onset may feel especially guilty about not being able to respond fully to the needs of their newborn. In women thought to be at risk, antidepressants can be given or psychotherapy can be started immediately after birth as a preventive measure. Hormonal treatments are ineffective. Depression with peripartum onset often recurs after subsequent pregnancies and often heralds **bipolar disorder**.

Anxiety often accompanies major depressive episodes and can also occur in mania or hypomania. **Anxious distress** is defined as at least two symptoms present during the most recent 2 weeks of the depressive episode, the most recent week of a manic episode, or the most recent 4 days of a hypomanic episode, such as feeling tense or restless, having difficulty concentrating because of worry, fearing that something awful might happen, or feeling like the individual might lose control.

Rapid cycling refers to distinct, sustained periods of mania, hypomania, or depression occurring **at least four times a year**, in the context of bipolar disorder. The cycles may be alternating sequences of highs and lows or frequent brief bouts of repeated depressions or manias, with only occasional excursions into the opposite pole. Rapid cycling bipolar

II disorder is a common pattern. Between episodes, patients with rapid cycling may have full, partial, or no recovery. Patients with no intervening recovery are said to be in continuous cycling and are very ill indeed. Rapid cycling is disabling because patients find it hard to carry out sustained activities. It is difficult to treat and may be initiated or made worse by antidepressants. Lithium treatment as monotherapy is relatively ineffective. Rapid cycling is more common in women and in patients who previously have had multiple bipolar episodes. Hypothyroidism comorbidity is common. Patients who exhibit mood changes over the course of hours or a day are usually considered to be experiencing mixed states, although the term *ultrafast rapid cycling* has also been used. Whether mixed and rapid cycling states are part of a continuum or are distinct states is unclear.

Mood episodes with **mixed features** are confusing mixtures of mood, thought, and behavioral symptoms that appear to be "out of synch" with one another. Mixed features are defined by the **simultaneous coexistence of depressive and manic symptoms** in the same mood episode. The DSM-IV designated a diagnostic category of mixed mood episode in the context of bipolar I disorder and required that patients meet all of the diagnostic criteria for mania and major depression simultaneously. By this strict definition, only about 10% of hospitalized patients with mood disorders met criteria for mixed states. Less strict definitions specified that only some of the criteria for depression and mania be met. Using such definitions, as many as 50% of hospitalized bipolar patients could receive the diagnosis of a mixed state. Because of the high prevalence of those subsyndromal presentations, the mixed episode category was removed from the DSM-5. Instead, the specifier "with mixed features" is applied to mood episodes that meet the full criteria for mania, hypomania, or major depression and have **at least three symptoms that belong to the opposite pole**, in both bipolar and major depressive disorders. In this way, mixed features are conceptualized as a dimensional approach that is added to a categorical diagnosis. This update allows the capture of those patients with subthreshold nonoverlapping symptoms of the opposite pole. Patients in this broader group tend to have a condition called **dysphoric mania**, which is characterized by a sad, tearful mood, often with suicidality, and motor and cognitive signs of mania, such as irritability, pressured speech, racing thoughts, insomnia, and excessive energy (described by patients as an unpleasant "wired" feeling). **Psychosis** is also common in mood episodes with mixed features.

Recognition of mood episodes with mixed features is especially important because patients with this condition respond more slowly to standard treatments for "pure" episodes and tend to become worse if treated with antidepressants in the case of bipolar disorder. Mixed features may occur at various times during a patient's mood cycle. They may be discrete episodes that occur as the predominant type of mood cycle that an individual experiences; they may be a particular stage during a mood episode, usually occurring after the episode has been going on for a while and the patient's functioning has deteriorated; or they may be a transitional phase in a cycle that is going from depression to mania or hypomania or vice versa. Patients with mixed features have a **high risk of suicide**, perhaps because they may simultaneously have a depressed mood and a high capacity for physical activity.

Some patients with bipolar disorder and major depressive disorder may develop **catatonic features**. The clinical picture is characterized by marked psychomotor disturbance that may include motoric immobility, excessive motor activity, extreme negativism, **mutism**, and **peculiarities of voluntary movement**, as well as echolalia (mimicking another's speech) and echopraxia (mimicking another's movements). Motoric immobility may be manifested by **catalepsy (waxy flexibility) or stupor**. The excessive motor activity is apparently purposeless and is not influenced by external stimuli. The diagnosis of catatonic features can be applied to a current major depressive or manic episode in major depressive disorder, bipolar I disorder, or bipolar II disorder. Some authors argue that racing thoughts can be so intense that a manic patient becomes locked into a catatonic state. In depressed patients, a catatonic state can be due to extreme psychomotor retardation. In patients being treated with antipsychotics, particular attention should be paid to the possibility that the catatonia is due to neuroleptic malignant syndrome (see Side Effects of Antipsychotic Agents, Chapter 16, Pharmacotherapy, ECT, and TMS).

The DSM-5 includes a specifier for the **level of concern of suicide** in all mood episode categories. Suicidal thoughts are common in depressed patients, and suicidal behaviors are the most lethal complications of depression (see Box 3.5). Suicidal thoughts are accompanied by varying degrees of intent. Many patients transiently wish that they would somehow disappear, not wake up from sleep, or be killed in an accident. Such feelings are referred to as

---

BOX 3.5
SUICIDE

Fifteen to twenty percent of patients with affective disorders severe enough to require hospitalization eventually die from suicide, and a diagnosis of depression is present in 45% to 70% of individuals who kill themselves. A number of associated clinical features of depression increase the risk of suicide: melancholia, psychosis, extreme hopelessness, mixed or transitional bipolar states, alcohol and drug use disorders marked impulsivity, a poor response to medication, definite plans for committing suicide, a history of prior attempts, and a family history of suicide.

Doctors and laypersons sometimes fear that asking about suicide will make it happen. In fact, the opposite is true. Patients may lose trust if they perceive doctors' reticence to discuss suicide as a sign of anxiety, much as they would not trust a surgeon afraid of blood. Talking about suicide, especially in detail with a new patient, can help defuse the intensity of the wish to act on it. Verbalizing the fantasy may bring some emotional relief, substituting for the act if suicide is seen as a way to communicate feelings that patients believe are unappreciated by others. Patients test doctors to find out if they are willing to listen to the patients' most disturbed feelings. The best rule is to ask the patient calmly and directly: "Do you have thoughts of hurting yourself?" "Are you suicidal?" This phrasing is much preferable to the following: "You wouldn't try hurting yourself, would you?" "You're not suicidal, are you?"

When depressed patients reveal suicidal intent, the following empathic but firmly optimistic approach is suggested: "Right now, you feel that your life is not worth continuing. My view is that your illness has greatly impaired your capacity to judge accurately your own self-worth and the external circumstances of your life. I will do everything I can to ensure your safety until the illness has been treated, because I think you will view your situation differently when you are well." Techniques for interviewing and managing suicidal patients are discussed in more detail in Chapter 12, Suicide.

passive suicidal thoughts. Others consider ending their lives more actively but feel restrained by attachments to loved ones or hopes of recovery. Of greatest concern is the patient who absolutely wants to die and makes plans to do so. Although the patient's functioning may be impaired in most other areas of life, he or she may be able to make detailed plans for committing suicide, which may include consulting medical references on lethal drugs and making plans to obtain a horde of such drugs or making arrangements, for example, to carry out carbon monoxide poisoning. Selecting a date, such as an anniversary, or writing a suicide note are clear warnings of serious intent. In patients with recurrent depressions, a history of suicide attempts is a strong predictor of future attempts. Serious attempts are usually preceded by thoughts and plans for suicide. The physician must ask all depressed patients about past and present suicidal ideas, attempts, and plans (see Box 3.5 and Chapter 12, Suicide).

Geriatric Issues

The aging of the U.S. population has made depression among the elderly a significant public health problem. Persistent depressive disorder affects up to 50% of residents in long-term care facilities. It is associated with considerable discomfort, disability, and risk of morbidity, as well as excessive use of non–mental health services.

Mood disorders beginning after approximately age 50 years are considered **late onset** and may have causes that are different from those beginning earlier. Recent studies with magnetic resonance imaging (MRI) suggest that many patients with late-onset mood disorder may have early subcortical **cerebrovascular disease**. MRI white matter hyperintensities have been found in these patients and are associated with apathy, psychomotor slowness, and retardation, a condition sometimes referred to as vascular depression. Late-life depression also seems to be a risk factor for Alzheimer's disease. While specific psychosocial factors, such as loneliness, poverty, and general medical debilitation, may be contributing factors to depression in the elderly, depression is not a normal or commonplace reaction to the events associated with aging, but instead is an illness requiring appropriate diagnosis and treatment.

Geriatric depression often occurs concurrently with a variety of **chronic medical illnesses**. Depression associated with the presence of chronic medical illness also increases the incidence of **premature mortality**, primarily from increased rates of cardiovascular and cancer deaths. Of note, the death rate 6 months after acute myocardial infarction is increased fivefold among depressed patients.

Between 10% and 20% of geriatric patients with mood disorders have **bipolar disorder**, as do 5% of those admitted to geropsychiatric units. Bipolar disorder in later life is a complex and confounding neuropsychiatric syndrome. While late-onset bipolar disorder is relatively rare, recurrence of remitted disease frequently occurs in late life. Elderly patients with late-onset bipolar disorder have been found to have higher cerebrovascular risk than that of patients with the early-onset disorder. Late-onset bipolar disorder is associated with a lower rate of familial illness than early-onset cases, a higher rate of medical and neurological comorbidity, and an increased vulnerability to relapse. In patients with a history of unipolar depression, mania may not develop until later life, and misdiagnosis is common, especially in type II bipolar disorder.

EPIDEMIOLOGY AND COURSE OF ILLNESS

Door-to-door surveys conducted over the past 20 years in many cities in the United States and in other countries have yielded relatively uniform findings regarding the

TABLE 3.2 Epidemiology of Mood Disorders

	Depressive Disorders	Bipolar Disorders
Prevalence	Major depression point: Men: 2.3–3.2% Women: 4.5–9.3%	Bipolar I lifetime: 0.4–1.6% Bipolar II lifetime: 0.5%
	Major depression lifetime: Men: 7–12% Women: 20–25%	
	Dysthymia lifetime: Men: 2.2% Women: 4.1%	Equal in gender and race High rates of divorce Cyclothymia lifetime: 0.4–1%
Age of Onset	Late 20s or 30s; childhood possible* May have much later onset† Individuals born after 1940 have greater rates and earlier onset than those born earlier‡	Late teens or early 20s; childhood possible* Cyclothymia may precede late onset of overt mania or depression
Family and Genetic Studies	Unipolar patients tend to have relatives with major depressive and dysthymic disorders and fewer with bipolar disorders Early onset, recurrent course, and psychotic depression appear to be heritable	Bipolar patients have many relatives with bipolar disorder, cyclothymia, unipolar depression, and schizoaffective disorder
Twin Studies	Concordance in monozygotic twins: 59% for recurrent depression, 33% for single episode only The concordance rates for monozygotic twins are 4 times greater than those found in fraternal (dizygotic) twins**	Concordance in monozygotic twins: 65–80%

*Childhood symptoms may not always be the same as adult symptoms; children may exhibit greater behavioral disturbance (e.g., as seen in family and school settings) and less expression of emotional symptoms.

†Careful evaluation may reveal special psychosocial factors, contributing medical conditions, or subtle earlier mood disturbances that escaped diagnosis and treatment.

‡In a phenomenon known as the "cohort effect," individuals born after 1940 are developing unipolar and possibly bipolar disorders at greater rates and with earlier ages of onset than those born prior to 1940. This is not an artifact of diagnostic trends but seems to represent a genuine epidemiological change that might reflect effects of the post–World War II social or physical environment on the expression of these disorders.

** Limited data on twins reared apart from each other (and from their parents) tend to show comparable results, strengthening the interpretation that familial illness is from shared genes, not only shared environment. However, molecular genetic studies of chromosomal material from large families with affective illness have not yielded replicable findings of markers. Researchers have not yet been able to implicate specific chromosomes or markers or to choose between single or multiple gene models.

lifetime prevalence of mood disorders in the industrialized world (Table 3.2). The point prevalence of depressive disorders in primary care practice settings was found to be about double that of the general population. This may reflect the increased help-seeking behavior in depressed patients. The National Comorbidity Survey Replication showed that the lifetime prevalence of major depressive disorder was 16.2% and the 12-month prevalence was 6.6%. Another recent survey, the National Epidemiologic Survey on Alcoholism and Related Conditions, demonstrated that the prevalence of 12-month and lifetime major depressive disorder was 5.3% and 13.2%, respectively. Being female; Native American; middle-aged; widowed, separated, or divorced; and low income increased risk. Being Asian, Hispanic, or African-American decreased risk. Women were significantly more likely to receive treatment than men. Both current and lifetime major depressive disorder were significantly associated with other specific psychiatric disorders, notably substance dependence, panic and generalized anxiety disorder, and several personality disorders.

Patients with bipolar disorder and the more recurrent forms of unipolar depression have a striking pattern of **decreasing cycle lengths** or increasing frequency of episodes over time. The average well period between the first and second episodes is 3 to 5 years. The cycle becomes progressively shorter, reaching a mean of less than 1 year after the sixth cycle (see Figure 3.3). Some patients develop classic **rapid cycling** (i.e., four or more episodes per year) as the illness progresses over time, entering a prolonged downhill course. This deterioration is not inevitable, however. There is also a group of patients who have a pattern of rapid cycling in which episodes cluster for a period of time and then diminish in frequency. The shortening of clusters may reflect

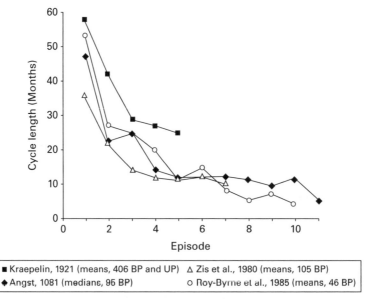

FIGURE 3.3 **Relationship between cycle length and episode number.** Episodes in recurrent mood disorders occur closer together over time. The first and second episodes are often several years apart. By the fifth episode, the average cycle is less than 1 year. References are to studies that collected data in unmedicated patients over long periods of time. BP, bipolar; UP, unipolar. (From Goodwin, F. K., and K. R. Jamison. *Manic-Depressive Illness.* New York: Oxford University Press, 1990. Reproduced with permission.)

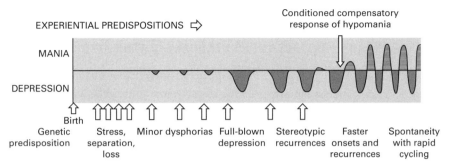

FIGURE 3.4 **Natural history of recurrent mood disorders: integrated model.** Genetic factors and early environmental stress may predispose an individual to develop a mood disorder. Early episodes are likely to be precipitated by environmental stress, whereas later episodes are more likely to occur closer together and spontaneously, without precipitants. (From Post, R. M., D. R. Rubinow, and J. C. Ballenger. Conditioning, sensitization, and kindling: implications for the course of affective illness. In *Neurobiology of Mood Disorders,* R. M. Post and J. C. Ballenger, eds. Baltimore: Williams and Wilkins, 1984. Reproduced with permission.)

neurobiological alterations in the brain caused by each successive episode, which result in a lowering of the threshold for illness (see Sensitization and Kindling Theory, later in this chapter).

Patients with mood disorders are more sensitive to emotional stress. The major life events with which most people are able to cope may precipitate episodes of illness in vulnerable patients. **Psychosocial stress** is especially likely to trigger episodes early in the course of the illness. These disorders often begin when patients first assume adult responsibilities, such as leaving home, going to college, getting married, or starting to work. While this association may be a coincidence, there is good evidence that these events are precipitating stresses for early episodes. After several recurrences, episodes are more likely to occur spontaneously, "out of the blue," with no apparent precipitants. These are autonomous, or endogenous, episodes (see Figure 3.4). Seasonal patterns that are not related to psychosocial stress may be apparent (e.g., wintertime depressions related to decreased light exposure). Precipitated and autonomous episodes are symptomatically indistinguishable, and individuals may, of course, suffer both.

Major Depression

Episodes of major depression usually begin **gradually**. If untreated, they last an average of **6 months**. Chronicity is a problem: about 20% of depressed patients remain depressed for up to a year or more and 12% for as long as 5 years. **Risk factors for chronicity** include a strong **family history** of depression, **older age**, **longer duration** of illness before treatment is sought, **alcoholism**, **medical illness**, disability of spouse, or multiple recent deaths of family members. From 50% to 70% of patients with major depression have **recurrent episodes** in their lifetimes. In those who have more than one episode, the average number is five to six. There is some tendency for individuals to have a recurrence of similar symptoms during each episode, such as melancholia, atypical symptoms, or psychosis, but there are many exceptions. One research group prospectively studied major depressive episodes occurring within 2 years to determine whether symptoms in

> **BOX 3.6**
> ## CASE EXAMPLE OF PROLONGED RECOVERY AFTER RAPID CYCLING
>
> One woman recovered fully from a 2-year stretch of rapid cycling complicated by frequent mood-incongruent paranoid delusions. She repeatedly failed makeup college courses, however, and could not sustain friendships because of persistent shyness and a vague tendency to make other people feel awkward around her. She remained slightly odd. It took her several years to regain enough cognitive capacity, social skill, and general self-confidence to complete her degree and begin dating.

the second episode could be predicted on the basis of symptoms in the first. The lack of robust consistency of symptoms or depressive subtype across episodes was striking. Persistent depressive disorder may be a prodrome to major depression, and it is likely to be associated with a less complete recovery after the major depression is over.

Bipolar Disorder

Patients with bipolar disorder are more likely than those with unipolar depression to have an **abrupt "switch"** of mood overnight or over a few days. This change is very striking when it occurs: patients behave normally one day and wake up the next day with rapid speech, altered behavior, and other manic symptoms. An episode is sometimes precipitated by **sleep deprivation**, resulting from travel or psychosocial stress, but it often occurs without explanation. Manic episodes are usually shorter in length than depressive episodes. Chronic mania, although rare, has been described. Indeed, the first patient to receive lithium had been manic for 5 years. Almost all patients with bipolar disorder have **recurrent episodes**. These episodes are more frequent and numerous than in unipolar depression. In some patients, continuous major and milder cycles are difficult to separate and count. Variation in the proportion and severity of the types of episodes is considerable. As mentioned earlier, about 10% of bipolar patients have little or no depression and can be considered to have unipolar mania. Patients with cyclothymia may remain stable or develop a full-blown bipolar disorder.

The degree of recovery between bipolar episodes varies. While many patients are able to resume normal activities within several weeks to months, approximately 40% of patients have significant social dysfunction for up to 2 years after an episode. Earlier in this century, before drug treatment became available, it was estimated that about one-third of bipolar patients had chronic, mild mood disturbances (i.e., persistent depressive disorder, hypomania, cyclothymia, or irritability). Current estimates of chronic symptoms are lower, although undertreatment of mild symptoms is widespread. Patients with mixed states, rapid cycling, mood-incongruent psychosis, or schizoaffective disorder (persistence of psychosis after resolution of mood symptoms; see Differential Diagnosis, later in chapter); substance abuse; or poor family support have an increased risk of **chronicity**. Even when they are apparently free of chronic symptoms, many patients have difficulty in functioning in work and family roles for long periods of time after episodes (see case example in Box 3.6). Neurobiological deterioration from repeated episodes may play a role in this phenomenon. Another factor is the **demoralization** patients experience for having their lives repeatedly interrupted by the illness, which derails friendships and interrupts education, work, and other activities. In general, depressive episodes and symptoms dominate the longitudinal course of bipolar disorder. On average, it takes about 10 years from onset of symptoms to diagnosis.

Even so, most patients with bipolar disorder function well, especially when they are taking the proper medication. Individuals with bipolar disorder are thought to be over-represented among successful individuals in the arts and other professions. This association is often attributed to mild, productive hypomanic characteristics, such as increased sociability, energy, and imagination, but it could be a result of the enhanced creativity or perceptiveness associated with an inherently greater range of moods.

THE INTERVIEW

Depressive Disorders

The depletion felt by a depressed patient requires the physician to be **active** in the interview, making greater efforts than with most other psychiatric patients to draw them out and show interest. Because the patient may feel so indecisive, helpless, and hopeless, the physician also needs to **take charge** in a tactfully firm way, urging a doubting patient to begin medication, making clear follow-up plans, and enlisting the family's support.

The demeanor exhibited by the patient during the interview can be very helpful in making a diagnosis of depression. Depressed patients characteristically appear with a deflected posture, bent shoulders, corners of the mouth and gaze looking downward. Gestural movements and facial mimic are reduced, and grooming may be neglected. Patients usually take more time to start answering questions, speak slowly, and speak in a lower tone of voice. The embarrassed smile that some depressed patients show, sometimes to conceal sadness, should not be confused with incongruity of affect that is more characteristic of schizophrenia.

When taking the history, the physician should ask the patient about normal patterns as well as variations, in order to **establish a baseline** and to assess persistent changes accurately. For example, it is helpful to ask patients with insomnia what time they usually get into bed, how long it takes to fall asleep, and the time at which they usually wake up and then get out of bed. It may emerge, for example, that a man who says he still gets up at his usual time of 7:00 a.m. in fact wakens an hour or two earlier than usual and lies in bed trying to fall back to sleep until the alarm goes off. It is also important to note physical illnesses, the use of sleeping pills and other medicines, and intentional weight loss diets that might mask or mimic vegetative signs.

Depressed patients are more trusting and cooperative when they feel that other people are accepting, not criticizing, them. Because these patients tend to feel blame from themselves and others, creating an atmosphere that feels **accepting** to them takes special skill on the part of the physician. Encouragement, however, can be a two-edged sword: while common sense might lead a physician to point out the positive aspects of the patient's life, for example, patients may interpret this optimism as a belittlement of their perceptions. Simplistic reassurances (e.g., "Don't worry. There's nothing to be that upset over.") may cause the patient to feel misunderstood and rejected. An empathic way to provide encouragement is to show appreciation of the patient's position by saying, for example, "I understand how bleak everything seems now. It must be very hard for you to believe that you once felt capable of functioning as well as you must have, judging from everything you have accomplished in the past."

Several factors may contribute to depressed patients providing an **incomplete or inaccurate history**. First, the cognitive or physiological aspects of depression may interfere: **poor memory** and concentration prevent recall or organization of historical material, and psychomotor retardation may make it difficult to convey information within the time allotted for the interview. Selective recall is also a common feature of depression. Patients tend to recall more readily negative past events than happy memories. This becomes especially important when assessing past hypomanic episodes, since depressed patients may be unable to recall them.

Second, the psychological aspects of depression can **alter perceptions** of reality on either a subtle level or at the more overt level of psychosis. For example, a patient whose depression is causing him to perform poorly at work may falsely assume that the boss has always disliked him. The physician may learn from a spouse, however, that the patient is a well-liked, hard-working employee whose lowered performance and failure to appreciate his normal strengths are in fact distinct features of the current depressive episode. Another psychological reason for misreporting is **shame**, which may cause patients to conceal their true concerns (see case examples in Box 3.7).

It may be useful to invite **family members** to attend the interview in order to overcome these conscious and unconscious sources of distortion. As a rule, the patient should be present when the family gives the history. Occasionally, however, a relative may want to speak privately with the physician, especially when the patient has told the relative a "secret," such as a suicidal or psychotic thought. In that situation, the physician should meet alone with the relative and then encourage the relative to meet with the patient and physician and express his or her concerns openly. This open communication usually reassures the patient of the family's concern and helps avoid infantilization of the patient. This joint meeting can also be a time for the physician to help the family understand that urging the patient to cheer up, even when it is done with the best of intentions, may have the opposite effect, especially if the patient already feels like a burden to the family.

The depressed patient's feelings of hopelessness, helplessness, and worthlessness tend to produce **characteristic responses to the physician**. Patients' initial reactions to the physician may be based on the **guilt** they feel about the depression and the **expectation**

BOX 3.7
CASE EXAMPLES OF SHAME AND DEPRESSION

It took the ward staff several weeks to discover that an isolated patient was having an olfactory hallucination that he smelled bad and a related delusion that he was being shunned by the other patients. In a more subtle example of shame, an elderly man said he was depressed because he felt guilty about continuing to socialize after his wife became ill. In an interview with the couple, it was clear that his wife was relieved that her husband was staying active. The interviewer then focused more profitably on the man's own fears of aging and loss, brought on by seeing his wife deteriorate. He had thought at first it would have been selfish to bring up his own concerns.

of being criticized or even punished for being depressed. One coping mechanism is to try to please the physician by **underreporting** symptoms so as not to seem like a complainer. Another reaction is to feel rejected and become inwardly **angry**. Some chronically depressed patients are paranoid just below the surface and are prone to struggle against expected punishment or other mistreatment. The physician who listens carefully may hear a subtle litany of disappointment toward previous physicians who have failed to cure symptoms, especially somatic ones such as unexplained pain or insomnia. The patient may use words of praise and thanks while at the same time using body language to criticize (e.g., saying, with raised eyebrows and a sigh, "All the doctors were very nice, but they were always in a rush to get me out, and, after all those pills, I still have stomach cramps.").

Helplessness and hopelessness may drive the patient to become very **dependent** on the physician, simultaneously expecting to be rescued while fearing that the physician, like the patient, is powerless to turn the tide. This conflict should be addressed by discussing the contradiction openly. To begin such a discussion, the physician might say, "I realize how much you want me to help you feel better and how scary it feels to hear me say it may take several weeks to gauge the effectiveness of the medicine. I can assure you that these are normal reactions in depression and that when it is all over, you'll look back on it like a bad dream." Another aspect of this reaction is the patient's fear that any expression of anger will cause the physician to think the patient is bad.

Physician responses often reflect the symptoms and defenses of particular patients. Compliant or excessively polite patients may make the physician feel omnipotent and elicit **rescue fantasies**, while more pessimistic or angry patients may cause the physician to feel threatened or **helpless**. The physician's awareness that such reactions are a response to opposing feelings helps to form a more complete picture of the patient's problems (see case example in Box 3.8). This example also illustrates the reactions of a

---

BOX 3.8

CASE EXAMPLE OF A SUICIDAL DEPRESSED PATIENT

A 54-year-old female outpatient readily described the recent onset of classic symptoms of major depression. She was extremely well groomed, polite, cooperative, and apologetic about crying. She repeatedly leaned toward the doctor and asked, "Do you think you can help me?" and complimented him on his understanding and sympathy. She began to describe a number of deprivations she had experienced in her life, beginning with child abuse and culminating in the recent refusal of her husband to pay for her to complete the college degree that she had foregone early in their marriage. Only when the physician began to probe her feelings of disappointment in important caretakers did she describe detailed plans to asphyxiate herself in the family garage, stating, "No one really cares what becomes of me." Had the physician assumed that the history was complete because of the patient's ingratiating, eager-to-please manner, he might have prematurely reassured her that everything would be all right. His initial pleasure in the patient's superficial faith in him would have prevented his discovery of her concealed, enraged wish for a vengeful suicide.

patient who is deeply ashamed of her angry feelings. The anger of depressed patients is often unconscious and is sometimes based on actual past life experiences of being punished or hated for expressing it. Prematurely urging patients to admit they are angry often makes them feel even more guilty and depressed. Usually, a better interview technique is to gradually explore situations in which assertive behavior is appropriate, using actual examples from the patient's current life or even his or her behavior with the physician. For example, once when the physician was late for a session with the patient described in Box 3.8, the patient smilingly apologized for making him rush. It proved fruitful for the physician to ask her in a sympathetic way if she had trouble acknowledging annoyance whenever she was inconvenienced.

Bipolar Disorder

The relationship between the patient with bipolar disorder and the physician can easily become **adversarial**. One reason for this tendency is that manic or hypomanic patients often seek treatment at the insistence of others, rather than because they feel that they are suffering. Additional history from family and friends is often necessary. The manic patient often appears excessively cheerful, with exaggerated movements, sometimes behaving theatrically and with excessive familiarity toward strangers, dressed with bright colors or extravagant clothing and accessories. In more severe, disorganized cases, patients can appear unkempt and disheveled.

The psychopathology of mania **blocks communication**, and patients may exert control through such means as humor, uninterruptible speech, sexual seductiveness, or flashes of intimidating anger. Interviewing a patient who is suffering from severe psychotic or thought-disordered mania is virtually impossible. It is usually counterproductive for the physician to spend time arguing with or countering the illogical thinking of the patient. A manic patient will try to **manipulate** the physician by bargaining to avoid limits or by forcing the physician to agree with any shred of truth in the patient's stories, in order to reinforce denial of his or her illness. Giving in to these manipulations only harms the patient and prolongs the destructiveness of the episode. The interview should be ended abruptly if the frustrated manic patient explodes into rage. For **safety** reasons, another person should be present when a patient with severe mania is being interviewed. It is dangerous to believe that one can "talk down" an agitated manic patient. Medication or involuntary hospitalization is often necessary. Many recovered manic patients retrospectively agree with such steps to restrict their freedom.

The manic patient's reaction to the physician is often the reverse of the reaction found in depressed patients. Depressed patients want help and they fear that the physician may not give it, whereas manic patients want to be left to their own devices and are afraid the physician will interfere. **Objection to treatment** is the rule, with the exception of grandiose patients, who want to have the physician listen to them and admiringly or sympathetically agree with them. The physician's responses to the patient may be marked by ambivalence. With hypomanic patients, it is often tempting to believe the patient's version of a situation, especially if the patient is in the coherent, euphoric, self-confident stage of the upswing. The physician may even **vicariously enjoy** the patient's enhanced energy and optimism. At the same time, the physician may respond to the patient's controlling and even frightening behavior with **anger, fear, or frustration**. It is understandably common to feel annoyed with severely resistant manic patients and to wish that they would get into deeper trouble, as though to teach them a lesson. Such a reaction should not, of course, be acted upon. The frustrated physician should remember that the

DEVELOPING AN ALLIANCE WITH A MANIC PATIENT

A manic businessman was spending excessive time and money working on a home computer, writing a program he thought would finally make him rich. He became enraged whenever his wife questioned the wisdom of buying more and more expensive equipment and staying up all night, disrupting the entire family. He finally admitted to his physician that he was terrified of losing a major account and was desperate to find a realistic way to embark on a different career. He was then able to see the danger of his current behavior and agreed to take medication and work seriously on the problems facing him.

patient has an illness and should not be blamed but helped, even if treatment must begin involuntarily.

The following techniques may engage patients more readily. It is helpful to find some aspect of patients' subjective inner worlds with which the physician can feel **agreement and sympathy**. The physician should listen to patients tell their side of the story, without interrupting too much, and should avoid challenging the patients' delusions or inconsequential distortions of history or common sense. Confrontations should be chosen extremely carefully (e.g., when it is important to determine if thoughts are delusional by offering possible alternatives). The physician should try to find areas in which patients' perceptions are reasonably accurate (e.g., understanding significant precipitants, such as family problems, serious losses, or life changes like leaving home for the first time). Any hints of **depression or low self-esteem** can help open the door. For some patients, it may be appropriate to ask whether they are "trying to reach for the stars" because they are unhappy with life as it exists, allowing them to express pain and ask for help without feeling embarrassed (see case example in Box 3.9).

Another area of common ground can be **psychophysiological symptoms**. Insomnia, racing thoughts, and overactivity eventually lead to feelings of exhaustion, and patients often admit to wishing that they could get some rest or "slow down the motor."

These guidelines are not needed in all cases. Many patients who have experienced previous bipolar episodes learn to recognize mania as dangerous to their well-being and form lasting partnerships with their physicians. Occasionally, first-time patients who are particularly self-observant and appreciative of stable, organized life patterns become frightened by the changes brought on by mania and actively seek help (see interviewing guidelines in Box 3.10).

Mild, **productive hypomania** deserves special comment. A small number of bipolar patients feel their best and function optimally during hypomanic states. They sometimes prefer to receive no medication and would rather keep the physician on "standby." They are willing to pay the price of episodic dysfunction in exchange for enhanced energy, sociability, sexuality, and creativity. The response of the physician to these patients can be complex. He or she may feel envy or frustration, which may lead to power struggles with the patient, or may vicariously enjoy the patient's exploits and seek to prolong the hypomanic state. Physicians who treat such patients flexibly (perhaps undermedicating them, according to some standards) need to pay careful attention to their own feelings in

---

BOX 3.10

INTERVIEWING GUIDELINES

FOR ALL PATIENTS WITH MOOD DISORDERS

- Ask about usual patterns in order to establish a baseline.
- Consult with family members for additional information.

FOR DEPRESSED PATIENTS

- Be active and directive.
- Try to strike an empathic balance, using encouragement, but avoid simplistic reassurance.
- Avoid premature exploration of the patient's unconscious anger.

FOR MANIC PATIENTS

- Avoid unnecessary confrontations.
- Try to elicit a complaint about some symptom or subjective experience with which the patient wants help.

---

order to act in the best interests of their patients. The physician who gets a "charge" out of a super-energetic patient may not act quickly enough to recommend an increased dosage of medication, for example. On the other hand, when a patient knows that the physician understands how enjoyable hypomania can be, the patient may accept help more readily and may be willing to collaborate with an "early warning system" (which often involves the family), in order to prevent extreme mood swings.

DIFFERENTIAL DIAGNOSIS

Although sadness is the core feature of depressive disorders, it is also a normal reaction to life adversity and can even be considered adaptive. Characteristics of normal sadness include adequate proportion to the provoking stimulus, brief duration, and lack of a major impact on the psychosocial functioning.

During **normal bereavement** following the death of a loved one, symptoms may be as severe as those found in major depression, with two important exceptions: low self-esteem is not pervasive (although there may be guilt about the relationship with the deceased person), and symptoms begin to resolve naturally within 2 to 3 months. Psychosis is absent. Culturally influenced symptoms, such as briefly seeing the image or hearing the voice of the deceased, can occur but are not truly psychotic in nature. Previous editions of the DSM required that the diagnosis of major depressive episode (MDE) not be made if the symptoms lasted for less than 2 months and were "better accounted for by bereavement." The majority of bereaved individuals do not meet criteria for MDE and recover without professional help. This so-called bereavement exclusion aimed to prevent "medicalization" of the normal phenomenon of grief but was removed in the latest edition of the DSM, for several reasons. First, bereavement can frequently last more than 2 months, sometimes as long as 1 to 2 years. Second, the loss of a loved one is a severe psychosocial stressor that can precipitate an MDE in vulnerable individuals, especially those with personal or family history of depression. Finally, bereavement-related MDE responds to the same psychosocial and medication treatments as non–bereavement-related depression.

Symptoms of depression are seen in patients with **adjustment disorder with depressed mood** (see DSM-5) after an identifiable psychosocial stress has occurred. These patients experience a spell of depression too mild or brief to be considered either major depression or a persistent depressive disorder. The symptoms resolve within 6 months once the stressor or its consequences are removed.

Although patients with **mood disorder due to another medical condition** may appear to be suffering from depression or bipolar disorder, they have, instead, a neurological or medical condition (not including those caused by substance abuse) that directly alters brain function (see Chapter 5, Neurocognitive Disorders and Mental Disorders Due to Another Medical Condition). In general, patients with such disorders tend to lack the sustained changes in self-esteem that are seen in depression and mania, such as extreme feelings of worthlessness or overconfidence, and may show evidence of subtle confusion or dementia. **Parkinson's disease** shares some symptoms with major depression, such as bradykinesia, decreased or even expressionless facial mimic, bradyphrenia, stooped posture, loss of interest and concentration, and reduced libido. Comorbidity between the two disorders is highly prevalent, around 40%. Features that help make a depression diagnosis in these patients include the presence of a pervasive low mood, sometimes with a diurnal variation, early morning awakening, pessimism (not proportional to the level of Parkinson's related disability), and suicidal ideation. Euphoria can be seen as well. Frontal lobe lesions with euphoria often present as silliness and lack of foresight. Extreme social disinhibition strongly suggests frontal lobe pathology. Common structural and physiological medical conditions that alter mood are summarized in Table 3.3. When evaluating a new patient, the physician's primary task is to exclude a medical etiology by obtaining a thorough medical history and, if necessary, by conducting a physical examination and ordering laboratory tests.

Patients suffering from **dementia** may present with manic-like agitation or with depression. Cognitive and behavioral changes mimicking depression, such as apathy and loss of concentration, are more common than those that mimic mania, such as restlessness and combativeness. The medical evaluation is most important in elderly patients because they are at the greatest risk of having another illness. Although "**pseudodementia**" may be a sign of depression in elderly persons, this assumption should be regarded as a diagnosis of exclusion. The appearance of a late-life affective disorder, especially in patients with no family history of such a condition, suggests a medical etiology.

Schizophrenia can resemble psychotic depression when patients have "negative symptoms" such as apathy, anhedonia, decreased motor activity, social withdrawal, and cognitive decline and can resemble mania when patients exhibit grandiose delusions and florid agitation. Euphoria can also be seen in schizophrenia, especially in the old subcategory of hebephrenia, wherein the patient presents as childish and silly. In contrast to manic patients, where mood elation can be contagious, mood elation in schizophrenic patients can provoke an uncomfortable feeling. Depressive symptoms can also be a prominent feature of the prodromal phase of schizophrenia, before the appearance of the full-blown psychotic first episode. In addition, depressive symptomatology commonly occurs in schizophrenia as an integral part of the disease, as a side effect of antipsychotic medication, or in the postpsychotic phase that, although controversial, some authors argue could be due to recovery of insight and recognition of the forthcoming difficulties. Thus, the diagnosis of an affective disorder or schizophrenia may not be accurate if it is

TABLE 3.3 Medical Conditions That Can Present With Mood Symptoms

Medical Conditions	Mania	Depression
Endocrine disorders		
Hypothyroidism		+
Hyperthyroidism	+	
Hypercalcemia		+
Addison's disease	+	
Cushing's disease	+	
Heart failure		+
Neurological disorders		
Multiple sclerosis	+	+
Alzheimer's disease	+	+
Stroke	+	+
Tumor	+	+
Temporal lobe epilepsy	+	+
Collagen vascular disease	+	+
Vitamin deficiencies		
B_{12}		+
Folate	+	
Malignant disease (especially of the lung and gastrointestinal tract)		+
Medications		
Sympatholytic antihypertensives	+	
Estrogen and progesterone		+
Excess thyroid hormone	+	
Adrenal steroids	+	+
Antineoplastics		+
Antiparkinson's	+	+

based on the symptoms present during a single cross-sectional period of an acute psychotic illness. A diagnosis based on a longitudinal evaluation is more reliable. A history of periodic psychotic illnesses with good return to functioning between episodes is more suggestive of an affective disorder, while a history of chronic or deteriorating functioning is more suggestive of schizophrenia. The family history can also help clarify the diagnosis. Finally, the diagnosis is sometimes based on the treatment response, either retroactively or pending the results of a "diagnostic" medication trial. For example, patients who respond well to lithium or who respond better to lithium than to antipsychotics are more likely to have bipolar disorder than schizophrenia.

Schizoaffective disorder is a condition in which a patient is psychotic during an episode of a mood disorder but continues to have psychotic symptoms (i.e., hallucinations or delusions) for at least 2 weeks after the mood disorder has resolved. This **persistence of psychosis during periods of more normal moods** characterizes the disorder. Researchers debate whether schizoaffective disorder is actually a combination of two separate diseases, schizophrenia and a mood disorder; a severe form of a mood disorder; or a different disease altogether. In any case, this syndrome is often disabling and difficult to treat.

Other psychotic syndromes, such as **delusional disorder**, **brief psychotic disorder,** or **schizophreniform disorder**, may resemble mania or psychotic depression. The main distinguishing factor between these disorders and mood disorders is that the patient's mood symptoms are not the most prominent feature of their illness. The physician must make a somewhat subjective judgment about this. The possibility of a mood disorder may be worth considering in patients with unexplained bouts of psychosis and good recovery between episodes, especially when there is a family history of mood disorder.

Substance abuse is a major problem in patients with mood disorders, affecting about one-half of depressed patients and bipolar patients. Most patients view substance use as "self-medication" (e.g., they use alcohol to quell agitation or insomnia). However, substance use can **cause or exacerbate** affective symptoms. Acute intoxication with stimulants, such as cocaine, "crack" cocaine, or amphetamines, produces a "high" that is indistinguishable from hypomania, except that it lasts from only a few hours to a few days and is followed by exhaustion and, sometimes, depression. Chronic stimulant misuse or intoxication with phencyclidine (PCP, angel dust) may produce a continuous state that mimics mania with paranoid psychosis. Hospitalization is often needed to stop the patient from using the drug long enough to clarify the diagnosis. Use of such drugs by individuals with underlying affective disorders or schizophrenia may result in a prolonged exacerbation that does not readily abate after the drugs are stopped. Chronic excessive alcohol use can cause feelings of depression, which may improve after several weeks of abstinence. Alcohol may also cause disinhibited behavior that resembles hypomania. Although this state is limited to the period of intoxication, if intoxication occurs frequently, it may produce diagnostic uncertainty, and prolonged abstinence may be necessary to make an accurate diagnosis. A person with problematic alcohol or drug use may not adhere to a regimen of prescription drugs, and this nonadherence may also precipitate depression or mania. Patients with mood disorders who also have alcohol and drug use disorders are more difficult to treat and have a high rate of suicide attempts and suicide. Alcohol is often used in suicide attempts and may be the factor that triggers impulsive, self-destructive behavior or that enhances the effects of an overdose of pills.

Generalized anxiety disorder and **panic disorder** can mimic depression. Patients show signs of worry, agitation, demoralization, and social withdrawal, and patients with panic disorder in particular commonly experience suicidal thoughts. Depressed patients often have severe anxiety and, sometimes, panic attacks as part of their illness. Predominance of either anxiety or depressive symptoms usually helps establish the correct diagnosis. Nevertheless, there is a high rate of comorbidity with depression and all of the anxiety disorders.

In patients with **personality disorders**, feelings of sadness, despair, hopelessness, and low self-esteem are often apparent. Patients with borderline, histrionic, or narcissistic personality disorders are especially prone to acute bouts of depressed mood and suicidal behavior. Manic-like, irritable hyperactivity and increased libido are also common. Episodes can usually be traced to psychosocial stressors and tend to resolve when external factors change. Borderline personality disorder can overlap significantly with bipolar disorder, especially bipolar II disorder, and indeed is often comorbid with it. Both conditions share features like affective instability, irritability, impulsivity, suicidal behavior, or social impairment. Patients with borderline personality disorder can even experience brief psychotic symptoms. They often have transient rapid changes in affect that can occur within just a few hours and that are usually precipitated by interpersonal events, such as perceived abandonment and extreme rejection sensitivity. The word *emptiness* may be used to describe their depressed feelings. Some patients can be diagnosed with both disorders in comorbidity, or present subsyndromal symptoms between bipolar disorders episodes, further complicating the differential diagnosis.

In contrast, a patient with a mood disorder who has healthy personality traits at the onset of the disorder may seem to deteriorate as the mood disorder progresses. For this reason, the patient may appear to have a personality disorder when first seen by the physician. For example, a depressed person may become unusually dependent, or a hypomanic patient may become extremely manipulative, suggesting antisocial traits. To make the diagnosis, the physician must take a careful history to learn as much as possible about what the patient's personality was like **before the onset of the affective symptoms**. The physician should ask how the patient has dealt in the past with important stresses and developmental stages and how he or she interacted with other people. Personality disorders are characterized by long-standing, consistent features of social functioning, fantasy life, and patterns in relationships and attitudes, whereas mood disorders are characterized by a more abrupt change in mental and social functioning at the time the illness begins. Patients with mood disorders may report that they are no longer themselves. Some patients have comorbid mood disorders and personality disorders and require treatment for both.

Patients may present with long-standing, mild mood symptoms, such as depression or irritability, that seem to have been caused by a personality disorder, but may resolve after treatment with antidepressant or mood-stabilizing drugs. This seemingly dramatic **change in personality** raises fascinating questions about the relationship between affective disorders and personality disorders. Such questions are of great interest to the general public. Physicians are often asked whether psychotherapy is necessary for certain kinds of ongoing life problems when medications such as fluoxetine can change so many aspects of personality. Conversely, some patients feel that if antidepressants are pushed upon them too aggressively, areas of personal concern will be ignored. It is valuable to acknowledge some of the uncertainties and to discuss these issues openly when patients raise them.

Sleep apnea, a common sleep disorder characterized by brief interruptions of breathing during sleep, can cause fatigue, diminished concentration, and other symptoms similar to those of depression. Sleep apnea is frequently associated with obesity. The diagnosis of sleep apnea requires a sleep laboratory assessment, that is, **polysomnography**, which is a comprehensive recording of the biophysiological changes that occur during sleep. Polysomnography of sleep apnea shows pauses in breathing that are followed by drops in blood oxygen and increases in blood carbon dioxide.

Children and adolescents with mood disorders pose special differential diagnostic problems. They may present primarily with **behavioral problems** at home and in school rather than with a clear, verbal description of their moods. Problem behaviors include withdrawal, sullenness, truancy, poor grades, and tantrums. Similar symptoms may occur in children and adolescents with learning disabilities, attention-deficit hyperactivity disorder, conduct disorder, and substance abuse. It can be difficult to distinguish extreme mood shifts from developmentally appropriate rebelliousness in teenagers. Adolescents with suicidal thoughts are often suffering from major depression rather than having an understandable reaction to social pressures felt from parents, friends, and schools. The longitudinal course of children and adolescents with bipolar disorder is manifested by rapid fluctuations in mood. Controversy concerning the diagnosis of pediatric bipolar disorder has focused attention on children with chronic irritability and hyperarousal. Children or adolescents previously diagnosed with bipolar disorder but who present persistent rather than episodic symptomatology are now eligible for the diagnosis of disruptive mood dysregulation disorder (DMDD) (see Chapter 15, Child and Adolescent Psychiatry). Psychotic symptoms resembling schizophrenia are often prominent in early-onset bipolar disorder.

MEDICAL EVALUATION

The medical evaluation of patients with mood disorders should include a physical examination and laboratory tests. The goals are to exclude mood disorders that are caused by another medical condition and to ensure the safety of treatment with medications. The history and physical examination usually uncover any major systemic illnesses. For patients with depression or mania, the standard laboratory tests are screening for **hepatic and thyroid function** (including thyroid-stimulating hormone, or TSH); studies of **electrolytes, calcium, blood urea nitrogen (BUN), creatinine**; a **complete blood count**; and a **urinalysis**. Urinary toxicological tests can be done to screen for drug abuse. An electrocardiogram may be obtained in patients over age 40 years because of the cardiovascular effects of some psychotropic drugs. The following tests are not part of routine screenings but may be useful under certain circumstances: electroencephalography, brain imaging by MRI or computed tomography (CT), assays of cobalamin (vitamin B$_{12}$) and ceruloplasmin, and screening for collagen vascular disease. Ideally, the medical workup should be completed before treatment is initiated, but the clinical condition of the patient often requires that treatment begin as soon as possible. In younger patients who appear to be physically well based on the history and physical examination, it is usually unnecessary to wait for laboratory results before starting treatment.

ETIOLOGY

The **biopsychosocial model** is useful for understanding the etiology of mood disorders, as it is for other psychiatric and medical disorders. One of the main assumptions of this model is that both normal and abnormal human functioning are produced by complex interactions between a number of biological, psychological, and social factors. Observations of diverse patterns of heredity, symptoms, course, and precipitating stresses suggest that the causes of mood disorders are multifactorial and heterogeneous. Furthermore, it has been difficult to match completely any biological or psychosocial variable proposed as causal with a distinct clinical group of patients. Instead, a variety of partial risk factors and correlations have emerged. Finally, even when biological and psychosocial abnormalities are discovered, it is not always possible to determine whether they are the causes or the effects of affective illness.

Neurobiological Theories

Genetics, early life experiences, and other factors combined determine different degrees of individual vulnerability to develop a mood disorder. Psychosocial factors may then act on this vulnerability to bring about mood episodes in susceptible individuals. It is possible that the higher the vulnerability load, the lower the amount of stressors necessary to trigger mood episodes and vice versa. Neurobiology offers crucial insights into the mechanisms whereby psychosocial experiences actually alter the brain at the cellular level, through epigenetic changes and/or in situations of early development and in adult life when there is neuronal plasticity.

Neurotransmitter Hypotheses

Early biochemical theories of mood dysregulation focused on the neurotransmitter norepinephrine. Several decades ago, it was observed that some patients became severely depressed while taking reserpine, an antihypertensive drug known to deplete norepinephrine. Tricyclic antidepressants (TCAs) coming into use at that time were found to increase the concentrations of **norepinephrine** and another neurotransmitter, **serotonin**. It was hypothesized that decreased levels of these two neurotransmitters in the brain caused depression and that excess amounts caused mania. Efforts to prove this theory by measuring the amounts of these substances or their metabolites in cerebrospinal fluid, urine, blood, and brain tissues (at autopsy) have yielded inconsistent results. The best evidence that serotonin contributes to the pathophysiology of depression comes from studies of **tryptophan depletion**, which show that lowering brain serotonin levels can induce acute symptomatic relapse in recovered depressed patients. Current research focuses on the interactions of these neurochemicals with a variety of other brain systems as well as on abnormalities in function and quantity of receptors for the transmitters. It is clear that there is a close interplay between serotonergic and dopaminergic neuronal systems at the anatomical and functional level. It has long been known, at least in mammals, that the central serotonergic system modulates the activity of dopaminergic neurons in both the nigrostriatal pathway and ventral tegmental area.

Conversion of tryptophan to serotonin is the rate-limiting step in the production of serotonin, and tryptophan metabolism appears to be the link between monoamines and other molecular abnormalities found in mood disorders, such as regulation in immune processes. An **increase in proinflammatory cytokines** has been documented in major depression, especially interleukin-6 (IL-6) and tumor necrosis factor alpha (TNF-α), and administration of therapeutic cytokines can cause significant depressive symptoms. Cytokines activate the enzyme indoleamine 2,3-dioxygenase (IDO), resulting in tryptophan depletion and thereby decreasing serotonin production. IDO also shunts tryptophan metabolism toward the kynurenin pathway with potential neurotoxic effects that contribute to the pathophysiology of depression. Cytokines also stimulate the hypothalamic–pituitary axis (HPA) and may influence noradrenergic activity.

Currently, chronic abnormalities of neurotransmission are thought to result in compensatory but maladaptive changes in the brain's regulation of itself, both at the level of **presynaptic autoreceptors** that provide feedback and possibly in the synaptic structure itself. Antidepressant drugs begin a process in which cells readapt as their exposure to neurotransmitters changes. The readaptation requires altered synthesis of receptor proteins, which may take several weeks to have effects. Also of recent interest is the discovery that norepinephrine may be increased initially in severe depression, mimicking a pathologically prolonged "fight or flight" stress reaction. There is also recognition that certain clinical subtypes of patients may have different abnormalities. For example, there appears to be a fairly specific decrease in serotonin concentration and a compensatory increase in serotonin receptors in the brains of people who have committed suicide by violent means. There is also evidence of decreased serotonin in the cerebrospinal fluid of certain violent criminals and suicide attempters. These and other observation have given rise to the notion that serotonin may play a role in impulsive or violent behaviors, as one piece of the larger puzzle of depression.

Additional neurobiological theories revolve around changes in neuronal plasticity, primarily in the hippocampus, at both the structural and the functional levels. Neuroimaging techniques have identified the hippocampus, the amygdala, and the prefrontal cortex as implicated in depression. Reductions in volume as well as in regional cerebral blood flow and glucose metabolism were described in these brain sites that are responsible for maintaining emotional stability. Chronic stress negatively regulates **hippocampal function,** whereas antidepressants ameliorate the effects of stress on neuronal morphology and activity, such as upregulation of hippocampal neurogenesis that is compromised in depression. Both stress and antidepressants have been shown to affect levels of brain-derived neurotrophic factor (BDNF), which is normally highly expressed in hippocampus and prefrontal cortex. BDNF plays a major role in neuronal growth, survival, and maturation. It has antidepressant-like actions and can induce transcription of a number of molecules.

In recent years, there has been growing evidence for a role of **glutamate** in the neurobiology of mood disorders. The majority of neurons and synapses in brain areas involved in emotion and cognition use glutamate for neurotransmission. Evidence implicating glutamate in the pathophysiology of mood disorders first came from postmortem and in vivo brain imaging studies. Altered glutamate levels in the prefrontal cortex, amygdala, and hippocampus are the main findings. Acute stress exposure in the prefrontal cortex and hippocampus appears to cause prolonged glutamate release. Additional evidence supporting the glutamate hypothesis comes from directly targeting glutamatergic neurotransmission. **Ketamine and other NMDA antagonists** have demonstrated rapid antidepressant responses (within hours of administration) in treatment-resistant depressed patients. Understanding the molecular and cellular changes that underlie the actions of neuropeptides and how these adaptations result in antidepressant-like effects may aid in developing drugs that target novel pathways for major depressive disorders.

Neuroendocrine Hypotheses

Peptides in the HPA are also active in cortical areas and may affect mood directly. The most striking neuroendocrine findings have been of **elevated serum cortisol** with **loss of normal diurnal variation** and dexamethasone nonsuppression of cortisol secretion, suggesting a model in which depression is seen as the result of a stress reaction that has gone on for too long. There is also evidence of increased adrenal mass in chronically depressed patients. Unfortunately, serum tests for hypercortisolemia are not sensitive or specific enough to be of clinical value in treating depression.

The **dexamethasone suppression test** (DST) is the most frequently used test to assess HPA-system function in psychiatric disorders. This neuroendocrine test normally suppresses cortisol secretion in by inhibiting adrenocorticotropic hormone (ACTH) pituitary release after administration of a low dose of dexamethasone, which acts by binding to specific glucocorticoid receptors. The parameter that is measured by this test is the capacity of the glucocorticoid receptors of pituitary corticotrophs to exert a negative regulatory effect on the release of ACTH and, consequently, cortisol. However, 50% of depressed patients fail to show cortisol suppression. Similar responses can be found in other disorders, such as bipolar disorder or schizophrenia, demonstrating the test's lack of specificity. Decreased glucocorticoid receptor mRNA expression has been documented in currently depressed patients and in remitted patients.

Early life experiences may confer vulnerability to develop a mood disorder, possibly through enduring abnormalities in the HPA axis. Although HPA-axis changes are usually regarded as state dependent, studies of depressed adults with a history of childhood abuse suggest increased HPA-axis responses to stress and attenuated adrenocorticotropin and cortisol responses to dexamethasone. These findings portend a possible trait component in vulnerable individuals.

Chronobiological Theories

Sleep disturbance is an important aspect of mood disorders, as described earlier. Sleep patterns appear to be regulated by an internal biological clock, or chronobiological center in the **hypothalamus**. Artificially induced sleep deprivation is known to alleviate depression or precipitate mania in some bipolar patients. Because a number of neurotransmitter and hormone levels follow circadian patterns of activity, it has been suggested that the brain's control of these may be related to brain events in sleep that, if disrupted, lead to biochemical abnormalities that affect mood.

Technological innovations that permit humans to extend daytime activities into the nighttime hours have eroded sleep. Such innovations include, most notably, artificial light, but also television, computers, telephones, and even central heating, which removes the incentive to stay in bed for warmth at night. These sleep disruptions are increasingly prevalent in society and can provoke mania in susceptible individuals. Such disruptions in sleep have also been linked to mood disorders with seasonal pattern and to light exposure. Seasonal changes in light exposure also trigger affective episodes in some patients, typically depression in the winter and hypomania in the summer in the northern hemisphere. The mechanism for this may involve retinal connections to hypothalamic nuclei that play a role in circadian regulation. Regulation of sleep in manic patients appears to have direct therapeutic effects.

Sensitization and Kindling Theory

Sensitization and the related phenomenon of kindling refer to animal models of recurrent affective disorders. In these models, repeated chemical or electrical stimulation of certain regions of the brain produces stereotypical behavioral responses or seizures. The amount of the chemical or electricity required to evoke the response or seizure decreases with each experience. When this reaction occurs with chemical stimuli, it is called sensitization; when it results from electrical seizure induction, it is known as kindling. In **kindling**, periodic spontaneous seizures occur after sufficient induction. These phenomena have been used as models to explain why, over time, affective episodes, particularly those seen in patients with bipolar disorder, **recur in shorter and shorter cycles** and **more autonomously** (i.e., with less relation to environmental precipitants). It appears that the threshold for certain types of abnormal brain activity drops progressively with repeated experiences of that activity. Researchers accurately predicted that the anticonvulsant drugs carbamazepine and valproic acid, which interfere with kindling, would have antimanic effects. In animals, kindling causes permanent synaptic changes mediated by altered genetic transcription of important neuronal proteins. It is hypothesized that repeated affective episodes may similarly be accompanied by progressive alteration of brain synapses that lower the threshold for future episodes and increase the likelihood of illness.

The mechanism of **sensitization** may also involve **genetic encoding**, the lasting alteration of gene expression as a result of a stimulus to the organism. Sections of the genome relevant to brain function are activated both by the sensitizing stress and by the animal's response to the stress. The result is learning, in the sense that long-term chemical and microanatomical changes in the brain cause lasting changes in behavior. Sensitization bears a key similarity to recurrent affective illness: infrequent, stress-precipitated episodes gradually change to more frequent, spontaneous episodes. Heritable factors in stress sensitivity and mood disorders could relate to the susceptibility of the gene to altered transcription of relevant proteins. Early life experience might play an important sensitizing role at a time in development when the brain is known to be more plastic; adult experiences that invoke conscious or unconscious memories of earlier stress could activate dormant neural pathways. Mirroring psychodynamic explanations, sensitization theory also suggests that mania may develop as a biologically overcompensated effort to regain equilibrium after depression, eventually becoming a conditioned response that may occur in the absence of depression.

Genetic Factors

Genetic studies using epidemiological samples validate the long-standing clinical impression that recurrent affective disorders tend to cluster in families. Relatives of patients with affective disorders are **two to three times** more likely to be ill than persons in the general population. Although families tend to aggregate in specific disorders along diagnostic lines (e.g., bipolar versus unipolar disorders), the overlap is considerable. Children of affectively ill parents are at especially high risk of developing several psychiatric problems. Up to 27% of children with one affectively ill parent become ill themselves, and many more develop personality or substance abuse problems. If both parents are ill, the rate of major affective illness in their children increases to 50–75%. The epidemiological evidence indicates that genetic vulnerability to mood disorders is somewhat **greater with bipolar disorder** than with unipolar depression. Studies of identical and fraternal twins also show impressive genetic links, which are somewhat greater for bipolar disorder than for unipolar depression. However, these studies do not show complete concordance in monozygotic twins, which indicates that environmental factors are involved in the expression of the disease. The pattern of inheritance is not Mendelian, and genetic or chromosomal markers have yet to be discovered. When couples with strong family histories of mood disorders seek genetic counseling before having children, it is important to point out the difficulty of making accurate predictions. Among candidate genes proposed, the 5-hydroxytryptamine transporter–linked polymorphic promoter region (5-HTTLPR) has been the most studied.

While genetic factors clearly play a role in the development of mood disorders in some patients, the presence of a **genetic predisposition** alone is not sufficient to cause a mood disorder, as evidenced by the **incomplete concordance** between identical twins. The occurrence of mood disorders in patients with no family history of them suggests that an acquired biological deficiency (e.g., genetic mutation, perinatal insult, viral or vascular disease of the brain) is involved, but it is not yet known exactly how important such a deficiency is to the development of mood disorders, especially in comparison to the effects that overwhelming psychosocial factors (e.g., psychological trauma in childhood, severe stress in adulthood) have on a person's life. The current view is that inherited or acquired biological vulnerabilities exist in most patients with recurrent or chronic mood disorders and that social and other environmental factors play various roles in triggering the onset of the disorders. Recent studies have provided new evidence of a gene-by-environment interaction, in which an individual's response to environmental insults is moderated by his or her genetic makeup.

A debate that runs throughout the search for the etiology of affective disorders is whether any particular **marker** is the cause or the result of the disorder. For example, is pessimism a learned behavior that results in depression, or does it reflect a specific effect of abnormal chemical activity in the area of the brain that controls mood? Similarly, does a biological finding such as elevated corticotropin levels merely reflect a primary defect in norepinephrine function, a defect that can both cause depressed feelings and produce alterations in the hypothalamus, or is the elevated corticotropin level itself toxic to the brain and therefore responsible for depressive symptoms? Another theme is to discover the links between specific clinical groups of patients and specific etiologies or markers.

For example, would the results of a specific biological test (e.g., serotonin receptor density) have predictive value in determining whether or not a patient will attempt suicide, or whether or not a particular drug will produce the best response in a particular patient? Preliminary results in some of these areas have emerged in research laboratories, but for the most part the answers to such questions remain speculative.

Psychosocial Theories

Most psychological and social theories of mood disorders focus on **loss** as the cause of depression in vulnerable individuals. Mania receives much less attention because it is considered more of a biologically rooted condition. Viewed from a psychological perspective, mania is usually regarded as a condition secondary to depression that arises from an attempt to overcompensate for depressed feelings rather than a disorder in its own right.

Research has underscored the role that early life experiences play in the formation of and vulnerability to depression. Studies range from those of children who were separated from parents in World War II to those of primates reared in isolation. However, many adults develop mood disorders with no discernible childhood trauma, or suffer traumas without becoming overtly depressed as adults.

Interpersonal Theory

Interpersonal theory maintains that social losses in a patient's current life contribute to depression and that improved interpersonal relations may alleviate the symptoms of depression. Social theories, amplified by epidemiological data of social risk factors for depression and bipolar disorder, are the basis of interpersonal theory. There is emphasis on the importance of **present relationships and coping skills**. The past is important because it reveals the ways in which a patient coped with earlier stresses and what social resources were available during those periods. A note of caution regarding this theory is that poor social relations can be the result of affective illness rather than the cause (e.g., a marriage collapses because a depressed spouse cannot meet the partner's needs).

Cognitive Theory

Cognitive theory, which developed from behavioral psychology, proposes that the primary defect in depressive illness is not a matter of mood but of incorrect cognition: depression results from **distorted thinking**, which causes unrealistically pessimistic and negative views of oneself and the world. The distorted thinking has three central maladaptive elements: negative views of oneself, the world in general, and the future (Beck's cognitive triad); distorted perceptions of new information and experiences; and logical errors that pervade the processing of new information. While cognitive theorists once thought that all of these distorted patterns were learned behaviors, they now allow for an etiological model that integrates biological, social, and psychological influences.

Psychodynamic Theory

Freud's classic treatise, "Mourning and Melancholia," was a seminal effort to explain why some individuals handle loss appropriately (mourning) while others go on to become depressed (melancholia). Subsequent psychodynamic theorists have refined this model, focusing on all the ways in which depression may reflect feelings of loss mingled with **dependency, anger** at the dependency, **shame** over the anger, and a personal sense of inadequacy. It has been hypothesized that individuals with a tendency toward depression may have more difficulty than others in achieving a secure sense of self-esteem and feeling comfortable about asserting their needs.

TREATMENT

To some extent, treatments of depression vary in their effectiveness depending on the severity of the illness. For patients with **severe depression**, pharmacological treatment is necessary. Psychotherapy alone, without medication, is usually ineffective. Although severely depressed patients may find it difficult to become engaged in psychotherapy, they may gain some much-needed emotional "breathing room" by meeting a caring, optimistic physician and seeing that their family has been mobilized to take care of them. A number of interventions should be considered, including a temporary respite from routine responsibilities. Major undertakings and decisions should be postponed because the patient's judgment and other psychosocial skills may be impaired. If the physician gives the order, the patient may feel less guilty about postponing plans or taking temporary sick leave. It may be helpful to gently talk over precipitating events and soften self-blame and hopelessness. Family therapy to defuse crises and support a household in stress may be helpful. A careful balance between the patient's initiative and the physician's encouragement may allow patients to return to normal activities even before they are completely well.

Hospitalization is sometimes necessary. In addition to providing physical protection, it may provide a welcome sense of being taken care of and relief from responsibility. About 10–20% of severely depressed inpatients improve without medication during the first or second week in the hospital. The physician must be wary of this improvement, however. The **milieu response** rarely lasts and should not preclude aggressive use of appropriate medication. In the hospital, measures to support physical health are important, as are gentle efforts to enhance patients' self-esteem by providing structured activities, such as creative arts, in which success is possible despite impaired cognitive functioning. Morale can also be boosted by the social support that patients receive in group therapy from those who are further along in recovery.

Pharmacotherapy

Antidepressant Agents
Numerous well-controlled studies have shown that patients with severe major depression, especially melancholia, are best treated with antidepressant drugs (see also Chapter 16, Pharmacotherapy, ECT, and TMS). Sixty to seventy percent of patients respond to antidepressants, whereas only 10% to 20% of severely depressed patients improve when given placebo.

Selective serotonin reuptake inhibitors (SSRIs) **are the usual first-line** choice because of their safety and tolerability. The SSRIs, as well as other newer antidepressants that have various effects on neurotransmitters (e.g., bupropion, venlafaxine, mirtazapine, see Chapter 16, Pharmacotherapy, ECT, and TMS), are as effective as the TCAs and MAOIs in **mild-to-moderate** depression. They have not been as definitively tested in relatively severe depression or melancholia.

The **tricyclic antidepressants** (TCAs) and **monoamine oxidase inhibitors** (MAOIs), the so-called first-generation drugs, have been used since the 1950s and 1960s. Although the efficacy of these medications is the best established in terms of empirical evidence gathered from controlled, double-blind studies, they have many unpleasant, dangerous side effects and may be lethal if used in a suicide attempt (see Chapter 16, Pharmacotherapy, ECT, and TMS). They are used mainly in patients who do not respond to one or more of the newer medications.

Patients with **atypical depression** may have a better response rate to SSRIs and MAOIs (55–75%) than to TCAs (35–50%). Because side effects are a drawback with both TCAs and MAOIs, many patients with atypical depression are now treated first with SSRIs. MAOIs may be used later in the sequence provided sufficient time is allowed to eliminate the SSRI, because lethal interactions may occur between these classes of drugs. Patients with **psychotic depression** rarely respond to antidepressants alone and require either the addition of an antipsychotic drug or a course of electroconvulsive therapy (ECT).

Although studies of the effects of medications in patients with persistent depressive disorders have not been as thorough as those for major depression, they suggest that antidepressants help most of these patients to a significant degree. Treatment should begin with SSRIs. Tapering of the medication is often attempted after 6 to 12 months of treatment, although many patients and physicians find it preferable to continue the medication indefinitely when its benefits are significant.

Antidepressants must be taken for **4 to 6 weeks** at the full therapeutic dosage before their complete effect is felt. A full response, however, may occur only after 8 to 12 weeks, because it sometimes takes several weeks for a patient's dosage to reach the therapeutic level. Therefore, unless the patient has severe side effects, the drug should not be stopped until it has been given at an adequate dosage for an adequate length of time. Only then can a patient be considered a nonresponder or partial responder. In general, nonresponders or partial responders suffering from any degree or subtype of depression will benefit from a different type of antidepressant. About 50% of melancholic nonresponders to TCAs achieve remission when they are given MAOIs instead. (These adjustments can bring the overall response rate to 80–90%.) It is common to try a sequence of antidepressants from **different classes** or to **combine two antidepressants**, such as adding venlafaxine or buproprion to an SSRI.

Augmenting agents should be added to antidepressants for patients with a partial response. **Lithium, stimulants** (e.g., dextroamphetamine or methylphenidate), buspirone, and thyroid hormone (levothyroxine or triiodothyronine) have been used successfully as augmenting agents. By themselves they are not very helpful in treating depression, but they seem to enhance the effects of standard antidepressants.

Thyroid hormone deserves special consideration as an augmenting agent in patients with low to normal thyroid function and should, of course, be used at the beginning of treatment in patients with unequivocal hypothyroidism as indicated by an elevated TSH level. There is now good evidence that the second-generation antipsychotics quetiapine and aripiprazole can be effective augmentation agents in treatment-refractory depression.

In the treatment of a single episode of major depression, **continuation treatment** at the full dosage that was used to resolve the depression should be maintained for at least **6 months** after the acute phase in order to prevent relapse. It has been shown that for patients who have discontinued treatment after their depression has gone into remission, relapse rates are at their highest level in the 6 months immediately following and then decrease. After 6 to 12 months of continuation treatment, the dosage should be gradually tapered and the patient should be observed for signs of relapse. When the medication should be stopped depends on individual factors. For example, it would be unwise to stop a college student's medication just before final examinations. If relapse occurs, the same medication is usually, but not always, effective.

If the patient has been depressed for a long time before receiving treatment or has a history of three or more recurrent episodes, the physician can assume that, without treatment, relapse is inevitable. Therefore, treatment may need to be continued for many years or life. Such long-term use of medication thus becomes a preventive, or prophylactic, phase of treatment. In deciding whether this **prophylaxis** is necessary, the physician needs to consider factors such as the degree of response to and side effects of the medication, the patient's life situation, and the severity and duration of previous episodes. The physician should explain to the patient that although his or her depression was effectively relieved by medication, these drugs do not cure depression or eliminate the tendency for depression to recur when the medication is stopped. In this sense, the preventive treatment of depression follows the same chronic disease model used for the treatment of hypertension and diabetes.

Adjunctive Drugs

Because antidepressant drugs usually take several weeks to begin working, adjunctive medications can be helpful at the beginning of treatment to provide immediate relief from insomnia, anxiety, and agitation. **Benzodiazepines**, which may be taken during the day and/or at bedtime), can help alleviate all of these problems. However, physical dependency may occur if they are used for more than a few weeks. **Trazodone**, given in a small dose (50–100 mg at bedtime), may be used as an alternative to benzodiazepines for the treatment of insomnia. Some antidepressants, especially the SSRIs and MAOIs, may cause insomnia, which is often alleviated by trazodone, zolpidem, or the benzodiazepines. Antipsychotics can be useful for severely agitated patients, but tardive dyskinesia may develop if they are continued for more than a few months (see Chapter 16, Pharmacotherapy, ECT, and TMS).

Treatment of Bipolar Depression

Acute bipolar depression has received little scientific study in comparison to unipolar depression. If antidepressant drugs are given for bipolar depression, without an antimanic on board, they may cause a switch to mania or a mixed state, or they may induce rapid cycling. Lithium and the anticonvulsants, which do not cause mania, are therefore safer for acute bipolar depression. Unfortunately, they are not as powerful against depression as they are against mania. In a few patients, lithium or anticonvulsants can be used alone with good antidepressant effects. However, the most common treatment for bipolar depression is an antidepressant combined with a mood stabilizer to prevent a manic switch. The antidepressant drugs are the same as those used in unipolar illness, although they are sometimes given in lower dosages and for shorter periods of time as a precaution. Many experts begin with bupropion or the SSRIs. The MAOIs may be most effective but also have the most side effects. The TCAs may be more likely to cause mania than other antidepressants.

Lamotrigine is an anticonvulsant that may be effective in treating bipolar depression, although the data are mixed. It has been associated with life-threatening skin reactions, including Stevens-Johnson syndrome and toxic epidermal necrolysis. Patients should be instructed to seek medical attention for any unexpected skin rash.

Olanzapine has been successfully used for the treatment of bipolar depression. One study examined the use of olanzapine and olanzapine-fluoxetine combination in the treatment of bipolar I depression. Olanzapine was more effective than placebo, and combined **olanzapine-fluoxetine** was more effective than olanzapine and placebo in the treatment of bipolar I depression, without increased risk of developing manic symptoms.

Quetiapine monotherapy is also an effective and well-tolerated treatment for depressive episodes in bipolar disorder.

Lurasidone, a novel antipsychotic drug, has been recently approved for the treatment of bipolar depression in monotherapy and as adjunctive therapy to lithium or valproate.

The management of bipolar depression in the **geriatric** population can be particularly challenging as there is a paucity of controlled pharmacological studies in this age group, and these patients tend to have substantial medical comorbidity.

Mood-Stabilizing Medication in Bipolar Disorder

Drug therapy is essential in the treatment of bipolar disorder to achieve two goals: rapid control of symptoms in acute episodes of mania and depression, and prevention of future episodes or, at least, reduction in their severity and frequency (see also Chapter 16, Pharmacotherapy, ECT, and TMS). The mainstays of somatic therapy are the mood-stabilizing drugs, or **bimodal** agents, that generally act on both mania and depression. Lithium and the anticonvulsants valproate and carbamazepine are considered the "traditional" non-antipsychotic mood stabilizers. All of the second-generation antipsychotic medications developed since the mid-1990s are also FDA-approved for mood stabilization in bipolar disorder, for acute mania, and, in most cases, for long-term prevention.

Lithium, in the form of **lithium carbonate**, is the most widely used mood stabilizer. It has potent effects in acute mania, allowing 60–70% of patients to achieve remission within several weeks. Lithium is most helpful in patients with **euphoric** mania and in those who have relatively **few or infrequent** episodes. When lithium is ineffective, or when medical problems prevent its use, the anticonvulsants are used. The **anticonvulsants** appear to be more effective than lithium in patients with **dysphoric** or **mixed mania**, in **rapid cyclers**, and possibly in patients who have had multiple episodes. Lithium and anticonvulsants may also be used in combination, in which they are sometimes more effective synergistically than alone.

A mood-stabilizing drug has certain limitations if it is used as the sole medication in acute mania. It may take a week or more before its effects are felt; it does not have sedative effects; and it cannot be given parenterally to uncooperative patients. Therefore, for the first few weeks of treatment, traditional mood stabilizers are usually combined with **antipsychotics or benzodiazepines for sedation**. The antipsychotics and benzodiazepines also have the advantage of being **injectable** when necessary. It is extremely important to sedate a manic patient in order to ensure the safety of the patient and others and because sleep is therapeutic against mania. Conventional antipsychotics such as chlorpromazine or haloperidol are rapidly effective in slowing down motor hyperactivity and in treating hallucinations and delusions in psychotic mania. The second-generation atypical antipsychotics, such as risperidone and olanzapine, may also be helpful and have fewer side effects. Improvements in grandiosity and psychotic symptoms usually occur within several days and symptoms are usually fully resolved within a few weeks. **Benzodiazepines**, such as lorazepam or clonazepam, are often used as the sole sedative in patients with milder symptoms or in combination with antipsychotics in those with more severe symptoms. They are not effective when used alone for severe or psychotic mania. When they are combined with antipsychotics, however, lower doses of the antipsychotics can be given, which helps reduce the potentially dangerous anticholinergic, hypotensive, and extrapyramidal side effects of the conventional antipsychotics.

Patients who are taking mood stabilizers require special medical monitoring. Blood levels of lithium must be measured regularly, especially in extremely agitated or medically compromised patients, because this drug can be severely toxic at levels only slightly higher than the usual therapeutic range (see Chapter 16, Pharmacotherapy, ECT, and TMS). The side effects of anticonvulsants are usually more benign than those of lithium.

Patients with the **rapid cycling** subtype, the acute **mixed** states, and **dysphoric mania** are difficult to treat. They may respond somewhat better to anticonvulsants or ECT than to lithium. Antidepressants tend to worsen these conditions. In fact, if a patient reports feeling worse after being given an antidepressant, this suggests that the apparent agitated depression may actually be a mixed state. Antidepressants should never be given to a patient who is manic.

Preventive Pharmacotherapy

After an initial manic episode, patients are usually treated indefinitely, although in some cases, such as those with no family history or modest severity, clinicians may consider tapering off the medication and monitoring them closely for future relapses. After patients have had two episodes of bipolar disorder, including depressive episodes, they are treated indefinitely because of the near certainty of relapse.

Prevention targets both manic and depressive episodes. Lithium has been the treatment of choice over five decades of international experience. Valproate and carbamazepine, given alone or in combination with lithium, are also often effective, although they have been less well studied. Almost all of the second-generation antipsychotics are also approved for long-term preventive use. Clinicians need to select a long-term medication regimen (monotherapy or a combination of medications) based not only on what worked acutely but also on potential side effects.

Patient responses fall along a spectrum: approximately one-third have no further episodes and are essentially cured; one-third have less frequent or less severe episodes and function reasonably well; and one-third continue to have relatively frequent and severe episodes, with ongoing disability. **Predictors of poor response** are mixed symptoms, rapid cycling, and multiple previous episodes. In patients with a poor response, it is especially important to try other treatments, including aggressive use of anticonvulsants.

Patients who experience **breakthrough episodes** of mania while they are taking mood stabilizers should be given an antipsychotic drug temporarily. Individuals who suffer breakthrough episodes of depression benefit from antidepressants. Patients with a tendency toward frequent or chronic breakthroughs may require a combination of multiple mood stabilizers, long-term antipsychotics, and antidepressants.

Electroconvulsive Therapy

Electroconvulsive therapy (ECT) is used for **depressed** patients who are **psychotic**, extremely **suicidal**, or medically ill because of **dehydration** due to severely decreased oral intake (see Chapter 16, Pharmacotherapy, ECT and TMS). It is also useful for other patients who have **not responded** to sequential trials of medication or who cannot tolerate the side effects of medications. Most patients with **melancholic** depression who have not responded to medication improve with ECT, particularly when it is administered earlier rather than later in the course of an episode. For patients with delusional depression, studies have shown that ECT is especially effective, making it the treatment of choice for some patients with this life-threatening condition.

Electroconvulsive therapy has powerful, rapid **antimanic** effects. It should be considered in life-threatening cases of manic violence, delirium, or exhaustion. It is also appropriate in patients who do not respond to medications after many weeks.

Psychotherapy

In patients with **mild to moderate depression**, psychotherapy can be quite useful, especially if it is a supportive form in which the therapist plays an active role in shoring up the patient's coping skills and makes suggestions for areas to work on. Patients suffering from the mildest forms of depression, especially if the episode has begun recently and is related to a specific stressor, may improve quite a bit with 1 or 2 months of regular sessions for advice, support, and encouragement delivered in a commonsense manner. For patients with somewhat greater difficulties in the mild-to-moderate range of severity, more specific psychotherapy is needed, often in combination with medication.

There are several well-defined approaches to psychotherapy for depression that can be quite helpful. **Cognitive therapy** and **interpersonal psychotherapy** have been extensively evaluated in well-designed studies of efficacy in depressed patients and have been codified in concisely written manuals. **Psychodynamic psychotherapy** is a less well-studied but nonetheless frequently used approach to the psychotherapy of depressed patients (particularly in conjunction with pharmacotherapy, see case example in Box 3.11). These therapies are similar in their examination of the patient's inner mental life (i.e., perceptions, cognitions, and feelings); reliance on a warm, empathic relationship between the patient and therapist; and education of the patient by the therapist, who makes explicit the diagnoses, explains the etiological theories of mood disorders, and discusses the patient's prognosis optimistically.

Cognitive Therapy

Cognitive therapy is based on the theory that incorrect cognitions (i.e., negative misperceptions of oneself and the surrounding environment) cause depression. Cognitive therapy is usually conducted **weekly for 3 to 4 months** and consists of stages, which take the form of specific therapeutic goals for the patient to meet. In the beginning, the therapist explains the theory behind cognitive psychotherapy and its efficacy. He or she then teaches the patient how to monitor systematically the thoughts that accompany depressing feelings and situations. The patient is asked to create a diary of **automatic thoughts** (given as written homework assignments), which the patient and therapist review together, looking for patterns of negative ideation. They then discuss ways in which these thoughts represent inaccurate self-appraisals. The therapist teaches the patient to question his or her own logic and has the patient try out **new cognitive strategies**. An improvement in the patient's mood results when his or her inaccurate, negative self-perception has been altered. For example, a patient's fear of not being able to finish a task may be overcome by completing a series of small subtasks, one at a time; if successful, the patient gradually reverses the conviction that the entire task is impossible (see case example in Box 3.12). Many self-help groups and popular books use cognitive and behavioral approaches to help people overcome depression by urging them to change the way they see themselves (e.g., passive, defective, victimized, or helpless).

Interpersonal Psychotherapy

The premise of interpersonal psychotherapy is that painful social experiences and troubled interpersonal relationships contribute to depression. In this form of therapy, physicians

BOX 3.11

CASE EXAMPLE OF PSYCHODYNAMIC PSYCHOTHERAPY FOR A DEPRESSED PATIENT

A 40-year-old businessman became depressed after receiving a promotion to head a division of his company. He had trouble eating and sleeping, began drinking more heavily, could not enjoy weekends with his wife and children, and felt sad and anxious most of the time. He reported that he "came to life" only when he made a sales presentation to a new client and could enjoy the client's positive response. It emerged that his father had been an angry and critical man and that the patient had always been frightened of speaking up against him. His parents had divorced when the patient was young, and he had always been more sympathetic toward his mother, who would reward him emotionally for good performances at school. Currently, in his new job, he often had to discipline recalcitrant coworkers and mediate disputes. He found this situation very unpleasant and realized it reminded him of the losing battles he had fought with his father and of his general feelings of intimidation around successful peers. He was afraid that his coworkers would hate him if he took a stand against anyone. He much preferred the sales talks because they were never confrontational.

His physician prescribed an antidepressant. As his symptoms remitted, he continued to explore these work issues. His physician suggested that his managerial job would become easier if he tried to assert himself more consistently. The coworkers might start to respect him if he could successfully address their problems by making firm decisions. This strategy worked. He began to enjoy his position after he was admired for getting results.

BOX 3.12

CASE EXAMPLE OF COGNITIVE THERAPY FOR A DEPRESSED PATIENT

A single female patient was depressed because she was unable to meet men. An examination of her automatic thoughts revealed that she felt unattractive, was afraid she would say something offensive, and expected to be rejected. Her first subtask was to simply say "hello" to male and female coworkers when she met them at the copying machine. After she discovered that doing so did not result in a catastrophe, she was told to ask a coworker to lunch. Soon she was going to lunch with a regular group at the office and began to feel better about herself. Although she was unable to set up a string of ideal dates during the 12 weeks of cognitive therapy, she had a marked improvement in her overall outlook.

help depressed patients deal more effectively with their current social and interpersonal problems. Interpersonal psychotherapy does not attempt to alter long-standing personality traits; instead, it addresses the **current context** in which the patients' symptoms developed. The goal of treatment is to help patients develop better mechanisms for coping with their particular problems, including developing a better understanding of their emotions and improving their interpersonal skills. Although early life experiences are discussed as influences on adult behavior and personality, the treatment of depression focuses on patients' current issues rather than looking extensively into their pasts.

As with cognitive therapy, interpersonal psychotherapy generally consists of **12 to 16 weekly sessions**. The first few sessions are devoted to identifying the patient's primary problem area, which is drawn from four possibilities: grief, role disputes, role transitions, and lack of interpersonal bonds. During this time, the therapist also educates the patient about the nature of depression and temporarily allows the patient to assume the sick role without guilt so as to facilitate his or her receptivity to help. During the middle stage, a strategy is worked out using a standardized approach to resolve the central problem. For example, if the problem involves interpersonal role disputes within a marriage or work setting, the therapist helps to define the stages of the dispute (i.e., complete dissolution, temporary impasse, or possibility of renegotiation). The patient is encouraged to view the situation from all possible perspectives (i.e., miscommunication, faulty perception, unrealistic expectations). The therapist then helps the patient consider alternative explanations or develop **new communication or negotiation skills**. The therapist also provides feedback to the patient about how he or she may be perceived by others. In the final stage, the patient deals directly with the impending loss of the therapeutic relationship and the need to consolidate the lessons learned in treatment.

Long-Term Psychotherapy and Preventive Treatment

After remission of the acute symptoms is achieved, psychotherapy may help to **prevent relapse and recurrence**. The use of monthly follow-up, or booster, sessions in interpersonal therapy has proved to be a successful tool in preventing relapse. For patients with more severe depression who were treated initially with aggressive pharmacotherapy and who have not been able to participate in meaningful psychotherapy, the continuation period can provide a first opportunity to consider the **psychodynamic effects of life stresses** and personality issues. For example, when a divorce precipitates a patient's major depression, a longer period of psychotherapy after the acute stage may enable the patient to establish a more successful relationship in the future. Dwelling on such factors during the acute period of recovery is not always helpful, however. Some patients benefit from raising their psychological defenses and avoiding too much exploration. Psychotherapy can also help patients cope with the **consequences of their illness**, such as time lost from family and work, weakened social ties, and damaged self-esteem.

Psychotherapy in Combination with Pharmacotherapy

Medication and psychotherapy are often combined in treating depression. Research and clinical experience suggest that the benefits are additive. Some patients in certain situations may respond best to only one treatment mode, however. Drug treatment alone may be best when the patient's time or finances are significantly limited or the history indicates that, in earlier depressive episodes, the patient has responded extremely well to medication. Psychotherapy alone is the best treatment if antidepressants are poorly tolerated or medically contraindicated or if earlier episodes resolved quickly without medication.

The personality styles of patients and their attitudes toward treatment modalities also affect the choice of treatment. Some patients, for example, are very interested in their inner psychological conflicts or the psychological meaning of external life events. Some feel that taking a medication is a "crutch" or an intrusion into their autonomous self. Patients who are disturbed at the prospect of opening up to a therapist are comforted by the notion that their depression may result from a "chemical imbalance" for which they are not to blame. These commonly expressed concerns reflect the various theories about the etiology of depression (i.e., the role of nurture versus nature). Although the physician cannot always define the cause accurately, it may be possible to do so for an individual patient after getting to know him or her in depth. Each viewpoint also reveals a personal meaning: patients want treatments that help them maintain a certain ideal image of themselves. For instance, to some people, medication means dependence and psychotherapy means independence, whereas to others, the reverse is true. It is usually appropriate to **respect the patient's choice** if he or she has strong feelings, because for many patients with milder depressions, either drug treatment or a specific psychotherapy may, by itself, be effective. If the patient does not improve, the therapist can later suggest an alternative type of treatment. Combining medication and psychotherapy may also have additive benefits in preventing recurrence. During preventive treatment, the physician must regularly review the patient's compliance with medication, any psychosocial stresses that have developed, and fluctuations in symptoms or functioning that indicate relapse. Breakthrough episodes often require a change in medication or a renewal of active psychotherapy.

Patients who have had **recurrent depressions** often want to know if they can ever stop taking medication. The physician can approach this concern in several ways. The combination of long-term intensive psychotherapy and antidepressants appears to allow some individuals to improve to the point where their personalities are stronger, more resilient, and less vulnerable to depression. This effect may be especially true for patients with depressions that clearly resulted from unique life stresses that are now safely past. If these patients are truly resituated (e.g., in an improved marriage or more stable career), it may be reasonable to **discontinue medications**. Careful attention must be paid, however, to any signs of recurrence. Other patients feel so much better when taking medication and tolerate it so well that they are willing to take it for life. These individuals should be encouraged to do so as warranted by the seriousness and frequency of the depressions they have suffered.

Bipolar Disorder

For patients with bipolar disorder, psychotherapy is always combined with medication, both during the acute episodes and for long-term prevention. Patients with acute mania find it difficult to engage in psychotherapy before the medication has taken effect; until it does, the therapist can apply the principles of psychotherapy to understand and manage the patient. Bipolar depression may be treated with the techniques for unipolar depressive disorders presented earlier, although little research has been conducted on the efficacy of such treatment. Nonetheless, it can be helpful to attempt psychotherapy as an alternative to antidepressants for individuals who switch easily into mania.

For patients with bipolar disorder, the major goal of psychotherapy is not so much to relieve acute symptoms as it is to **enhance long-term psychosocial stability**. A practical focus on maintaining healthy interpersonal relationships, managing stress, and following healthy habits of sleeping regularly, eating nutritious food, and exercising may promote in patients an overall stability of lifestyle that is thought to decrease their chances of full-blown relapses. Research into this treatment, called **interpersonal and social rhythm therapy (IPSRT)**, has been shown it effective.

Teaching patients about the importance of complying with their medication schedule and recognizing early signs of relapse are central tasks. Bipolar patients tend to deny their illness more than patients with depression because they enjoy the enhanced energy, sociability, sexuality, and creativity that they believe they experience in the manic state. For some patients, these enhancements are objectively true as well, at least early in the course of hypomania. Complaints about the side effects of medication (e.g., patients often complain of feeling dull) pose a complex problem. It is important for the physician to find out whether the patient's true "complaint" is that he or she misses feeling "high" and is having trouble accepting the need for medication.

Because of its earlier age of onset, erratic symptoms, frequent recurrences, and tendency to cluster in families, bipolar disorder has different effects on the patient's life than recurrent depression. Particularly if the illness begins during the adolescent years, interruption of developmental tasks may occur, such as solidifying a sense of identity, forming lasting relationships outside the family, and establishing a career path. Learning to discriminate normal from abnormal moods may present problems. Patients may fear strong emotions and believe them to be abnormal; this fear may cause them to avoid emotionally charged or intimate life experiences. In addition, recurrent episodes take an exhausting, cumulative toll on the patient, resulting in prolonged demoralization.

Bipolar disorder also affects the patient's family and other relationships. Patients feel guilty and lose relationships because of what they do during manic episodes and what they do not do during depressive episodes. They may also feel angry and guilty about, or identify too closely with, affected parents, siblings, or offspring. Patients may have concerns about genetic transmission and may face the painful decision of whether or not to have children.

Finally, patients often suffer losses during treatment. For those patients who truly are more creative or productive during hypomanic episodes or who experience significant cognitive and physical side effects from lithium, the losses are genuine. For others, the losses are symbolic. Having a chronic illness and needing lifelong medication can lead to lowered self-esteem and feelings of defectiveness. Patients may blame the physician or the medication for their failures in life (e.g., blaming the loss of a job on a tremor caused by medication rather than their erratic, manic behavior).

REFERENCES CITED

Angst J. Unsolved problems in the indications for lithium prophylaxis in affective and schizoaffective disorders]. Bibl Psychiatr, 161:32–44. (German), 1981.

Kraepelin E. *Manic depressive insanity and paranoia*. Edinburgh, Scotland E & S Livingstone,1921.

Olfson, M., S. Shea, A. Feder, M. Fuentes, Y. Nomura, M. Gameroff, and M. M. Weissman. Prevalence of anxiety, depression, and substance use disorders in an urban general medicine practice. *Archives of Family Medicine* 9:876–883, 2000.

Rost, K., M. Zhang, J. Fortney, J. Smith, J. Coyne, and G. R. Smith. Persistently poor outcomes of undetected major depression in primary care. *General Hospital Psychiatry* 20:12–20, 1998.

Roy-Byrne, P, Post RM, Uhde TW, Porcu T, Davis D. The longitudinal course of recurrent affective illness: life chart data from research patients at the NIMH. Acta Psychiatr Scand Suppl. 317:1–34, 1985.

Wells, K. B., R. D. Hays, M. A. Burnam, W. Rogers, S. Greenfield, and J. E. Ware, Jr. Detection of depressive disorder for patients receiving prepaid or fee-for-service care: results from the Medical Outcomes Study. *JAMA: Journal of the American Medical Association* 262:3298–3302, 1989.

Zis, AP, Grof P, Webster M, Goodwin FK. Prediction of relapse in recurrent affective disorder. *Psychopharmacology Bulletin* 6:47–49, 1980.

SELECTED READINGS

American Psychiatric Association. *Treatment of Patients with Bipolar Disorder. Practice Guideline*, 2002. DOI: 10.1176/appi.books.9780890423363.50051. http://www.psychiatryonline.com/pracGuide/pracGuideTopic_8.aspx

American Psychiatric Association. *Treatment of Patients with Major Depressive Disorder. Practice Guideline*, 2010. DOI: 10.1176/appi.books.9780890423363.148217. http://www.psychiatryonline.com/pracGuide/pracGuideTopic_7.aspx

Deshauer, D., D. Moher, D. Fergusson, E. Moher, M. Sampson, and J. Grimshaw. Selective serotonin reuptake inhibitors for unipolar depression: a systematic review of classic long-term randomized controlled trials. *Canadian Medical Association Journal* 178:1293–1301, 2008.

Duman, R. S., N. Li, R. J. Liu, V. Duric, and G. Aghajanian. Signaling pathways underlying the rapid antidepressant actions of ketamine. *Neuropharmacology* 62: 35–41, 2012.

Goodwin, F. K., and K. R. Jamison. *Manic-Depressive Illness*, 2nd ed. New York: Oxford University Press, 2007.

Jamison, K. R. *An Unquiet Mind: A Memoir of Moods and Madness*. New York: Alfred A. Knopf, 1995.

Karasu, T. B. *Psychotherapy for Depression*. Northvale, NJ: Jason Aronson, 1990.

Kendler, K. S., R. C. Kessler, E. E. Walters, C. MacLean, M. C. Neale, A. C. Heath, and L. J. Eaves. Stressful life events, genetic liability, and onset of an episode of major depression in women. *American Journal of Psychiatry* 152:833–842, 1995.

Kessler, R. C., K. A. McGonagle, S. Zhao, C. B. Nelson, M. Hughes, S. Eshleman, H. U. Wittchen, and K. S. Kendler. Lifetime and 12-month prevalence of DSM-III-R psychiatric disorders in the United States: results from the National Comorbidity Survey. *Archives of General Psychiatry* 51:8–19, 1994.

Leonard, B. E. The concept of depression as a dysfunction of the immune system. *Current Immunology Reviews* 6(3):205–212, 2010.

MacKinnon, R. A., R. Michels, and P. J. Buckley. The depressed patient. In *The Psychiatric Interview in Clinical Practice*, 2nd ed. Arlington, VA: American Psychiatric Publishing, 2009.

Murphy, J. M., N. M. Laird, R. R. Monson, A. M. Sobol, and A. H. Leighton. A 40-year perspective on the prevalence of depression. The Stirling County Study. *Archives of General Psychiatry* 57: 209–215, 2000.

National Guideline Clearinghouse. *Major Depression in Adults in Primary Care*. Rockville, MD: Agency for Healthcare Research and Quality (AHRQ), 2012. http://www.guideline.gov/content.aspx?id=37277

Nugent, T. R., A. R. Tyrka, L. L. Carpenter, and L. H. Price. Gene–environment interactions: early life stress and risk for depressive and anxiety disorders. *Psychopharmacology (Berlin)* 214:175–196, 2011.

Oquendo, M. A., A. Barrera, S. P. Ellis, S. Li, A. K. Burke, M. Grunebaum J. Endicott, and J. J. Mann. Instability of symptoms in recurrent major depression: a prospective study. *American Journal of Psychiatry* 161:255–261, 2004.

Post, R. M. Transduction of psychosocial stress into the neurobiology of recurrent affective disorder. *American Journal of Psychiatry* 149:999–1010, 1992.

Rosenthal, N. E. Diagnosis and treatment of seasonal affective disorder. *JAMA: Journal of the American Medical Association* 270:2717–2720, 1993.

Rush A. J., W. E. Golden, G. W. Hall, et al. *Depression in Primary Care: Clinical Practice Guideline, Vol. 1: Detection and Diagnosis*. AHCPR Publication No. 93-0550. Rockville, MD: U.S. Department of Health and Human Services, Public Health Service, Agency for Health Care Policy and Research, 1993.

Rush A. J., W. E. Golden, G. W. Hall, et al. *Depression in Primary Care: Clinical Practice Guideline, Vol. 2: Treatment of Major Depression*. AHCPR Publication No. 93-0551. Rockville, MD: U.S.

Department of Health and Human Services, Public Health Service, Agency for Health Care Policy and Research, 1993.

Trangle, M., B. Dieperink, T. Gabert, B. Haight, B. Lindvall, J. Mitchell, H. Novak, D. Rich, D. Rossmiller, L. Setterlund, and K. Somers K. *Health Care Guideline: Adult Depression in Primary Care.* Bloomington, MN: Institute for Clinical Systems Improvement (ICSI), September 2013.

Sanacora, G., G. Treccani, and M. Popoli. Towards a glutamate hypothesis of depression. An emerging frontier of neuropsychopharmacology for mood disorders. *Neuropharmacology* 62:63–77, 2012.

Sher, L., M. A. Oquendo, and J. J. Mann. Risk of suicide in mood disorders. *Clinical Neuroscience Research* 1:337–344, 2001.

Solomon, A. *The Noonday Demon: An Atlas of Depression.* New York: Scribner, 2001.

Vieta, E., and M. Valentí. Mixed states in DSM-5: implications for clinical care, education and research. *Journal of Affective Disorders* 148:28–36, 2013.

Weissman, M. M., and M. L. Bruce. Affective disorders. In *Psychiatric Disorders in America: The Epidemiologic Catchment Area Study*, L. Robins and D. Reiger, eds. New York: Free Press, 1990.

Schizophrenia and Other Psychotic Disorders

MATTHEW D. ERLICH, THOMAS E. SMITH, EWALD HORWATH, AND FRANCINE COURNOS

The syndrome of psychosis is the hallmark of several psychiatric disorders, including schizophrenia. Schizophrenia is of particular importance because it strikes people in the prime of their lives, usually in late adolescence or young adulthood (see Table 4.1). It tends to have a debilitating and long-term course, interfering with school, work, marriage, and parenthood. Although schizophrenia can be a devastating illness, the degree of disability and functional impairment is widely variable. Many individuals with psychotic illnesses manage their symptoms well and live full and satisfying lives. Some achieve great things despite their illness, such as the Nobel Prize winning mathematician John Nash, whose story has been told in the book (Nasar, 1998) and movie, *A Beautiful Mind*.

DIAGNOSTIC AND CLINICAL FEATURES

Historically, the term *psychotic* described conditions that grossly interfered with patients' functioning (see Box 4.1, Historical Perspectives on Schizophrenia). The current definition is more precise: individuals are considered to be **psychotic** when they demonstrate a loss of reality testing as manifested by delusions, hallucinations, or a formal thought disorder, which involves disruptions or disorganization in the style and presentation of thoughts. The presence of these psychotic symptoms requires a diagnosis, since, by definition, they are not part of normal mental functioning (see Chapter 1, Psychiatric Assessment and Treatment Planning). A useful analogy is the symptom of fever, which requires a more specific diagnosis such as pneumonia, endocarditis, or strep throat. Merely describing a patient's symptoms as psychotic does not confer a specific diagnosis on the patient. The differential diagnosis of psychosis includes schizophrenia and other closely related disorders (i.e., brief psychotic, delusional, schizophreniform, and schizoaffective disorders) as well as mood disorders with psychotic features, substance/medication-induced psychosis, and psychotic disorders due to another medical condition.

TABLE 4.1 Epidemiology of the Schizophrenia Spectrum and Other Psychotic Disorders

Disorder	Lifetime Prevalence	Age of Onset	Course of Illness
Schizophrenia	0.3-0.7%	Late adolescence to young adulthood	Waxing and waning illness with many individuals remaining chronically ill
Schizophreniform disorder	0.2%	Late adolescence to young adulthood	About one-third of individuals recover within a 6-month period. Many of the remaining two-thirds will eventually receive a schizophrenia or schizoaffective diagnosis
Schizoaffective disorder*	0.3%	Typically, early adulthood; ranges from adolescence to late adulthood	Better prognosis than schizophrenia but significantly worse than mood disorder
Delusional disorder	0.2%	Typically adulthood, middle age and later	Ranges from remission without relapse to remission alternating with relapse to chronic waxing and waning
Brief psychotic disorder	Uncommon	Late 20s to early 30s	Can resolve within a few days; may account for up to 9% of cases of first-onset psychosis
Schizotypal personality disorder**	0.2%	Emergence in childhood and adolescence	Relatively stable course with few developing schizophrenia

*More common in women than in men; all other psychotic disorders are equally prevalent among males and females.

**Schizotypal personality disorder is considered in DSM-5 to be a "schizophrenia spectrum" disorder because of evidence that these individuals share common genetics and neuropsychiatric characteristics with patients with schizophrenia, suggesting that the personality disorder likely represents an attenuated form of the illness.

Symptoms of Schizophrenia

Symptoms of schizophrenia can be grouped into three broad categories: positive, negative, and disorganized. The positive/negative symptom distinction was originally developed in the 19th century by the neurologist Hughlings Jackson, with positive symptoms consisting of abnormal "superimposed" behaviors, and negative symptoms representing the loss of normal mental and neurological functions with the onset of illness. Disorganized symptoms are sometimes referred to as positive symptoms, though research suggests they are an independent domain of psychopathology.

Positive Symptoms

Positive symptoms typically include delusions and hallucinations (see Table 4.2). **Delusions are fixed** ideas based on **incorrect perceptions** of reality that **do not stem from a shared system of cultural beliefs,** such as religious convictions. Delusions are commonly paranoid or persecutory and may also be bizarre, somatic, grandiose, or referential (i.e., referring to events in the environment that the patient believes has special

BOX 4.1
HISTORICAL PERSPECTIVES ON SCHIZOPHRENIA

Morel, a European psychiatrist, first used the term *demence precoce* in 1856 to refer to an illness with severe intellectual deterioration beginning in late adolescence. Later, several other psychiatrists described specific variations in presentation or course. In 1871, Hecker delineated a hebephrenic type with a "silly" affect and a deteriorating course, and in 1874, Kahlbaum described catatonia as a mental illness characterized by stupor in the absence of gross neurological disease.

In his landmark textbook of 1896, Emil Kraepelin, a distinguished German psychiatrist, used the term *dementia praecox* to unify these disorders, which were previously considered separate diseases. He specifically referred to a disabling, often deteriorating condition with an onset in young persons. In the most severe cases, it resulted in a dementia-like outcome. He emphasized the distinction between dementia praecox, which resulted in deterioration, and manic-depressive psychosis, which had a more favorable outcome, in his view. Neo-Kraepelinian revivals of his ideas (e.g., in DSM-III and DSM-IV) have emphasized the deteriorating course and poor outcome. In the early 20th century, the German psychiatrist Schneider considered specific psychotic symptoms, such as delusions of thought control, thought broadcasting, and thought insertion, to be pathognomonic. Although these symptoms are still considered characteristic of schizophrenia, they are also observed in other psychotic disorders.

In 1911, Eugen Bleuler named the disorder *schizophrenia* and described what he believed were specific psychological features: loosening of associations, blunting of affect, autism, and ambivalence (i.e., indecisiveness). Bleuler viewed schizophrenia as having a variable outcome, being either chronic or intermittent in its course, and resulting always in a defect in personality, however slight.

Bleuler's ideas were widely taught in schools of psychiatry in the United States and contributed to a fairly broad, perhaps over inclusive, concept of the illness. It should be noted that even narrow, specific definitions of schizophrenia are likely to include a group of disorders with similarities in symptomatic presentation and response to current psychopharmacological therapies. Disagreements about the nature of the core psychopathology have been significant barriers to determining the true prevalence, predictors of outcome, core neurobiological disturbance, and genetic pattern of inheritance of schizophrenia. The DSM-5 has eliminated the previously included categorical subtypes of schizophrenia (paranoid, disorganized, catatonic, undifferentiated, and residual) after two decades of clinical and academic research that raised questions about their validity, reliability, and diagnostic utility.

TABLE 4.2 Positive Symptoms of Schizophrenia

Hallucinations: auditory more common than visual		
Delusions:		
Persecutory	Thought insertion	Religious
Grandiose	Thought withdrawal	Thought broadcasting
Erotomanic	Thought control	Somatic
Referential	"Made" thoughts, feelings, actions	

significance for him or her). The case example in Box 4.2 illustrates these different types of delusions, which often occur in combinations.

Some delusional beliefs, commonly referred to as **Schneider's first-rank symptoms of schizophrenia,** were once considered pathognomonic of schizophrenia. However, recent studies have shown that these symptoms may also occur in other psychotic disorders, such as psychotic mood disorders. Schneider's first-rank symptoms include thought broadcasting, thought insertion, and thought withdrawal. Patients with **thought broadcasting** believe that their thoughts can be perceived by others (i.e., as though the thoughts are being broadcast aloud). One such patient insisted on leaving the hospital because he was convinced that everyone knew his thoughts and that he could have no privacy. Patients with **thought insertion** believe that their thoughts are not their own but are instead the thoughts of another person who has inserted them into their heads. A young male patient, for example, was convinced that his brother transmitted to him a thought telling him to kill their mother. Patients with **thought withdrawal** believe that their thoughts are somehow being removed from their heads.

Paranoid patients feel frightened or enraged in response to a perceived threat or a delusion of persecution. They can be extremely hostile and guarded or exquisitely sensitive to any perceived slight. These patients may feel convinced that they have discovered the source of their persecution and have "caught on" to their persecutors, as in the case of one man who felt clever when he saw a fellow worker winking at someone else because he was sure that this was proof of a plot against him. **Grandiose** patients may be indignant if they feel that they are not receiving the level of respect that is in keeping with their

---

BOX 4.2

CASE EXAMPLES OF DELUSIONS

A young man believed that he was the son of a famous popular singer (grandiose) and thought that his mother was lying to him about his paternity (paranoid). At one point, he saw a limousine driving through his neighborhood, and he became convinced that the singer had sent someone to keep an eye on him (referential). A Dominican woman believed that she was the daughter of the deceased former President of the Dominican Republic and that he would come and rescue her from the hospital (grandiose). A man who was convinced that his brain was leaking out of his head wore a tight cap that he refused to remove because he was sure that it kept his brain in place (bizarre somatic).

inflated sense of personal status. Some patients feel perplexed and distressed about their strange perceptual experiences. Such patients experience emotional relief when they have formed a delusional explanation for their perceptions. For instance, a woman felt quite perplexed and worried by a sense that her apartment had somehow changed. As her symptoms evolved, she became convinced that the superintendent of her apartment building was entering her apartment and deliberately moving the furniture to retaliate against her for a complaint she had lodged. The delusional conviction was accompanied by both a sense of relief that she now understood the problem and by feelings of rage at the superintendent.

Patients with schizophrenia often have unusual perceptual experiences and may develop delusional interpretations of these experiences. **Auditory hallucinations**, in which sounds are heard in the **absence of any real auditory stimulus**, are the most common type of perceptual disorder in these patients. They may hear the sounds of bells, whistles, whispers, rustlings, and other noises, but, most often, the sounds are of voices talking. Patients may hear several voices talking to each other in a critical or disparaging way about themselves or a single voice making threatening or other persecutory comments. One adolescent girl constantly heard the voices of several women calling her a "dirty bitch" and making other nasty remarks about her; one young man heard a voice telling him that he was going to be killed. He was so convinced of this that he ran away from his home and hid in abandoned buildings for weeks. Command hallucinations, in which the individual hears a voice telling him or her to engage in a behavior, vary from the benign to the dangerous. They are especially important to assess for, as patients may be at risk to harm themselves or others to oblige the command.

Patients with schizophrenia may have hallucinations that involve other sensory modalities as well, but these are less common. **Visual hallucinations** are more indicative of delirium, a general medical condition or the effect of a substance, such as a drug of abuse or even a prescribed medication, than they are of schizophrenia. Such hallucinations indicate that a workup is necessary to exclude an acute medical disorder. When visual hallucinations occur in schizophrenia, they are often accompanied by delusional ideas and other sensory perceptions. For example, a religiously preoccupied woman reported that she heard a voice calling and then saw "the Virgin Mary beckoning to me."

Patients with schizophrenia may have **tactile hallucinations** (involving sensations of touch or pain) that may be accompanied by paranoid interpretations of perception: one woman with schizophrenia often wailed loudly in pain because she felt a cutting sensation in her head; she was convinced that a group of social workers was hacking at her brain with knives. **Olfactory and gustatory hallucinations** (of taste or smell) have also been described in schizophrenia: a middle-aged man reported that he smelled a foul odor and was convinced that his organs were rotting because a neighbor had slipped a white powder under his door. Tactile, olfactory, and gustatory hallucinations also require an assessment of possible medical causes such as alcohol withdrawal, temporal lobe epilepsy, and brain tumors.

Negative Symptoms

The most common emotional change in schizophrenia is a **general "blunting" or "flattening" of affective expression** (Table 4.3). Patients may seem to be emotionally detached or distant, and their expression of feelings may be limited both in terms of vocal intonation and facial movement. They may describe extremely disturbing experiences with little apparent emotional reaction. They may appear quite wooden and robot-like, and lacking in warmth or spontaneity. The emotional blunting may be accompanied by

TABLE 4.3 Negative Symptoms of Schizophrenia*

Affective flattening	Avolition
Asociality	Alogia (poverty of speech)
Anhedonia	Attentional disturbance
Poverty of content of speech	

*Note the distinction between "primary" negative symptoms (i.e., direct manifestations of the illness) and those "secondary" to (or caused by) positive symptoms, depression, or antipsychotic medication side effects, such as pseudoparkinsonism.

a change in the patient's sense of self. One man reported that he had no feelings whatsoever and that he felt "dead" inside. It is important to recognize that such symptoms may be due to or exacerbated by the side effects of antipsychotic medications, particularly in patients who present with a shuffling gait, tremor, or cogwheel rigidity (see Chapter 16, Pharmacotherapy, ECT, and TMS).

A gradual **loss of volition (avolition),** accompanied by **apathy** and decreased emotional expression, is a core symptom in many patients with schizophrenia. These patients often have a history of remaining at home, separating themselves off from loved ones, and doing little except watching television. In the most severe cases, patients seem to lose interest in all activities and progressively withdraw into an isolated, inactive, almost vegetative state. These patients usually deny feeling depressed, however.

Disorganized Symptoms

Many people with schizophrenia have significant cognitive and behavioral disorganization symptoms, which are among the most disabling features of the disorder (Table 4.4). Their thoughts may be strung together by incidental associations, and the connection between one idea and the next may not be readily apparent. Some patients with schizophrenia have **bizarre or idiosyncratic thought processes,** whereby thoughts and ideas have obvious meaning to the patient while being extremely difficult for others to discern. For example, when asked why he was in the hospital, one patient replied that his mother had "clogged up" his kitchen sink, which made his thoughts flow out of his head. The most characteristic type of formal thought disorder exhibited by patients with schizophrenia is **loosening of associations,** in which thoughts seem completely unrelated, or only obliquely related, to each other. When asked what had brought him to the hospital, one

TABLE 4.4 Disorganized Symptoms of Schizophrenia

Derailment (loose associations)
Illogicality
Thought blocking
Neologisms
Clang associations
Incoherence (word salad)
Idiosyncratic speech
Catatonic behaviors: mutism, stupor, negativism, bizarre postures, stereotypic movements, excitement, echolalia, echopraxia

patient with schizophrenia replied, "I was home when a drum began beating. I flew too low." Another type of formal thought disorder is **clanging,** in which conceptual connections between words or thoughts are replaced by sound associations (e.g., cycle and psycho; Pepto-Bismol, peptobismuth, and petrobismuth). Patients with the most severe form of loosening of associations express themselves in a **word salad** (i.e., incoherent patterns of words with no apparent connection or meaning that are strung together). In one case, a young woman approached a nurse and asked for "the thing that goes, the nails that made me barf."

Patients with schizophrenia may use words in peculiar ways. These **disturbances in word choice** are another sign of a formal thought disorder. When a woman, for instance, was asked why she was in the hospital, she replied, "Being unhealthy. In my head I feel like I'm a bleed." The use of **neologisms,** which are made-up words with meanings known only to the patient, is common. For example, a man with schizophrenia used the term "fumebook," which he defined as "a special temple to protect you."

Psychotic patients may also experience **thought blocking,** which is a sudden derailment of their train of thought with a complete interruption in the flow of ideas. A young woman trying to explain her school history said that she "took courses…" but she could not proceed any further with her thought. Thought blocking may leave patients quite perplexed or embarrassed.

Individuals with a formal thought disorder often have good vocabularies and other evidence of an intellectual capability that is more advanced than their low level of conceptual organization would suggest. A college student with schizophrenia may use sophisticated technical terms, for example, to express a completely confusing, disorganized idea.

Patients with schizophrenia may have profound psychomotor retardation or excitement, engage in bizarre acts, or have a gradual diminution of volitional activity. **Schizophrenia with catatonia,** in particular, is marked by episodes of bizarre behavior in which patients assume and maintain strange postures. They may also be unresponsive to questions or other stimuli, or might repeat an examiner's words (**echolalia**) or behaviors (**echopraxia**). One man sat fixedly staring at his hand, which he held almost directly over his head. Such patients may have a peculiar rigidity. They may allow their limbs to be moved but may then hold them in the position in which they are placed (**waxy flexibility**). Such bizarre posturing may alternate with extreme psychomotor agitation. Catatonic posturing is sometimes accompanied by delusions that relate to the behavior. For example, in describing his thoughts, one young man who had been admitted to the hospital with catatonic posturing reported that a remark he made to someone on the street had caused a commercial airplane crash in which many people had died. He was afraid to move or talk because he was convinced that he would cause another crash.

Of note, according to the DSM-5, catatonia may be diagnosed as a specifier for psychotic or mood disorders; it may also be a separate diagnosis on its own or a manifestation of another medical condition. Delineating catatonia as its own category reflects decades of research indicating catatonic symptoms to be just as likely, if not more likely, associated with mood disorders and other medical conditions, rather than merely a subtype of schizophrenia or psychosis.

Bizarre behavior in patients with schizophrenia is often influenced by delusional fears. In one case, an immigrant who was found running naked down the street later explained that the KGB and the FBI were chasing him. In another case, a man jumped from a window because he was convinced that people who wanted to kill him were pursuing him.

Diagnosis of Schizophrenia

According to the DSM-5 definition, schizophrenia is diagnosed when an individual has two or more of the following symptoms present for at least 1 month: hallucinations, delusions, disorganized speech, grossly disorganized or catatonic behavior, and negative symptoms. In addition, an individual's social or occupational functioning must have deteriorated (see DSM-5). Continuous signs of illness, which may include symptoms from the prodromal and residual phases of the illness that do not meet a level of severity to be considered psychotic, must be present for at least 6 months.

Patients with schizophrenia may exhibit thought, perceptual, emotional, and behavioral disturbances simultaneously. Catatonic patients, for example, may hear voices commanding them to assume bizarre bodily postures, which they then maintain for hours. Patients' symptoms usually wax and wane. Some patients have florid hallucinations early in the course of the illness and develop progressive emotional blunting (i.e., negative symptoms) at a later stage. Symptoms may occur in clusters and interact in complex ways, as in the case of one young man who hallucinated that he heard his mother's persecuting voice and gradually became convinced that his real mother had been replaced by an imposter.

Severity in Schizophrenia

The DSM-5 has introduced severity specifiers for the core symptoms on a five-point scale from 0 (symptoms are not present) to 4 (symptoms are the most severe). Quantifying the symptoms is consistent with the more dimensional approach of the DSM-5 and is an effort to better capture the heterogeneity of symptom type, severity, and overall functioning of patients with schizophrenia.

Other Psychotic Disorders

Schizophreniform Disorder
The signs and symptoms of schizophreniform disorder are essentially the same as those of schizophrenia, with two key differences (see DSM-5). In schizophreniform disorder, the duration of illness must be **at least 1 month but less than 6 months**. Although impaired social and occupational functioning may be present, it is not required for the diagnosis. For example, a man was able to continue to work for 2 months after he began having auditory hallucinations accusing him of wrongdoing. It was not until he had a heated argument with a fellow worker who he believed was persecuting him that his occupational functioning became impaired.

Schizoaffective Disorder
The key feature of schizoaffective disorder is that a **major depressive or manic episode is present concurrently with the core symptoms of schizophrenia** (see DSM-5). In addition, the diagnosis requires that psychotic symptoms are present **without prominent mood symptoms** for at least **2 weeks**. This distinguishes a schizoaffective diagnosis from a mood disorder in which psychotic symptoms occur only in the setting of depression or mania. For example, one young man was hospitalized twice for acute episodes of mania. After the second episode resolved, he had a persistent delusion that his mother was lying to him about the identity of his true father.

Delusional Disorder

The essential feature of delusional disorder is the prominence of a persistent but relatively circumscribed **delusion** of at least **1-month duration** in the absence of other symptoms typical of schizophrenia (see DSM-5). For instance, a young assistant television producer was convinced that a cameraman was in love with her, surreptitiously watching her with his camera, and following her. She was able to continue working and had no other psychotic or mood symptoms.

Brief Psychotic Disorder

In patients with brief psychotic disorder, delusions, hallucinations, or disorganized speech or behavior are present for **at least 1 day but for less than 1 month** (see DSM-5). After this brief period, patients **return to full premorbid functioning**. In one case, an adolescent girl began to have auditory hallucinations in which she heard a voice calling her a "sinner" after one of her brothers had murdered another brother. The hallucinations, as well as agitation, continued for several weeks, but the symptoms then resolved. Brief psychotic disorder is often, but not always, seen in the context of a severe emotional stressor (see case example in Box 4.3).

Psychotic Disorder Due to Another Medical Condition

The diagnosis of psychotic disorder due to another medical condition is made when hallucinations, delusions, or gross disorganization are caused by the **direct effects of a medical illness**. Medical illnesses that can cause psychotic symptoms include, but are not limited to, neurological disorders (e.g., brain tumors, cerebrovascular disease, Huntington's disease, dementias), central nervous system infections (e.g., meningitis, encephalitis, HIV), endocrine disorders (e.g., thyroid or parathyroid disease, Addison's disease), metabolic disturbances (e.g., hypoglycemia, hypoxia), hepatic encephalopathy, renal failure, autoimmune disease involving the central nervous system, and fluid and electrolyte disturbances. Delirium, including that caused by alcohol withdrawal, is a common condition that is frequently associated with psychotic symptoms. Delirious patients are more likely to experience visual hallucinations, unlike in schizophrenia,

---

BOX 4.3

CASE EXAMPLE OF BRIEF PSYCHOTIC DISORDER

A maintenance worker who was separated from his wife had waited in line for gasoline for 3 hours during an oil shortage and was told, when his turn came, that the gasoline had just run out. He became agitated and shouted at the attendant. He also became physically threatening, and the police brought him to the emergency room. The man was incoherent, spat at the staff, cursed, and paced wildly. He failed to respond to haloperidol given intramuscularly and was admitted to the acute inpatient unit. In a few days, he had completely recovered his normal behavior and was apologetic for his agitated behavior. The man's prior history of good social and occupational functioning and the brief duration of symptoms with complete resolution suggested that he was suffering from a brief psychotic disorder.

where auditory hallucinations are more common. Also, a hallmark of delirium is a fluctuating level of alertness and orientation. Patients with schizophrenia usually do not present with acute changes in alertness, and are typically well oriented in spite of their psychotic symptoms.

Some medications used for medical illnesses can also induce psychosis (e.g., adrenocorticosteroids, atropine, anticholinergics, ketamine, or other NMDA receptor antagonists). In one case of psychotic disorder due to another medical condition, a lawyer was admitted to the hospital with persecutory auditory hallucinations and the delusion that his law partners wanted to kill him. A physical examination indicated that he was tachycardic and restless, and laboratory studies confirmed that he had thyrotoxicosis.

Substance/Medication-Induced Psychotic Disorder

The diagnosis of substance/medication-induced psychotic disorder is made when hallucinations or delusions are the **result of illicit or prescribed substance intoxication or withdrawal**. Substances associated with psychotic symptoms include alcohol, amphetamines, cannabis, cocaine, hallucinogens, inhalants, opioids, phencyclidine, and sedatives. For example, an adolescent boy was brought to the emergency room in a wildly agitated state, screaming that devils were trying to mutilate him. His friends reported that they had attended a party where he was smoking crack cocaine. The symptoms cleared when he was no longer intoxicated.

Course of Schizophrenia

Schizophrenia is characterized by prodromal and residual phases in addition to the active phase of psychotic symptoms. Prodromal and residual symptoms consist of negative symptoms or "attenuated" psychotic experiences and thoughts similar to those observed in patients with **schizotypal personality disorder** (see Chapter 8, Personality Disorders). By definition, **prodromal symptoms** occur prior to the onset of the disorder. Usually, the label of prodromal symptoms is applied retrospectively, after the patient has developed florid signs of psychosis. The prodromal designation relies on clinical observations of subthreshold symptoms and remains an important area for neurobiological and clinical research. The prodrome can persist for several years. **Residual symptoms** tend to last as long as the disorder is present. Acute exacerbations of psychotic symptoms may occur periodically, particularly when patients do not take their antipsychotic medications, and are superimposed on the residual symptoms.

In addition, the DSM-5 includes specifier subtypes to demarcate the illness's chronicity. A **first episode** is the initial manifestation of the illness, in contrast to the **multiple episodes** specifier, applied when a patient has had a minimum of two episodes, such as a first episode followed by a remission and then a minimum of one relapse of psychosis. These episodes are further specified by the acuity of symptoms, for example, partial to full remission of symptoms. A diagnosis of schizophrenia, first episode, currently in full remission indicates that a patient had a first episode warranting a diagnosis and has experienced an extended period of time without the presence of psychotic symptoms. The specifier **continuous** applies to patients with an extended duration of psychotic symptoms and extremely brief, if any, periods of remission. This distinction acknowledges that for many patients, schizophrenia is an episodic illness with flare-ups and remissions, rather than a chronic disease of steady deterioration.

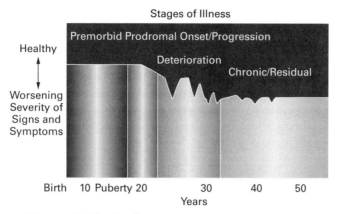

FIGURE 4.1 Natural History of Schizophrenia. Although the course of schizophrenia is highly variable, a pattern of prodromal, deteriorating, and chronic phases is characteristic. (Adapted from Figure 1 in Lewis D. A., and J. A. Lieberman. Catching up on schizophrenia: natural history and neurobiology. *Neuron* 28:325–334, 2000.)

The natural history of schizophrenia is variable, although Figure 4.1 shows a typical course of illness. The prodrome is typically followed by illness onset and **progressive worsening** of symptoms and functional impairment during the early phase, which is often manifested as a failure to return to previous levels of functioning. College students, for example, may have their studies interrupted by the illness and then be unable to resume school successfully. Most patients, however, have an initial period of deterioration and then reach a plateau in their level of functioning. Many patients stabilize to a degree by the third decade of the illness, although usually at a functional level significantly below that predicted by premorbid function.

Longitudinal follow-up studies in Europe and North America found that about one-fourth of patients with schizophrenia have **full remission** of symptoms, about one-fourth have **mild residual** symptoms, and about one-half have **moderate to severe symptoms.** A long-term follow-up study of patients released from the Vermont State Hospital found that 5 to 20 years after the onset of the illness, many patients had made a significant recovery in social functioning (Harding et al. 1987; Harding 2005).

Long-term studies of schizophrenia have identified several **predictors of good outcome. Women** tend to have a somewhat better outcome than men with respect to social and marital functioning. Premorbid factors such as poor social functioning and schizoid personality predict a worse social outcome, while premorbid factors such as being **married** and having **higher intelligence** (as measured by standardized intelligence tests) predict a more favorable outcome. Several studies have found that a **family history** of affective disorder is associated with a better outcome, while a family history of schizophrenia is associated with a worse outcome.

Two prospective multinational studies conducted by the World Health Organization in the 1980s–1990s found that patients with schizophrenia in nonindustrialized developing countries tended to have better outcomes than those in developed countries. Recent studies suggest, however, that these differences may not be as pronounced. Nonetheless, there has been speculation that course and outcome in schizophrenia may be affected by factors such as the degree of social isolation or support, nature of employment, family milieu, and social stigma.

THE INTERVIEW

The first goal in interviewing psychotic patients is to establish an **alliance**. Inexperienced interviewers may feel uncomfortable when they first meet with psychotic patients. Several specific guidelines may be helpful in the initial approach to these patients (see Box 4.4, Interviewing Guidelines). In psychotic disorders, paranoid symptoms may hamper the formation of a trusting relationship. Physicians should **listen attentively and respectfully** to these patients. Psychotic patients often feel alienated, misunderstood, and unappreciated. They are aware that most people react to them with disbelief, and they benefit from **acceptance and empathy** for their distress. It is particularly important that physicians be professional in their interactions with these patients. They should introduce themselves, using their full names and titles, and explain what their role is and what they would like to do for the patient. Psychotic patients easily feel intruded upon and require some additional space to feel comfortable, so the physician should remain at least beyond arm's reach (see Chapter 13, Violence).

Physicians should meet with patients only for as long as the patient can tolerate it. For hospitalized patients, brief contacts once or twice a day may be better tolerated than fewer lengthier meetings (e.g., several 45-minute sessions per week). The patient's reaction to the interview should be used as a guide to the duration and frequency of the sessions.

Providing a **structure** for the interview is also important. Open-ended questions such as "What problems do you think you are having?" often do not produce informative answers. Closed-ended questions, such as "How old are you? Whom do you live with? Were you seeing a psychiatrist before this hospitalization?" usually help put patients and interviewers at ease and make it easier to progress to questions about patients' symptoms. Although the patient may say bizarre things that will make the physician feel uneasy, some areas of patients' intact reality testing will almost always be revealed. This becomes apparent if the physician steers the interview toward neutral subjects.

The physician should be direct without being confrontational. It is helpful to listen respectfully to what patients have to say without agreeing or disagreeing with their

---

BOX 4.4

INTERVIEWING GUIDELINES

- Listen attentively and respectfully to the patient in order to establish an alliance.
- Provide structure, keep interactions brief, and steer the interview toward neutral subjects when interviewing a disorganized and severely delusional patient.
- Avoid arguing with a patient about delusional beliefs, but at the same time, do not agree with or encourage them.
- Take an educational approach and label psychotic symptoms as reactions to stress.
- Do not remain in a situation that feels dangerous.

> ### BOX 4.5
> ## CASE EXAMPLE OF INTERVIEWING TECHNIQUES WITH A HOSPITALIZED DELUSIONAL PATIENT
>
> When asked what had brought him to the hospital, a paranoid man stated that it was a big mistake caused by his father's overreaction to him. The physician replied that he understood the patient's feeling but that it would be best for the patient to take medication to help him control his anger and that a meeting would be arranged with his father to try to resolve their differences. The meeting revealed that the son had felt persecuted by neighbors and had attempted to smash their door with a hammer.

unrealistic beliefs. Many patients with schizophrenia claim that they are fine and that others are persecuting them. These psychological defenses of denial and projection, which are prominent in psychotic patients, help them reduce feelings of anxiety and low self-esteem. Contradicting them often cannot change these ideas. On the other hand, it is helpful for the physician to inform patients about their assessment of the reasons for hospitalization, the diagnosis, the purpose of medication, and the treatment plan, even if patients are unlikely to agree with everything, as illustrated in the case example in Box 4.5. Resistance to accepting an illness and medical advice about it is common in all patients, not just psychiatric patients, and it helps to be tolerant when it surfaces.

Perceptual disturbances, such as auditory hallucinations that are outside the realm of common human experience, can be anxiety provoking for both patients and interviewers. An **educational approach** that labels the experience as a symptom of the illness can be reassuring to patients. The physician might suggest that the hallucinations are a symptom of stress and that medication may help the patient to cope more effectively. Paranoid patients may not feel reassured at first but are often able to respond to reassurance gradually as their reality testing improves.

Learning to work with psychotic patients can be an intense, emotionally overwhelming experience. Patients may be only partially aware that interviewers are health professionals and may see them as intrusive, seductive, hostile, or dangerous. This misperception is symptomatic of the paranoid psychological process, in which patients attribute their own aggressive or sexual impulses to those around them, including the physician, as illustrated in the case example in Box 4.6. In such situations, the physician's appropriate response is to reassure the patients that he or she is a health professional who wants to be helpful and has no intention of harm.

The physician's initial response to a psychotic patient may be one of **anxiety, fear, bewilderment, or amusement**. Extremely paranoid and hostile patients may be quite frightening. The degree of fear that the physician feels is an important measure of the hostility that the patient may be feeling and expressing nonverbally. A common error for the physician is to try to overcome or deny being afraid, which may cause the physician to miss the patient's hostility or to continue the interview even after the patient has become increasingly upset or threatening. One resident was struck when he continued to interview a patient who started pacing in circles around his chair, making wild gestures.

> **BOX 4.6**
>
> ## CASE EXAMPLES OF PATIENTS WITH DELUSIONS ABOUT THEIR PHYSICIANS
>
> A young woman with schizophrenia became convinced that her physician was making a sexual advance when he came to her hospital room to see if she was free to meet with him. This belief occurred despite his waiting for a response after knocking on her door and asking her to come out of the room. In another case, a man accused a psychiatry resident of being in league with the FBI to lock him up and force him to divulge certain information.

When a patient is acting in an extremely disorganized or bizarre way, the physician may feel bewildered and not know how to proceed. Asking a structured set of simple, direct questions may restore a sense of order and control to the interview. The physician may ask the patient to describe his or her work history, education, or place of residence: "When is the last time you were working?" "How far did you go in school?" "Where do you live?" A disorganized patient may become sidetracked and pursue bizarre or irrelevant topics. The physician can **refocus the interview** by simply telling the patient that it is time to move on to another subject. For example, when a grandiose patient described her close connection to the British royal family and provided a litany of their lineage, the physician thanked her and then inquired about the people who were living with the patient in her apartment.

A psychotic patient may express bizarre thoughts or feelings, and the physician's emotional responses to a patient can provide important clues as to any unstated feelings the patient may be communicating. The impulse to laugh may be the interviewer's attempt to feel superior and distant from disturbing primitive impulses that a psychotic patient can stir up within the physician. Fear on the part of the physician usually indicates that the patient feels angry and hostile. If the physician feels perplexed, this reaction usually indicates that the patient's thought processes are disorganized. With increasing experience, a physician can learn to gather important information by being aware of his or her own emotional responses but not overwhelmed by them.

DIFFERENTIAL DIAGNOSIS

The differential diagnosis of the schizophrenia spectrum disorders includes other disorders characterized by psychosis, disorganized thinking, inappropriate or blunted emotional responses, and catatonia. The following symptoms are more characteristic of patients who have **delirium** or a **psychotic disorder due to a another medical condition:** a fluctuating level of consciousness; poor motor coordination; incontinence; inability to perform simple mental tasks (e.g., following commands, naming objects, doing arithmetic, or copying simple geometric designs); disorientation as to person, place, or time; confusion; and memory impairment (see Chapter 5, Neurocognitive Disorders and Mental Disorders Due to Another Medical Condition). Because delirium is often a manifestation of a life-threatening medical condition, physicians who assume abnormal behavior is always indicative of a psychiatric disorder rather than another medical condition can lose the opportunity to institute life-saving measures, as is illustrated in the case example in Box 4.7.

BOX 4.7

CASE EXAMPLE OF MEDICALLY ILL PATIENT MISDIAGNOSED WITH SCHIZOPHRENIA

A 53-year-old woman appeared in the emergency room crying and confused. She stated that she was unable to find her way home and gave a history of taking a psychiatric medication. A medical intern completed a physical assessment and reported no abnormal findings. The case was referred to a psychiatrist, with the intern stating, "This woman is a schizophrenic if ever I saw one." The psychiatrist learned that the patient had been working as an accountant until recently and that her symptoms had been present only for several months. She had been feeling depressed and forgetful, and her internist had given her an antidepressant. In addition to getting lost in her own neighborhood, the patient reported urinary incontinence, which is usually a sign of nonpsychiatric illness. A neurologist who subsequently evaluated the patient discovered that she had papilledema (swelling of the optic nerve head) and, eventually, the diagnosis of glioblastoma was made. The psychiatrist reviewed the emergency room intern's report to see if he had examined the patient's fundi. He had done so and had noted that the margins of the optic disks were sharp. Although it seems remarkable, the intern's prejudicial belief that this woman had schizophrenia and was, therefore, not medically ill apparently caused him to miss the papilledema. In addition, he knew little about the diagnostic criteria for schizophrenia, which is unlikely to have an onset at age 53 years and is usually not associated with urinary incontinence or disorientation as to place.

Intellectual disabilities and **communication disorders** are usually associated with a limited capacity for verbal expression. These disorders can often be confirmed by inquiring about the patient's school history and psychometric test results, which will document long-standing impairments. An onset of illness in early childhood or later adult life should also raise the index of suspicion for a disorder other than schizophrenia. The absence of a history of impairment in social or occupational functioning weighs against the diagnosis of schizophrenia. Patients with **neurodevelopmental disorders**, such as **autism spectrum disorders**, can exhibit negative symptoms with deficits in communication, impaired cognition, and strange behaviors—all of which may resemble schizophrenia, but they lack the core symptoms of schizophrenia (see Chapter 15, Child and Adolescent Psychiatry). It is also possible for patients with neurodevelopmental disorders, including intellectual disabilities, communication disorders, and autism spectrum disorder—all diagnoses made before adulthood—to later develop schizophrenia.

A prominent mood disturbance suggests **depression or mania.** However, the differentiation of schizophrenia, schizoaffective disorder, and **bipolar disorder** may be difficult. It is important to assess whether psychotic symptoms are accompanied by prominent mood disturbances, as is illustrated in the case example in Box 4.8.

Closely related to delusional disorders are illnesses characterized by persistent, intrusive, and unrealistic concerns (e.g., persistent fears of contamination in

> ### BOX 4.8
> ## CASE EXAMPLE OF SCHIZOAFFECTIVE DISORDER
>
> A 38-year-old man had been given a diagnosis of bipolar disorder. He was hospitalized several times for acute manic episodes, with symptoms of elated mood, incessant talking, energetic pacing, and loud singing of operatic arias. The staff found his mood to be infectious and endearing. During his worst episodes, he had the delusion that he was a close friend of a famous operatic tenor and had to be released from the hospital in order to join him on a world tour. After approximately 10 years of intermittent manic episodes, the psychotic symptoms became more persistent and often remained after the mood disturbance had resolved. At that point, the diagnosis was reevaluated and changed to schizoaffective disorder.

obsessive-compulsive disorder) or misinterpretations of bodily appearance, as in eating disorders and body dysmorphic disorder. Even if individuals with these disorders have no insight, the diagnosis of delusional disorder is not indicated. Instead, their psychosis is acknowledged by adding a specifier for "absent insight/delusional beliefs." (See Chapter 6, Anxiety, Obsessive-Compulsive, and Stress Disorders, and Chapter 10, Somatic Symptom and Related Disorders.)

A history of substance use should suggest the possibility of **substance-induced psychosis** (see case example in Box 4.9). Psychotic symptoms may be caused by the use of cocaine, amphetamines, and phencyclidine (PCP, angel dust). Acute onset, rapid improvement in symptoms, a history of recent substance use, and a positive urine toxicology screening test support the diagnosis of a substance-induced disorder. Patients will often deny their substance use, and family members or friends may need to be contacted for additional information (see Chapter 7, Substance-Related and Addictive Disorders). Abrupt discontinuation of certain substances or medications that are taken regularly by the patient can also cause psychotic symptoms. Alcohol withdrawal is the most common of these conditions and may be accompanied by visual, tactile, or auditory hallucinations.

Observing the patient at a single point in the course of the illness may not fully clarify the diagnosis. Physicians should keep in mind that the diagnosis of schizophrenia

> ### BOX 4.9
> ## CASE EXAMPLE OF SUBSTANCE-INDUCED PSYCHOSIS
>
> A 26-year-old man with a history of cocaine use began to smoke crack daily. Two days before he was admitted to the hospital, he began to read the Bible constantly and hear the voice of God speaking to him. He believed that his mother and brother were out to hurt him and became agitated. After he was admitted to the hospital, his urine was tested and found to be positive for cocaine. His psychotic symptoms resolved within several days.

requires that the patient is ill for 6 months. The differentiation of schizophrenia from other psychotic disorders may remain unclear until the patient has been observed and followed for an extended period of time.

MEDICAL EVALUATION

When a patient presents with an acute problem or when the duration of illness cannot be established, it is essential to obtain a thorough account of the psychiatric symptoms, their duration, recent life events, alcohol and other substance use, physical symptoms, and medical history, including any use of prescription or over-the-counter medications. It may be necessary to speak to family members or others to obtain such information.

In addition, a thorough physical examination and appropriate laboratory tests are needed to rule out another medical condition. The following tests should be performed as soon as possible: routine blood tests (e.g., **complete blood count, electrolytes, blood urea nitrogen, and creatinine**), **toxicology screening**, **thyroid and liver function tests, vitamin B$_{12}$ and folate levels**, and tests for sexually transmitted infections. When the neurological examination reveals a focal abnormality, imaging studies (e.g., computerized tomography [CT] or magnetic resonance imaging [MRI]) are also indicated. In addition, a **brain MRI** should be obtained as part of the evaluation for any new-onset psychotic disorder. Olfactory hallucinations are often clinically associated with temporal lobe epilepsy; an electroencephalogram (EEG) may be necessary to rule out this disorder.

Patients with schizophrenia have higher rates of comorbid substance-related disorders and other serious medical conditions than those in the general population. Whether due to pathophysiologic processes, lifestyle differences, failure to follow through with primary care treatment recommendations, discriminatory treatment by health care providers, and/or the adverse effects of antipsychotic medications, patients with schizophrenia commonly struggle with serious physical illnesses that are easily overlooked, as the case example in Box 4.10 illustrates. Fortunately, there is increasing attention to this matter (see Physical Health Comorbidity, later in this chapter).

BOX 4.10

CASE EXAMPLE OF PATIENT WITH DELIRIUM

A 35-year-old woman became severely agitated during her clinic appointment. She was brought to the emergency room, where she became totally out of control and was placed in restraints on a stretcher. The examining medical resident learned that she was registered as a patient at the psychiatry clinic and assumed that her agitation was a nonmedical problem. The psychiatry resident examined her, found her to be agitated and disoriented, contacted her clinic, and learned that she had a history of diabetes mellitus. Blood was quickly drawn and the serum glucose level tested, and an ampule of 50% dextrose solution was given intravenously. Within a few minutes, the patient calmed down completely and became oriented. Laboratory results showed an initial serum glucose level of 27 mg/dL, which confirmed the diagnosis of hypoglycemia-induced delirium.

TABLE 4.5 Neurobiology of Schizophrenia

Level of Investigation	Potential Etiological Contribution
Genetic	Multiple susceptibility alleles have been defined
Cellular programming	Disrupted genetic and protein expression
Cellular development	Abnormal induction, patterning, and synaptogenesis
Neural systems	Disrupted connectivity in local and macro circuits

ETIOLOGY

Several avenues of investigation have shown promise in revealing the cause(s) of schizophrenia. Research advances indicate it is likely a neurodevelopmental illness with clear heritable risk factors.

Neurobiology

A number of neurobiological abnormalities have been identified in schizophrenia (Table 4.5).

Genetic and Neurodevelopmental Factors

Evidence for a genetic contribution to the etiology of schizophrenia comes from family, twin, and adoption studies. Family studies have shown that the risk of developing schizophrenia is 10% in siblings of patients with schizophrenia and 13% in children with one parent with schizophrenia. In children with two parents with schizophrenia, the risk rises dramatically to 30–40%. The overwhelming majority of relatives of people with schizophrenia do not develop the disorder, however.

Twin studies have found that the **concordance** for schizophrenia in monozygotic twins of a schizophrenic proband approaches 50%, compared with a concordance of approximately 15% in dizygotic twins. These studies suggest that there are **vulnerability** genes for schizophrenia that are passed down from generation to generation. Another possibility is that new genetic mutations occur in schizophrenia vulnerability genes, conferring risk when there is no significant family history. **Advancing paternal age** is a major cause of new mutations in humans, and studies have shown that paternal age at conception is a significant risk factor for schizophrenia. Segregation and linkage studies have identified a number of candidate genes that may confer susceptibility to schizophrenia, but to date, no single gene or combination of genes has been identified that is causally linked to schizophrenia.

Recent research indicates that many patients with schizophrenia had delayed development as infants and children. A small subgroup of such offspring has been identified in whom the most severe motor deficits were related to obstetric complications, "pandysmaturation" (i.e., stunted cranial development in the first year of life), and low birth weight. Findings such as these have stimulated interest in the possibility that schizophrenia may result from a primary developmental lesion that occurs during fetal life, results in subtle developmental delays in infants, and is manifested as frank psychotic symptoms in late adolescence.

Genetic researchers have proposed that a significant proportion of the development of the brain is under genetic control. There is a growing body of research focusing on synaptic density and neuronal connectivity in the hippocampus and prefrontal cortex in schizophrenia. There is evidence indicating disruption in neuronal migration, development, and connectivity in these regions of the brain that may begin as early as the second trimester of pregnancy in individuals who ultimately develop schizophrenia.

Other interesting findings have emerged as well, including a higher rate of schizophrenia spectrum disorders among individuals with **velocardialfacial syndrome** (or DiGeorge's syndrome), a 22q11.2 deletion syndrome with the more commonly recognized symptoms of facial, endocrine, and heart defects. Moreover, individuals with schizophrenia—and their clinically unaffected first-degree relatives—often have **abnormalities with ocular smooth pursuit movements** and saccades. Such findings indicate promise regarding a neurogenetic explanation for etiology, clinical diagnosis, and prevention strategies in the future.

Neurochemical Factors

The predominant biological hypothesis for a neurophysiological defect in schizophrenia has been the **dopamine hypothesis**, which holds that the psychopathology found in schizophrenia is caused, in part, by a disturbance in the dopamine-mediated neuronal pathways in the brain (see Figure 4.2). This theory is supported by the blocking effect that most antipsychotic drugs have on the postsynaptic dopamine receptors and by the increase in dopamine activity in the dopamine-mediated pathways that psychotomimetic agents (e.g., amphetamines) usually cause.

The human brain has four principal dopamine tracts: the nigrostriatal, mesolimbic, mesocortical, and tuberoinfundibular tracts. The nigrostriatal tract is involved in the regulation of extrapyramidal motor activity. Excess dopamine activity in this tract is responsible for certain stereotypic behaviors seen in animals given dopamine-stimulating agents such as amphetamine or apomorphine. Deficient dopamine activity in this tract is responsible for the characteristic motor symptoms of Parkinson's disease; the postsynaptic

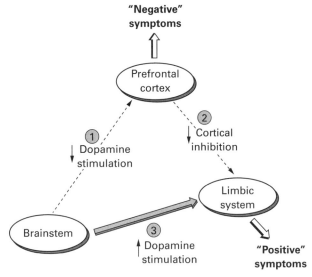

FIGURE 4.2 Neurobiology of schizophrenia. Current evidence suggests that diminished dopaminergic stimulation of the prefrontal cortex (1) may be responsible for the "negative" symptoms of schizophrenia, whereas the limbic system may produce "positive" symptoms in response to decreased cortical inhibition (2) and increased dopaminergic stimulation (3).

dopamine blockade in this tract accounts for the extrapyramidal side effects of antipsychotic drugs. The role of the nigrostriatal tract in the pathophysiology of schizophrenic symptoms is not clearly understood. This system may play a role in mediating various appetitive behaviors and responses to environmental stimuli, which are often impaired in schizophrenia.

The tuberoinfundibular dopamine tract has its cell bodies in the hypothalamus and exerts an inhibitory effect on prolactin secretion from the posterior pituitary gland. It is not known whether this tract plays a role in the pathophysiology of schizophrenia. The dopamine blockade of this pathway is responsible for several important neuroendocrine side effects of antipsychotic drugs, however.

Disturbances in the dopamine functioning of the mesolimbic and mesocortical tracts are hypothesized to play a central role in mediating the disorders of thought, affect, and symbolic processes seen in schizophrenia. There is evidence that patients with schizophrenia have a primary deficiency of dopamine activity in the mesocortical tracts, which results in loss of feedback inhibition and a secondary increase in dopamine activity in the mesolimbic tracts. According to this model, **hypodopaminergic cortical activity** underlies the negative symptoms of schizophrenia (e.g., avolition), whereas **hyperdopaminergic mesolimbic activity** accounts for positive symptoms including hallucinations and delusions.

Recently, the dopamine hypothesis has been amended with improved neuroimaging that can isolate other neuropeptides and neural circuits. Research has implicated the excitatory glutamate neurotransmitter system in schizophrenia, suggesting that hypofunction involving the NMDA subtype of central nervous system glutamate receptors may underlie the dopamine neurotransmitter abnormalities that are the hallmark of the illness. There are other potential pathological processes that could yield cognitive deterioration and the negative symptoms associated with schizophrenia. Abnormalities of GABA, an inhibitory neuropeptide, in the dorsolateral prefrontal cortex may negatively impact memory and cognition. The very high association of tobacco smoking and schizophrenia has been well known, but the properties of nicotine may stimulate cholinergic signaling that may also improve memory and negative symptoms (Karam et al., 2010). Clearly, exploring the role of non-dopamine neural circuits is an exciting area of study for better understanding the course, diagnosis, and, hopefully, treatment options for the illness.

Environmental Factors

The fact that the concordance between monozygotic twins, who are genetically identical, is no more than 50% is also convincing evidence for a significant environmental role in the etiology of schizophrenia. Adoption studies support the broad genetic hypothesis of a predisposition to schizophrenia, but their main contribution has been to show that sharing an environment with someone who has schizophrenia does not account for the familial aggregation of cases. While environmental factors undoubtedly contribute in some way to the etiology of schizophrenia, studies have ruled out the possibility that schizophrenia in the rearing family is a primary environmental cause.

A number of studies have described a seasonal pattern in the birth rates of people who develop schizophrenia. More patients with schizophrenia are born during the **winter and spring** months than at other times of the year. In the United States, people with schizophrenia are more likely to be born between December and May. Seasonal differences are most marked in the northeastern and Midwestern states and less marked in the southern states. A variety of theories, invoking nutritional, genetic, and infectious factors, have attempted to relate the birth pattern to the etiology of schizophrenia. Perhaps the most widely disseminated theory is that a **viral** infection occurring in the mother during gestation may cause schizophrenia in the offspring. Epidemiological studies have shown that incidence rates of schizophrenia increased in populations of individuals born in times of **extreme famine** and during **influenza** outbreaks.

Psychosocial Factors

Psychosocial factors may play a role in the etiology of schizophrenia, but it remains unclear what that role might be. Researchers hoping to identify any characteristics that might contribute to the development of this disorder have examined the family and social environment of patients with schizophrenia. Thankfully discarded, historical theories had pointed to the negative impact of a "schizophrenogenic mother," or the presence of grossly deficient early emotional nurturing of patients with schizophrenia. These theories were seriously flawed by the retrospective, unsystematic observations upon which they were based. They were destructive to the families and loved ones of patients, and are counter to current research and clinical evidence. Ongoing prospective studies of individuals who are genetically at higher risk for schizophrenia may reveal valid psychosocial factors that influence whether or not a particular person will develop the disorder.

Clinical observations and research data suggest that **stressful life events** can adversely affect the long-term course of patients with schizophrenia and that family and social factors can influence the prognosis as well (see Psychosocial Treatment, including the discussion of expressed emotion, later in this chapter). Sometimes patients will suffer an exacerbation of their psychotic symptoms in response to an isolated event, such as the death of a caretaking parent. A consistently chaotic psychosocial environment may contribute to other patients' unremitting course of chronically severe symptoms.

Schizophrenia is more common among persons in the **lower socioeconomic classes.** A debate continues as to whether this phenomenon is due to social causation (i.e., that specific risk factors in persons of lower social class precipitate the illness) or "social drift" (i.e., that people with schizophrenia "drift" into the lowest social class because of the disability caused by the illness). A separate risk factor is the chronic stress of poverty, which may have an adverse effect on the outcome of the illness.

TREATMENT

Psychopharmacology has made the most dramatic contribution to controlling the symptoms and improving the quality of life of patients with schizophrenia and other psychotic disorders. Psychotherapy and other psychosocial treatments, however, are also important, because they provide patients with the human connections that help them to improve social skills, become educated about their illness, and engage in "psychiatric rehabilitation," wherein patients can learn or relearn skills necessary to live independently and work competitively. Today, most patients with schizophrenia who need hospitalization stay for only brief periods of time (see Hospital Treatment, later in this chapter).

Pharmacotherapy

Beginning in the early 1950s, antipsychotic medications became available to treat the hallucinations, delusions, thought disorders, and behavioral agitation associated with schizophrenia. In some respects, the success of these agents revolutionized the management of this disorder. Before they became available, a diagnosis of schizophrenia often resulted in chronic institutionalization. With the advent of antipsychotic medications, the symptoms of many patients significantly improved, allowing them to live outside the confines of mental hospitals.

Antipsychotic Medications

The first-generation antipsychotics are similarly efficacious in treating schizophrenia (see Chapter 16, Pharmacotherapy, ECT, and TMS). The second-generation antipsychotic **clozapine** is notably more effective in patients with schizophrenia who do not respond to other antipsychotic drugs. Approximately half of such patients improve with clozapine (Leucht et al. 2013). Clozapine binds to both dopamine and serotonin receptors, and it has a much lower incidence of extrapyramidal side effects than that of first-generation dopamine-blocking-only antipsychotic drugs. Clozapine carries a risk of agranulocytosis, which led to fatal outcomes for a small number of patients involved in early trials in the 1970s. However, reintroduction of clozapine with strict hematological monitoring, guidelines for careful titration, and a national registry greatly improved the safety of the medication and led to its approval for use in the United States and elsewhere. Clozapine has been found in multiple trials to be the most effective medication for treatment-resistant schizophrenia, and it also reduces the risk of suicide. As clozapine has a serious side effect profile, it should be considered after a patient has failed to respond adequately to monotherapy trials of two antipsychotics from different chemical classes.

After clozapine was approved for market use in 1990, other second-generation antipsychotics were developed to mimic clozapine's activity while avoiding the risk of agranulocytosis. Like clozapine, these newer agents have a lower affinity for binding to D_2 receptors and a lower risk for extrapyramidal side effects when given at low dosages, as compared to the first-generation antipsychotics. Unfortunately, the second-generation antipsychotic agents have not proved to have the superior efficacy in the treatment of persistent positive symptoms that is seen with clozapine. Initial studies suggested that these agents were more effective than first-generation antipsychotics in the management of cognitive deficits and negative symptoms, such as lack of volition and motivation, and for several years the second-generation agents were widely accepted as first-line treatments for schizophrenia. A series of large, prospective, well-controlled studies that were conducted between 2001 and 2007 and recent meta-analyses reveal that a meaningful difference in efficacy between first- and second-generation agents is much less than originally thought. For example, when lower doses of first-generation agents are used in combination with medications that limit extrapyramidal symptoms, first-generation agents have been shown to be as effective as second-generation agents in controlling both positive and negative symptoms. Moreover, the low cost of the first-generation medications is another advantage, and these medications remain the mainstay for treatment of psychotic disorders in low- and middle-income countries.

The value of having many different choices of antipsychotic medications lies in the fact that each patient has very individual responses to the therapeutic and side effects of particular antipsychotic medications. It is important to work diligently to find the best possible fit for each person in treatment.

Pharmacotherapy for Acute Episodes

Antipsychotic medications are the treatment of choice for acute psychotic symptoms, whether associated with an acute exacerbation of schizophrenia or schizoaffective disorder or with brief psychotic disorder, schizophreniform disorder, or delusional disorder.

Improvement in agitation and hallucinations may occur within a few days, whereas improvement in delusions and thought disorder often requires several weeks of medication. Antipsychotics are also effective for patients suffering from a psychotic disorder due to another medical condition, although careful consideration must be given to potentially dangerous side effects and medication interactions (see Chapter 16, Pharmacotherapy, ECT, and TMS). Often low doses of antipsychotic medications are appropriate for patients who are medically ill or elderly.

Although a number of studies have shown that all first- and second-generation antipsychotics are effective in the treatment of acute psychotic symptoms, their effectiveness in treating the negative symptoms, such as blunted affect and social withdrawal, is less well established. Early studies indicated that some patients showed improvement in some negative symptoms such as social withdrawal, but this may have resulted from the decrease in paranoid delusions and thought disorder. More recently, clozapine and other second-generation antipsychotics have shown some promise of greater efficacy in treating negative symptoms and may have benefits for residual functional impairments as well. Primarily because of their lower incidence of extrapyramidal side effects (and in spite of their cardiometabolic side effects and higher cost), second-generation antipsychotic agents are more commonly prescribed than first-generation agents in the United States. In clinical practice, higher doses of antipsychotics are sometimes used for patients with agitated psychosis or for patients who do not respond to lower doses. In patients with severe agitation or other dangerous, disabling symptoms that fail to respond to standard doses, the risks involved in increasing the dosage are sometimes justified in the attempt to relieve the symptoms. An alternative to high dosages of antipsychotics is the use of safe **adjunctive sedatives** (e.g., lorazepam). For agitated psychotic patients whose behavior continues to be difficult to manage when they are taking standard doses of antipsychotics, adding lorazepam, 2–4 mg/d, given in divided doses, is a safe, practical way to provide sedation until the patient responds to an antipsychotic.

It is recommended that patients continue to take antipsychotic medications for at least 6 to 12 months following an initial diagnosis of schizophrenia, as research has demonstrated markedly higher rates of relapse for individuals who discontinue antipsychotic medications following recovery from an initial episode. The length of an antipsychotic medication trial depends on the acuity of the episode, the response to the medication, and the existence of psychosocial supports, among other factors. In other words, each treatment is patient centered.

Long-Term Use of Antipsychotics

Most people with schizophrenia do best with lifelong medication management using the lowest possible doses to prevent relapse. However, a subgroup of patients can eventually discontinue their medications and do well without them. One study (Harrow, Jobe, and Faull, 2012) showed that patients with schizophrenia who do well off antipsychotic medications for prolonged periods of time are a self-selected group with better premorbid developmental achievements and other skills that allow them to do as well or better after medication discontinuation. This must, of course, be differentiated from those patients who would improve on medication but have either never received treatment or have discontinued needed treatment.

Several antipsychotic agents carry a significant risk of **cardiometabolic side effects**, including weight gain, elevated fasting glucose and cholesterol, and type 2 diabetes mellitus. These side effects are more commonly seen with second-generation antipsychotics as well as with the low-potency first-generation agents (see Chapter 16, Pharmacotherapy,

ECT and TMS). In addition to obesity and diabetes, smoking, hypertension, sedentary lifestyle, and elevated cholesterol levels comprise the major risk factors for **cardiovascular disease**. Studies have shown a threefold increase in the risk of cardiovascular disease in subjects with the metabolic syndrome as compared with healthy subjects, and it is estimated that 40% to 50% of patients with chronic schizophrenia meet criteria for the metabolic syndrome, approximately twice the prevalence in the general population. More than two-thirds of patients with schizophrenia, compared to one-half in the general population, die of cardiovascular disease, and it has been estimated that patients with chronic mental illness die, on average, a decade to two earlier than the general population.

Of special concern is that patients with schizophrenia are less likely to receive appropriate monitoring and treatment of metabolic abnormalities associated with antipsychotic medications. In a large national study, 30% of patients with schizophrenia who met diagnostic criteria for diabetes were not receiving treatment with antidiabetic agents, 88% of those with elevated cholesterol were not receiving a lipid-lowering agent, and 62% of those meeting criteria for hypertension were not receiving antihypertensive medications (Nasrallah et al. 2006). Given the substantial long-term health complications of these conditions, it is imperative that behavioral health treatment plans incorporate efforts to identify, monitor, and address metabolic disturbances.

Pharmacotherapy for Other Psychotic Disorders

For patients with schizoaffective disorder or a mood disorder with psychotic symptoms, a **mood stabilizer** is often an important component of the treatment (see Chapter 3, Mood Disorders, and Chapter 16, Pharmacotherapy, ECT, and TMS).

Treatment Adherence

It is estimated that more than 50% of patients with schizophrenia have difficulties following their medication regimens. There are several reasons for this: (a) concerns about **side effects** commonly experienced with antipsychotic medications; (b) **poor awareness** of having an illness and needing medications; (c) **cognitive limitations** that make it difficult for patients to follow complicated medication regimens; and (d) the general tendency of people with any chronic illness to discontinue their medication regimens over time. It is imperative that physicians and family members pay careful attention to adherence issues, as nonadherence is a leading contributor to relapse in patients with severe psychotic disorders. Prescribing physicians should always aim to simplify patients' medication regimens, work collaboratively with patients to achieve the most tolerable regimens, and carefully and continuously educate patients regarding side effects and how they can be successfully managed. Structured group and individual psychotherapeutic approaches can help educate patients about how to manage medications and enhance adherence.

Long-acting injectable (depot) antipsychotic medications are available for patients who are not able or willing to take medications orally on a daily basis. There are some patients who find these periodic injections acceptable even though they do not adhere to oral regimens. Of course, adherence remains a concern, as patients need to show up for the injections. Families and key support persons should be engaged as needed to assist and monitor patients who have histories of poor adherence or are taking multiple medications at a time.

Treatment of Prodromal and First-Episode Schizophrenia

Although the onset of schizophrenia is typically in the late-teenage years or early 20s, research has shown that "high-risk" individuals (e.g., individuals with first-degree relatives who have schizophrenia) often show subtle social, cognitive, and neuropsychological deficits in early childhood and teenage years. This has led to efforts to identify individuals with schizophrenia prodrome or "attenuated psychosis syndrome" (a condition included provisionally in DSM-5 as requiring further study), that is, those individuals (usually teenagers) who display subtle cognitive deficits or attenuated psychotic symptoms (illusions, odd thinking), who are at significant risk for developing schizophrenia. Studies suggest that treatment interventions including psychoeducation, social cognition skills training, and the use of antipsychotic or antidepressant medications may be helpful for this population and may lower rates of conversion to psychosis.

Psychosocial Treatment

Medication alone is rarely sufficient for the treatment of patients with schizophrenia. The reasons for this include (1) the relapse rates for patients taking medications average 40% during the first year after hospital discharge and 15% each subsequent year for the next several years; (2) the improvement in symptoms is often only modest even in patients who take adequate doses of medication; (3) patients' social and occupational impairments typically persist despite a good symptomatic response to medication; and (4) there are high rates of nonadherence to medication recommendations. Thus, patients with schizophrenia, like many psychiatric illnesses, are best treated using multiple modalities and psychosocial treatments in conjunction with medication improve outcome.

Today's approaches are **recovery oriented**—that is, they aim to help patients achieve the highest possible level of functioning. For many years, psychosocial treatments focused primarily on maintaining patients in the community without relapse and rehospitalization. Recovery-based practices are person centered, in which health care providers are collaborators in identifying an individual's goals and promoting shared decision making. **Shared decision making** means that the individual's goals and the provider's recommendations are aligned to foster self-determination and empowerment. With a recovery orientation, therefore, medications are merely a part of treatment. Instead, self-management, relapse-prevention strategies, improving medication adherence, cognitive and social skills training, peer and family support, and psychoeducation, among others, are the vanguard of managing schizophrenia and similar illnesses.

Optimizing individualized recovery-based goals is especially important for individuals with schizophrenia, as quality of life and improved self-esteem are essential to successful treatment. In fact, recovery is a federally recognized priority of the National Institute of Mental Health (NIMH) and the Substance Abuse and Mental Health Services Administration (SAMSHA), with a multitude of resources for patients, families, providers, and policymakers alike (Mueser et al. 2013).

In applying recovery-oriented approaches to a patient with schizophrenia, clinicians must be careful to provide the appropriate type and level of therapy. Treatment that is too intensive may place demands on the patient that can worsen psychotic symptoms and lead to relapse. On the other hand, lack of sufficient stimulation and expectations can lead to the patient's withdrawal and poor functioning, a situation that occurred in the past in large custodial state hospitals, in which patients who were left idle became increasingly socially dysfunctional. The optimal level of intervention varies with each individual and is usually discovered only by trial and error in the context of good working relationships between the patient and the treating staff.

Individual Psychotherapy

Supportive, structured psychotherapies aim to help patients manage their illness by learning about their symptoms, medications, and side effects, as well as how to improve their social and occupational functioning. Cognitive-behavioral therapy (CBT) has been shown to be effective for persistent psychotic symptoms. Using a highly structured approach, patients can learn to identify the circumstances that trigger symptom exacerbation and develop alternative coping strategies.

Group Therapy

Group therapy for patients with schizophrenia teaches **self-care, social cognition**, and **occupational skills**. Through group therapy, the clinician may be able to evaluate effectively patients' abilities to concentrate and get along with others. It can also be an efficient way of educating patients about physical and mental health issues.

Family Therapy

One of the most critical strategies in the treatment of schizophrenia is to preserve a patient's existing support network, which is most often the family. Family therapists concentrate on helping family members develop more effective ways of relating to a relative with schizophrenia. Studies suggest that patients do best when families have realistic expectations of patients and can provide emotional support while minimizing criticism and hostility. The term "high expressed emotion" has been coined to refer to a hostile or overly demanding family environment that can increase the chances of relapse in patients with schizophrenia. Family therapy is often essential to **reduce expressed emotion** and provide support for family members who are coping with ill relatives. Many studies have shown that family therapy aimed at reducing high expressed emotion substantially lowers relapse rates in schizophrenia. This therapy can be provided in a variety of ways, including through use of multiple-family groups, whereby members of different families share their struggles and problem-solving approaches.

Psychoeducation

Psychoeducation, initially developed to help family members learn more about schizophrenia and its management, is now a core component of most treatment plans for schizophrenia. Patients and family members are educated about the signs and symptoms of the illness; the medical nature of the unusual phenomena that patients experience; the course and outcome of the illness; the somatic and psychosocial treatments; the strategies for reducing the chances of relapse; and the techniques for handling residual symptoms. Psychoeducation takes place in both clinical and nonclinical settings. The National Alliance on Mental Illness (NAMI) and other advocacy groups formed by people with mental illness and their family members usually include psychoeducation as part of their mission. A growing number of books and online evidence-based sources of information about mental illness, including first-person accounts by people living with schizophrenia, can serve as sources of both education and inspiration.

Peer Support and Self-Help Groups

Peer support and self-help groups provide a forum for patients and their families to talk about common experiences, exchange advice about illnesses and their management, and offer each other support. In recent years, the self-help movement has undergone a significant expansion among patients with schizophrenia, influencing not only the development of support groups but also of patient-operated vocational and leisure programs and counseling activities. These multidisciplinary programs are recovery oriented and may collaborate with medical treatment, thus achieving the dual goal of enhancing an individual's self-esteem and improving the level of functioning of these patients.

Vocational Programs

Up to 75% of patients with schizophrenia have difficulty obtaining and maintaining competitive employment. Comprehensive vocational support programs, however, have been shown to have a dramatic impact. Supported employment programs using the Individual Placement and Support (IPS) model, which emphasizes rapid and direct job placement and continuing support to patient and employer, are viewed as one of the most effective evidence-based vocational interventions. Supportive employment programs provide such services as job placement, job coaching, intensive support, counseling, and medication management in the context of real-world experiences and stressors to facilitate success in the workplace.

Cognitive Remediation

Cognitive remediation (CR) approaches that identify and address a patient's primary deficits in short-term memory, cognitive functioning, and skills for establishing relationships in employment and community settings are a recent innovation. CR programs often include computer programs, coaching, and virtual as well as counselor-led feedback. Studies have shown that this approach—when combined with psychosocial skills training—improves functional capacity and provides better outcomes for patients.

Self-Management Techniques

Patients may develop their own self-management techniques to manage psychotic symptoms that have not responded well to medication. One woman with schizophrenia had continuous auditory hallucinations that did not remit on any antipsychotic medication, including clozapine. She held a job running a human service agency and drowned out her voices by rehearsing lists of what she needed to do each day. She reported that she never wrote down any of these tasks because that would interfere with her self-management technique. A college professor with schizophrenia commuted to work by car and had to pay a toll at a manned booth every day. He heard the toll taker cursing at him each time he went through the booth, but reminded himself that these were auditory hallucinations and ignored them. An operating room nurse with schizophrenia observed that at times of stress she had days when her mind was too disorganized to follow all of the operating room procedures. She learned to reduce the sources of her stress but also called in sick on the occasional days that felt she might be impaired. Many patients show great courage in the face unremitting symptoms and strive to function well despite them.

THERAPEUTIC SETTINGS

Institutional and Residential Care

Hospital Treatment

Today, most patients with schizophrenia who need hospitalization stay in the hospital for only brief periods. Inpatient hospitalization is usually reserved for diagnostic or medical assessments and treatments that would be difficult to perform on an outpatient basis; severe psychiatric symptoms that endanger patients or others; and the management of crises, such as the loss of housing or social supports, that interfere with living in the community. An attempt is made by the staff to resolve the immediate problems and discharge patients as soon as possible.

Although it was common at one time, long-term hospitalization is now reserved for patients with the most severe unremitting symptoms that are incompatible with living outside of a hospital setting (see Box 4.11 for a description of deinstitutionalization). For a small minority of patients with schizophrenia, this approach remains the best one available.

Housing Resources

Supervised community settings for mentally ill persons provide housing with varying degrees of supervision and have largely replaced long-term hospital care. Supervised living programs help patients who live apart from their families but cannot live completely independently. These programs may provide help with taking medication; keeping

---

BOX 4.11

CHRONIC MENTAL ILLNESS AND THE PUBLIC MENTAL HEALTH SYSTEM

Most people associate the label "chronic mental illness" with schizophrenia. This is valid, up to a point. However, the term *chronic mental illness* refers primarily to any severe, persistent mental illness, with continuous or intermittent psychotic symptoms and associated functional disability. This may be true of a number of other serious mental disorders, including schizoaffective disorder, bipolar disorder, and major depression with psychotic features. Patients with chronic mental illness often have more than one disorder. The most frequent coexisting condition is substance use, but intellectual and neurological impairment are also common.

Most patients with chronic mental illness are cared for in the public mental health system. The number of state hospital beds for such patients was dramatically reduced during the 1960s and 1970s, a phenomenon known as deinstitutionalization. Homelessness became a significant problem in the 1980s, primarily for social and political reasons such as family fragmentation, poverty, diminished public funds for housing, reduced entitlement benefits for the poor and disabled, and economic downturns. Deinstitutionalization is actually a misnomer, because the reduction in state hospital beds was offset by the creation of homes for the aged and dependent in the community. Nonetheless, some mentally ill persons have become homeless, and they require extensive outreach efforts by the mental health system.

For most patients, the shift from long-term hospitalization to a community-based system of care has been beneficial. At peak occupancy, typical state hospitals were usually overcrowded and poorly staffed and had little to offer in the way of treatment. Antipsychotic medications, residential programs in the community, and psychoeducational and rehabilitation approaches have improved the outcome of patients with schizophrenia. Patients themselves report that the quality of life outside of a hospital is better.

medical appointments; arriving on time for school, work, or day programs; structuring time; grooming; preparing meals; using leisure time; and relating to other residents.

Some community settings, such as nursing homes, may be almost as restrictive as hospitals. Others, such as adult homes and board-and-care homes, have limited supervision. In recent years, the connections between supervised housing and mental health treatment have been strengthened in some states, so that patients living in these settings now receive more effective mental health services while living in the community.

There are different housing models. **Congregate supportive housing** is a residential facility where people with mental illness among others share a building. In **scatter-site housing**, an agency or municipality may lease a single apartment to a patient in a building among other community dwellers, reducing the stigma of a residential treatment facility and promoting acclimation into the community. Both of these models share a common goal: individuals with a severe mental illness living within the community.

Community-Based Psychosocial Rehabilitative Programs

Surveys show that many patients with schizophrenia experience the lack of productive activity as their greatest source of dissatisfaction. Social isolation is also common. Community-based psychosocial rehabilitation programs focus on introducing more productive activity and socialization by improving self-care, social skills, occupational skills, and use of leisure time. Approaches include various day programs; vocational rehabilitation; social skills training; and helping patients obtain volunteer positions, paid part-time or fulltime jobs, or further education. Some rehabilitation programs now take place in whole or in part outside of clinical settings (e.g., in schools or places of employment), such as the supported employment programs already described, and may refer to participants as "clients," "students," "employees," or "consumers" in order to enhance "nonpatient" identity.

Clubhouse Programs

Psychosocial clubs, of which the international Fountain House program is the best-known example, are usually operated by patients (often referred to as "clients" or "consumers"), peers (consumers who are trained to provide clinical support), and other nonmedical staff working as a team. These recovery-oriented programs provide socialization, recreation, and a variety of different types of support and are often run by peers who have lived experience with a chronic illness.

Assertive Community Treatment

Assertive Community Treatment (ACT) is a model for providing comprehensive psychiatric services in the community, including medication, through the use of well-staffed **multidisciplinary teams**. Although ACT has been shown to be a cost-effective approach with good outcomes for cooperative patients, ACT teams are more commonly used to reach out to patients who do not voluntarily come to treatment.

Crisis Intervention, Emergency Services, Outreach Services, and Case Management

Relying less on long-term hospital care and more on a system of community-based services has certain consequences. Disengagement in treatment is a concern, and some patients avoid the treatment system altogether. Others remain in treatment but continue to suffer episodes of relapse that require urgent intervention. Most patients face the problem of coordinating their own care and entitlement benefits in an increasingly fragmented service delivery system; this has led to an expansion of certain services to help rectify these problems.

Crisis intervention and emergency services are useful during periods of acute psychosis, when the possibility of hospitalization is imminent. Outreach services are most often targeted toward patients who resist needed treatment or are homebound. Case management provides a linkage function, assisting patients with access to mental health services, health care, and entitlement benefits. With implementation of the Affordable Care Act (2010), case management and patient navigation services are increasingly being introduced for the management of all chronic illnesses.

Overcoming Barriers to the Care of People with Schizophrenia

Stigma

Schizophrenia is a highly stigmatized illness, and people who have this disorder experience discrimination in many settings. This includes medical settings, where it has been repeatedly shown that physicians are less likely to provide adequate medical care to people who have a serious mental illness. Such attitudes contribute to the increased morbidity and mortality seen among people with schizophrenia. One of the major goals of the recovery movement, among patients and providers alike, is to reduce stigma to thus enhance support to patients and their families.

Advocacy

The stigma of schizophrenia and other mental illnesses has also been manifested in discriminatory reimbursement for mental health care. There has been an ongoing effort to change this by such organizations as the National Alliance on Mental Illness. Recently, very significant gains have been made in achieving **parity** such that health insurance for mental illnesses is expected to match that available for other medical disorders.

Inpatient and Outpatient Commitment

Statutes vary from state to state to allow for both involuntary inpatient care and involuntary outpatient treatment. People with schizophrenia, their family members, the physicians who care for them, and the lawyers who protect their rights have had many disagreements about how to best balance the autonomy of a patient against the need to provide care to severely disabled people who lack insight or pose a danger. Involuntary commitment, whereby a patient is mandated to treatment, or voluntary (self-elected) commitment is most often used for patients who are repeatedly brought to hospitals, often by the police, because they pose a risk of harm to themselves or others.

Substance Use Comorbidity

Research shows that approximately half of people with schizophrenia will at some time in their lives also meet criteria for an alcohol or other drug use disorder. Hazardous substance use is associated with many negative outcomes, including an increased risk for violence and higher rates of HIV, hepatitis B, and hepatitis C infections than rates in the general population. There is currently insufficient funding and integration of services to provide good care to many people with schizophrenia and comorbid substance use problems.

Physical Health Comorbidity

Outside of some hospital inpatient settings, psychiatric and nonbehavioral medical care services have long coexisted separately, in parallel realms. Nonetheless, there is increasing recognition that the physical care health needs of patients with schizophrenia and severe mental illnesses are often poorly met, contributing to poor health outcomes and constituting a public health crisis for these patients. Also, worsening physical health may trigger a relapse of psychosis and vice versa. Studies estimate that a person with a diagnosis of schizophrenia may die as much as two decades younger than the general population from illnesses related to hypertension, obesity, asthma or chronic obstructive pulmonary disease (COPD), and myocardial infarctions (Druss 2007).

Patients with schizophrenia have multiple risk factors for early mortality, including decreased physical activity; cardiometabolic side effects of psychotropic medications; high rates of smoking; comorbid substance abuse; discriminatory care in medical settings; and impaired cognition and negative symptoms that contribute to poor adherence and reduced communication with health care providers.

Health care in the United States is undergoing dramatic transformation under the Affordable Care Act. This includes broad attempts to integrate mental health and substance use services with physical health care. The aim is to improve system-wide care coordination, reduce disparities, and address the irrefutable connection between diseases of the mind and body. Collaboration among psychiatrists, primary care physicians, and other clinicians improves both medical and psychiatric outcomes, saves lives and money, and improves engagement of patients across the medical spectrum. Models for care integration already exist, but barriers to implementation have prevented their wide dissemination. Models include building primary care services into mental health or substance use programs or, more commonly, building mental health and substance use services into primary care programs. Methods of approaching integration in cost-effective ways include collaborative care, stepped care, and the use of telemedicine to reach rural health care providers. Most of the work on integrating medical and mental health care has focused on common mental disorders, most often depression, with fewer initiatives focused on people with schizophrenia and other psychotic disorders

Jails and Prisons

There is a growing concern that because the number of psychiatric inpatient beds in the United States has progressively diminished, many people with schizophrenia are now imprisoned when they behave in disruptive ways and commit misdemeanors such as disorderly conduct and trespassing (a deleterious form of **trans-institutionalization**). There is also concern that mentally ill inmates who are in prison for more serious crimes are not receiving needed treatment. States vary greatly in their approaches to these problems, but almost everyone involved agrees that better mental health care in forensic settings and more jail diversion programs are needed.

REFERENCES CITED

Druss, B. Improving medical care for persons with serious mental illness: challenges and solutions. *Journal of Clinical Psychiatry* 68(Suppl 4):40–44, 2007.

Harding, C. M. Changes in schizophrenia across time: paradoxes, patterns, and predictors. In Davidson, L., Harding C., Spaniol L. (eds.) *Recovery from Severe Mental Illnesses: Research Evidence and Implications for Practice*. Boston University: Center for Psychiatric Rehabilitation, 2005.

Harding, C. M., G. W. Brooks, T. Ashikaga, J. S. Strauss, and A. Breier. The Vermont Longitudinal Study of Persons with Severe Mental Illness, II: long-term outcome of subjects who retrospectively met DSM-III criteria for schizophrenia. *American Journal of Psychiatry* 144:727–735, 1987.

Harrow, M., T. H. Jobe, and R. N. Faull. Do all schizophrenia patients need antipsychotic treatment continuously throughout their lifetime? A 20-year longitudinal study. *Psychological Medicine* 42:2145–2155, 2012.

Karam, C. S., J. S. Ballon, N. M. Bivens, Z. Freyberg, R. R. Girgis, J. E. Lizardi-Ortiz, S. Markx, J. A. Lieberman, and J. A. Javitch. Signaling pathways in schizophrenia: emerging targets and therapeutic strategies. *Trends in Pharmacological Sciences* 31(8):381–390, 2010.

Leucht, S., A. Cipriani, L. Spineli, D. Mavridis, D. Orey, F. Richter, M. Samara, C. Barbui, R. R. Engel, J. R. Geddes, W. Kissling, M. P. Stapf, B. Lässig, G. Salanti, and J. M. Davis. Comparative efficacy and tolerability of 15 antipsychotic drugs in schizophrenia: a multiple-treatments meta-analysis. *Lancet* 382(9896):951–962.

Mueser, K. T., F. Deavers, and D. L. Penn. Psychosocial treatments for schizophrenia. *Annual Review of Clinical Psychology* 9:465–497, 2013.

Nasar, S. *A Beautiful Mind.* New York: Simon and Schuster, 1998.

Nasrallah, H. A., J. M. Meyer, D. C. Goff, J. P. McEvoy, S. M. Davis, T. S. Stroup, and J. A. Lieberman. Low rates of treatment for hypertension, dyslipidemia and diabetes in schizophrenia: data from the CATIE schizophrenia trial sample at baseline. *Schizophrenia Research* 86:15–22, 2006.

SELECTED READINGS

Barber, M. E. Recovery as the new medical model for psychiatry. *Psychiatric Services* 63:277–279, 2012.

Bleuler, E. *Dementia Praecox or the Group of Schizophrenias.* New York: International Universities Press, 1950.

Cannon, T. D., K. Cadenhead, B. Cornblatt, S. W. Woods, J. Addington, E. Walker, L. J. Seidman, D. Perkins, M. Tsuang, T. McGlashan, and R. Heinssen. Prediction of psychosis in youth at high clinical risk: a multisite longitudinal study in North America. *Archives of General Psychiatry* 65:28–37, 2008.

Deegan, P. E., and R. E. Drake. Shared decision making and medication management in the recovery process. *Psychiatric Services* 57:1636–1639, 2006.

Hirsch, S. R., and D. R. Weinberger, eds. *Schizophrenia,* 2nd ed. Oxford: Blackwell Science, 2003.

Johnstone, E. C. *Searching for the Causes of Schizophrenia.* Oxford: Oxford University Press, 1994.

Lieberman, J. A., T. S. Stroup, J. P. McEvoy, M. S. Swartz, R. A. Rosenheck, D. O. Perkins, R. S. Keefe, S. M. Davis, C. E. Davis, B. D. Lebowitz, J. Severe, and J. K. Hsiao. Clinical Antipsychotic Trials of Intervention Effectiveness (CATIE) Investigators: effectiveness of antipsychotic drugs in patients with chronic schizophrenia. *New England Journal of Medicine* 353:1209–1223, 2005.

Lieberman, J. A., T. S. Stroup, and D. O. Perkins, eds. *The American Psychiatric Publishing Textbook of Schizophrenia.* Washington, DC: American Psychiatric Publishing, 2006.

McGrath, J. J. Variations in the incidence of schizophrenia: data versus dogma. *Schizophrenia Bulletin* 2006 32:195–197

Mueser, K. T., and S. Gingerich. *The Complete Family Guide to Schizophrenia. Helping Your Loved One Get the Most Out of Life.* New York: Guilford Press, 2006.

Newcomer, J. W. Metabolic considerations in the use of antipsychotic medications: a review of recent evidence. *Journal of Clinical Psychiatry* 68(Suppl 1):20–27, 2007.

Picchioni, M. M., and R. M. Murray. Schizophrenia. *British Medical Journal* 335:91–95, 2007.

Saks Elyn, R. *The Center Cannot Hold: My Journey Through Madness.* New York: Hyperion, 2007.

Substance Abuse and Mental Health Services Administration. SAMHSA news release. SAMHSA announces a working definition of "recovery" from mental health disorders and substance use disorders. http://www.samhsa.gov/newsroom/advisories/1112223420.aspx, 2011.

Tamminga, C. A., and H. H. Holcomb. Phenotype of schizophrenia: a review and formulation. *Molecular Psychiatry* 10:27–39, 2005.

Neurocognitive Disorders and Mental Disorders Due to Another Medical Condition

JENNIFER M. RUCCI AND ROBERT E. FEINSTEIN

Neurocognitive disorders are common syndromes with multiple etiologies affecting cognition. Patients with neurocognitive disorders experience a decline in cognitive functioning as the defining feature of their illness. Patients with mental disorders due to another (i.e., nonpsychiatric) medical condition have symptoms that appear to result from a psychiatric disorder but the symptoms are caused by the direct physiological consequences of medical conditions with known biological etiologies. For example, an adrenal tumor can produce a "secondary" panic disorder that is clinically indistinguishable from the "primary" panic disorder seen in psychiatric patients. For all of these patients, a balanced biopsychosocial-cultural approach to the evaluation, differential diagnosis, and treatment of symptoms is complex but of critical importance.

DIAGNOSTIC AND CLINICAL FEATURES

Historically, neurocognitive disorders, mental disorders due to another medical condition, and substance-induced disorders were grouped together under the heading "organic mental disorders." A decision was made to reclassify this group of "organic" disorders in the DSM-IV into two separate groups of disorders, to remove the implication that primary psychiatric disorders, such as schizophrenia, do not have a biological basis. The DSM-5 continues this classification and elaborates further on the need to determine the specific etiologies of these syndromes. It has replaced the term *dementia* with *neurocognitive disorder* to emphasize the neurological etiologies and cognitive effects. The terminology of the category of mental disorders due to another medical condition has been updated for the DSM-5 as well. The DSM-IV labeled this category of illnesses as due to a general medical condition. The new terminology better reflects the fact that psychiatric disorders are indeed medical illnesses.

Neurocognitive Disorders

Delirium

Patients suffering from delirium experience an **acute change** in mental status that often leaves them feeling bewildered. The hallmarks of delirium are **fluctuating levels of consciousness** and an **inability to acquire new information** (see DSM-5). The typical signs include **confusion, disorientation**, periods of **sleepiness alternating with periods of agitation, difficulty using and understanding language**, and **deficits in attention, memory, and concentration**. **Perceptual disturbances** may occur, including misinterpretations, illusions, or frank visual or auditory hallucinations (see Table 5.1 for epidemiological information).

The case example in Box 5.1 illustrates a typical clinical presentation of delirium, characterized by orientation throughout the day and confusion in the evening. The evening nursing staff felt that the patient was quite sick, whereas the patient appeared reasonably lucid to the morning staff. This short-term fluctuation in orientation and sensorium is referred to as **waxing and waning**. Because delirium can come and go, the syndrome may not be easily recognized or diagnosed. Serial evaluations on different occasions are sometimes required to make the diagnosis.

Course

Certain patient characteristics increase the likelihood of delirium: age over 65 years, preexisting neurocognitive disorder, and severe medical illness. Delirium can occur very rapidly over seconds to minutes, for example due to dehydration or high altitude. It often develops over a period of hours to days. Delirium can be a life-threatening condition that is reversible with treatment, or it can result in irreversible brain damage (see Table 5.2). Rapid diagnosis with emergency intervention may in some cases be essential to prevent permanent brain damage or death (see case example in Box 5.2). With proper diagnosis and prompt treatment, recovery is often possible within hours or days, depending on the underlying etiology. However, delirium carries a high risk of morbidity and mortality. Studies indicate that geriatric hospitalized patients with delirium have a mortality rate of 20% to 75% during their hospitalization (Adamis et al. 2006). Fifteen percent of those discharged with a diagnosis of delirium die within 1 month and 25% within 6 months.

Major and Mild Neurocognitive Disorders (Dementia)

Major neurocognitive disorder (NCD) is characterized by **significant cognitive decline** over time, **causing impairments in function and cognitive testing** (see DSM-5). The decline should be documented by objective assessment, in addition to subjective report, and should be present in at least one of the following cognitive domains: complex attention, executive function, learning and memory, language, perceptual-motor, or social cognition.

Patients with major NCD may not wish to acknowledge or may not be able to recognize their mental deficits, declining intellectual abilities, memory problems, or emotional and behavioral changes. The changes caused by major NCD usually have a slow or **insidious onset** and, therefore, are often first recognized by the patient's family, friends, or coworkers (see case example in Box 5.3). Frequently, patients cannot acknowledge their deficits and may go out of their way to **conceal** them from others. When one patient with major NCD was asked, "Who is the governor of your state?" she tried to conceal a memory lapse with the retort, "Who cares? He's just another idiot politician, anyway." Other changes associated with major NCD may include **perseveration** of speech (i.e., repeating an idea,

TABLE 5.1 Epidemiology and Course of Delirium and Major Neurocognitive Disorder

Disorder	Prevalence	Age of Onset	Course	Risk Factors
Delirium	10–30% of hospitalized patients	Any age; most common after age 40 years	Variable, depending on etiology	Increases with age
Major neurocognitive disorder (NCD)	Age 65–69, 1–2% Age 85+ 15–30%	Most common after age 40 years	65% chronic, 25% partially treatable, 10% reversible	Increases with age and positive family history
Major NCD due to Alzheimer's disease	Represents 2/3 of all major NCD 24 million people worldwide. From age 70, prevalence doubles every 5 years; from age 90, almost 50%	Typically after 65, but an early onset form exists	Progressive downward deterioration, starting with isolated memory deficits	Increases with age; female gender; positive family history of first-degree relative with disorder; head trauma increases risk 3–4 times; Down's syndrome; defects in apolipoprotein E4 allele
Major NCD due to Lewy body disease	10–20% of major NCD; second most common cause of major NCD	Usually 50+	Cognitive decline and visual hallucinations	Family history, males and females equal
Major NCD due to vascular disease	5–20% of patients with major NCD	Earlier age than Alzheimer's disease	Stuttering course: deterioration and destabilization	Cardiovascular disease (hypertension, abnormal lipid profiles, smoking, history of arrhythmia, diabetes); more common in men
Major NCD due to traumatic brain injury (TBI)	1.7 million TBIs annually	Any age, most occur in early childhood, late adolescence, or old age	Acute change after acute injury. Can worsen with repeated TBIs	Falls, risk-taking behavior, young and old age
Major NCD due to HIV disease	33% of hospitalized HIV patients	Any age, typically much younger than other major NCDs	Chronic course: deterioration over time	HIV risk factors (sexual contact, transfusions, intravenous drug use)
Major NCD due to frontotemporal lobar degeneration, including Pick's disease	7 per 100,000	50–60 years old most common	Change in social interactions and personality before cognitive decline	Family history accounts for 40% of cases with autosomal dominant transmission; linked to amyotrophic lateral sclerosis
Major NCD due to prion disease, including Creutzfeldt-Jakob disease	1 in 1 million, most common prion disease	Most commonly 45–60 years old	Very rapid course, typically death within 1 year of diagnosis	Contact with infected nervous tissue; family history

> **BOX 5.1**
> ## CASE EXAMPLE OF DELIRIUM
>
> A previously cognitively intact 78-year-old man was brought to the emergency department (ED) by the staff of his nursing home because they had observed him becoming confused and aggressive toward his roommate in the evenings for the past week. They had not brought him in sooner because he was back to his normal self by the next morning after each incident. In the ED he reported the year as 1955 and his location as the grocery store. He appeared to be hallucinating and responding to internal stimuli, yelling at someone who was not physically present. Physical examination was significant only for tachycardia, while a standard laboratory investigation included an abnormal urinalysis with multiple white blood cells, blood, and leukocyte esterase. The diagnosis was delirium due to urinary tract infection. He was prescribed antibiotics and his cognitive functioning returned to baseline within 48 hours.

TABLE 5.2 Symptoms and Causes of Life-Threatening Deliriums

Disease Category or Agent	Clinical Presentation
Structural CNS Damage	Headache or focal neurological signs.
Intracranial bleeding	Bleeding occurs in 25% of strokes. In young persons, berry aneurysm is the most common cause. In general, increased risk of bleeding with advancing age and presence of hypertension.
Subdural bleeding	Often due to head trauma. Increased risk for alcoholics. It can occur long after acute head trauma.
Infectious Disease	
Bacterial meningitis	Headache, stiff neck, meningeal signs, sudden fever, and increased white blood cell count; epidemics.
Encephalitis (due to virus or opportunistic infection)	Initial flu-like prodrome of headache, rhinorrhea, sore throat, fever blisters. Then delirium, neurological symptoms, or seizures. Slight increase in white blood cell count. It can be caused by self-infection or epidemics.
Metabolic and Nutritional Disease	
Decreased cerebral perfusion causing hypoxemia; hypovolemia, hypoglycemia	Decreased blood pressure, glucose, pO_2, or hematocrit; signs and symptoms of cardiac failure (myocardial infarction, congestive heart failure, arrhythmia) diabetes, respiratory distress (COPD, asthma, pulmonary embolism)
Hypertensive encephalopathy	Hypertension, papilledema
Wernicke's encephalopathy	Ataxia, neurocognitive effects. Seen in 3% of alcoholics; 17% mortality rate
Substance Related	
Drugs of abuse	Delirium due to alcohol or cocaine intoxication (most common); delirium due to withdrawal of alcohol, sedative-hypnotics. Status seizures secondary to withdrawal are often life-threatening.
Over-the-counter or prescription drugs	Delirium due to use of anticholinergics, benzodiazepines, or narcotics. At risk for arrhythmias
Poisons (environmental)	Delirium and symptoms specific to poison (e.g., household products such as pesticides, solvents, carbon monoxide, lead)

BOX 5.2

CASE EXAMPLE OF LIFE-THREATENING DELIRIUM

A 26-year-old man who regularly ran 6 miles every day did not return home from his run one evening. The next day he was found wandering on a nearby highway by the police and was brought to the emergency room in a confused state. He could not remember what had happened, nor did he know where he was or where he had been. He had a fluctuating level of consciousness and attention. He was paranoid, illogical, and seemed to be listening to voices. He felt that others wanted to kill him. He had some of the cardinal symptoms of delirium. He subsequently had a seizure, then lapsed into a coma, and later died. The postmortem diagnosis was delirium due to a ruptured berry aneurysm.

---

question, phrase, or word over and over again) and **alterations in personality** (preexisting personality traits may change or become exaggerated or rigid).

Patients with **mild neurocognitive disorder** have clear cognitive decline that is determined to be outside of normal aging, but only to a modest degree. The neurocognitive domains and etiologies are the same as for major NCD, but patients do not have functional limitations hindering their independence in everyday activities. It has

---

BOX 5.3

CASE EXAMPLE OF MAJOR NEUROCOGNITIVE DISORDER DUE TO ALZHEIMER'S DISEASE

A 63-year-old male retired pilot came to see his physician at the insistence of his wife. She had become frightened by his driving, as he would stop in the middle of intersections and appear lost, nearly causing several accidents. He denied any concerns about his ability to function, his memory, or his thinking. She was also concerned about his new inability to pay bills (he paid the same one multiple times and didn't pay others at all), his lack of interest in doing things with her, and his need to be told the same thing multiple times. She was especially worried that he was planning to renew his pilot's license and return to flying a small plane. On mental status examination, the patient had clear deficits in orientation, naming, and memory. His clock drawing was grossly abnormal with an inability to set up the clock or properly set the time. Angry with his wife for insisting on the evaluation, the patient showed the characteristic lack of concern for his losses, whereas his wife was terrified about the potential dangers of his still driving and flying. She had good reason to be concerned, and the physician counseled him to avoid driving and flying. Although he was resistant, this restriction may have been lifesaving for him and others. The roles in the family changed as his wife became responsible for the driving and the finances. Psychoeducation and family therapy helped the patient and his wife to adjust to the changes and enjoy the time they had left with each other.

---

been estimated that 20% of the population over 70 has mild NCD. Not all of these individuals go on to develop major NCD. There is ongoing research to identify potential differences that might predict which individuals are most likely to progress to major NCD.

Course

A common initial symptom of major NCD is a simple lapse in memory, such as forgetting names, neglecting to turn off lights, or becoming confused about directions. Some individuals cannot remember whether they have locked the door and repeatedly get out of bed to double-check the lock. Patients with major NCD experience a gradual decline in several domains of cognitive functioning (e.g., they cannot calculate the correct change when shopping, they cannot balance a checkbook, they get lost when driving, or they don't recognize some family members). They may become accusatory or paranoid and blame others for their own mistakes. For example, a man may accuse his wife of stealing his keys when in fact he has forgotten where he has placed them. In general, **long-term memory remains intact** until late in the illness. As major NCD progresses, problems with orientation occur in the following typical sequence: patients first lose track of the time of day, next their geographic location, and in severe cases patients may not remember their family or even their own identity.

As the cognitive decline continues, patients with major NCD may appear **apathetic, dull, or depressed**. Patients with severe NCD involving the frontal lobe may present with **fluctuating or labile moods, disinhibition**, and deteriorating social graces, including inappropriate lewdness. Severely affected patients are generally calm but may be easily startled if they are suddenly disturbed. They are comforted by familiarity and stability and are particularly vulnerable to change. This vulnerability can result in exaggerated emotional outbursts or occasional episodes of violent or unpredictable behavior. At the end stages, memory, intellect, and cognitive capacities may decline to the point of complete disorientation. Patients may be unable to care for themselves or carry out their normal daily activities, such as cooking, shopping, dressing, eating, and toileting. Many patients eventually become bedridden. At this stage, individuals are susceptible to other illnesses, such as infections and accidents, which often become the immediate cause of death.

The course of major NCD varies largely depending on its type (see Table 5.1). Major NCD due to Alzheimer's disease typically presents with an insidious onset and a **slow, steady, deteriorating** course with a downward progression in functioning. Patients can be expected to decline 10–20% per year on standard cognitive assessments. Vascular disease follows a **stepwise or stuttering** course. Patients may have stable mild deficits for years, with discrete incidents of new vascular injury and rapid deterioration as new mini-infarcts develop. Some patients with vascular disease may regain stability with decreasing capacity and remain stable for years.

Major NCD due to traumatic brain injury (TBI) is often sudden in onset, has a variable recovery course, and can become permanent (see Box 5.4).

Lewy body disease follows a course similar to Alzheimer's disease but often includes visual hallucinations and, late in the course, motor symptoms similar to Parkinson's disease. The rigidity and bradykinesia characteristic of patients with Parkinson's disease may cause them to appear to have a more severe cognitive loss than they actually do. Frontotemporal lobar degeneration often begins with a change in personality and social interaction due to localized damage in the frontal lobes, which are the centers of inhibition.

BOX 5.4

CASE EXAMPLE OF MAJOR NEUROCOGNITIVE DISORDER DUE TO HEAD TRAUMA

A 20-year-old male college student suffered a severe concussion in a skiing accident. He presented to his student health service because he was failing his classes. In the 3 months since his accident he had been unable to learn any new subject material presented in his classes. Although his short-term memory was severely impaired, his long-term or retrograde memories were intact, with the exception of the accident, which he could not remember. His intellectual capacities that were based on pre-accident learning were also unimpaired. An MRI of the head revealed bilateral damage of the mamillary bodies.

Creutzfeldt-Jakob disease is a unique and devastating prion illness that is associated with characteristic myoclonic jerks; affected individuals rapidly progress to death over several months.

Mental Disorders Due to Another Medical Condition

Mental disorders due to another medical condition are classified on the basis of their predominant feature. Each of the major diagnostic categories has a corresponding diagnosis due to another medical condition. Patients with these disorders can experience psychotic, mood, or anxious symptoms or a personality change. **Intellectual functioning usually remains intact** in all of these disorders.

Psychotic Disorders Due to Another Medical Condition

Patients with psychotic disorder due to another medical condition have another clearly identified medical illness (not a psychiatric illness such as schizophrenia) that is etiologically responsible for the development of delusions, hallucinations, or other psychotic symptoms, such as disorganized thinking. Patients may present with delusions or with isolated hallucinations, but only rarely will they have both. In the case example in Box 5.5, the patient was already diagnosed with a medical problem before developing a psychotic illness, making the medical etiology of his psychosis more evident. Patients may present with typical paranoid delusions such as a belief that the CIA is after them or fear that the medical staff is trying to

---

BOX 5.5

CASE EXAMPLE OF PSYCHOTIC DISORDER TO SYSTEMIC LUPUS

A 47-year-old man was admitted to the hospital with complaints of fever, weakness, butterfly rash, diffuse joint pain, anemia, and renal failure. The diagnosis was systemic lupus erythematosus. One week later, he became psychotic, with loosening of associations, disorganized behavior, and delusions that the nursing staff wanted to kill him. The most likely cause of his new-onset psychosis was lupus cerebritis.

---

harm them. They also may have grandiose delusions. Typical hallucinations are manifested as commanding voices that direct the patient to take action or respond to directions. Some patients have frightening visual hallucinations while others may have tactile or olfactory hallucinations. Certain hallucinations can be a sign of a particular illness. For example, olfactory hallucinations of burning rubber are highly suggestive of partial complex seizures.

Depressive and Bipolar Disorders Due to Another Medical Condition

Mood disorders due to another medical condition can resemble depression, mania, or mixed features (see Chapter 3, Mood Disorders). Symptoms of these medically induced mood disorders can be missed when the symptoms are mild or are incorrectly attributed to the medical condition. For example, a mild depression may be the first sign of Parkinson's disease, but the depressive symptoms may be incorrectly attributed to the rigidity and bradykinesia of Parkinson's (depression associated with Parkinson's disease is thought to be caused by the disease itself rather than a reaction to having the disease). A case example is presented in Box 5.6.

Anxiety Disorders Due to Another Medical Condition

Anxiety disorders due to another medical condition can present with generalized anxiety, panic attacks, or phobias (see case example in Box 5.7).

Personality Change Due to Another Medical Condition

Patients with a personality change due to another medical condition display atypical behaviors or ways of interacting, which may range from an exaggeration of preexisting personality traits to an entirely new personality style or behaviors. For example, a sloppy person may become sloppier, and a shy person may become reclusive or gregarious. Often family members will say that an individual "just isn't the same person anymore," as the case example in Box 5.8 illustrates.

There are five subtypes of personality change due to another medical condition (see DSM-5). Patients with the **labile** subtype may display stormy affects and irritability in association with manic, depressive, or rapidly cycling moods. **Disinhibited** patients may have the appearance of someone with an antisocial personality disorder, characterized by newly impulsive or unpredictable behaviors, distractibility, and poor judgment. Some patients exhibit euphoria and express their emotions inappropriately. The **aggressive** subtype of personality change is characterized by irritability and anger, as well as aggression. Minor stress may precipitate impulsive and violent verbal or physical outbursts. **Apathetic**

BOX 5.6

CASE EXAMPLE OF DEPRESSIVE DISORDER DUE TO PANCREATIC CARCINOMA

A 50-year-old female former alcoholic began awakening early every morning over the course of 3 weeks. She inexplicably felt depressed and tearful and had intermittent thoughts of killing herself. She was hospitalized with additional complaints of anorexia, abdominal pain, constipation, and weight loss. Her medical workup revealed jaundice, and ultrasound studies showed an abdominal mass. At surgery, she was found to have pancreatic cancer.

CASE EXAMPLE OF ANXIETY DISORDER DUE TO PHEOCHROMOCYTOMA

A 35-year-old woman complained of the sudden onset of severe anxiety and fear of impending doom that made her unable to leave the house without help from a friend. She also had headaches, excessive sweating, palpitations, and occasional chest discomfort, which she associated with severe work stress. Her physician found that she had diastolic hypertension of 140 mm Hg and abnormally high levels of urinary catecholamines. Ultrasound studies and an intravenous pyelogram suggested a right adrenal gland tumor, which was confirmed surgically. Her panic attacks were due to the pheochromocytoma.

---

patients appear to have depression with psychomotor retardation and may have problems initiating, organizing, planning, and executing tasks. It is often difficult to differentiate apathy from major depressive disorder. Patients with **paranoid** personality changes are suspicious, mistrustful, and secretive but, by definition, do not have frank loss of reality testing. (Paranoid patients with loss of reality testing should be classified as having a psychotic disorder due to another medical condition rather than a personality change.)

Course
The course of mental disorders due to another medical condition varies greatly depending on the specific medical condition that is responsible for the psychiatric symptoms. As a general rule, the psychiatric symptoms do not remit until the underlying other medical condition is treated or otherwise resolves.

THE INTERVIEW

Brain deficits may commonly be expressed during the interview, and the physician may notice inattention, poor concentration, poor comprehension, memory loss, fluctuating

---

CASE EXAMPLE OF PERSONALITY CHANGE DUE TO ANOXIC BRAIN INJURY

Following global hypoxia during a cardiovascular surgery, which produced anoxic brain injury, a 52-year-old woman's husband reported she was never the same. Although he had trouble describing specific changes, he said "her eyes have a different look" and she was "a different person" after the surgery. Specifically, she was less outgoing, more irritable about small changes in her usual routine, and less emotionally connected to him. She even had different interests, now reading scientific and engineering books for hours a day, whereas before the surgery she preferred fiction.

levels of consciousness, confusion or befuddlement, inability to focus, the appearance of being "lost," or impairment in learning, speech, hearing, or vision. Falling asleep during the interview or an inability to sit still may be also observed.

Patients with neurocognitive disorders and mental disorders due to another medical condition frequently require special considerations during the interview (see Box 5.9). In particular, physicians should be **sensitive to the patient's limitations**, modifying their usual interviewing style to accommodate the patient's needs. For example, to communicate effectively the physician may have to speak louder than usual, use more hand gestures, express a stronger affect, or write with pen and paper. It may be necessary for the physician to get close enough to see the patient's lips moving or to speak directly into the patient's "good" ear. To focus attention, the physician may need to hold the patient's hand or repeatedly touch the patient's arm or shoulder. These techniques should be used only if the physician believes that they will improve the therapeutic relationship or help to elicit relevant information.

It is important for physicians to note their **emotional reactions** toward patients with cognitive impairment, who may elicit feelings of pity, hopelessness, helplessness, disgust, or fear. Physicians who are unaware of such reactions may make errors, such as keeping cognitively impaired patients at an emotional distance, talking down to patients as if they were children, or overextending themselves in offering special care to a fragile patient. When patients or their families express feelings of hopelessness and helplessness, the physician may become unduly pessimistic about the patient's capacity to benefit from treatment. Physicians who are aware of this reaction can empathize with the patient's or the family's frustrations and further the therapeutic alliance. Similarly, the physician's anger or embarrassment in response to a disinhibited patient's cursing or sexually inappropriate comments may further the physician's understanding of the challenges facing the family at home with the patient.

BOX 5.9
INTERVIEWING GUIDELINES

- Adjust your interview style so the patient can see, hear, and touch you.
- Maintain a calm, private, and confidential environment.
- Begin the interview with open-ended questions, which help establish rapport as well as begin to identify the patient's deficits.
- Move to closed-ended questions to assist the patient with difficult answers or to gather vital information quickly.
- Help modulate the patient's anxiety level by avoiding long silences and by explaining the need for all of your questions.
- Bolster the patient's self-esteem with realistic reassurance.
- Be sensitive to patients' shame about their deficits.
- Minimize the test atmosphere by telling the patient that he or she cannot fail a mental status examination.
- Interview the patient's family for information as well as to assess their emotional state and ability to assist in the treatment.

Interview Setting

The interview setting should be as private as possible, to preserve the patient's confidentiality and dignity. When privacy is not possible, the physician should maintain confidentiality by not asking sensitive questions or raising personal topics (e.g., HIV status) in a setting such as a curtained-off area of the emergency room in which others might overhear.

To ease the distress of the interview situation and to facilitate communication, the patient's physical comfort should be considered. The immediate physical environment might require adjustment (e.g., rearranging the furniture, raising the bed, seating the patient in a chair, or suggesting that the patient lie down) so that it is easier for the patient to speak. The physician should also be comfortably situated. Environmental noise and distractions should be kept to a minimum. When the environment does not have enough normal sensory stimulation, as in some intensive care units (ICU), normal sounds may need to be introduced. For example, turning on the radio in an ICU can mediate the sensory deprivation of the milieu and may improve the quality of the interview.

Interview Questions

The interview can begin in the standard manner with open-ended questions such as "What brings you here today?" and "How are you feeling?" Such questions allow patients to feel that they are being understood and are free to express their concerns. Open-ended questioning builds rapport and trust and allows the physician to observe the patient's behaviors and emotional tone while attending to the patient's responses. The physician can observe deficits such as slurred, dysarthric, or aphasic speech, as well as abnormal movements, gestures, or grimaces. By carefully listening and observing, the physician can begin to differentiate brain deficits from primary psychiatric disturbances. If the patient's level of consciousness, attention, concentration, and intellectual ability appear to be normal, the physician can follow the guidelines of a basic psychiatric interview (see Chapter 2, The Psychiatric Interview).

When patients appear to be confused or bewildered or are suffering from intellectual decline, it may be necessary to switch from open-ended to **closed-ended questions**. Closed-ended questions give the patient several possible answers from which to choose. They may be simple "either-or" questions or questions that require only "yes or no" answers. Closed-ended questions may be helpful if patients have a restricted capacity because of focal brain deficits or if the physician is trying to obtain specific information quickly (e.g., from a patient who is delirious). The physician might ask, "Did you take drugs? Answer yes or no." "Did you fall down or lose consciousness?" Focal questions such as "Do you know today's date or time?" "Do you recall my name?" "Do you know where you are?" may help the physician establish the patient's orientation and capacity for immediate recall.

Therapeutic Interventions

Patients may need help **modulating their level of anxiety** during the course of the interview. Long silences or pauses during the interview are stressful to many patients with cognitive deficits and should be used judiciously. Patients with neurocognitive disorder often try to conceal their deficits because they are ashamed of appearing stupid. They may deny, even to themselves, that they have a serious brain disease or may try to protect their families from seeing their deficits. Physicians need to find a balance between respecting patients' needed defenses and obtaining the information necessary for diagnosis and treatment. Reassuring patients that they cannot "fail" the interview and acknowledging their efforts to respond to questions are usually sufficient to avoid defensive responses.

Before beginning formal mental status testing, the physician might offer **reassurance** with comments such as "This is not a test to see how smart you are, but, rather, I will be asking you some questions that will help me learn how you think and what you can remember." The physician should avoid making patients feel as though they are taking a "brain test" that can be passed or failed. One way to build confidence is to start with easy problems so that the patient can get several answers correct. For example, "Please add 1 plus 1, 2 plus 2," and so on, building in complexity with each question. Patients with a neurological condition may have a low anxiety tolerance and may only be able to tolerate several brief episodes of testing before they become agitated and confused. Excessive anxiety may make patients seem more neurologically impaired than they really are. However, when mental status deficits are subtle, they are easier to detect if patients' anxiety level is increased. Excessive repeated testing should be avoided to protect the self-esteem of these highly vulnerable patients.

Patients who realize that they cannot remember things or suddenly become fearful that they are losing their intellectual capacity may develop a **catastrophic reaction**. This reaction is a sudden outburst of extreme, intense emotion (e.g., anger, rage, or tears or violence) that may occur when patients first realize, on an emotional level, that their mental capacities are deteriorating rapidly. Patients will later describe a mixture of fear and intense shame. Such reactions are more likely when the patient's self-esteem is grounded in intellectual abilities and prowess. Most catastrophic reactions can be managed with empathy and support.

Family Interview

Family members should be consulted early in the evaluation process of cognitively impaired individuals. Families are invaluable sources of information because they are usually the best observers of patients' baseline, deficits, or problems. Interviewing the family as a unit typically allows the most important information to emerge quickly and provides access to information that the patient may wish to conceal or may not be able to remember or communicate.

Family interviews should follow the same basic pattern as individual patient interviews. The family interview can progress from open-ended to closed-ended questions as required. During the interview, the physician should observe the interactions between the patient and the various family members, keeping the following questions in mind: Does the family understand the illness? Are the patient's deficits highlighted or concealed in the presence of family members? Can the spouse or children help? Are some members frightened of the illness? Are some members good observers and capable of helping?

Families are often the best resources for implementing a treatment plan and follow-up care. They may be able to provide most of the physical care for patients, assist in educating the patient about the illness, and help with specific rehabilitative tasks, such as relearning how to drive or read. A family can be a wonderful source of emotional support and hope as well, and can give the patient a sense of normalcy. If the family is too overwhelmed by the illness to be helpful, they may need the support of a professional caregiver or agency.

DIFFERENTIAL DIAGNOSIS

There are three steps in the differential diagnosis of neurocognitive disorders and mental disorders due to another medical conditions: (1) differentiate neurocognitive disorders, mental disorders due to another medical condition, and substance-induced disorders from all other primary psychiatric disorders; (2) differentiate among these three specific syndromes (i.e., neurocognitive disorder, a mental disorder due to another medical condition, or a substance-induced disorder); and (3) identify the specific etiology that has produced the psychiatric symptoms.

A detailed medical history will help to determine whether the patient has another medical or neurological illness or is suffering with a primary psychiatric disorder. The following signs strongly suggest that psychiatric symptoms are caused by another condition with anatomical or physiological disruption in the central nervous system: (1) an **acute onset** of symptoms (i.e., within hours or days); (2) the development of psychiatric symptoms in a patient **over 40 years** of age with **no prior psychiatric history**; and (3) recent use or abuse of psychoactive **drugs**. Almost all of the major psychiatric illnesses have a slow, insidious onset over a period of weeks, months, or even years, although some exceptions to this general principle exist. For example, major NCD due to Alzheimer's disease has a slow, insidious onset, while brief reactive psychoses and some dissociative states may occur immediately after a catastrophic psychological trauma.

A patient presenting with a first episode of psychiatric or neurological symptoms and no prior history of psychiatric symptoms should be evaluated for acute medical problems causing psychiatric symptoms. Many medical and neurological illnesses present with disturbances in thinking or mood, changes in behavior, or subtle neurological symptoms, such as tremors, tics, or other abnormal movements. It is vital to obtain a detailed medical history from both the patient and the family (see also Medical Evaluation later in this chapter). With this information, a thorough differential diagnosis can be made that sets the foundation for further workup and treatment. Assuming that psychiatric symptoms are caused by a psychiatric disorder can lead to mistakes in diagnosis in which major life-threatening medical illnesses are not recognized. The case example in Box 5.10 illustrates the pitfalls of assuming that new psychiatric symptoms result from a primary psychiatric illness.

BOX 5.10

CASE EXAMPLE OF ALCOHOL WITHDRAWAL MISTAKEN FOR BIPOLAR DISORDER

A single 38-year-old female attorney became confused and agitated 2 days after an endoscopic retrograde cholangiopancreatography (ERCP) to evaluate her for chronic pancreatitis. The medical team suspected bipolar illness, as her physical exam, laboratory studies, and head CT were normal except for slightly elevated liver enzymes. The psychiatrist asked the family to check the patient's home. Multiple empty alcohol containers were found, and a diagnosis of delirium tremens was made. In retrospect, alcohol withdrawal should have been suspected sooner given the patient's pancreatitis and lack of any previous psychiatric history. Faster recognition would have allowed prompter treatment and a faster recovery.

Once it has been determined that psychiatric symptoms are caused by another medical condition, the specific syndrome and etiology should be identified. In some cases, the neurocognitive syndrome can be identified (e.g., delirium or dementia) but the medical condition that has caused it cannot be determined. In other cases, a specific medical cause (e.g. hypothyroidism) may be the clear cause. In still other cases, the exact relationship between the psychiatric condition and the medical illness may be difficult to determine. For example, is a brain tumor causing depression or is the patient's depression a psychological reaction to having a brain tumor? When suspicion is high that the psychiatric symptoms are caused by another known medical condition, but a causal relationship cannot be proven, the diagnosis of a mental disorder due to another medical condition should still be made. The patient's recreational drug use history, signs and symptoms of drug intoxication or withdrawal, and urine drug testing can help differentiate substance-related disorders (see Chapter 7, Substance-Related and Addictive Disorders).

The case example in Box 5.11 illustrates the complexity of diagnosing medical illnesses that present with psychiatric symptoms, as this patient's long history of symptoms was incorrectly explained by multiple psychiatric diagnoses. Diagnostic parsimony should have raised the possibility that one illness explained all of her psychiatric and medical symptoms.

Special Areas of Concern in Differential Diagnosis

The steady intellectual decline or cognitive loss over months to years and the absence of acute or variable confusion can help to differentiate major or minor **NCD** (i.e., **dementia) from delirium**. Patients with neurocognitive disorder have an increased risk of a superimposed delirium. In that situation, delirium must first be identified and treated before a diagnosis of major or mild NCD can be made.

The timeline of cognitive issues can also be used to differentiate neurocognitive disorders from intellectual disabilities. Whereas acute onset of symptoms should raise concern for another medical condition, lifelong symptoms are likely indicative of an intellectual disability. Of course, it is important to remember that individuals with intellectual disabilities can also have a superimposed disorder due to another medical condition or a subsequent neurocognitive disorder. These individuals should always be compared to their own baselines in order to determine if these additional etiologies may also be present.

Depression can present as **pseudodementia**, particularly in the elderly. Patients may appear to have a true neurocognitive disorder when in fact they have a primary depression associated with cognitive deficits that are typically reversible with treatment. Patients with pseudodementia often have **"patchy" memory loss**, and their intellectual deficits tend to be inconsistent. Patients with neurocognitive disorder have more global memory loss, and their intellectual deficits persist and decline over time. Pseudodementia should be considered in the differential diagnosis if a patient's confusion or a memory problem is **triggered by a loss** (see case example in Box 5.12). Patients with pseudodementia tend to **complain about their deficits** and exaggerate the severity of their symptoms, while patients with neurocognitive disorder often try to minimize or conceal their deficits. Patients with pseudodementia typically seek help and tend to behave in a dependent or demanding manner. They often make little effort to respond to mental status questions, and repeatedly say "I don't know," whereas those with a true neurocognitive disorder will often be distressed and struggle to answer mental status questions. When differentiation is not possible, a trial of antidepressants can be helpful, as those individuals with

BOX 5.11

CASE EXAMPLE OF DEPRESSIVE DISORDER AND NEUROCOGNITIVE DISORDER DUE TO WILSON'S DISEASE MISTAKEN FOR MULTIPLE PRIMARY PSYCHIATRIC DISORDERS

An 18-year-old college freshman presented to the student health service with sadness, irritability, and inability to concentrate on her schoolwork. She was diagnosed with an adjustment disorder related to conflicts about leaving home. Her symptoms resolved after a brief period of psychotherapy. In her junior year, she again experienced irritability and a depressed mood, as well as intermittent crying spells that began after she learned that her sister was suffering with a chronic liver disease. The symptoms resolved quickly after another brief period of psychotherapy and several visits with her sister. At age 25 years, she missed several menstrual cycles and began to "feel different." Her gynecologist was unable to explain the etiology of her amenorrhea. Two years later the patient developed a depressed and labile mood accompanied by episodes of rage and anxiety that did not seem to be connected to any particular precipitants. She began to abuse alcohol and gained 60 pounds. A neurologist, an internist, and a psychiatrist all felt that her problems were caused by depression, alcoholism, and a personality disorder. She returned to psychiatric treatment for several years. At age 30 years, the patient had an episode of slurred speech when she was clearly sober. A neurological workup, which included a serum ceruloplasm level, a slit-lamp ophthalmic exam, and a head CT scan, confirmed a diagnosis of Wilson's disease. This disease's insidious onset explained most if not all of her medical and psychiatric complaints over the past 12 years.

Wilson's disease is caused by a rare genetic defect in copper metabolism that affects the liver and brain. The patient's initial psychiatric symptoms were not evaluated for medical causes, and none of the physicians made a connection between the sister's liver disease and the patient's psychiatric and other medical symptoms. The sister had the chronic form of liver disease caused by Wilson's disease, while the patient had the psychiatric and central nervous system symptoms of the same illness.

Once this unfortunate woman had been given a diagnosis of a psychiatric disorder, consideration was no longer given to the possibility that another medical illness might have been causing her psychological symptoms. Her psychiatric symptoms were approached with a psychological bias that attributed her symptoms to conflict, loss, displaced anger, and problems in social adjustment. Because the correct diagnosis was delayed, she sustained significant brain damage and enjoyed only a partial recovery. In hindsight, this tragic result could have been entirely prevented if Wilson's disease had been diagnosed and treated earlier.

BOX 5.12
CASE EXAMPLE OF PSEUDODEMENTIA

A 72-year-old woman told her physician that she was extremely distressed about her "severe memory loss." Her memory had changed 3 weeks earlier, after a close friend passed away. She was afraid that she had Alzheimer's disease, like her mother, who had suffered with dementia for the last 5 years of her life and died at the age of 75 years. The patient appeared distressed, but was also irritated by the physician's questions and made little effort to answer them. Her response to most of the mental status questions was "I don't know." Her demeanor and responses were typical of a patient with pseudodementia, as was the rapid onset of her symptoms.

---

pseudodementia will often experience full remission of their symptoms, whereas those with a true neurocognitive disease may be minimally helped, if at all. Once all of the symptoms of depression have been treated, the individual suspected to have pseudodementia should have his or her cognition reassessed to be sure a true neurocognitive disorder is not also present.

Substance-induced disorders are the great imitators of other psychiatric illnesses. The wide array of symptoms and syndromes due to drug use are frequently indistinguishable from those of primary psychiatric disorders and psychiatric disorders due to another medical condition (see Chapter 7, Substance-Related and Addictive Disorders). Any type of prescription or over-the-counter drug, as well as herbal preparations and drugs of abuse, may induce psychiatric symptoms. Therefore, it is important to take a detailed drug history of all patients that includes drugs, vitamins, herbs, and supplements that are currently being used, the frequency with which they are taken, the typical daily dosage, and the time of last ingestion. Illegal drug use can be the most difficult to uncover, although many patients are reluctant to discuss their use of herbal preparations or supplements as well. Urine drug screening can be helpful in uncovering drug use, but it can be misleading in that a negative drug screening test does not rule out drug withdrawal syndromes, past abuse of drugs, or use of many herbal supplements that are not routinely tested by a urine drug screen.

Commonly prescribed medications that may produce an **iatrogenic delirium** include anticholinergic agents (diphenhydramine, tricyclic antidepressants) and benzodiazepines. Corticosteroids can precipitate a manic episode, and anti-Parkinson's agents such as amantadine, which affect the dopamine system, may produce psychotic symptoms, especially visual hallucinations.

Partial complex seizures consist of focal cerebral seizure activity that results in an altered state of consciousness, flashbacks, and feelings of déjà vu. These seizures can be associated with **psychotic symptoms**, including paranoid and grandiose delusions, that are distinguished from symptoms of schizophrenia only by the presence of seizure activity on EEG. Psychotic symptoms can appear between seizure episodes (i.e., interictally) or during seizures. The focal seizures may produce olfactory hallucinations or may affect visual perception such that size or shape of objects may appear distorted.

Personality changes resulting from focal seizures may be characterized by a **deepening of emotions, a preoccupation with moral or religious issues,** and an **unusual speaking**

> **BOX 5.13**
>
> ## CASE EXAMPLE OF PERSONALITY CHANGE DUE TO PARTIAL COMPLEX SEIZURES
>
> The wife of a 45-year-old man with a past history of alcoholic seizures and an obsessional personality style reported that her husband had become more emotional and irritable, less obsessive, and less interested in having sexual relations over the past year. He had also developed stringent religious beliefs that did not correspond to his religious upbringing and a habit of recording everything in his diary. The patient did not recognize any changes in his personality. A 72-hour ambulatory electroencephalogram (EEG) revealed new temporal abnormalities.

style often described as tedious, didactic, verbose, and circumstantial. Men often have decreased **libido**, but women may have increased libido (see case example in Box 5.13).

MEDICAL EVALUATION

Patients who present with a first episode of major psychiatric symptoms should receive a complete medical evaluation that includes the following elements: (1) medical history with a thorough review of risk factors; (2) detailed psychosocial history with special emphasis on the patient's current living situation, including family and other social supports, work, finances, and relevant cultural or religious factors; (2) a detailed accounting of prescribed and over-the-counter medication, use of herbal supplements, and recreational drug use and abuse; (3) medical review of systems; (4) physical examination, including a detailed neurological examination; (5) assessment of the patient's mental status and neurobehavioral symptoms; (7) laboratory testing; and (8) head CT and/or brain MRI scan, as well as EEG, lumbar puncture, and other sophisticated laboratory tests as clinically indicated.

Neurological Review of Systems

The neurological review of systems should specifically include headaches, seizures, syncope, head trauma, central nervous system (CNS) infections; weakness, paresthesia, and paralysis; atrophy, involuntary movements, tremors, gait disturbances, and incoordination; pain or sensory loss; loss of control of urination or defecation; sweating; and changes in vision, speech, hearing, equilibrium, swallowing, and taste.

Physical Examination

The vital signs are often the earliest objective evidence that a medical condition is producing a change in mental status. The heart and respiratory rates, blood pressure, and temperature should be routinely evaluated in all patients. An increased heart rate and slightly bulging eyes might suggest hyperthyroidism; an upper respiratory tract infection, fever, and confusion might suggest encephalitis; and an increase in heart rate, respiratory rate, and blood pressure in the absence of fever might suggest pheochromocytoma.

Neurological Examination

A detailed focal neurological examination should be performed in all patients presenting with psychiatric symptoms for the first time, including testing of the cranial nerves, motor system, sensory system, cerebellum functions, deep tendon reflexes, and gait. Possible significant findings include brisk deep tendon reflexes, increased muscle tone, and bilateral Babinski signs associated with neurocognitive disorder, and impaired coordination and peripheral neuropathy suggestive of alcohol-induced changes.

An adjunctive neurological examination may uncover **abnormal primitive reflexes** or **frontal release signs**, such as the snout, sucking, rooting, and grasping reflexes; Hoffmann's sign (elicited by pressing on the fingernail of the patient's middle finger to elicit abnormal flexion and adduction of the thumb); the palmomental reflex (or Radovici's sign, elicited by scratching the thenar eminence to elicit contraction of the contralateral mentalis muscles of the chin); or the glabellar tap (elicited by tapping repeatedly on the patient's forehead to elicit repetitive eye closings that do not extinguish with time). Appearance of these reflexes typically indicates loss of frontal lobe volume to some disease process, typically major NCD.

Laboratory Tests

General laboratory screening tests may help to confirm or uncover a diagnosis of a medical condition producing psychiatric symptoms. Helpful laboratory studies include a complete blood count, an electrolyte panel, blood glucose, urinalysis, a toxicology screen, liver function tests, sedimentation rate, and thyroid function tests. In the setting of cognitive decline, the following tests should be considered, depending on the history: a rapid plasma regain (RPR) screen for neurosyphilis, a thiamine level for Wernicke-Korsakoff syndrome, testing for HIV, and antibody screens for Lyme disease.

Neuroimaging

MRI and CT are both options for neuroimaging, although MRI is more sensitive to subtle changes. Global cortical **atrophy** is associated with major NCD due to Alzheimer's disease, whereas localized atrophy is seen with frontotemporal lobar degeneration. Vascular disease, previously referred to as multi-infarct dementia, is characterized by multiple small cerebral ischemic infarcts. Large structural changes such as neoplasms or normal-pressure hydrocephalus can also be identified. The case example in Box 5.14 illustrates the importance of a thorough workup that includes neuroimaging in patients with new cognitive deficits. Without a CT scan, the patient in this case could have been improperly treated for major NCD instead of receiving curative surgery for his meningioma. Positron emission tomography (PET) scans are now being used to detect some of the early neurological changes of Alzheimer's disease, even before any measurable cognitive impairment.

Electroencephalogram (EEG)

The electroencephalogram can be used to diagnose delirium, seizures, and certain forms of NCD. EEG changes associated with **delirium** include diffuse cortical slowing of the alpha waves, which directly correlates with fluctuations in attention and the incapacity to acquire new information. Patients with diffuse alpha-wave slowing usually have a somnolent and anergic clinical delirium (Pro and Wells 1977). Some delirious patients can also

CASE EXAMPLE DEMONSTRATING THE UTILITY OF NEUROIMAGING IN EVALUATION OF NEW COGNITIVE DEFICITS

A 65-year-old landscaper became lost while driving his car and was unable to find his way home. He called his wife, who had to go and pick him up because he was so afraid. His wife took him to his physician. She said that her husband had recently been irritable and harshly critical of her for mistakes that he had made (e.g., forgetting to turn off the gas burner on the stove at night, bouncing several checks). The patient said, "I feel like someone is slowly draining my mind of my personality, my thinking, changing my feelings…reducing me to rubble." He could not remember the exact date or the day of the week. He could remember only four numbers in sequence and only one out of three objects after 5 minutes. He was unable to solve simple mathematical problems, even though he had graduated from high school. The medical history and physical examination were normal, except for frontal release signs (i.e., the Babinski reflex, rooting reflex, and snout reflex) and soft neurological symptoms, such as left–right confusion, mixed dominance, and drift. While the clinical findings suggested neurocognitive disorder due to Alzheimer's disease, a head CT scan revealed a bilateral frontal brain tumor. Biopsy indicated a benign meningioma.

have a hyperactive, hyperaroused, or agitated clinical presentation, with an EEG pattern of low-voltage, rapid-activity theta waves. As a patient passes from delirium into coma, the EEG may progress to high-voltage delta activity in a bilaterally synchronous or random pattern.

When using EEG to diagnose delirium, two or more EEGs may be necessary to obtain a recording during a period of confusion. Alternatively, a computerized EEG that has a database of recordings for comparison can determine whether or not a single EEG recording is abnormal. The EEG of patients with **Creutzfeld-Jacob disease** is characterized by the gradual loss of normal brain electrical rhythms; generalized biphasic or triphasic **periodic sharp wave complexes** appear with a frequency of approximately 1–2 per second and are diagnostic.

Sleep Studies

The case example in Box 5.15 illustrates the value of sleep studies in specific situations. Symptoms of a sleep disorder can sometimes be confused with depression.

Mental Status Testing and Neurobehavioral Assessment

A complete, formal mental status examination should be performed in all patients who have changes in behavior, thinking, or mood. The presence of a neurological or other condition affecting the brain is often first identified by such an examination. Tests that are most helpful in differentiating a primary psychiatric disorder from a neurocognitive disorder or a mental disorder due to another medical condition are described in Boxes 5.16 and 5.17.

BOX 5.15
CASE EXAMPLE OF DEPRESSIVE DISORDER DUE TO OBSTRUCTIVE SLEEP APNEA

A 55-year-old male had been struggling with depression for several years. His main complaints were fatigue, depressed mood, anhedonia, and poor sleep. He had been treated with multiple antidepressants to no avail. The patient was able to fall asleep easily, but woke up multiple times during the night. He would then be so tired during the day that he fell asleep while driving on multiple occasions. He was obese and had diabetes and asthma. A sleep study confirmed the diagnosis of obstructive sleep apnea. The patient was treated with a continuous positive airway pressure machine (CPAP), which produced restful sleep, and his depression resolved.

BOX 5.16
MENTAL STATUS TESTING

Full mental status testing includes the assessment of level of consciousness, orientation (to time place and person), memory (four spheres: immediate recall, short-term memory, intermediate memory, and long-term memory), and cognitive ability.

LEVEL OF CONSCIOUSNESS
1. Observe whether the patient is awake and alert or confused and befuddled.
2. If the patient is awake and alert, note whether the level of consciousness remains the same or fluctuates (waxes and wanes). Fluctuations in the level of consciousness suggest that the patient is delirious.
3. If the level of consciousness fluctuates, note the length of the cycles of fluctuation. The cycles may be short (i.e., apparent during the interview) or long (i.e., occurring over the course of hours or days).
4. Note whether the fluctuations occur at certain times of the day. It is not uncommon for elderly persons to be fully alert during the day but to become delirious in the evening. This phenomenon is referred to as **sundowning** and is often seen in geriatric patients in hospitals and nursing homes.
5. Assess the patient's ability to learn new information by offering information about the patient's condition and then evaluating what is remembered. Asking the patient to read a paragraph in the newspaper and then discuss it is an alternative approach.

ORIENTATION TO TIME, PLACE, AND PERSON
1. Time: Ask, "What time of the day is it?" "Do you know what day of the week it is?" "What is the date today?" "What year is it?" "Do you know the current season?"
2. Place: Ask, "Do you know exactly where we are right now?" "What is the name of this place?" "In what institution, city, state, and country are we currently located?"

(continued)

3. Person: Ask, "What is your name? What do you do for living? Who is in your family?"
4. Correct answers to all of the questions about time, place, and person are summarized as "oriented × 3."
5. Disorientation caused by another medical condition typically occurs in the following sequence: time is lost first, place is lost second, and person is lost third. A different sequence of emerging deficits suggests a primary psychiatric disorder.

MEMORY: IMMEDIATE RECALL

1. Introduce yourself, and then ask if the patient remembers your name. If the patient does not, repeat your name several times, show the patient your ID badge, and ask again.
2. Ask the patient to repeat a span of digits: "I would like you to repeat immediately after me some numbers that I want you to recall. For example, if I say 1 and 3, then I want you to repeat 1 and 3. Let's try it." Start with two digits, then three digits, and so on, up to seven digits. Speak with a fixed tone, as rhythms add a memory cue.Most patients can recall a digit span of at least seven digits as is required for a typical phone number.

MEMORY: SHORT-TERM

Test One: Three-Item Verbal Recall

1. Give the patient three words to remember (usually, the names of two concrete objects and one abstract idea): "Please remember and repeat the following: ball, telephone, and charity." Ask the patient to repeat the three words immediately, which tests immediate recall and also shows whether the patient can attend, concentrate, and understand instructions. Go on to other interview questions. After 5 minutes, ask the patient to repeat the three words again.
2. If the patient can only remember two of the three (2/3) items, repeat the test. If the patient has a primary psychiatric disorder, the memory should improve. If the patient has a neurological deficit, the memory will remain impaired. The patient can be given a categorical hint (i.e., a round object) or a list of multiple-choice answers, which provides additional cues and uses recognition memory (which is less readily impaired than short-term recall).
3. If the patient can only recall 0/3 or 1/3 items after 5 minutes, provide three evocative or colorful things to remember. "Please remember these things that I love: The Beatles, fast red cars, and chocolate ice cream." If the patient can recall these after 5 minutes, it means that the poor score on Test One was probably due to anxiety, inability to attend (secondary to delirium), poor concentration, or lack of effort.

Test Two: Visual and Tactile Recall

1. Place three objects, such as a pen, a quarter, and a set of keys, in front of the patient. Ask the patient to look at the objects and name each one. Hide the objects and ask the patient to recall them after 5 minutes.

(continued)

2. If the objects are not recalled, the patient can be instructed to examine and touch the objects while repeating their names out loud. Hide the objects and ask the patient to recall them after 5 minutes. The addition of auditory and tactile sensory input should make it easier to remember the three objects. If the memory deficit persists, it is probably due to a severe neurophysiological disorder.

MEMORY: INTERMEDIATE-TERM

1. Ask the patient to recall events that have happened over the last day or week.
2. Ask the patient what was for dinner the day before (if what the patient had can be confirmed).
3. Alternatively, ask the patient about current events or recent changes in the news or weather.

MEMORY: LONG-TERM

1. Ask the patient to recall events that happened years ago.
2. Ask, "Where and when were you born?" or "Where did you live prior to your current residence?" if the answers to these questions can be confirmed.
3. Alternatively, ask the patient to name past presidents of the United States (after confirming that the patient has had enough education to know about the presidents or has had easy access to information about the presidents in daily life).

COGNITIVE ABILITY

1. Cognitive ability is tested by asking the patient to do a complex operation (e.g., solve a mathematical problem) that can be performed accurately only if the sensorium is clear and the patient is fully conscious and oriented, has an intact memory, and is able to concentrate. Simple mathematical problems (e.g., adding numbers) or word problems (e.g., spelling the word "world" backward) are examples of cognitive tests.
2. Before testing begins, find out how much education the patient has had in order to choose the appropriate level of difficulty of the first cognitive test.
3. A good starting test is serial 7 subtractions. Instruct the patient, "Beginning with 100, keep subtracting 7 until I tell you to stop." If the patient completes this task without difficulty, steadily increase the complexity of the mathematical problems.
4. If the patient performs poorly on the first test, switch immediately to a drastically simpler test at which the patient is likely to succeed with no difficulty. It is important to make it easy for the patient to answer the next few questions correctly to minimize anxiety, increase confidence, and improve performance on subsequent tests. If the patient makes many mistakes in serial 7 subtractions, ask, "Can you count backward from 21 to 10?" If the patient still has difficulty, switch to an easy calculation with money, such as "If you have a nickel and a penny, how much money do you have?" Money problems are easier for most patients.
5. Gradually increase the degree of difficulty, until the cognitive deficits appear again. A more complex money question might be, "If an orange costs 50 cents, and you give the grocer $5.00 to buy four oranges, how much change would you receive?"

BOX 5.17
ADJUNCTIVE MENTAL STATUS TESTING

CLOCK TEST

The clock test (Tuokko et al. 1992) can be administered with a pencil and paper. There are three parts to this test: clock drawing, clock setting, and clock reading. Clock drawing is primarily a visual-spatial skill located in the nondominant (usually right) cerebral hemisphere. Clock setting and clock reading require comprehension of the concept of time. They are primarily a function of the dominant (usually left) cerebral hemisphere. In other words, the clock test is a simple way of evaluating the gross cognitive function of both cerebral hemispheres.

1. Clock drawing: Ask the patient to draw a circle with a clock face, placing all the numbers in the proper location within the circle.
2. Clock setting: Have the patient add hands to the clock to indicate a specific time. Try several different times.
3. Clock reading: Show the patient several drawings of clocks. The clocks should have hands, but no numbers, indicating several different times. Ask the patient to read the times.
4. Normal elderly persons may have some difficulties with clock drawing but can easily do clock setting and clock reading. About 80% of patients with major neurocognitive disorder due to Alzheimer's disease have difficulty in performing all three tasks.

SET TEST WITH WORD INTRUSION

The set test with word intrusion (Fuld 1983) is easily administered.

1. Ask the patient to name 10 objects in each of three general categories, or sets (e.g., "Name 10 cities, 10 foods, and 10 animals.")
2. The maximum score is 30 out of 30 (30/30). A score of 25–30/30 is considered normal. A score of 15–25/30 indicates that either a primary psychiatric disorder or a neurocognitive disorder is present. A score of less than 15/30 strongly suggests that the cause is a neurocognitive disorder rather than a primary psychiatric condition.
3. A word intrusion occurs when the patient adds an object from one category to a different category (e.g., when the patient is asked to name 10 animals, the patient includes the name of a city or a food). The more word intrusions, the greater is the likelihood of a neurocognitive disorder due to Alzheimer's disease, as compared with other causes of neurocognitive disorder.
4. This test does not have much validity if it is used alone, but it is helpful as an adjunctive test when other mental status deficits have already been detected. A score of less than 15/30 with word intrusions increases the probability of major neurocognitive disorder due to Alzheimer's disease by 10–20%. Patients who score less than 15/30 without word intrusions are likely to have another cause of major neurocognitive disorder.

(continued)

FRONTAL ASSESSMENT BATTERY

The frontal assessment battery (Dubois et al. 2000) was developed to detect specific deficits related to the frontal lobes, which can be helpful when evaluating for a frontal-temporal disease. The test has six subtests that evaluate both cognitive and behavioral function of the frontal lobe, including abstract reasoning, verbal fluency, temporal organization, execution of specific actions, sensitivity to interference, inhibition of response, impulsivity, and overriding environmental cues.

STANDARDIZED OUTCOME MEASURES

There are many research scales that are becoming more useful in clinical practice given their increasing availability. Some of the more commonly used cognitive assessments are the Brief Cognitive Rating Scale (BCRS), Delirium Rating Scale (DRS), Alzheimer's Disease Assessment Scale (ADAS), and Wechsler Adult Intelligence Scale (WAIS). Functioning can also be assessed formally with the Functional Assessment Staging Tests (FAST) and the Bristol Activities of Daily Living Scale. A neuropsychologist will often include these tests as part of a detailed cognitive assessment (Bucks et al. 1996; Doraiswamy et al. 1997; Reisberg 1988; Sclan and Reisberg 1992; Trezepacz 1999; Wechsler 1939).

One commonly used test is the **Mini Mental Status Exam** (MMSE). It consists of a series of questions testing the areas of orientation, attention, immediate recall, short-term recall, and language skills (Folstein et al. 1975). Box 5.18 includes sample test items. A perfect score is 30/30 and a score of 25/30 or above is usually within the normal range, although there are specific norms for each age. A score of 20–25/30 is probably indicative of cognitive impairment, and a score below 15/30 is clearly abnormal. The test takes only 10 minutes to administer and can be done at the patient's bedside with paper and a writing utensil. The MMSE score can be followed over time to assess a person's improvement or decline.

Use of the Montreal Cognitive Assessment (MoCa) and the Frontal Assessment Battery (FAB) are other tests commonly used for a more detailed assessment for neurocognitive deficits.

ETIOLOGY

Neurocognitive disorders and mental disorders due to another medical condition may have one cause or multiple causes.

Neurocognitive Disorders

Delirium

Most forms of delirium are clinically indistinguishable from each other, and they are all thought to be due to dysfunction of the reticular activating system (RAS) at the level of the brainstem. A person with a normally functioning RAS is awake,

---

MMSE SAMPLE ITEMS

ORIENTATION TO TIME

"What is the date?"

REGISTRATION

"Listen carefully. I am going to say three words. You say them back after I stop.

Ready? Here they are...APPLE (pause), PENNY (pause), TABLE (pause). Now repeat those words back to me."

[Repeat up to five times, but score only the first trial.]

NAMING

"What is this?" [Point to a pencil or pen.]

READING

"Please read this and do what it says." [Show examinee the words on the stimulus form.]

CLOSE YOUR EYES

---

alert, and capable of learning, with a good memory, attention span, and concentration. When the nervous system becomes impaired, for example by severe dehydration, the RAS can malfunction and the person becomes confused. Diverse medical conditions with different etiologies can impact the RAS, causing the syndrome of delirium.

Delirium may be caused by a wide array of pathological processes (Engel and Romano 1959). **Medication-induced** delirium is by far the most common delirium. Some additional common causes include structural damage of the central nervous system (e.g., seizure or head trauma); metabolic or endocrine disorders (e.g., thyroid disease, hepatic or renal failure); infectious diseases (e.g., HIV infection, Lyme, herpes simplex encephalitis, or pneumococcal or meningococcal meningitis); primary brain tumors or metastatic neoplastic disease (e.g., breast cancer); and autoimmune disorders (e.g., systemic lupus erythematosus or polyarteritis nodosa). In addition, it is a helpful to classify the etiology of delirium as either (1) life-threatening within minutes and requiring emergency intervention or (2) must be recognized immediately but can be treated over a period of hours to days (see Table 5.2).

Major and Mild Neurocognitive Disorders

Major and mild NCD can be caused by primary diseases of the central nervous system or by secondary involvement of the central nervous system by systemic diseases. Neurocognitive disorder can be classified by six different etiologic subtypes: (1) structural damage to the central nervous system (e.g., Alzheimer's disease, vascular disease, frontotemporal lobar degeneration, or Lewy body disease); (2) infectious diseases (e.g., HIV infection, tuberculosis meningitis, or chronic cryptococcus meningitis); (3) metabolic or nutritional disorders (e.g., hypothyroidism, hyperthyroidism, Wilson's disease, thiamine or niacin deficiency); (4) neoplastic diseases (e.g., glioma, astrocytoma, or breast or lung cancer that has metastasized to the brain); (5) autoimmune disorders (e.g., systemic lupus erythematosus); and (6) drug or poisonous reactions (e.g., alcohol intoxication, gasoline inhalation, or glue sniffing).

Alzheimer's Disease

Patients with Alzheimer's disease have the typical histopathological landmarks on postmortem examination of **neuritic plaques and neurofibrillary tangles**. Genetic research has linked the main component of these structures, the proteins beta-amyloid and tau, with several chromosomal mutations present in families with strong presence of Alzheimer's dementia. Genetic tests are now available for three of these variants: amyloid precursor protein, and presenillin 1 and 2. Other genetic research in Alzheimer's has focused on apoprotein E, typically known for its relevance to lipid transport. Although the mechanism is unclear, the E4 allele increases the risk of disease, and the E2 allele decreases it. Abnormalities of neurotransmitters have also been recognized in Alzheimer's disease. Decreased serotonin, imbalance in the noradrenergic system, and presynaptic cholinergic brain deficit have all been found in dementia and are the basis of many current treatments.

Vascular Disease

Neurocognitive disorder due to vascular disease is produced by the **occlusion of small vessels** secondary to damage from hypertension or arteriosclerosis, which leads to **focal or lacuna brain infarctions**. Vascular damage in the basal ganglia, thalamus, and subcortex have been linked with this major neurocognitive disorder. These lesions are sometimes missed on neurological examination because they are too small to produce focal neurological findings. CT or MRI scans will reveal the infarcts.

Parkinson's Disease and Lewy Body Disease

Major NCD due to Parkinson's disease and that due to Lewy body disease **are** associated with abnormal protein deposits in the brain referred to as **Lewy body formation**. In Parkinson's disease, Lewy bodies are found in the **substantia nigra**, whereas in Lewy body disease there are Lewy bodies in the **limbic and neocortical** areas (McKeith et al. 2004). Both of these illnesses may be caused by the same imbalance between dopaminergic inhibition and cholinergic stimulation but starting in different areas of the brain. In Parkinson's disease, the process starts in the basal ganglion, and in Lewy body disease it starts in the cortex. In both illnesses, patients lose nerve cells and pigmentation, and cellular Lewy bodies form.

Frontotemporal Lobar Degeneration
The brains of patients with frontotemporal lobar degeneration, including Pick's disease, have large numbers of neurofibrillary tangles in the absence of amyloid plaques. These tangles are concentrated in the frontal and temporal lobes and are associated with abnormal tau proteins.

Human Immunodeficiency Virus (HIV) Infection
Major NCD in patients with HIV infection has a number of etiologies, including direct pathophysiological effects of the HIV infection, as well as secondary causes. The HIV virus directly infects the brain shortly after seroconversion (positive testing for the infection). The virus is probably carried by macrophages that cross the blood–brain barrier and often produces mild or subclinical **meningoencephalitis** and delirium, which may be the earliest signs of HIV infection. The CNS infection may later produce **subcortical** disease through an autoimmune reaction. These deficits usually present years after seroconversion and probably coincide with the gradual deterioration of the immune system. The earliest symptoms of major NCD due to HIV disease include memory loss, depressive symptoms, decreased flexibility in thinking, personality changes, and difficulty in performing complex actions.

The secondary causes of HIV-related NCD include illnesses that develop as a consequence of **immunosupression**, such as tumors and opportunistic infections, or the **effects of the drugs** used to treat the illness. The opportunistic illnesses caused by HIV immunosuppression may include brain lymphomas, Kaposi's sarcoma, toxoplasmosis, cryptococcus, cytomegalovirus infection, herpes virus infection, or chronic hypoxia due to opportunistic lung infections. Reverse transcriptase inhibitors used in treating HIV infection may produce adverse mental effects, including depression, hallucinations, and drowsiness.

Huntington's Disease
Huntington's disease results from a mutation in the autosomally dominant inherited huntington gene, with insertion of multiple repeats of a specific genetic sequence (CAG). This mutation is responsible for symptoms of psychosis, depression, and neurocognitive disorder, as well as personality changes.

Prion Disease
Sporadic Creutzfeldt-Jakob disease is the most common neurocognitive disorder due to prion disease. A **prion** is an abnormal transmissible protein. Most cases of prion disease occur sporadically, but some are hereditary. The illness can be acquired through contact with the brain tissue of affected individuals. Cross-species acquisition through a prion known to affect cattle seems to cause a variant of Creutzfeldt-Jakob disease known as mad cow disease.

Traumatic Brain Injury
Neurocognitive disorders may be caused by any illness that damages the deep brain structures associated with memory, especifically the **mammillary bodies, hippocampus**, and **fornix**. Head trauma victims are at particular risk. Traumatic brain injuries due to motorcycle or motor vehicle accidents, falls, or violent assault are usually

coup-contra-coup lesions (e.g., a blow to the back of the head that injures the frontal or temporal cerebral lobes).

Major or Mild NCD Due to Another Medical Condition
Normal-pressure hydrocephalus is caused by excessive cerebral spinal fluid displacing cerebral tissue without an increase in intracranial pressure. Possible etiologies include a previous subarachnoid hemorrhage or subclinical encephalitis or meningitis. Classically, it presents with the **triad of** neurocognitive disorder, **gait disturbance,** and **urinary incontinence**. It can be reversed with periodic removal of cerebrospinal fluid or an indwelling cerebral shunt.

Thiamine deficiency results from poor nutrition and is often seen in alcoholics. Neurocognitive disorder due to **thiamine deficiency**, also referred to as **Korsakoff's disease**, is associated with severe short-term memory deficits.

Other causes of neurocognitive disorder include structural lesions, such as tumors; partial complex seizures; infections, such as neurosyphilis; hypoxia (e.g., from drowning or surgical intervention); drugs (e.g., phencyclidine); and autoimmune disease, such as multiple sclerosis or vasculitis affecting the posterior cerebral artery.

Mental Disorders due to Another Medical Condition

Figure 5.1 outlines the common etiologies of mental disorders due to another medical condition.

Psychotic Disorders Due to Another Medical Condition
The most common medical causes of hallucination and delusions are **substance-induced** psychotic disorders. Cocaine, methamphetamines, and stimulants commonly produce an acute psychosis that may be clinically indistinguishable from acute paranoid schizophrenia. Chronic abuse of large amounts of crack cocaine or methamphetamine may also produce a persistent psychosis that is probably a result of brain kindling caused by intermittent low-level irritation of the cerebral cortex. Hallucinations may also be caused by acute withdrawal from alcohol, barbiturates, benzodiazepines, ecstasy, or LSD.

Other etiologies include seizures, Huntington's disease, neoplasms, hypoxia, hypoglycemia, and hepatic disease. Involvement of the posterior nondominant cerebral hemisphere often produces visual hallucinations, whereas lesions of the subcortex and temporal lobe are associated with delusions.

Sensory-deprivation hallucinations may develop when a person is in an environment with inadequate sensory stimulation, such as an intensive care unit or solitary confinement. These hallucinations may also occur in elderly patients with cataracts or otosclerosis, who have radically reduced visual and auditory sensory input. In medically ill patients, sensory deprivation should be an etiology of exclusion to avoid missing other reversible causes, such as medication reactions.

Mood Disorders Due to Another Medical Condition
The leading medical causes of depression are medications and endocrinopathies. Other causes are often neurological, including **Parkinson's disease, Huntington's disease**, and **stroke**. Manic symptoms, such as euphoria, talkativeness, irritability, increased energy, and grandiose plans, are commonly observed and can be caused by hyperthyroidism,

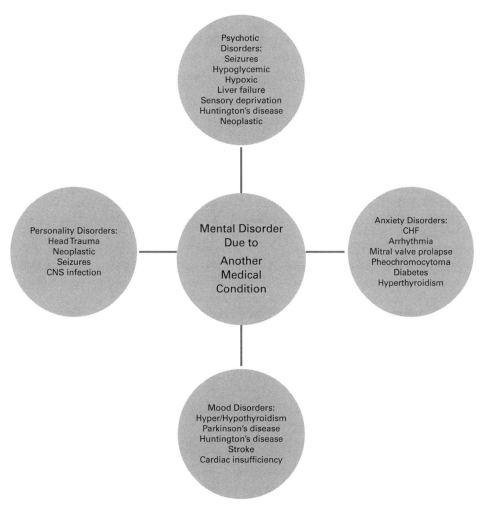

FIGURE 5.1 Common etiologies of mental disorders due to another medical condition. CHF, congestive heart failure; CNS, central nervous system.

seizures, steroid use, stimulant abuse, brain injury, liver disease, and nondominant hemispheric strokes.

Patients with **hyperthyroidism** often present with fatigue, weight loss, sweating, heat intolerance, scant menstruation, tachycardia, tremor, and bulging eyes (proptosis). Frequent neuropsychiatric manifestations are insomnia and crying episodes that are easily confused with depression and anxiety. The most common causes of hyperthyroidism are Graves' disease, inflammatory thyroiditis, excessive thyroid hormone replacement therapy, and, rarely, thyroid or ovarian cancers. The diagnosis is confirmed by high thyroid hormone levels and low thyroid-stimulating hormone (TSH).

Patients with **hypothyroidism** often present with fatigue, weight gain, constipation, cold intolerance, menorrhagia, goiter, reflex delay, and myxedema (i.e., dryness, hair loss, edema, hoarseness, and muscle weakness). When hypothyroidism is mild, it may present with depression, suicidality, or psychosis. When it is severe and long-standing, it commonly presents as neurocognitive disorder. The most common causes of hypothyroidism are iatrogenic, due to lithium use or treatment of hyperthyroidism by surgery or irradiation, as well as autoimmune thyroid disease. Rarely, it may be caused by pituitary or hypothalamic disease. The diagnosis is confirmed by low thyroid hormone levels and high TSH levels.

Cardiovascular diseases have emerging associations with depression. Multiple small infarcts in the areas of the brain that control mood may result in a depressive syndrome referred to as vascular depression. Vascular lesions in the medial frontal cortex are most highly associated with depression (Alexopoulos et al. 1997).

The list of **prescription drugs** that may cause depression as a side effect is long. Among the common offenders are disulfiram, benzodiazepines, opiates, antihypertensive drugs (beta blockers, calcium channel blockers), statins, and hormonal agents such as estrogen replacement and oral contraceptives. Withdrawal from medications such as steroids may also cause depressive symptoms. Prescription drugs that may produce mania as a side effect are the corticosteroids, antidepressants, stimulants, and thyroid hormone. St John's Wort, an herbal medication with antidepressant effects, has been known to induce mania as well. Individuals who have a predisposition toward affective illness are more likely to be affected by these drugs.

Illicit substances are also common offenders in producing mood disorders in either the intoxication or withdrawal phases. Depressive symptoms are common in persons who abuse alcohol, opiates, phencyclidine, sedatives, or hypnotics and also in those who are in withdrawal from stimulants or alcohol. Manic symptoms are common in patients who are acutely intoxicated with cocaine or other stimulants, phencyclidine, marijuana, hallucinogens, caffeine, inhalants, alcohol, or anabolic steroids.

Anxiety- and Obsessive-Compulsive-Related Disorders Due to Another Medical Condition

Many medical conditions may produce anxiety symptoms. Endocrine disorders such as diabetes or hyperthyroidism can result in generalized anxiety symptoms such as tremulousness, "butterflies" in the stomach, and uneasiness. Some hormonally secreting tumors or cancers can cause symptoms of panic or agoraphobia, including palpitations, shortness of breath, or feelings of doom. Panic symptoms may occur after a patient develops a cardiac arrhythmia or a respiratory illness. Infectious agents such as streptococcus can cause pediatric acute-onset neuropsychiatric syndrome (PANS), which presents with obsessive-compulsive symptoms in children that may include repetitive worrying, fears, or compulsive behaviors such as excessive hand-washing. Disorders of adrenal function may produce symptoms of social phobia or agoraphobia. Anxiety symptoms may also be caused caffeinism, nicotine withdrawal, and intoxication or withdrawal from a wide range of substances (see Differential Diagnosis, and Chapter 7, Substance-Related and Addictive Disorders). A **pheochromocytoma** is a catecholamine-secreting tumor of the adrenal medulla or other abdominal paraganglionic sites. It may produce symptoms of panic attacks and, rarely, agoraphobia. Additional physical symptoms include malignant hypertensive episodes, headaches, and severe abdominal, back, or pelvic pain. The tumor may be definitively diagnosed by a 24-hour urine sample that shows high levels of catecholamines or derivatives.

Prescription drugs that may produce anxiety symptoms include bronchodilators, thyroid replacement hormone, antihistamines, and antidepressants. Excessive caffeine intake and nicotine withdrawal can produce symptoms of generalized anxiety and panic disorder. Cocaine intoxication or withdrawal, marijuana abuse, and alcohol and opiate withdrawal can also cause anxiety symptoms.

Personality Changes Due to Another Medical Condition

The specific personality changes are generally related to the location of the brain lesions. Many personality changes are associated with pathological changes in the frontal lobes, especially in the right hemisphere. It has been estimated that 90% of patients with frontal lobe lesions have personality changes. By far the most common cause of personality change is traumatic brain injury. Other etiologies include CNS neoplasms, epilepsy, and CNS infections.

Patients with disinhibition frequently have pathological damage to the orbital-frontal part of the brain from trauma or a brain tumor. Apathy tends to be caused by tumors or trauma to the frontal cortex convexities or dorsal lateral frontal cortex. Lability is usually associated with lesions of the nondominant cerebral hemisphere, usually the right hemisphere. Aggression is frequently caused by head trauma or other damage to the frontal, prefrontal, or temporal cortex, or to the hypothalamus, amygdala, or limbic region. Diffuse brain lesions due to structural diseases and hyperthyroidism can also produce lability and personality changes.

TREATMENT

The treatment of neurocognitive disorders and mental disorders due to another medical condition often begins with treatment of a medical condition. Psychiatric treatment using a biopsychosocial-cultural approach can often help restore an optimal level of brain function and improve quality of life.

Psychotherapy

Psychoeducation and supportive psychotherapy can help patients and their families to understand their deficits and adapt to their illness. The physician can offer a caring, emotionally supportive, and safe environment in which patients and their families can talk about their deficits, feelings, stresses, and attempts at adaptation. Psychosocial support from the family or other social groups may be mobilized. In general, the physician will make suggestions, give guidance, provide reassurance, and encourage reality testing. A combination of these efforts will usually improve patients' ability to function and decrease their vulnerability to everyday stresses.

Some brain deficits require specific adaptations in psychiatric techniques. For example, a patient with attention deficits will need the physician to use simple sentences with clear evocative language. Physicians may teach patients to accommodate for their deficits through demonstration, for example, by emoting strongly and accentuating feelings with hand gestures when working with a patient who has a blunted affect.

Behavior Therapy

Three behavioral approaches can be used to promote recovery from specific brain deficits: operant-behavioral treatment, social learning treatment, and cognitive-behavioral treatment (see also Chapter 17, Psychotherapy).

Operant-Behavioral Treatment

Operant-behavioral treatment is a traditional behavioral approach that evaluates the sequence of events that lead up to a specific maladaptive behavior and the consequences that result from the behavior, often characterized as the *ABCs*. The **a**ntecedent refers to the stressor that precipitates a maladaptive behavior, the **b**ehavior is the event or action desiring modification, and the **c**onsequences are the resulting effects of that behavior. The physician can modify the triggers, the behavior itself, and can determine whether the consequences of a behavior are reinforcing (encouraging a repetition of the behavior) or extinguishing (causing a decrease in the maladaptive behavior) in order to develop effective interventions (see case example in Box 5.19).

A token economy system (often used in inpatient settings) of rewards encourages preferred behaviors with the positive reinforcement of receiving tokens that can be accumulated for privileges. For some patients more immediate reinforcements, such as praise, are more effective. Identifying and eliminating any triggers in the environment that may precipitate maladaptive behavior is also important. For example, if crowds trigger agitation in a brain-injured patient, crowds should be avoided. The focus of behavioral treatment is to reduce the frequency and intensity of maladaptive behaviors, as complete elimination is often not possible.

Social Learning

Social learning is often used in combination with other treatments and is typically offered in a group setting. This approach helps neurologically impaired patients who have maladaptive behaviors to model themselves after others who have more socially appropriate behaviors. For example, a social skills group can help patients relearn how to

---

BOX 5.19

CASE EXAMPLE OF OPERANT-BEHAVIORAL TREATMENT

A patient with major NCD due to Alzheimer's disease developed violent outbursts. The outbursts occurred after his wife attempted to groom him. The consequence of his outbursts was that his wife would leave in disgust and his favorite nurse would come to console him. His behavior was modified by having the nurse do the regularly scheduled grooming (positively reinforcing the nonviolent behavior) instead of the spouse (removing the negative reinforcement of the violent behavior) and having the spouse bring the patient a favorite food during her visit (positively reinforcing the nonviolent behavior). These changes were successful in reducing the frequency and intensity of his violent episodes. In this case, the antecedent to violence was being groomed by his wife, the behavior was physical outbursts, and the consequences were disgust for the wife and a visit from the patient's favorite nurse. In this situation, the maladaptive behavior was reinforced by the wife's departure and the arrival of the nurse. The behavioral therapy involved developing a set of different **a**ntecedents and **c**onsequences, resulting in less aggressive **b**ehavior (A-B-C).

groom themselves and reestablish their manners. These groups rely heavily on modeling, role-playing, and positive reinforcements.

Cognitive-Behaviorial Therapy (CBT)

Cognitive-behaviorial therapy focuses on changing distorted or irrational thought processes that cause pathological emotions and drive problematic behaviors (see case example in Box 5.20).

There is a wide array of specific **cognitive techniques** that are aimed at specific deficits. Memory can be enhanced by teaching patients to use reminders, cues, or mnemonics. Making lists on paper or with a handheld digital device may also be helpful. Problems of orientation may be ameliorated by having caregivers repeat the day, date, time, and place. Patients can also be taught to orient themselves through frequent use of a calendar or daily newspaper or by using a watch or computer. Specific language deficits can be improved through speech therapy, cognitive retraining, and comprehension exercises. Some intellectual deficits can be compensated for through a reeducation process that breaks down an intellectual task into small, manageable steps that can be learned anew by using alternative brain capacities. These techniques may be used to teach patients how to drive, do mathematical problems, or read.

Family Therapy

Psychoeducation

Many families with a patient suffering from a cognitive disorder or a medically caused psychiatric disorder need to learn about their family member's illness and discuss the impact of the illness on the family. Families need help in understanding the signs and symptoms of the disease, and the probable course toward remission or progression. Families should be advised about available treatments, how they can be involved in the treatment, and how they can get help with the daily routine care of the patient. When necessary, a family may need help in preparing for a patient's death.

BOX 5.20

CASE EXAMPLE OF COGNITIVE-BEHAVIORAL THERAPY (CBT)

A young man with a neurocognitive disorder due to traumatic brain injury thought that everyone could tell that he was gravely ill just by looking at him. When he met people at a party, he thought they knew about his illness and did not want to be his friend. As a result of this cognitive distortion, he got more depressed, stopped bathing, and remained in pajamas all day. This behavior reinforced the possibility that others would see him as ill, thus diminishing his opportunity to make friends. CBT challenged and corrected his irrational beliefs, leading him to change his behaviors, including bathing and getting dressed, which will hopefully result in his making friends.

In the opening family sessions, it is especially helpful to teach families about patients' specific deficits and behaviors and help them to differentiate the true neuropsychiatric deficits from the psychological conflicts or reactions to the illness. This information frequently ameliorates anger toward the patient and fosters a more supportive family attitude (see case example in Box 5.21). In addition, it is important to focus on making realistic changes that will increase hope and promote new family coping strategies. There is often an element of grief counseling, as everyone in the family is likely experiencing some loss due to the patient's deficits. The stages of grief usually include denial, anger, bargaining, and, eventually, mourning and resolution.

Structural Family Therapy

Family therapy can be a particularly effective form of treatment for patients with cognitive deficits. A neurocognitive disorder may precipitate changes in the entire family structure. Most patients with a neurocognitive disorder lose some prestige and power and function differently within the family. As a consequence, some family members may assume new leadership positions and others may define or assume new roles. Assistance with this process can decrease family stress and improve a family's cohesiveness and capacity for problem solving.

BOX 5.21

CASE EXAMPLE OF PSYCHOEDUCATIONAL FAMILY THERAPY

A 45-year-old man suffered right cerebral hemispheric damage from a severe automobile accident, which resulted in paralysis of his left arm and inattention to the left side of his body. His wife was becoming increasingly angry with him as he insisted that he could dress himself but would only partially complete the task. His wife would try to finish dressing him, but he would insist that he was finished, become furious, and shout until she left the room. He would remain only partially dressed, and his wife would be ashamed to take him out of the house. Supportive psychotherapy was begun 3 months after the accident. The physician explained to both of them that the patient's inability to finish dressing himself was based on a persistent neurological syndrome called hemi-neglect, such that the patient did not realize that he was partially undressed and argued with his wife because he thought that she was unnecessarily babying him. His wife had thought his refusal to dress himself was a stubborn denial of his illness rather than a cortical deficit. The patient cried as he began to accept and grieve his neurological losses. Once the couple understood the situation, they were less angry and could work together toward dressing the patient. Thus, supportive psychotherapy helped the patient and his wife to understand better his neurological deficits and loss of capacity, to formulate realistic expectations, and to develop ways to adapt. As a result, this patient had improved functioning and a better relationship with his wife.

The structure that existed prior to illness should be compared with the one that has developed since the patient became impaired. Box 5.22 contains a set of questions that can be used in ascertaining the family structure. As a picture of the family structure emerges, specific interventions can be designed to help family members reorganize and adapt to new roles and positions of power. After several sessions, the entire family may be mobilized to be the major caregiver for a patient (see case example in Box 5.3).

Strategic Family Therapy

Strategic family therapy focuses on problem identification and a familial approach to problem solving. The first step is to establish open, honest, direct lines of communication within the family. Interventions and homework assignments improve communication skills and break vicious circles of poor communication. Once good communication is established, families can identify specific conflicts or problems and then develop unique solutions that involve the impaired family member. Individual strategies and solutions to particular problems of everyday life are emphasized.

Pharmacotherapy

Psychoactive drugs may be used to target specific psychiatric symptoms or a constellation of symptoms associated with neurocognitive disorders, although psychotherapeutic techniques and other solutions can be offered first. For example, a person with major NCD who seems agitated may be in pain, frustrated by an inability to communicate due to a cerebrovascular incident, or afraid because the person doesn't know where he or she is. None of these situations would be improved with psychiatric medications.

Sometimes psychiatric medications are appropriate, but they may need to be used differently in older or neurologically impaired individuals. Doses are likely to be different, and mode of delivery may need to be altered. For example, a patient may be unable

---

BOX 5.22

SUGGESTED QUESTIONS TO EVALUATE FAMILY STRUCTURE

The physician should ask the following questions in order to assess the family's structure before and after the illness: Who was the head of the household before? Who is the head of the household now? Who made and enforced the family rules? How have these rules changed since the illness? How did and does the family negotiate with the outside world? How were family disputes settled, and how are they negotiated now? What were and are the roles of the parents and children? Do the children now need to take on more of a parental role as their parents became ill? How did the parents get along as a couple before, and how are they getting along now? What were and are the different roles of each parent? How do the children interact as siblings? What were and are the different roles of each child?

to swallow pills and may need to use dissolvable or liquid medications, patches, or, as a last resort, injections. When prescribing drugs for elderly or debilitated patients, the following principles should be kept in mind: (1) lower dosages of all medications should be used, as patients may have slower hepatic or renal clearance or increased sensitivity to medications; (2) interactions with other medications should be carefully considered; and (3) prescription of multiple drugs should be avoided, or at least kept to a minimum, whenever possible.

Cognitive Enhancers

Several medications directed at the cognitive effects of dementia have become available in the past few years. The first on the market were **anticholinesterase inhibitors**. These medications counteract the loss of cholinergic neurons associated with Alzheimer's disease and Lewy body disease. Currently, there are several available anticholinesterase agents: donepezil, galantamine, and rivastigmine. Unfortunately, studies indicate that these medications do not reverse the disease process, but they can slow the rate of decline (Trinh et al. 2003, Qaseem et al. 2008). At this point, there are no medications that reverse Alzheimer's disease or help patients regain lost functioning. Anticholinesterase inhibitors are commonly associated with nausea, vomiting, and resulting weight loss, but are otherwise usually well tolerated.

Memantine is an **N-methyl-D-aspartate (NMDA) antagonist** with similar effectiveness. It was developed on the principal that glutamate, which acts on NMDA receptors, is an excitatory neurotransmitter that in excess can cause cell death. A combination of memantine and an anticholinesterase inhibitor is frequently prescribed in Alzheimer's disease; the combination has been shown to be safe and possibly more effective than either medication alone (Qaseem et al. 2008).

Some studies indicate that treatment as well as prevention of Alzheimer's disease may be facilitated by high-dose vitamins, especially vitamin E and the B-complexes or omega fatty acids. Individuals who regularly take nonsteroidal anti-inflammatory drugs (NSAIDs) may have a lower risk of Alzheimer's disease (Etminan et al. 2003). Estrogen is known to be neuroprotective, and the possibility of estrogen replacement therapy as a treatment for Alzheimer's is underway. Gene therapy is also under early investigation, with possible alterations of the genes for amyloid and nerve growth factor.

Antidepressants

Antidepressants can be used to treat depressive and anxiety symptoms seen in patients with neurocognitive disorder as well as psychiatric syndromes due to other medical illnesses. Caution must be used in that patients with neurocognitive disorders may respond differently to antidepressant treatment than patients suffering with primary psychiatric disorders. There is good evidence to support the use of antidepressants in depression associated with Alzheimer's disease, and emerging evidence that they may be useful for the behavioral symptoms as well. Depression associated with neurocognitive disorder due to vascular disease is known to respond poorly to antidepressant medications.

The antidepressants most commonly used are the **selective serotonin reuptake inhibitors** (SSRIs). Side effects are often limiting factors in older patients or those with complex medical conditions (see Chapter 16, Pharmacotherapy, ECT, and TMS). Caution should be exercised in the use of serotonin norepinephrine reuptake inhibitors

(SNRIs) in patients with cardiovascular disease (because of their tendency to elevate blood pressure) and the use of bupropion in patients with neurological illnesses (because of its tendency to lower the seizure threshold). Mirtazapine's side effects of sedation and weight gain can be desirable for some medically ill individuals. The older tricyclics and monoamine oxidase inhibitors may be used, but they tend to be less well tolerated and can induce delirium in the elderly.

Antipsychotics

Recent evidence suggests that all antipsychotics are associated with an **increased risk of sudden cardiac death in the elderly,** and they all have FDA-mandated black-box warnings for use in psychosis associated with dementia (major NCD) (Ray et al. 2009). The potential benefit should be carefully weighed against the possible risk before prescribing antipsychotics in this population (Schneeweiss and Avorn, 2009). Although antipsychotic medication is sometimes required to control agitation associated with delirium, appropriate medical treatment directed at the cause of the delirium should be the first priority (Carson et al. 2006.)

Patients with psychotic symptoms and movement disorders such as Parkinson's disease are most vulnerable to extrapyramidal side effects, thus antipsychotics should be avoided, if possible. Interestingly, antipsychotics worsen psychosis in patients with neurocognitive disorder due to Lewy body disease.

Anxiolytics

Benzodiazepines can provide immediate relief for patients with anxiety symptoms due to another medical condition. Their long-term use should generally be discouraged because of the risk of physiological dependence. In addition, benzodiazepines can cause impaired cognition in the elderly, and their use increases the risk of accidents and falls. **Buspirone** can be useful for long-term anxiolytic treatment.

Lithium

Acute manic symptoms in patients with a mood disorder due to another medical condition can be treated with lithium. Medications that may be producing manic symptoms (e.g., steroids, antidepressants, and thyroid hormone) should be discontinued, if possible. If the mania-inducing medication is medically necessary, the mood disorder can be treated with lithium. Lithium is also useful as an adjunct to boost the antidepressant effects in patients with depression secondary to another medical condition. Many medically ill patients cannot take lithium because of impaired renal function, thyroid abnormalities, or medication interactions. Geriatric patients are more sensitive to the effects of lithium and can become toxic at much lower levels, making close blood level monitoring essential.

Anticonvulsants

Anticonvulsants, including valproate, carbamazepine, and lamotrigine, have a wide range of uses in patients with mood disorders due to another medical condition, as well as in those with violent behavior resulting from severe neurological deficits and agitation associated with neurocognitive disorder. This class of medications is being prescribed more frequently given the increasing concern about the use of antipsychotics in geriatric individuals. Patients with brain disease frequently have epileptic disorders as well, allowing the convenient use of the anticonvulsant for two indications.

Potential adverse reactions include hepatotoxicity and blood dyscrasias with valproate, drug interactions and blood dyscrasias with carbamazepine, and somnolence and rash with lamotrigine.

Preventative Measures

As current treatments for cognitive disorders have limited efficacy, the research focus has shifted to include prevention. Physical and mental exercise may help prevent age-related dementias. Several studies indicate that physical exercise and intellectually stimulating activities, such as crossword puzzles, social involvement, and formal education, are associated with a lower incidence of Alzheimer's disease. Controlling known medical risk factors is also helpful, such as maintaining a healthy weight and blood pressure.

REFERENCES CITED

Adamis, D., A. Treloar, F. C. Martin, and A. J. Macdonald. Recovery and outcome of delirium in elderly medical inpatients. *Archives of Gerontology and Geriatrics* 43:289–298, 2006.

Alexopoulos, G. S., B. S. Meyers, R. C. Young, T. Kakuma, D. Silbersweig, and M. Charlson. Clinically defined vascular depression. *American Journal of Psychiatry* 154:562–565, 1997.

Bucks, R., D. L. Ashworth, G. K. Wilcock, and K. Siegfried K. Assessment of activities of daily living in dementia: development of the Bristol Activities of Daily Living Scale. *Age and Aging* 25(2):113–120, 1996.

Carson, S., M. McDonagh, and K. A. Peterson. systematic review of the efficacy and safety of atypical antipsychotics in patients with psychological and behavioral symptoms of dementia. *Journal of the American Geriatrics Society* 54:354–361, 2006.

Doraiswamy, P., F. Bieber, L. Kaiser, K. R. Krishnan, J. Reuning-Scherer, and B. Gulanski. The Alzheimer's Disease Assessment Scale: patterns and predictors of baseline cognitive performance in multicenter Alzheimer's disease trials. *Neurology* 48(6): 1511–1517, 1997.

Dubois, B., A. Slachevsky, I. Litvan, and B. Pillon. The FAB: a Frontal Assessment Battery at bedside. *Neurology* 55:1621–1626, 2000.

Engel, G. L., and J. Romano. Delirium: a syndrome of cerebral insufficiency. Journal of Chronic Diseases 9(3):260–277, 1959.

Etminan, M., S. Gill, and A. Samii. Effect of non-steroidal anti-inflammatory drugs on risk of Alzheimer's disease: systematic review and meta-analysis of observational studies. *British Medical Journal* 327:128–132, 2003.

Folstein, M. F., S. E. Folstein, and P. R. McHugh. "Mini-Mental State": a practical method for grading the cognitive state of patients. *Clinical Journal of Psychiatric Research* 12:189–198, 1975.

Fuld, P. A. Word intrusion as a diagnostic sign in Alzheimer's disease. *Geriatric Medicine Today* 2(41):33–41, 1983.

McKeith, I., J. Mintzer, D. Aarsland, D. Burn, H. Chiu, et al. Dementia with Lewy bodies [Review]. *Lancet* 3:19–24, 2004.

Pro, J. D., and C. E. Wells. The use of encephalogram in the diagnosis of delirium. *Diseases of the Nervous System* 38:804–808, 1977.

Qaseem, A., V. Snow, J. T. Cross Jr, M. A. Forciea, R. Hopkins Jr, et al. Current pharmacologic treatment of dementia: a clinical practice guideline from the American College of Physicians and American Academy of Family Physicians. *Annals of Internal Medicine* 148:37–378, 2008.

Ray W. A., C. P. Chung, K. T. Murray, K. Hall, and C. M. Stein. Atypical antipsychotic drugs and the risk of sudden cardiac death. *New England Journal of Medicine* 360:225–235, 2009.

Reisberg, B. Brief Cognitive Rating Scale (BCRS). *Psychopharmacology Bulletin* 24(4):629–636, 1988.

Schneeweiss, S., and J. Avorn. Antipsychotic agents and sudden cardiac death—how should we manage the risk? *New England Journal of Medicine* 360:294–296, 2009.

Sclan, S. G., and B. Reisberg. Functional assessment staging (FAST) in Alzheimer's disease: reliability, validity, and ordinality. *International Psychogeriatrics* 4(Suppl 1):55–69, 1992.

Trinh, N., J. Hoblyn, S. Mohanty, and K. Yaffe. Efficacy of cholinesterase inhibitors in the treatment of neuropsychiatric symptoms and functional impairment in Alzheimer disease. *JAMA: Journal of American Medical Association* 289(2):210–216, 2003.

Trzepacz, P. The Delirium Rating Scale. Its use in consultation-liaison research. *Psychosomatics* 40:193–204, 1999.

Tuokko, H., T. Hadjistavropoulos, J. A. Miller, and B. L. Beattie. The Clock Test: a sensitive measure to differentiate normal elderly from those with Alzheimer's disease. *Journal of the American Geriatrics Society* 40:579–584, 1992.

Wechsler, D. *The Measurement of Adult Intelligence*. Baltimore: Williams & Wilkins. 1939.

SELECTED READINGS

Blazer, D., S. Steffens, and E. Busse. *Essential of Geriatric Psychiatry*. Arlington, VA: American Psychiatric Publishing, 2007.

LeBlond R., and D. Brown. *DeGowin's Diagnostic Examination*, 9th ed. New York: McGraw-Hill, 2009.

Moore, D. P. *Textbook of Clinical Neuropsychiatry*, 2nd ed. Livre, UK, Oxford University Press, 2008.

Yudofsky, S. C, and R. E. Hales, eds. *The American Psychiatric Press Textbook of Neuropsychiatry and Behavioral Sciences*, 5th ed. Arlington, VA: American Psychiatric Press, 2008.

6

Anxiety, Obsessive-Compulsive, and Stress Disorders

FRANKLIN R. SCHNEIER, HILARY B. VIDAIR,
LESLIE R. VOGEL, AND PHILIP R. MUSKIN

Anxiety is a normal human emotion, characterized by a state of apprehension that has physiological, psychological, and behavioral components. Anxiety most commonly reflects concern about a situation that is perceived as potentially dangerous and threatening. For example, planning to walk down a dark, deserted alley may trigger anxious apprehension. Hearing footsteps then intensifies this state into a physical readiness that will facilitate escape if it is necessary. Acute fear and a fight-or-flight reaction will ensue if that potential threat is realized. A moderate level of anxiety in anticipation of a threat can therefore be highly adaptive. Anxiety is a powerful motivator; low levels of it can produce increased attention and improved performance.

Anxiety becomes maladaptive when it occurs with an intensity that is out of proportion to the threat, persists after the threat has resolved, becomes generalized to benign situations, or occurs in the complete absence of a stressor. The mental disorders known as anxiety disorders are generally considered to be examples of **ineffective adaptations to naturally occurring threats**, including dangers from predators, social conflicts, germs and disease, and other environmental hazards. The case example in Box 6.1 illustrates three forms of anxiety in one individual: a chronic form, an acute but adaptive form, and an acute but maladaptive form.

The experience of anxiety can range from predominantly psychological (e.g., worry) to largely somatic (e.g. cardiac, respiratory, gastrointestinal, or neurological symptoms) with distress limited to concern about such symptoms. These elements of anxiety may interact in complex ways—for example, mental distress can give rise to physical symptoms, such as sweating, palpitations, diarrhea, or shortness of breath, which may then potentiate the psychological distress and lead to avoidance of a perceived stressor. Avoidance may, in turn, interfere with constructive adaptation to the stressor, leading to greater anxiety when it is next encountered. Anxiety may be triggered by an exogenous environmental cue or a change in the internal milieu due to a physical disease state or the effects of a drug, or it may occur in the absence of any identifiable stressor.

Anxiety reaches the threshold for a clinically recognized disorder when it is **persistent** and **impairs a person's occupational, social, or familial functioning** or causes

---

BOX 6.1

CASE EXAMPLE OF THREE FORMS OF ANXIETY SYMPTOMS

A 23-year-old male medical student had experienced chronic anticipatory anxiety about his school performance since he was a child. The anxiety was tolerable and of a low grade. He experienced a mild conscious feeling of tension; he frequently worried about his grades and was hyperalert in classroom situations and perfectionistic about his homework. The anxiety increased before his first series of national board examinations, creating more discomfort for him but also motivating him to study for hours in a highly organized, effective way. During a clerkship he experienced a qualitatively different anxiety while giving an oral presentation to the attending physician. He suddenly experienced stammering, palpitations, sweating, dyspnea, and tremor of his hands and head. After this panic attack, he called in sick on the day of his next anticipated presentation, and showed up late to another, manifesting phobic avoidance for the first time.

---

the person a significant amount of **distress**. Anxiety can manifest as an array of physical symptoms, including tachycardia, palpitations, chest pain, difficulty breathing, restlessness, insomnia, headaches, difficulty in swallowing, gastrointestinal complaints, frequent urination, paresthesias, blurred vision, lightheadedness, dizziness, and sexual dysfunction. Many people find that they can temporarily reduce or prevent their anxiety by avoiding situations they associate with feeling anxious; however avoidance may lead to difficulties completing work and cause opportunities for social or family interaction to be missed. Such impairment can lead to secondary depressive symptoms. In some cases people use alcohol, prescription drugs such as benzodiazepines or opiates, or illicit substances in an attempt to manage their anxiety.

DIAGNOSTIC AND CLINICAL FEATURES

Historically the category of anxiety disorders included panic disorder, social anxiety disorder, agoraphobia, specific phobias, generalized anxiety, substance-induced anxiety, acute and posttraumatic stress disorders, and obsessive-compulsive disorder. Based on a growing body of clinical and research experience, the DSM-5 now emphasizes distinctions within this grouping, separating posttraumatic stress disorder and acute stress disorder into a category of trauma- and stressor-related disorders, and obsessive-compulsive disorder into a category of obsessive-compulsive and related disorders. In addition, the anxiety disorder category in DSM-5 now includes two disorders that had previously been classified with disorders of childhood onset: separation anxiety disorder (see DSM-5) and selective mutism (see DSM-5), in recognition of the observation that these disorders can persist or evolve into other anxiety disorders in adulthood (see Chapter 15, Child and Adolescent Psychiatry). The trauma- and stressor-related disorders and obsessive-compulsive disorder are usually associated with prominent anxiety and avoidance symptoms. Therefore, despite the organizational changes of the DSM-5, this chapter includes coverage of these other disorders, which were historically grouped as anxiety disorders.

Panic Disorder

Recurrent panic attacks are the hallmark of panic disorder, although panic attacks can also occur in other conditions. A **panic attack** is characterized by the abrupt onset of intense fear or discomfort (see DSM-5). One patient described it this way: "It feels...like hot all through me, and shaky. And my heart just feels like it's pounding, and I'm breathing really quick." The terror is experienced as a feeling of impending doom, with a fear of dying, "going crazy," or losing control. Physical symptoms such as trembling, sweating, and shortness of breath commonly occur. A key feature of panic is the adrenergic surge that resembles the normative **fight-or-flight response,** a sympathetic nervous system response characterized by tachycardia, sweating, and a sense of distress. An inherent feature of this response is preparation to confront or escape from a perceived threat or challenge. In panic disorder this response occurs repeatedly in the absence of a real threat.

Panic attacks may be expected or unexpected. **Unexpected panic attacks** occur without any apparent precipitating factor. **Expected panic attacks** occur upon exposure to or in anticipation of a specific obvious trigger, such as traveling over a bridge or leaving home. Many people report that they are not aware of any specific life stressors preceding the onset of panic disorder, although some recall an emotional stressor, such as the breakup of a relationship or the use of a mind-altering substance, such as cocaine, LSD, or marijuana.

Although panic attacks can be isolated events, they sometimes evolve into the **triad** of panic disorder: the acute panic attack, anticipatory anxiety, and phobic avoidance (see DSM-5). Following the experience of an **acute panic attack**, individuals often fear a recurrence. Their fear of getting another attack or of entering a situation that might trigger panic symptoms is called **anticipatory anxiety**. These individuals often start to avoid situations in which they anticipate experiencing panic. This **avoidance** often begins with specific situations where prior attacks occurred, but it may rapidly generalize to many situations in which it might be difficult to get help in the event of a panic attack (see case example in Box 6.2).

Approximately 9% of adults in the general population will have a panic attack at least once during their lives. The lifetime prevalence of panic disorder is 1.5–3.5%, and the prevalence in **females** is approximately twice that in males. The onset is usually **between late adolescence and the mid-30s** but may occur at any age. The course of panic disorder ranges from **episodic outbreaks** with several years of remission between them to continuous symptoms, with **waxing and waning** over a number of years. Other anxiety disorders co-occur in approximately 20% of individuals with panic disorder. Major depression frequently accompanies panic disorder (40–70% of patients over their lifetime), and about 20–25% of depressed patients have a lifetime history of panic disorder. Panic disorder is also a risk factor for suicide. Comorbid substance abuse occurs in about 15% of panic disorder cases.

Triggering situations such as taking public transportation produce anxiety because they symbolically represent to the individual something that is traumatically overwhelming. Whether or not such situations are inherently dangerous is not the issue. The person with panic attacks who fears flying on an airplane, for instance, is typically afraid of being confined in a space or situation from which escape is not possible in the event of getting a panic attack. The level of anxiety that is experienced is similar to the emotional reaction that most people would have if the plane were about to crash.

BOX 6.2

CASE EXAMPLE OF PANIC DISORDER

A 34-year-old woman began to experience recurrent and unexpected panic attacks. During these attacks she experienced the abrupt onset of sweating, shortness of breath, nausea, and dizziness. She noticed that these attacks often occurred when she felt she could not escape from a situation, such as when she was on a train, bus, or an airplane. Her hands would begin to tremble. Within seconds, her heart rate seemed to accelerate so fast that she felt light-headed. She would often become extremely short of breath, and although she realized that she was hyperventilating, she could not slow down her breathing. The more she hyperventilated, the dizzier she felt. She soon began to anticipate these attacks and avoided public transportation to try to prevent them from occurring. When she did have an attack, she could not control the episode, and her panic would increase in intensity. During the last attack, she felt like she was going to have a heart attack and feared going crazy. After suffering with this for 15 minutes, which felt like 5 hours, she made an emergency call to her internist. His reassuring voice and episodic prescriptions for diazepam had always helped her in the past, although she had never taken the medicine. She felt somewhat better after talking to him, and, after 20 minutes, the panic began to subside on its own.

Agoraphobia

Phobias are excessive fears of specific objects, situations, or experiences. The phobic disorders have been divided into agoraphobia, specific phobias, and social anxiety disorder (or social phobia), based on the type of feared situation and associated characteristic patterns of age of onset, course, comorbidity, and familial distribution.

Persons with agoraphobia have **intense fear or anxiety in two or more places or situations from which escape might be difficult or in which help might not be available** (e.g., shopping in a crowded supermarket, using public transportation, or being outside of the home alone). The anxiety is out of proportion to the actual threat of the situation or the sociocultural context. They may or may not give a history of panic attacks in these situations. A person with agoraphobia might fear a crowded supermarket and feel compelled to leave abruptly, even if it means leaving packages and money at the cash register. The person then may become too anxious to go to the supermarket for fear of having a panic attack or other physical symptoms (e.g., vomiting), or fear of embarrassment should he or she feel the need to actually escape from the cashier line. People with agoraphobia avoid their anxiety-provoking situations, endure them with significant distress, or manage them only when accompanied by a **"phobic companion"** or a person with whom they feel secure. Active avoidance of these situations may escalate to the point that individuals become housebound and are dependent on others to perform every task and activity that involves going outside the home (see DSM-5). Approximately half of patients with agoraphobia also have panic disorder, and either disorder can precede the other. In contrast with prior editions of the DSM in which agoraphobia was always linked to the presence or absence of panic disorder, agoraphobia can be diagnosed as a separate entity according to the DSM-5.

Social Anxiety Disorder (Social Phobia)

Social anxiety disorder, also known as social phobia, is characterized by a persistent **fear of social interactions, being observed, or performance situations**, due to concerns about **embarrassment or humiliation**. Persons with social anxiety disorder may feel intensely self-conscious in a wide variety of social interactions (e.g., going to parties, talking to a boss, or asking someone for a date), observable activities (e.g., eating and drinking), or performance activities (e.g., public speaking). During the feared situation, or in the anticipation of it, symptoms may include **fear of negative social evaluation, blushing, sweating, tachycardia, trembling, and a desire to escape**. The fear is out of proportion to the actual danger in the social situation or the sociocultural context. Persons with social anxiety disorder tend to marry later and to achieve below their potential at work. The ramifications of severe social anxiety disorder can include social isolation and avoidance of school and employment (see DSM-5). There is a **performance specifier** of social anxiety disorder, which is characterized by fear restricted to public speaking or performing that interferes with individuals' career or schooling. This specifier was added in the DSM-5 and the prior specifier for a "generalized type" of social anxiety disorder was removed.

The prevalence of social anxiety disorder in adults in the United States is 5–13%, with a slightly higher female-to-male distribution. The onset is usually in the **mid-teens**, and often emerges out of a history of childhood shyness. Social anxiety disorder is characterized by a **chronic** course, which may be complicated by depression or self-medication with alcohol or other substances, leading to greater impairment (see case illustration in Box 6.3).

Specific Phobia

Specific phobia is characterized by intense **fear or anxiety and avoidance of a specific object or situation**. Several specifiers of phobias exist, including phobias of animals (e.g., dogs, spiders), the natural environment (e.g., heights, storms), blood, injection, or injury, and other (e.g., vomiting, choking). A "situational" phobia is similar to a focused form of agoraphobia (e.g., taking elevators, airplanes, claustrophobia). People with phobias experience anxiety when confronted with their feared stimulus, and they often have somatic symptoms such as palpitations and lightheadedness. Blood, injection, and injury phobias are uniquely related to a **vasovagal** physiological response, which includes similar

---

BOX 6.3

CASE EXAMPLE OF SOCIAL ANXIETY DISORDER

A 42-year-old man was promoted to a new job requiring that he give small, informal luncheon lectures. As he began to speak at his first lecture, he suddenly experienced profuse sweating, palpitations, and a feeling of faintness, and he was unable to continue. His boss was taken aback but promptly took over the talk. After that experience, the employee began drinking before giving a lecture, because it "calmed him down." Eventually, he needed more and more alcohol and was fired after giving a lecture while he was visibly intoxicated.

somatic symptoms but is accompanied by a decrease in heart rate and blood pressure, often resulting in fainting.

Although the fears are irrational or excessive for the particular situation and sociocultural context, individuals are unable to overcome them. They may be aware that the chances of being stuck in an elevator are very low, yet they continue to be afraid to the point where they will take the stairs instead, even when doing so is extremely inconvenient. Specific phobia features include the **anticipatory anxiety** provoked by worrying about or confronting the feared object and the resulting **avoidance behavior** (see DSM-5).

As with any anxiety disorder, the diagnosis of specific phobia is made only when fear, avoidance, or other symptoms result in functional impairment or extreme distress. A hospital worker, for example, who has a fear of needles, may be seriously impaired at work because of constant exposure to the phobic situation. In contrast, a person living in Alaska who fears snakes has little opportunity to encounter one or experience impairment related to snakes, and, therefore, should not receive a diagnosis of specific phobia. Because of their circumscribed nature, specific phobias are often less impairing than other anxiety disorders.

Specific phobias are among the most **common** anxiety disorders; the lifetime prevalence of specific phobia in the United States is 10–11%. This disorder has a **peak onset in childhood** and a **second peak in the mid-20s**. Phobias that continue into adulthood have a **spontaneous remission** rate of about 20%.

Generalized Anxiety Disorder

Persons with generalized anxiety disorder experience **frequent, excessive** anxiety and **worry** and **autonomic nervous system hyperarousal**, which causes significant distress and/or impairment in functioning (see DSM-5). Symptoms include **restlessness, fatigue, irritability, muscle tension, and impaired sleep and concentration** (see case illustration in Box 6.4). These individuals may report **constant anxiety** without discrete episodes of panic, or obsessions or compulsions. Unlike phobias, the worries in generalized anxiety disorder encompass **multiple domains** that are typically part of life, such as work or school performance, finances, intimate and social relationships, and health. The worries take up significant energy and time, which impairs the individual's ability to function efficiently at home or at work. Mild depression is often present, and persons become demoralized as the anxiety interferes with their ability to enjoy life. **Major depression** frequently co-occurs. The anxiety usually precedes full-blown depression but may also co-occur or persist after a depressive episode has resolved.

Generalized anxiety disorder has a lifetime prevalence of approximately 5% and two-thirds of individuals diagnosed with this disorder are **female**. It frequently makes its initial appearance when people are in their **early 20s**, although it can occur at any age. The course is **chronic**, with **waxing and waning** of symptoms and exacerbations during times of stress. Many individuals develop other syndromes, such as panic disorder, major depressive disorder, or substance use disorders. Those patients with generalized anxiety disorder who focus predominantly on their somatic symptoms may not associate them with anxiety and often consult nonpsychiatric physicians, such as cardiologists, neurologists, and pulmonologists.

Anxiety Disorder Due to Another Medical Condition

Anxiety and panic attacks can also occur from the direct effects of another medical disorder, mimicking a variety of "functional" anxiety syndromes (i.e., anxiety for which no

BOX 6.4

CASE EXAMPLE OF GENERALIZED ANXIETY DISORDER

A 40-year-old married woman with two high school–aged children complained of chronic anxiety and worry that were making it difficult for her to sleep or focus on her work. She worries about a variety of situations, including her relationship with her spouse, her finances, her performance at work, and her children's health. She reports having difficulty relaxing because her mind "never stops" and she cannot "turn it off." Her worries often feel uncontrollable and have led to difficulty concentrating. She feels fatigued every morning at the thought of what she has to accomplish that day. She often feels restless, with frequent stomachaches and muscle tension. Because of these physical symptoms, she went to her physician, who did not find anything physically wrong.

medical cause is known), sharing symptoms of **sympathetic nervous system overactivity** that include tachycardia, palpitations, hypertension, sweating, tremor, and subjective feelings of nervousness (see Chapter 5, Neurocognitive Disorders and Mental Disorders Due to Another Medical Condition); vasovagal reactions and syncope may also occur. For this psychiatric diagnosis, the physical illness must be evidenced by history, physical examination, and laboratory findings; precede the onset of the anxiety or panic symptoms; and be commonly known to precede the type of anxiety experienced. It is crucial to consider a full medical differential diagnosis before assuming that a patient has a psychiatric disorder, although both can coexist.

Numerous medical, neurological, endocrinological, and toxic conditions can cause anxiety (see Table 6.1). Some medical diagnoses that precede anxiety and panic symptoms include various respiratory illnesses, cardiovascular disorders, and endocrine disease. Because of the anxiety-like symptoms they produce, myocardial infarction, angina pectoris, hyperthyroidism, pheochromocytoma, carcinoid syndrome, autoimmune encephalitis, and the adrenergic response to hypoglycemia in diabetic patients can be mistaken for anxiety disorder (see case example in Box 6.5). Panic-like symptoms, such as a sense of dread, dizziness, or shortness of breath, can also accompany pulmonary embolism and transient ischemic attacks of the brain.

Substance/Medication-Induced Anxiety Disorder

Substance- or medication-induced anxiety disorder is a syndrome in which symptoms of anxiety result from the use of, or withdrawal from, substances such as alcohol, caffeine, tobacco, marijuana, and other illicit drugs, or medications such as benzodiazepines, amphetamines, diethylpropion, methylphenidate, phendimetrazine, and thyroid medications. A substance- or medication-induced anxiety disorder is diagnosed only if the anxiety symptoms are severe enough to elicit clinical attention, are a **consequence of the substance itself** (evidenced by history, physical examination, or laboratory findings), and do not represent an independent anxiety disorder (see also Chapter 5, Neurocognitive Disorders and Mental Disorders Due to Another Medical Condition, and Chapter 7, Substance-Related and Addictive Disorders).

TABLE 6.1 Medical Causes of Anxiety

Endocrine Disorders
Pheochromocytoma
Thyroid dysfunction
Pituitary dysfunction
Adrenal disorders
Neurological Disorders
Head trauma
Neurosyphilis
Seizure disorders
CNS neoplasms
Cerebrovascular disease
Encephalitis and meningitis
Huntington's disease
Multiple sclerosis
Toxic and Metabolic Disorders
Alcohol or sedative withdrawal
Stimulant intoxication (cocaine, amphetamines, caffeine)
Sympathomimetic agents
Cannabis
B_{12} deficiency
Hypoxia
Ischemia
Anemia
Autoimmune Disorders
Systemic lupus erythematosus
Temporal arteritis
Polyarteritis nodosa

BOX 6.5

CASE EXAMPLE OF ANXIETY DISORDER DUE TO HYPERTHYROIDISM

A 32-year-old woman presented with anxiety, sweating, and weight loss over a 6-month period. She was prescribed a benzodiazepine, which had no effect on her symptoms. Eventually, thyroid function tests were conducted, which led to a diagnosis of hyperthyroidism due to Graves' disease. The patient was given the antithyroid medication methimazole, but she did not consistently take it. She continued to take the benzodiazepine episodically. Although some of her symptoms were masked by the medication, the hyperthyroidism was left untreated. Gradually, she developed exophthalmos, which became more and more pronounced; ptosis; and severe hair loss. She eventually agreed to take a stable regimen of methimazole; once she did, her thyroid function tests became normal, her symptoms disappeared, and she no longer needed the benzodiazepine.

The presentation of substance- or medication-induced anxiety disorders is as varied as the substances themselves. With some exceptions, the anxiety most likely results from either intoxication with stimulant drugs or the withdrawal of depressants and opioids from the central nervous system.

Stimulant Intoxication

Anxiety may be caused by acute intoxication with stimulant drugs, which include **cocaine** and **amphetamines**. The effects of stimulants can be affected by their **route of administration** and the **amount** of stimulant used. As the euphoria induced by cocaine becomes progressively more difficult to achieve, users take increasingly larger amounts, which produce an anxiety syndrome that includes the psychophysiological signs and symptoms of adrenergic stimulation. Panic attacks may also occur in acutely intoxicated cocaine users who have no previous history of panic disorder. They may continue to have panic attacks even when they are not intoxicated. The same is true of marijuana users.

Common stimulants such as **caffeine** and **diet pills** can also be anxiogenic. The spectrum of symptoms they can produce ranges from generalized anxiety or discrete panic attacks to obsessive-compulsive symptoms or phobic symptoms. Autonomic nervous system arousal may be evidenced by tachycardia, hypertension, mydriasis, and diaphoresis. The case example in Box 6.6 illustrates a case of caffeinism.

Alcohol Withdrawal

Two types of alcohol withdrawal may lead to an anxiety syndrome. **"Classic" alcohol withdrawal**, which is seen most often in a hospital setting, occurs in alcoholics who either **stop or sharply reduce** their alcohol intake for several hours to one day. Withdrawal usually occurs 24–48 hours after the last drink but may occur up to a week later and can be delayed by administration of cross-reactive medications, such as those administered in a hospital setting (benzodiazepines, barbiturates, opiates, general anesthesia). Symptoms of withdrawal include jitteriness, nervousness, mild tremor, and a mild increase in the heart rate and blood pressure. Panic attacks may also occur. Even an experienced interviewer may mistake a patient's withdrawal from alcohol as panic disorder or another anxiety syndrome, since the clinical presentations are similar. Thiamine depletion in malnourished alcoholics,

---

BOX 6.6
CASE EXAMPLE OF CAFFEINISM

A 38-year-old man was referred to a nutritionist for advice regarding weight loss. He was 40 kg overweight and had a history of poor sleep, dysphoric mood, and restlessness. He complained of headache, tachycardia, frequent urination, and an inability to lose weight. His dietary history was significant because he drank 10–12 cans of caffeinated cola daily. He was advised to discontinue the cola intake and make other dietary changes. He also arranged an appointment with a therapist and complained of fatigue, dysphoria, and an intense headache. The therapist arranged for a psychiatric consultation, in which it was determined that the patient's anxiety symptoms were the result of ingesting too much caffeine. Abruptly discontinuing the habit then produced a transient withdrawal syndrome.

as well as magnesium wasting, which potentiates thiamine deficiency, may also lead to mental status changes that some clinicians may mistake for severe "anxiety." Replenishing magnesium is essential for the thiamine supplementation to be effective.

The second type of alcohol withdrawal, **nocturnal withdrawal syndrome**, is also characterized by anxiety but involves **a milder, less prolonged** process, occurs in non-alcoholics, and is not a function of addiction. Since a small amount of alcohol (e.g., a few glasses of wine) can produce a sedative effect, it is often used as a sleep aid. Initially, alcohol inhibits rapid eye movement (REM) sleep but, because alcohol is rapidly metabolized, its inhibitory effect soon abates, causing a **rebound increase in REM**. This rebound effect results in insomnia, anxiety, and a sense of unease, symptoms that the individual may try to relieve by drinking more alcohol, thus reinforcing the habit of drinking alcohol.

Withdrawal from Benzodiazepines and Barbiturates

The **shorter-acting benzodiazepines** tend to produce a more rapid onset of symptoms and a more intense withdrawal syndrome, characterized by **jitteriness**, a sense of **unease**, **insomnia**, mild **tremulousness**, and increased pulse and blood pressure. As with alcohol, there is a concomitant rebound increase in REM during sleep. "Rebound anxiety" may occur as soon as a few hours after the last dose of a short-acting benzodiazepine such as alprazolam is taken. "Rebound insomnia" may occur in the early morning hours with triazolam, a benzodiazepine used as a sleep aid. Benzodiazepine withdrawal can mimic symptoms of anxiety disorders such as generalized anxiety disorder or panic disorder.

Patients withdrawing abruptly from the prolonged use of high dosages of **short-acting barbiturates** become anxious, tremulous, nauseated, and weak within approximately **24 hours** of taking the last dose. The syndrome peaks around the second or third day of abstinence. Patients who use large doses of butalbital, found in Fiorinal/Fioricet, may experience withdrawal when they run out of medication or are admitted to a hospital and do not disclose their Fiorinal use.

With **longer acting** benzodiazepines and barbiturates, signs and symptoms of withdrawal may appear within **several days** of the last dose. There may be a mild withdrawal syndrome consisting of anxiety, or a more severe syndrome consisting of frightening dreams, insomnia, visual hallucinations, delirium, hyperthermia, cardiovascular collapse, exhaustion, and even death. The resolution of the delirium may take several days or more, even when the patient is promptly given large dosages of replacement benzodiazepines or barbiturates.

Withdrawal from Opioids

Anxiety syndromes are also caused by withdrawal from opioids, such as morphine, heroin (which is converted to morphine in vivo), methadone, fentanyl, meperidine, and codeine. Acute **heroin** withdrawal causes marked anxiety that **begins 8–12 hours** after the last dose is taken. During this phase, the addict has intense cravings for the drug. The subjective anxiety is accompanied by tachycardia, raised blood pressure, mydriasis, restlessness, and tremor. The withdrawal syndrome peaks at 48–72 hours after the last dose, with piloerection, yawning, sneezing, nausea, vomiting, and diarrhea.

Abrupt **methadone** withdrawal also causes anxiety and a psychophysiological cascade similar to that produced by heroin withdrawal, although it is generally **milder and more prolonged** because the longer half-life of methadone allows blood levels of the drug to fall less rapidly after it has been discontinued. The syndrome begins 24–48 hours after the last dose, and mild symptoms may occur up to 6 weeks later. Withdrawal from **meperidine** begins approximately 3 hours after the last dose, peaks in about 8 hours, and usually lasts approximately 4 days.

Paradoxical Reactions

Certain pharmacological agents that normally cause calming and sedation occasionally have a paradoxical effect in specific groups of patients, such as **elderly persons, children**, and patients with **dementia**. **Benzodiazepines** and **barbiturates** may occasionally cause anxiety, disinhibition, confusion, and agitation. Such central nervous system depressants should be avoided in these individuals or, if used, should be given in minimal dosages, and the patients should be carefully monitored for agitation and confusion. In addition, **marijuana** may cause anxiety and irritability in some susceptible individuals.

Obsessive-Compulsive Disorder

The cardinal features of obsessive-compulsive disorder (OCD) are obsessions and compulsions (see DSM-5). **Obsessions** are **intrusive, recurrent, and persistent thoughts, urges, or images experienced** that an individual tries to ignore or suppress. Most individuals with obsessions find that they cause them marked anxiety or distress. Common obsessive themes include fear of **contamination, dirt, or germs**; disturbing **sexual, religious, or violent** obsessions; and thoughts about **need for orderliness**. An obsession such as "I may have forgotten to lock my door" commonly leads to **compulsions** or **repetitive behaviors** that the individual **feels driven to perform in response to the obsession**. Examples of compulsions include repeated checking to see if the door has been locked or complex cleaning rituals. Compulsions can also be mental acts such as counting, praying, or silently repeating words performed to "neutralize" the obsession.

Some people with OCD have good or fair insight, recognizing that their OCD beliefs are irrational. Others have poor insight and think their OCD beliefs are probably true. More rarely, some patients lack any insight and are convinced their OCD beliefs are true. In recognition of such cases the DSM-5 has added a delusional beliefs specifier. For example, a person may insist that if certain thoughts or rituals are not repeated over and over again, they or a loved one will surely be punished by a catastrophic event. The urge to complete a compulsion can sometimes be resisted, but the delay often causes increased anxious tension, which is relieved only by performing the compulsive act. Because these rituals may become extremely **time-consuming** (e.g., more than 1 hour per day), individuals with severe OCD often have little time for work or family relationships, and, consequently, their functioning and quality of life can be dramatically impaired. The OCD diagnosis also includes a tic specifier to indicate if the person has a current or past history of tic disorder.

The lifetime prevalence of OCD is approximately 2.5%. It occurs with equal frequency in adult males and females. OCD usually begins in **adolescence or early adulthood**, although it can begin as early as childhood. Generally, the age of onset is 6–15 years for males and 20–29 years for females. The onset is most often gradual but can be acute, and the course tends to be **chronic**, with waxing and waning of symptoms. About 15% of these individuals experience a progressive decline in occupational or social functioning. Box 6.7 provides a case example.

Posttraumatic Stress Disorder (PTSD)

Posttraumatic stress disorder (PTSD) is a **psychophysiological syndrome** that follows **exposure to a traumatic event such as threatened or actual death, sexual violence, or serious injury**. Examples include combat exposure, rape, an automobile accident, or a civilian disaster such as a hurricane (see DSM-5). Exposure to the trauma may be experienced by a direct experience, witnessing it happening to someone else, learning about it

---

BOX 6.7

CASE EXAMPLE OF OBSESSIVE-COMPULSIVE DISORDER

A 16-year-old high school track star had had various rituals and obsessions since early adolescence. He counted to himself, over and over again from 1 to 3, and he had various touching rituals, which if resisted caused vague but intense distress. He also traveled a circuitous route to high school, avoiding hospitals, physicians' offices, dentists' offices, and funeral homes, because of a fear that he could be exposed to AIDS, which he rationally knew was not possible. Although this added about 30 minutes each way to school, he explained it to his friends as part of his training for running. Unfortunately, his running began to be involved in his obsessive-compulsive symptoms as well. As he raced down the track, he had to move his feet in a rapid sequence of three beats, slight pause, and three beats again. His coach was furious and thought of kicking him off the team. This was devastating to the patient because his major source of self-esteem was the feeling of strength he experienced while running.

---

occurring to a close family member or friend, or repeated or extreme exposure to aversive aspects of a trauma (e.g., a first responder continually exposed to human remains). The latter does not include exposure via electronic media or pictures unless such viewing is work related. PTSD was first defined as an official psychiatric diagnosis in 1980, but post-traumatic symptoms had been described in the United States as early as the Civil War, and the Vietnam War heightened awareness of this disorder. While the original accounts of PTSD were based on experiences of soldiers in combat, the syndrome is now recognized to occur after a wide variety of traumas.

The **four cardinal features** of PTSD are intrusive reexperiencing of the initial trauma, avoidance, persistent negative alterations in cognitions and mood, and alterations in arousal and activity. **Reexperiencing** includes recurrent flashbacks to the scene of the trauma, intrusive and involuntary distressing memories, or recurrent nightmares. **Flashbacks** are often triggered by cues that provide a reminder of the trauma (e.g., a sudden loud noise that recalls the explosive sound of the battlefield). The diagnosis of PTSD may be specified as "with dissociative symptoms" if the person experiences persistent depersonalization (feelings of unreality or being detached from oneself) or derealization (experiencing surroundings as unreal or distorted). Persons may also try to **avoid all reminders of the trauma**, including distressing memories and feelings as well as external reminders (e.g., people, places). **Negative alterations in cognitions and mood** represent a new criterion in DSM-5, and include inability to recall important aspects of the trauma; persistent distorted cognitions about themselves, others, and causes or consequences of the traumatic event; a persistent negative emotional state (e.g., fear, guilt); and feelings of detachment from others. **Alterations in arousal and reactivity** include **irritable behavior and angry outbursts, self-destructive behavior, hypervigilance, an exaggerated startle response, and sleep difficulties**. Box 6.8 provides a case example.

The prevalence of PTSD in the general population is 3–4%. Subgroups exposed to trauma more frequently, such as inner city residents or combat veterans, have much higher rates. PTSD can occur in **childhood or adulthood**. Although over one-third

> ## BOX 6.8
> ## CASE EXAMPLE OF POSTTRAUMATIC STRESS DISORDER
>
> A 30-year-old war veteran was exposed to heavy combat and multiple episodes of attacks while on patrol. He witnessed the violent deaths of several men in his company. After his return home, the patient had had flashbacks, terrifying nightmares, chronic anxiety with episodic panic attacks, and a feeling of being numb and unconnected to his family, his friends, and the joys of life that he so looked forward to during military service. He refused to get treatment because he believed that to do so would be cowardly, especially when he compared his situation with that of his comrades who died. He rationalized this refusal by saying that he could simply avoid things that he knew would trigger flashbacks. He avoided, therefore, all movies with violence, television news programs, written reminiscences about war, and discussions of his wartime experiences. However, he could not avoid abrupt noises, such as the occasional car backfire, the explosion of Fourth of July fireworks, or the thump when his wife or children occasionally dropped something. Any such noise would trigger intense autonomic arousal, with hyperventilation, rapid heart rate, tremulous hands, profuse sweating, and flashbacks of one of the many times he had witnessed bomb blasts.

of the civilian population has been exposed to a catastrophic stressor, less than 10% of exposed persons develop a full posttraumatic stress syndrome, which suggests that the development of PTSD also depends on **individual vulnerability and resilience**.

The course of PTSD is variable, both in terms of the duration of the disorder and the delay between the initial trauma and the emergence of symptoms. Symptoms usually begin within 3 months of the trauma, but in some people, years may go by before symptoms appear. For example, women who are sexually assaulted may experience a posttraumatic syndrome immediately after the assault, or after a delay of several years. The PTSD diagnosis includes a specifier for delayed expression, which means that full diagnostic criteria are not met until at least 6 months after the traumatic event.

Factors predictive of a positive outcome include a **solid social support system**, **good psychiatric and medical health** before the trauma occurred, and a **rapid onset** of symptoms. The course is often complicated if the risk of trauma is ongoing (e.g., an abused spouse continues to be threatened) or if the person attempts to alleviate symptoms through self-medication with alcohol or drugs.

Acute Stress Disorder

Acute stress disorder occurs after experiencing or being **exposed to a traumatic event** (directly or indirectly, as in PTSD). This disorder has specific signs and symptoms resembling those of PTSD (e.g., intrusion, negative mood, avoidance, arousal, dissociation), although they occur more rapidly after the trauma and are shorter in duration (see DSM-5). Specifically, a patient must experience at least nine symptoms within the following five categories: intrusive symptoms, negative mood, dissociative symptoms, avoidance symptoms, and arousal symptoms. The symptoms often begin immediately after the trauma is experienced and must persist for between **3 days and 1 month** to meet diagnostic criteria. The likelihood of developing acute stress disorder depends on the severity of the trauma and the degree of exposure. Symptoms persisting more than 1 month are classified as having evolved into PTSD.

THE INTERVIEW

When interviewing a patient who is complaining of anxiety, it is important that the physician elicit the specific thoughts, behaviors, and physical symptoms that comprise the **experience** of anxiety, as well as the **pattern** of symptoms over time, and the **social** and **cultural context** (see Box 6.9, Interviewing Guidelines). The interviewer should explore what triggers the anxiety and what relieves it, and if there are any medical conditions or treatments that may be contributing to anxiety-like symptoms.

Patients with anxiety disorders may initially describe their symptoms in great detail, or focus on a single aspect of their anxiety or a secondary manifestation like depression, or report only vague unease. The interviewer must elicit specific information about the symptoms, such as the **onset**, **duration**, **distribution**, **quality**, and **intensity** of the symptoms; the **past history** of anxiety symptoms; the **family history** of anxiety symptoms; and whether any other symptoms are associated with the anxiety. Common anxiety disorder features such as panic attacks, obsessions and compulsions, excessive fears of embarrassment, and exposure to traumatic events should be queried. Persistent but gentle questioning by the interviewer may be needed to obtain the details. An effective approach to interviewing patients with anxiety disorders is to alternate between listening carefully to the patient's elaboration on various topics and asking specific questions.

BOX 6.9

INTERVIEWING GUIDELINES

- Ask about the specific symptoms of anxiety, including the following characteristics of the thoughts, behaviors, and physical symptoms:
  - Onset
  - Duration
  - Distribution
  - Quality
  - Intensity
- Inquire about associated symptoms, including depression and suicidal ideation.
- Inquire about the patient's life history, and listen for psychosocial triggers of anxiety and the context in which they have occurred.
- Ask whether the patient has any theories about the origin of the symptoms.
- Obtain a complete medical history.
- Maintain a calm, reassuring demeanor.
- Avoid expressing irritation with the patient.

Because depressive symptoms often coexist with anxiety symptoms, the interviewer should ask specifically about symptoms of **depression** and presence of **suicidal ideation**. The interviewer should also ask about other conditions that are sometimes associated with anxiety disorders, such as substance abuse, eating disorders, bipolar or psychotic disorders, or medical disorders such as thyroid disease.

The **life history** is an important part of the interview because it may suggest psychosocial causes of anxiety. Since patients do not necessarily consider such information to be relevant to their symptoms, they may not spontaneously provide an integrated life history that reveals the juxtaposition between their symptoms and what is going on in their lives. Alternatively, some patients will want to focus exclusively on precipitating events and must be coaxed to provide information on their symptoms. The interviewer should take a parallel history, which is divided into two parts according to time sequence: the first part is the history of the symptoms; the second part is the life history. The interviewer might say to the patient, "Please tell me what was going on in your life at the onset of your symptoms." If the patient responds by saying, "Not much," the interviewer should ask the patient to elaborate. The patient's starting point may give the interviewer the first clues about the relevant context in which the symptoms have occurred. Events that might seem negligible to the patient might be identified by the interviewer as stressors or precipitating events.

Some patients may initially withhold information because of embarrassment or shame, such as obsessive-compulsive patients who fear their rituals will be viewed as bizarre, patients with social anxiety disorder who fear their symptoms will not be taken seriously, or trauma victims who believe they should have just "gotten over it." The interviewer should maintain a calm, accepting demeanor and may need to juggle the pursuit of specific data with expressions of empathy that help foster an environment in which the patient feels safe enough to divulge distressing information.

Interviewing anxious patients can elicit a variety of **emotional experiences in physicians**, who may feel rewarded by the patient's appreciation of their listening, empathy, and attempts to understand. But empathy carried to the extreme can inadvertently reinforce the patient's fears. "It is understandable that you have been afraid to drive since your sister's car accident," expresses empathy; however, adding a statement such as, "I, too, would probably never drive again," is not appropriate. It is more therapeutic to empathize with both the experience of anxiety and the patient's desire to overcome it.

Sometimes a patient's anxiety can seem contagious, leading the interviewer to feel pressured to offer a hasty solution to what is typically a chronic problem. It can feel frustrating to hear a patient's fears and vulnerability, and to realize that it may not be possible to reassure the patient fully. This may lead the interviewer to grasp hold of a more manageable, perhaps medical aspect of the patient's problem, although doing so may lose sight of the main issue or even be counterproductive ("You mentioned that over the past 10 years, with each new panic episode, you fear a heart attack is occurring. The biggest problem we see with heart attacks is that people tend to ignore early symptoms, and rapid treatment in the ER is critically important."). It may be more helpful to simply acknowledge the patient's difficulty ("So with each new panic attack, it's hard for you to recognize the symptoms as anxiety.")

At the other extreme, another common experience is annoyance with a patient who fears something that seems trivial, such as worries about schoolwork in an A student with generalized anxiety disorder. The urge to tell a patient, "That's ridiculous, just get over it," signals the need for self-reflection on the part of the interviewer. It can be helpful to remind oneself that such patients already know that their anxiety is irrational, but they are coming for treatment because this knowledge does not reduce their level of distress. Staying calm and empathic during the interview while offering psychoeducation about anxiety and explaining types of treatment available will provide a structured, therapeutic environment for the patient without overwhelming the physician.

DIFFERENTIAL DIAGNOSIS

Most individual symptoms of anxiety are nonspecific, occurring in a variety of psychiatric conditions and in healthy individuals, so making the correct diagnosis requires consideration of their pattern and context. In addition, the pattern of anxiety is a critical differentiating factor in the various anxiety disorders (see Table 6.2).

Generalized Anxiety Disorder

Anxiety in generalized anxiety disorder is related to multiple areas such as work, finances, illness, and other stressors. The anxiety may increase in intensity over hours or days and may reach a peak level of extreme intensity, but discrete panic attacks are uncommon and, if they occur, they are not the main focus of concern, as is the case in panic disorder. Similarly, worries may encompass fears of embarrassment in social situations, but unlike social anxiety disorder, here they are not the predominant focus and occur with or without evaluation. Persons with generalized anxiety disorder worry across **multiple domains** of stressors. It is the excessive worry about future problems that is considered abnormal, as opposed to the inappropriate ideas found in the thoughts, urges, and images characteristic of OCD. Nonpathological anxiety differs from generalized anxiety disorder in that it is easier for the person to control and is less pervasive, has a shorter duration, and is less impairing. The common medical condition of **hyperthyroidism** should not be overlooked in the patient presenting with nervousness.

TABLE 6.2 Overview of Characteristic Symptom Patterns Across Anxiety and Obsessive-Compulsive Disorders

	Panic Disorder and Agoraphobia	Social Anxiety Disorder	Generalized Anxiety Disorder	Obsessive-Compulsive Disorder
Panic Attacks	Yes, initially unexpected	If present, limited to social situations	If present, related to worry	If present, related to obsessive fears
Anticipatory Anxiety	For situations that trigger panic or make escape difficult	For social or performance situations	Across many types of situations	For situations that trigger obsessions and compulsions
Typical Cognitions	During panic: worry dying, losing control, having a heart attack	Fear of embarrassment, negative evaluation	Worries about money, safety, future, relationships	Obsessive fears of contamination, causing harm to others, not doing something "just right"
Typical Physical Symptoms	Dyspnea, palpitations, lightheaded	Blushing, sweating, trembling	Tension, insomnia, restlessness	Nonspecific
Typical Behaviors	Avoid closed spaces, being alone. Seek reassurance	Avoid public speaking, social interactions	Avoid reminders of worry, seek reassurance	Washing/cleaning, checking, ordering Avoid contaminants

Panic Disorder

The differential diagnosis of panic disorder includes anxiety disorder due to another medical condition, **substance/medication-induced** anxiety disorder, and **depression**. Panic attacks can occur as part of a social anxiety disorder, but those are predictably related to social situations and do not occur unexpectedly, as is required, at least initially, for the diagnosis panic disorder. In addition, people with panic disorder tend to manage better in a feared situation when another person accompanies them, while those with social anxiety disorder may be distressed by the thought of additional evaluation from a companion.

Specific Phobia

The differential diagnosis of specific phobia includes panic disorder, other phobias, PTSD, and OCD. In panic disorder, at least some unexpected attacks occur unrelated to a specific phobia object or situation. Anxiety in agoraphobia is related to at least two situations rather than a specific stimulus. In social anxiety disorder, anxiety is related to negative evaluation during social or performance situations rather than another type of object or situation. PTSD requires exposure to a traumatic event. Finally, people with OCD must have obsessive thoughts specifically related to the feared situation or object that are more typical to an OCD presentation.

Social Anxiety Disorder

Social anxiety disorder must be distinguished from other disorders that may involve social anxiety and the avoidance of social situations, including panic disorder, other phobias, generalized anxiety disorder, major depression, autism spectrum disorders, and avoidant personality disorder. Persons with social anxiety disorder may have panic attacks, but unlike in panic disorder, these attacks are elicited only by social situations in which they fear embarrassment. People with **generalized anxiety disorder** will worry about a variety of situations rather than predominantly focus on social situations. **Depressed** patients typically avoid social situations out of disinterest rather than fear of embarrassment. In addition, concern about negative evaluation focuses on feeling that they are unworthy of social interaction instead of fear of their social performance or physical appearance. Individuals with autism spectrum disorders typically have social-skills deficits as opposed to performance anxiety, whereas those with social anxiety disorder typically have communication abilities and age-appropriate relationships; however, they may struggle in initial interactions with new people. Social anxiety disorder should also be differentiated from common normative responses such as milder forms of stage fright and shyness that do not cause substantial distress or interference. **Avoidant personality disorder** overlaps greatly with more severe forms of social anxiety disorder, but it typically includes a broader pattern of avoidance. Finally, disorders such as **schizoid** and **schizotypal personality disorders** include avoidance of social interaction; however, this is due to lack of interest rather than a desire to be social that is inhibited by fear of evaluation.

Obsessive-Compulsive Disorder

Obsessive-compulsive disorder should be distinguished from other mental disorders involving recurrent or intrusive thoughts, images, impulses, or behaviors. The differential diagnoses include anxiety disorder due to another medical condition (e.g., autoimmune-based compulsions that are generally rapid in onset after an infection), substance/medication-induced anxiety disorder, and phobias in which there is a preoccupation with a feared object or situation. Persons with persistent brooding in major **depression** or excessive worry in **generalized anxiety disorder** do not find their ruminative thoughts absurd or attempt to suppress the thoughts through rituals. **Obsessive-compulsive personality disorder** describes a rigid and orderly personality style but does not include actual obsessions and compulsions. OCD should not be confused with superstitious and checking behaviors that do not cause distress and may be within the realm of normal, everyday behavior. In addition, although individuals with OCD may have poor insight or even delusional beliefs, they do not have other features of schizophrenia, such as hallucinations or formal thought disorder.

Posttraumatic Stress Disorder

The differential diagnosis of PTSD includes adjustment disorder, acute stress disorder, and OCD, when these disorders include recurrent intrusive thoughts that are experienced as inappropriate but are not related to an experienced traumatic event. **Adjustment disorder** may be the appropriate diagnosis when a person experiences a milder traumatic event (e.g., break-up of a relationship) (see DSM-5). The flashbacks in PTSD must be distinguished from perceptual and dissociative disturbances that occur in other disorders, such as psychotic disorders, substance/medication-induced disorders, and **dissociative disorders** (see description of dissociative phenomena in Box 6.10).

Acute Stress Disorder

The differential diagnosis between acute stress disorder and PTSD is that the former must occur **within 1 month** while the latter occurs only when symptoms have

---

BOX 6.10
DISSOCIATIVE PHENOMENA

Dissociation is a ubiquitous human psychological phenomenon. Acutely, it tends to relieve anxiety by separating the mental content of a thought that produces anxiety from the unpleasant feeling of anxiety. It may be a mild phenomenon that is a common response to daily life experiences or a severe, incapacitating psychiatric disorder, with various gradations between these two extremes. Biological factors seem to play a role in severe dissociation.

Depersonalization/derealization disorder is characterized by repeated experiences of depersonalization and/or derealization (see DSM-5). **Depersonalization** is a dissociative phenomenon in which a person feels **somewhat removed** from his or her body. For example, a 40-year-old business executive was mildly uncomfortable during airplane travel, but he had to fly frequently because of his job. He would feel quite relaxed and happy as he walked down the ramp to the airplane, but he then he would begin to feel mildly anxious, with a sensation of being "slightly out of

(continued)

my body." He describes the sensation as a hyperobjective experience of watching himself. In his mind, he is describing his motions to himself as if he were observing another person. "Now he's walking down the ramp, now he's entering the airplane, now he's showing his ticket to the stewardess." These are merely thoughts. He is aware that they are due to anxiety.

Derealization is a dissociative state in which a person experiences his or her surroundings as **strange or unreal**. For example, a soldier in his first experience of combat was being flown by helicopter into a forward area. As the chopper quickly skirted a line of trees and came down in the landing zone, he saw flare markers shooting into the sky, artillery rounds landing 200 yards away, and infantry troops that had previously landed running into the trees to form a skirmish line. He felt as if the scene were in a movie and not actually real. He had a dual emotional experience of anxiety and of great interest and excitement. He watched the unfolding battle scene as if he were not about to be plunged into its center.

Dissociative amnesia is a disorder in which past events that are usually of a traumatic nature are forgotten, in a way that is inconsistent with ordinary forgetting (see DSM-5). When the patient retrieves the information during the course of psychotherapy, the patient is often interested and enlightened but not surprised, because the patient has the feeling that he or she has known the information all along in some way. Traumatic episodes that pass in and out of consciousness over many years are more common than complete repression. Examples of such episodes are combat experiences in young adulthood, or sexual, abusive, or abandonment traumas of childhood. **Dissociative fugue** may accompany dissociative amnesia and is characterized by apparently purposeful travel or bewildered wandering that is associated with amnesia. The syndrome presents as the patient suddenly travels away from home, often far away, and sheds his or her personal identification. It is sometimes associated with some degree of stupor and mild confusion. The patient may be brought to the emergency room by the local police after being found wandering. Some patients may retain their ability to interact superficially with people and to work and may set up a new life. The differential diagnosis of dissociative amnesia and fugue should include malingering about the symptom of amnesia as well as a mental disorder due to a general medical condition or a substance/medication-induced disorder.

Dissociative identity disorder is the current term for multiple personality disorder. It is characterized by the presence of two or more subjectively felt, distinct personality states, or an experience of possession (see DSM-5). There are recurrent gaps in the recall of everyday events, important personal information, and/or traumatic events. It is associated with childhood trauma or abuse.

been present for more than 1 month. Acute stress disorder should also be differentiated from an anxiety disorder due to another medical condition, substance/medication-induced disorder, brief psychotic disorder, and an exacerbation of a pre-existing mental disorder.

Anxiety disorder due to another medical condition should be differentiated from delirium, substance/medication-induced anxiety disorder, the primary anxiety disorders, and adjustment disorder, which would be diagnosed when an individual has an anxious response to the stress of having a medical condition as opposed to anxiety that is a physiological consequence of the condition. **Substance/medication-induced anxiety disorder** should be classified as substance intoxication or substance withdrawal, and it should be diagnosed instead of a substance disorder if the anxiety symptoms are more severe than typically encountered with such a diagnosis and are the focus of clinical attention. This diagnosis should also be differentiated from a primary anxiety disorder, delirium, or an anxiety disorder due to another medical condition.

MEDICAL EVALUATION

Anxiety disorders are occasionally mimicked by medical conditions, especially endocrine, cardiac, and neurological disorders (see case illustration in Box 6.11). Excessive focus on possible medical etiologies can unnecessarily delay appropriate psychiatric treatment of anxiety disorders, as the case example in Box 6.12 demonstrates.

The medical evaluation of patients complaining of anxiety must strike a balance between avoiding excessive workups that delay the prescription of appropriate psychiatric treatment and investigating possible physiological explanations for the anxiety symptoms. A crucial first step is to take a careful, thorough medical history; review of systems; and review of medications (including prescription drugs and over-the-counter drugs) and other agents (including recreational drugs, alcohol, nicotine, and caffeine) that have recently been consumed by the patient. Taking the patient's vital signs and doing a physical examination that focuses on the signs of endocrine, cardiac, pulmonary, and neurological diseases are the next steps. Useful laboratory tests may include a complete blood count and tests of thyroid function, blood glucose levels, and arterial blood gas levels. An assessment of cardiac functioning, which may include an ECG, chest x-ray, 24-hour Holter monitoring test, and echocardiogram, should be considered in patients with a recent onset of anxiety

---

BOX 6.11
ANXIETY DISORDER DUE TO A PHEOCHROMOCYTOMA

A 38-year-old mother and businesswoman complained of sudden, unpredictable brief attacks of tachycardia, pounding headaches, and dizziness. The symptoms did not correspond to a change in her mood or circumstances. Her family physician advised her to see a psychiatrist for treatment of "anxiety attacks," but she never did. A friend referred her to an endocrinologist, who discovered an epinephrine-secreting pheochromocytoma. After the tumor was removed, the woman had no more attacks.

BOX 6.12

CASE EXAMPLE OF DELAYED DIAGNOSIS OF PANIC DISORDER

A 43-year-old woman presented to the emergency room with the chief complaint of "palpitations." An electrocardiogram (ECG) revealed that the sinus rhythm was normal, with occasional premature atrial contractions. She was reassured that "nothing was abnormal" and was sent home. The following year she again presented to the emergency room with the same chief complaint. On that occasion, the ECG showed a normal sinus rhythm with occasional premature ventricular contractions, and an echocardiogram revealed "marked to moderate-late systolic posterior prolapse of the mitral valve." Another year later she presented to the emergency room complaining of palpitations and dizziness. She did not complain of chest pain, syncope, or dyspnea. Twenty-four-hour Holter monitoring revealed a mean heart rate of 97 beats per minute and 326 premature ventricular contractions per hour. She was again diagnosed with mitral valve prolapse and was given propranolol. Over the following 10 years, she presented to the emergency room about once a week complaining of palpitations. By that time, she had stopped working because the palpitations were so bothersome. Finally, a psychiatric consultation was requested for treatment of her anxiety and she was diagnosed with panic disorder. She took the antipanic medication sertraline and her anxiety and panic remitted. At a follow-up visit, 24-hour Holter monitoring revealed a normal sinus rhythm with a mean heart rate of 78 beats per minute and no premature ventricular contractions.

---

symptoms with physical symptoms suggesting cardiac ischemia (e.g., crushing chest pain), particularly in individuals over age 40 years.

Mitral valve prolapse appears to occur more frequently in patients with **panic disorder** than in people without panic disorder, although there does not appear to be an elevated frequency of panic disorder in patients with mitral valve prolapse. Mitral valve prolapse and panic disorder share some characteristics, such as palpitations, light-headedness, and chest pain. In patients who have both mitral valve prolapse and panic disorder, the "cardiac symptoms" resolve when they are taking antipanic medication, even though there are continued findings of mitral valve prolapse (i.e., the prolapse has not resolved). The treatment may be addressing a neurochemical defect common to both mitral valve prolapse and panic disorder, and the "cardiac symptoms" may not stem strictly from the mitral valve prolapse.

ETIOLOGICAL ISSUES ACROSS ANXIETY, OBSESSIVE-COMPULSIVE, AND STRESS DISORDERS

The etiology and pathophysiology of anxiety, obsessive-compulsive, and stress disorders can be considered at multiple levels of organization, which have complementary implications for treatment. Genetic predisposition, which may be phenotypically expressed at levels including protein expression, brain neurotransmitter system function, and functional neurocircuitry, interacts with environmental stressors and protective experiences to influence the emergence of symptomatology. Anxiety manifests itself as autonomic nervous system activation, thoughts, and behaviors, which all interact with each other. These features, in turn, interact with the contexts of intrapsychic, familial, and sociocultural dynamics. Effective treatments may target neurotransmitters, cognitions, behaviors, and/or relationships. Brain systems mediating anxiety and stress interface with other hormonal systems, and other primary medical conditions may initially present as anxiety, affording other avenues for intervention.

Neurobiological Concepts

Genetic Predisposition and Interactions with Environment
The biological vulnerability to develop specific anxiety disorders varies from person to person. In some persons, the vulnerability may be so great that symptoms occur in the absence of any detectable stressors. Others will develop symptoms only after a sufficiently stressful trigger, such as smoking marijuana, loss of a close relationship, or a traumatic experience. Finally, others are so resilient that they will not develop an anxiety disorder even when exposed to extreme chronic stressors.

The effects of genes and environment on vulnerability for anxiety disorders have been estimated by family studies and twin studies. Each of the anxiety disorders is to some extent **familial**, with first-degree relatives carrying a 10–30% risk of developing the same disorder. Most estimates of heritability for each anxiety disorder fall in the **30–50% range**, suggesting that both genes and environment make major contributions. Other studies suggest that rather than *directly* conferring risk for specific anxiety disorders, genes may more directly influence **trait features** that in turn confer risk for the development of specific disorders. Relevant heritable traits include behavioral inhibition (a tendency to withdraw from novelty) and neuroticism (a stable tendency to experience negative emotional states).

Candidate gene association studies have not found any single gene to be responsible for more than a small percentage of the heritability of anxiety disorders. Early studies focused on polymorphisms of genes regulating neurotransmitters known to be relevant to psychopathology, including serotonin (5-hydroxytryptamine$_{2A}$ receptors, serotonin transporter), monoamine metabolism (catechol-O-methyltransferase, monoamine oxidase A), dopamine (dopamine D_4 and D_2 receptors, dopamine transporter), and G-protein signaling. These studies have been limited by the available knowledge base for selecting candidate genes, patient samples with ethnic and racial heterogeneity, and deficiencies in the definition and measurement of phenotypes. Genome-wide association studies, which do not require hypothesized candidate genes, hold promise for future identification of genetic factors. Recently, the first genome-wide association studies (GWAS) aiming to identify common variants have been published for the anxiety-related personality trait neuroticism and panic disorder. These studies suggest involvement of a large number of small effect size variants in the predisposition to anxiety disorders, a characteristic shared with other psychiatric disorders.

There has been growing investigation of the mechanisms of gene–environment interaction in the development of anxiety disorders. The findings have been inconsistent, with some animal and human studies suggesting that polymorphisms, such as those of the promoter region of the serotonin transporter gene, interact with environmental stressors to increase the risk of anxiety and depressive disorders.

Animal and human studies suggest a role for **epigenetic** phenomena, involving modification of gene function as a mechanism of gene–environment interaction, in the development of anxiety disorders. In one relevant animal model, rodent pups receiving low levels of maternal licking and grooming (whether from their birth mother or a foster mother) developed into fearful adults, with heightened startle responses and intense adrenocortical responses to stress. The differences in adrenocortical responses to stress were linked to differential synthesis of hippocampal receptors. This synthesis was regulated by genes whose rates of expression were in turn modified by epigenetic variation (histone methylation and deacetylation) induced by normally occurring levels of maternal behaviors. The adrenocortical changes could be reversed by specifically blocking these epigenetic modifications.

Neurotransmitters

Several neurotransmitter systems have been implicated in the pathophysiology of anxiety disorders and their treatments, including serotonin, norepinephrine, dopamine, γ-aminobutyric acid (GABA), and glutamate. **Serotonin** is the most-studied neurotransmitter in anxiety disorders, in part because of the ubiquitous efficacy of selective serotonin reuptake inhibitors (SSRIs) for most of the anxiety disorders. Serotonergic neurons project from the raphe nuclei and act through a diverse array of receptors spread throughout the brain. Although SSRIs appear to have a net effect of increasing serotonergic transmission, it does not appear that a general deficiency of serotonin is a primary cause of anxiety, although more subtle abnormalities in the serotonin system may be present. One of the major postulated mechanisms of SSRI function is the downregulation of the 5-HT_{1A} autoreceptors and the subsequent relaxation of negative feedback on the serotonergic neuron. Stimulation of these receptors activates neurogenesis, which appears partially responsible for anxiolytic effects. Serotonin also has been shown to act during development to establish normal anxiety behaviors.

The **locus coeruleus** is a brainstem structure that contains the majority of **noradrenergic** neurons in the central nervous system. It projects to several important brain structures thought to be involved in human emotion, particularly the limbic system, amygdala, hippocampus, and cerebral cortex (see Figure 6.1). The central noradrenergic neurons in the locus coeruleus appear to alert and alarm an individual to potentially threatening environmental factors; in situations of potential "danger," the locus coeruleus sets off a sympathetic discharge that may facilitate responses, ranging from an alerting and adaptive response to one that is anxiogenic and disabling. Pharmacological agents that increase locus coeruleus discharge, such as the α_2-antagonist yohimbine, can mimic both the psychic and physical sensations of anxiety, particularly in persons who are vulnerable to anxiety. Conversely, agents that decrease central noradrenergic release (e.g., the α_2-agonist clonidine) partially or completely alleviate the physiological components of anxiety.

The specific effectiveness of benzodiazepine medications in relieving anxiety suggested some connection between anxiety and the function of **benzodiazepine receptors**, first discovered in 1977. The central nervous system benzodiazepine receptor shares a chloride ionophore complex with the GABA receptor. The binding of a benzodiazepine such as diazepam to the benzodiazepine receptor facilitates the action of **GABA** as an inhibitory neurotransmitter. On the neuronal surface, the GABA receptor is linked to a chloride channel in the neuronal membrane. When the benzodiazepine binds to its receptor, chloride channels open, sending chloride into the cell. This causes hyperpolarization of the cell membrane and, therefore, inhibition of neuronal firing.

The β-carbolines are found in plants and are present in coffee. These chemicals act as inverse agonists at the benzodiazepine receptor and are anxiogenic. Abnormalities in

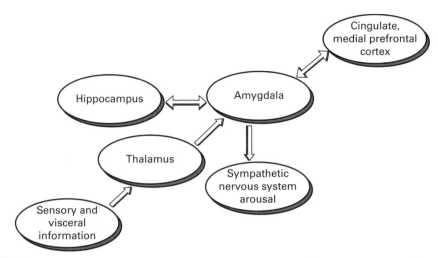

FIGURE 6.1 Schematic diagram of the neurocircuitry involved in fear responses in anxiety disorders. Sensory and visceral information about a threat is conveyed to the amygdala, where it is integrated with contextual information from the hippocampus and regulatory input from the prefrontal cortex, leading to expression of a fear response.

GABA and benzodiazepine receptor function have been associated with panic disorder and other anxiety disorders.

Glutamate is a major excitatory neurotransmitter in the brain. Drugs modulating glutamate have shown activity and animal models of anxiety, and glutamate receptors mediate the acquisition and extinction of fear conditioning, believed to be key processes in the development of and recovery from anxiety disorders. In humans, abnormal regional brain glutamate levels have been reported for several anxiety disorders.

The neurotransmitter **dopamine** has been shown to be important in animal models of **fear conditioning**. Originating in the ventral tegmental area, the mesolimbic dopamine system targets the amygdala and nucleus accumbens, which are structures constituting the fear-related circuitry. Stress can enhance dopamine release preferentially in the medial prefrontal cortex, a critical region for conditioned fear responses.

The Hypothalamic–Pituitary–Adrenal (HPA) Axis
The HPA axis is an important part of the **stress response system**, and it interacts functionally with noradrenergic neuronal systems. Acute stress results in the release of corticotropin-releasing factor (CRF) from the paraventricular nucleus of the hypothalamus, which increases peripheral adrenocorticotropic hormone (ACTH) and cortisol levels. **Cortisol**, along with activation of sympathetic and parasympathetic systems, orchestrates the body's stress response. Dysregulation of the HPA axis has been hypothesized to be associated with anxiety and stress disorders, particularly PTSD.

Neurocircuitry, Attention, and Learning
One element common to most of the anxiety disorders (including PTSD, panic disorder, and phobias) is an elevated sensitivity to threat, which appears to involve brain systems that have been identified to mediate **"fear" responses** in animals and healthy humans. Visual threat information rapidly passes from the retina to the thalamus and immediately to the amygdala (LeDoux 2000), providing a quick but rough estimate of threat. Slower

cortical pathways provide a more detailed representation of threat features and allow modulation of the threat response. The **amygdala** thus plays a central role in processing sensory stimuli in order to assess risk of threat, and its activity is regulated "top-down" by the prefrontal cortex. Detection of threat by the amygdala triggers a cascade activating the sympathetic nervous system for a fight-or-flight response.

For most of the anxiety disorders, **conditioned responses** to feared stimuli appear to play some role in the development or maintenance of the disorder. In PTSD, for example, fear of a particular threat generalizes to non-dangerous reminders of the original trauma (e.g., an earthquake victim avoids news reports about any natural disasters). Fear of these non-dangerous situations may persist even if the person with PTSD has repeated exposure to the newly feared situation, unlike the normal process of exposure to a non-dangerous situation leading to extinction of fear.

Animal studies of fear learning, in which learned fear-like responses develop to cues that have been paired with aversive events in a conditioning procedure, have identified essential neurocircuitry for the learned fear responses. The expression of conditioned fear involves a pathway from the basolateral amygdala (BLA) to the central nucleus in the superior portion of the amygdala, which projects to the periaqueductal gray (PAG) and hypothalamus. Stimulation of the PAG produces coordinated patterns of physiological and behavioral changes consistent with a fear reaction. Projections to prefrontal cortex, thalamic "association" nuclei, and neuromodulatory systems—such as the noradrenergic system—govern arousal and regulate behavior. The **hippocampus** plays a key role in distinguishing between safe and dangerous contexts. Extinction of fears involves the laying down of new memories; the process is mediated by the amygdala, hippocampus, and medial prefrontal cortex.

The application of brain imaging techniques of positron emission tomography (PET) and functional magnetic resonance imaging (fMRI) to anxiety disorders has led to a rapid expansion of knowledge of brain regions and circuits that appear associated with the pathophysiology of anxiety and anxiety disorders. A meta-analysis (Etkin and Wager 2007) compared processing of negative emotional stimuli in patients with PTSD, social anxiety disorder, and specific phobia, as well as in healthy individuals who through experimental fear conditioning had developed anxiety to discrete cues. Common to patients with all three disorders was consistent **hyperactivation of the amygdala and insula** (a region involved in dysphoric bodily sensations). A similar pattern of activation was noted during fear conditioning in healthy volunteers, which suggests that amygdala and insula hyperactivation in patients shares common features with fear-conditioning experiences in healthy subjects.

Neuroimaging studies of the treatment of anxiety and stress disorders have shown that improvement in symptoms of social anxiety disorder is accompanied by decreased activity in the amygdala and the medial temporal lobe, and that improvement in OCD is accompanied by normalization of caudate hyperactivity. Early studies of neural predictors of treatment response have reported that increased rostral anterior cingulate activation to fearful faces at baseline predicts a better response to venlafaxine in generalized anxiety disorder and predicts a favorable response to cognitive-behavioral therapy in patients with PTSD.

Increased understanding of the mechanisms of fear and anxiety acquisition and extinction appears to have important implications for diagnosis and treatment of anxiety disorders. Cognitive-behavioral therapies specifically engage extinction mechanisms that counteract the excessive generalization of fears that is seen in anxiety disorders. Understanding of the neurocircuitry and associated neurotransmitters has informed research efforts to more efficiently change fear memories, by combining cognitive-behavioral techniques with modulation of relevant neurotransmitters.

Psychosocial Concepts

Cognitive-Behavioral Approach

The cognitive behavioral model for the etiology of anxiety disorders integrates behavioral and cognitive concepts. Behaviorists explain anxiety through empirically validated principles of learning, such as **classical conditioning**. Classical conditioning, as it applies to the anxiety and stress disorders, is the process by which a person learns to associate a neutral object or situation with something that naturally results in a fear response. In the first case study of classical conditioning in humans, the behaviorist Watson taught a child to be afraid of a rat by presenting the rat immediately before a loud and startling noise. Over time the child associated the rat with his experience of being startled and became afraid of the rat.

Another learning theory central to the development of anxiety is **operant conditioning**. Operant conditioning occurs when a response is rewarded or punished by the environment and thus results in an increase or decrease of that response. One example of operant conditioning is negative reinforcement, which occurs when a person is reinforced for escaping from a situation (i.e., feels temporarily relieved) and thus increases the tendency to avoid the situation. Both classical and operant conditioning may be important in the development or maintenance of anxiety disorders. For example, a person riding an elevator that gets stuck between floors might, through the process of classical conditioning, begin to fear elevators. Subsequently, when the person tries to take the elevator, she experiences fear and walks out before the doors closed. Walking out of the elevator results in a calm feeling, thus negatively reinforcing her avoidance of elevators. If the person were then repeatedly re-exposed to elevators without getting stuck again, the association between the conditioned and unconditioned stimulus would likely become extinguished, thus reducing the anxiety related to riding in an elevator.

Cognitive theory suggests that thoughts are interconnected with emotions and behavior. **Negative automatic thoughts**, often referred to as **cognitive distortions** because they are usually inaccurate, mediate the relationship between an event and anxiety. A person who is socially anxious and about to give a speech may focus on the thought that he will make a fool of himself, thus intensifying his fears. A variety of cognitive distortions commonly occur in patients with anxiety disorders, including **catastrophizing** (exaggerating a potential problem into a catastrophe), **generalization of danger** ("if one person doesn't like my speech, I'll never be a good speaker"), and **overestimating the likelihood of a negative outcome (fortune telling)**. Once anxiety is elicited, these distortions help to maintain the anxiety, which often results in a cycle that patients temporarily stop by engaging in avoidance (e.g., as in specific phobia) or compensatory behavior (e.g. compulsions, as in OCD).

Psychodynamic Approach

Psychodynamic approaches to anxiety focus on discovering the frightening unconscious emotional meanings that are associated with real-life stressors and with the conscious thoughts and feelings that mediate anxiety states. Many patients with symptomatic anxiety states are consciously aware that certain situations have an exaggerated emotional meaning for them. A patient with panic attacks triggered by arguments with family members may recognize that his fear of dying and loss of control has meaning beyond the immediate constellation of physical symptoms. Psychodynamic theories of anxiety consider mechanisms of symbolic representation that attach frightening emotional significance to real-life events. This perspective views anxiety as a signal of unconscious, intrapsychic conflict. For example, patients with panic often have conflicts and insecurities regarding dependency. These conflicts may derive from early childhood and may be based on actual deprivation, a heightened sensitivity to normal environmental deprivation experiences, or a combination of the two. These dependency issues of early childhood may continue throughout life and become commingled with later issues of competition and achievement, making patients with anxiety vulnerable to situations that symbolically represent these issues.

Evidence for the involvement of unconscious processes in anxiety comes from fMRI imaging studies. In one study, a group of normal subjects viewed a series of fearful faces that were presented either within conscious awareness or using a backward masking technique that prevented conscious awareness of the emotion presented. Only the unconscious processing of the faces was associated with an increase in amygdala activity that was directly correlated to the baseline severity of anxiety (Etkin 2007).

TREATMENT

General Principles of Pharmacotherapy

The **selective serotonin reuptake inhibitors** (SSRIs) and **serotonin norepinephrine reuptake inhibitors** (SNRIs) have emerged as the **first-line** pharmacotherapy treatment for obsessive-compulsive disorder as well as most of the anxiety and stress disorders, based on numerous randomized, controlled trials for the specific disorders. The preference for SSRIs is based on a combination of good efficacy, safety, and tolerability (see Chapter 16, Pharmacotherapy, ECT, and TMS). Rates of satisfactory clinical response range from 40% to 80% in most single trials. The SNRIs at lower doses appear to have a mechanism of action identical to that of SSRIs, and there is no strong evidence for superiority of SNRIs or of any single SSRI over others. An optimal trial of SSRIs should last 8–12 weeks to assess acute efficacy; this is somewhat **longer than for the treatment of depression**, although improvement may occur sooner. Antidepressant medications should be initiated at a low dose for patients with panic disorder, who may be vulnerable to initial stimulating effects. The ultimate dosages of antidepressants for the effective treatment of anxiety and stress disorders are generally in the same range as those used for major depression, and patients with OCD often require doses at the high end of this range. For responders to an acute trial, maintenance treatment of at least **6–12 months** is generally indicated to reduce risk of relapse upon medication discontinuation.

If a single trial of an SSRI is ineffective, **switching** to another SSRI may still be effective, although this recommendation is based on limited data. Alternatives include switching to a different class of medication, such as an SNRI, or adding a second medication with a complementary mechanism of action, such as adding benzodiazepines to SSRI treatment of panic disorder or social anxiety disorder. Because there is more heterogeneity of response to second-line treatments among different anxiety disorders, these will be discussed later in the chapter, under specific anxiety disorders.

Benzodiazepines remain widely used in the treatment of anxiety disorders, with benefits including rapid onset of effect; well-substantiated efficacy in panic disorder, social anxiety disorder, and generalized anxiety disorder; and safety in overdose. Although these medications are widely used on an as-needed basis, they are most effective for anxiety disorders when taken on a regular schedule. Drawbacks of benzodiazepines include risk of abuse and dependence, dose-related side effects of sedation, and impairment of cognition and coordination. Unlike the SSRIs, they are not an effective treatment for the depression that often co-occurs with anxiety disorders.

Medication and psychotherapy treatments are often combined to maximize benefit, although research to date suggests that this approach may be superior mainly for selected patients who do not respond completely to a first treatment.

General Principles of Psychotherapy

Cognitive-Behavioral Therapy

Cognitive-behavioral therapy for anxiety, obsessive compulsive, and stress disorders is an empirically validated treatment that is **directive** and **time limited** (typically involving 12–20 weekly sessions). Therapy sessions are structured and often include a combination of empirically validated cognitive and behavioral techniques. Several meta-analytic studies on the efficacy of CBT for adult anxiety disorders have demonstrated medium to large effect sizes for this treatment in comparison to control conditions. Recently, a meta-analysis of 27 studies comparing CBT for adult anxiety disorders to placebo treatments (e.g., supportive counseling, a relaxation condition, pill placebo) found that CBT was significantly more efficacious (Hofmann and Smits, 2008).

CBT targets specific symptoms or problems and sets **specific goals** (e.g., increasing social interactions to twice per week; being able to remain in the presence of a previously feared situation or stimulus; making five calls to seek a new job; tolerating obsessive thoughts without resorting to compulsive behaviors). Types of intervention are then related to specific goals, with therapy often focusing on changing thoughts and behaviors that interfere with these goals. The clinician works with the patient to identify problems, hypothesize solutions, and experiment with different treatment strategies. This method is often referred to as **collaborative empiricism**. Therapists initially teach their patients techniques and gradually coach them to independently apply skills learned in treatment. Patients are assigned homework to help facilitate continued use of CBT skills between sessions. A typical CBT session includes a brief assessment of symptoms, review of the status of the presenting problem and homework assigned, setting the agenda for the current session, learning and practicing a new CBT technique, assigning new homework, and a summary of the session, including a review of goals, progress, and feedback from the patient.

Some common components of CBT include psychoeducation, somatic management, mindfulness, cognitive restructuring, exposure therapy, problem solving, and relapse prevention (see also Chapter 17, Psychotherapy). **Psychoeducation** addresses the causes and maintenance factors of anxiety as well as understanding of the cognitive-behavioral model. Patients are taught basic cognitive and behavioral theory (e.g., how their perception of an event leads to their anxiety and ultimately their behavior). Patients also learn how to monitor their anxiety throughout the week by identifying situations in which they notice that they are experiencing anxiety.

Somatic management typically includes progressive muscle relaxation, breathing retraining, and other self-soothing techniques (e.g., visualizing positive imagery, changing physiological temperature). **Mindfulness** techniques can teach patients to focus their awareness on thoughts, sensations, and emotions in the present moment without avoiding or purposefully changing them. As part of anxiety treatment, mindfulness can help patients learn to observe, tolerate, and accept these occurrences without judgment.

The cognitive component of CBT focuses on helping patients **identify distorted automatic thoughts** and **restructure** them so that they are more adaptive, thus leading to reductions in negative emotions and increases in adaptive behavior. First, they are trained to identify automatic thoughts that lead to their anxious symptoms. The therapist then works with the patient to examine the accuracy of their thoughts by looking for evidence that they are realistic and considering other possibilities. Cognitive distortions are identified by asking questions such as, "Am I magnifying the importance of things or catastrophizing about a situation's consequences?" Once patients recognize that a thought is distorted, they work with the therapist to reframe it by developing a more rational response. Later in the course of therapy, patients work to change their intermediate and core beliefs.

The goal of **exposure therapy** is to have patients approach a feared situation and remain in it until they habituate to the situation, thus reducing anxiety. Patients receive positive reinforcement for engaging in proactive behavior (e.g., by the therapist praising them for their effort, by feeling good once they realize they can do it, and by rewarding themselves). Before beginning exposure therapy, therapists review the rationale with their patients, explaining that avoidance leads to the maintenance of anxiety, which exposure will help reduce. Patients' concerns are addressed, and therapists strive to obtain their commitment to the treatment (Leahy et al. 2012).

Therapists typically work with their patients to create a **fear and avoidance hierarchy**, which lists objects or situations in order of the degree to which they are feared and/or avoided. Patients are taught to rate their fear of each situation or object on a **Subjective Units of Distress (SUDS) scale** from 0 to 10. The information provided by the patient will be the basis for future exposure exercises. For example, a patient diagnosed with OCD who has obsessions and compulsions related to cleanliness may report that walking by a garbage can would result in a SUDS score of 3, while touching the garbage can for 20 seconds would be a 7, and touching the garbage inside the can for 20 seconds without washing their hands for 15 minutes would be a 10. Once the therapist has gathered this information, exposure typically begins with an activity thought to elicit a moderate amount of anxiety (e.g., a SUDS scale score of 4).

During an exposure task, SUDS scores typically increase and are maintained before they decrease. Therapists prevent patients from leaving the situation until their SUDS score has dropped by at least 50%, to ensure that their anxiety has habituated. Otherwise, the connection between the situation and the anxiety may be reinforced. The exposure exercise is repeated in and between sessions until anxiety becomes minimal or nonexistent. Patients then continue working up their hierarchy in a graduated fashion, making modifications with the therapist as clinically indicated. Some therapists may choose to have the patient engage in flooding, which involves beginning with the most feared activity in the hierarchy and preventing the patient from escaping the situation; however, graduated exposure is more likely to engage a patient in treatment.

Some therapists teach their patients **coping skills** such as deep breathing, relaxation, or coping statements to use during the exposure. Others think that this prevents the patient from fully experiencing the anxiety and therefore prevents them from fully habituating. Therapists may begin with imaginal exposure, having patients close their eyes and imagine the situation as they listen to the therapist provide a detailed account of what it would be like to be in the feared situation. This is particularly common when there is no realistic way to confront the feared stimulus (e.g., patients diagnosed with PTSD after a war cannot actually return to the field of battle where they saw someone shot). However, in vivo techniques are optimal when possible. Cognitive restructuring techniques can also be part of exposure therapy. For example, therapists can identify a patient's negative automatic thoughts about engaging in this technique, work to test and reframe these thoughts, and review the patient's thoughts after an exposure exercise.

Problem solving is typically used to help patients clarify their goals, brainstorm and evaluate solutions to problems, assess outcomes, and address related obstacles. Finally, a central feature of CBT is **relapse prevention**, which teaches patients to essentially be their own therapist by identifying changes in their mood, challenging their thoughts, examining their behavior, assessing their progress, and setting goals to prevent or reduce further symptoms and manage problems before they become exacerbated (Beck, 1995).

Psychodynamic Psychotherapy

Psychoanalytically based treatments for anxiety disorders uncover ingrained and largely unconscious patterns from childhood that are active in current anxiety-provoking situations. As the patient's **emotional conflicts** are identified and resolved, the current stimulus may lose its power to inflict anxiety. Treatments involve varying measures of exploration, support, and positive suggestion, depending on the phase of the treatment, the severity of the symptoms, and the availability of the underlying emotional themes. A small number of recent controlled trials have suggested possible efficacy for psychoanalytic-based therapies for specific anxiety disorders, improving on the previous literature of anecdotal case reports.

ETIOLOGY AND TREATMENT OF SPECIFIC ANXIETY DISORDERS

Panic Disorder and Agoraphobia

Etiology

Attention to the neurobiology of panic was stimulated in the 1960s by the observation that a panic attack can be reproduced by infusion of chemical agents such as lactate. This paradigm was extended to the study of carbon dioxide inhalation as a "panicogen," and developed into a theory of panic disorder as a dysfunction of an adaptive **suffocation alarm mechanism** that, in response to a physiologic misinterpretation, leads to respiratory distress, hyperventilation, and a desire to escape (Klein 1993). Recent studies suggest that laboratory panicogens cause peripheral somatic sensations resembling those in natural panic attacks, sensations which patients misinterpret as an impending catastrophic event, a phenomenon known as anxiety sensitivity. Brain imaging studies have suggested amygdala hyperactivity and decreased prefrontal cortical regulation of fear circuitry.

Pharmacotherapy

While **SSRIs** and **SNRIs** have emerged as the first-line pharmacotherapy for panic disorder on the basis of multiple randomized, controlled trials, benzodiazepines, of which clonazepam and alprazolam have been best studied, are also often used on a daily basis. For the panic disorder patient who presents in crisis, **benzodiazepines** have the advantage of rapid onset of action. Sometimes both classes of drugs are started initially and benzodiazepines are later tapered off. The older class of tricyclic antidepressants, particularly imipramine and clomipramine, have also appeared effective in controlled trials, but these are less commonly used because of higher rates of adverse effects.

Cognitive-Behavioral Therapy

CBT for panic disorder typically begins with psychoeducation about the cognitive-behavioral model of panic (i.e., maladaptive interpretations of physiological symptoms), related physiological arousal, including the fight-or-flight response (activation of the sympathetic nervous system), and the physiological effects of hyperventilation. Treatment includes techniques such as breathing retraining, progressive muscle relaxation, and challenging and restructuring distorted thoughts (e.g., catastrophizing the meaning of symptoms) to reduce anxiety. "Interoceptive exposure," or exposure to the induction of bodily sensations (e.g., via vigorous exercise or induced hyperventilation), is typically conducted to teach patients how to cope with experiencing somatic symptoms. Developing a hierarchy of in vivo exposure activities for avoided situations in which patients fear they will panic is also typical, particularly for patients who are diagnosed with agoraphobia. Goals include the elimination of safety behaviors (e.g., companion while driving, sitting down to prevent fainting from anxiety) (Leahy et al. 2012). A meta-analysis of 124 CBT and pharmacotherapy studies for panic disorder demonstrated efficacy for both approaches (Mitte 2005a).

Social Anxiety Disorder (Social Phobia)

Etiology

Social anxiety disorder often develops out of childhood traits of shyness and behavioral inhibition, a tendency to avoid novel people and situations that can be assessed in toddlers and is moderately heritable. Less frequently, specific social traumas appear to have etiological importance. From an evolutionary perspective, this disorder has been conceptualized as a misadaptation related to **submissive behaviors** that are seen across group-living species. Persons with social anxiety disorder have been shown to have increased vigilance for social threats, as exemplified in studies assessing response to threatening facial expressions, and hyperactivity of the amygdala and associated fear circuitry in response to social threats. Other studies have suggested abnormalities in serotonin, dopamine, GABA, and HPA-axis systems.

Pharmacotherapy

SSRIs and the SNRI **venlafaxine** are well established as treatments for social anxiety disorder, based on multiple randomized, controlled trials. Single randomized, controlled trials have also supported the efficacy of the benzodiazepine clonazepam, the alpha-2-delta calcium channel agents gabapentin and pregabalin, and the antidepressant mirtazepine. Monoamine oxidase inhibitors (MAOIs) have also appeared highly effective in several randomized, controlled trials, but these are rarely used because of the higher risk of adverse effects. Most clinical trials have not specifically studied the subgroup with fear limited to **performance situations**, although small trials have suggested that either beta-adrenergic blockers or benzodiazepines can be useful when taken on an as-needed basis for performance fears.

Cognitive-Behavioral Therapy

CBT for social anxiety disorder focuses on restructuring distorted thoughts related to social evaluation and performance as well as exposure to social situations that have been avoided or that result in intense anxiety. A fear hierarchy is created to use during exposure tasks. Typically, role-playing, imaginal exposure, or both are conducted before patients practice exposures repeatedly in vivo. During in vivo exposure, patients are encouraged to eliminate safety behaviors, such as drinking alcohol, and to engage in avoidance behaviors, such as disagreeing with someone in a conversation. They often learn how to shift their focus from internal physical sensations of anxiety to external cues, such as the conversation with the person they are speaking to or their physical environment. Social skills training may also be warranted (Leahy, Holland, & McGinn 2012). Comparative studies of CBT and medication for social anxiety disorder have shown roughly similar response rates, and the efficacy of both approaches has been supported by meta-analyses.

Obsessive-Compulsive Disorder

Etiology

The specificity of response to serotonergic medications in OCD has led to a focus on serotonin in its etiology, but evidence remains conflicting. Neuroimaging studies have identified a distinct pattern of dysfunction that appears to differ from the abnormalities in fear circuitry described for panic disorder, PTSD, and the phobias. OCD is instead associated with dysfunction in the **corticostriatal circuit** linking the orbitofrontal cortex, caudate nuclei, and globus pallidus, and with resolution of these abnormalities upon response to treatment with medication or CBT. Support for the role of basal ganglia in OCD also comes from evidence of obsessive-compulsive symptoms in neurological disorders that involve the basal ganglia, such as Huntington's disease and PANDAS (pediatric autoimmune neuropsychiatric disorders associated with streptococcus), which in some cases are characterized by antistriatal autoantibodies.

In addition, OCD occurs with greater frequency in patients with Sydenham's chorea or ischemic injury to the caudate. The repetitive nature of obsessions and compulsions has been associated with neurobehavioral concepts of difficulties filtering stimuli, and with animal models involving stereotypies or excessive grooming behaviors.

Pharmacotherapy

Serotonergic reuptake inhibitors (**SSRIs** and **clomipramine**) have been well established as first-line pharmacotherapy, based on numerous randomized, controlled trials. Although the SSRIs and clomipramine are clearly helpful for OCD, relatively high doses are often required, and the magnitude of benefit is sometimes limited. The only other medications found helpful in replicated randomized, controlled trials are **second-generation (atypical) antipsychotics** when used as augmentation to ongoing SSRI treatment. These medications have appeared useful for patients who do not respond completely to SSRIs, even in the absence of any psychotic symptoms. However, because of potential serious adverse effects (e.g., extrapyramidal symptoms, tardive dyskinesia, and metabolic syndrome), the risks and benefits of antipsychotics must be weighed carefully.

Cognitive-Behavioral Therapy

CBT for OCD focuses on exposure to obsessions while resisting engagement in compulsions or other kinds of avoidance. Typically, the patient and therapist work together to develop a hierarchy of obsessions and avoided situations and stimuli, from least to most anxiety provoking. Exposure to each step on the hierarchy is then conducted, via imaginal and/or in vivo techniques, while patients prevent their ritualized response (e.g., refrain from washing their hands after riding a train while thinking about the likelihood that they have contracted a disease).

Some patients diagnosed with OCD will need to participate in imaginal exposure to their thoughts (e.g., their loved ones getting hurt) without engaging in mental rituals such as counting or praying. Often, exposure exercises are continued beyond the top of a patient's hierarchy to reinforce the idea that if they can engage in an exaggerated activity (e.g., dig through garbage without washing their hands for 30 minutes afterward), they can manage situations that occur in daily life (e.g., brush against a garbage can) (Leahy et al. 2012).

Studies comparing medication and CBT treatments of OCD have suggested that patients who are able to comply with CBT tend to show greater benefit and are less likely to relapse after treatment is discontinued.

Posttraumatic Stress Disorder

Etiology

Neurophysiological alterations found in patients with PTSD include hyperresponsive fear circuitry, increased sympathetic activity, and abnormal HPA function. The stress hormone cortisol, which is increased acutely post-trauma, is often persistently low and nonresponsive to stressors in chronic PTSD. Several studies have reported reduced volumes of anterior cingulate cortex and hippocampus volume, either as an antecedent predisposing factor or possibly as a consequence of PTSD. As only a minority of persons exposed to a traumatic event go on to develop chronic PTSD, some research has viewed PTSD as a failure of the normal fear extinction processes.

Pharmacotherapy

SSRIs are the only medications with an FDA indication for PTSD, based on multiple randomized, controlled trials. The magnitude of their benefit as monotherapy is often inadequate, however, and their efficacy for PTSD in the absence of concomitant psychotherapy has been questioned. A small number of randomized, controlled trials have demonstrated efficacy for the alpha-adrenergic blocker prazosin as an adjunctive medication that targets sleep disturbance, although side effects of hypotension may occur. Benzodiazepines have generally not appeared efficacious in PTSD. Studies of civilian-related PTSD have tended to demonstrate greater responsiveness to treatment than that shown in studies of combat-related PTSD, but the reasons for this are unclear. Pilot studies have suggested possible efficacy for pharmacological strategies administered immediately post-trauma (e.g., beta blockers) to interfere with consolidation of traumatic memories.

Cognitive-Behavioral Therapy

CBT for PTSD typically focuses on coping with trauma-related anxiety, exposure to memories of the trauma, and cognitive restructuring. First, patients are taught to manage their anxiety regarding the traumatic experience via techniques such as progressive muscle relaxation or controlled breathing. Imaginal exposure then focuses on specific details of the trauma, such as the various sensations and emotions that were experienced. Exposures to feared internal and external cues (e.g., dizziness, sounds of helicopters) should also be incorporated into treatment. Patients may be asked to write narratives or draw pictures of their traumatic experiences and discuss them in therapy. In vivo exposure is also typically conducted to return the patient to situations that have been avoided since the traumatic event (e.g., returning to the area one experienced an earthquake).

Emotion regulation and mindfulness skills may benefit patients with complex or severe PTSD or those who have difficulty engaging in exposures. Finally, cognitive restructuring may be used to reframe distorted thoughts, such as "I should have been able to prevent it" or "Something terrible could happen at any minute." Cognitive techniques can also be used to help engage patients in exposure exercises (Leahy et al. 2012). In a meta-analysis of 38 randomized, controlled trials focused on psychosocial treatment for PTSD, the strongest evidence was found for trauma-focused CBT (Bisson et al. 2007).

An alternative trauma-focused psychotherapy for PTSD is eye movement desensitization and reprocessing (EMDR), although it is unclear whether its therapeutic effects are due to specific eye movement techniques or to more general elements in common with cognitive-behavioral therapies.

Generalized Anxiety Disorder

Etiology

Generalized anxiety disorder appears to share genetic risk factors with depression, and depression and other disorders frequently co-occur with this condition. Worry in generalized anxiety disorder may function physiologically to dampen autonomic nervous system arousal.

Pharmacotherapy

The **SSRIs** and **SNRIs** have been shown effective for generalized anxiety disorder in multiple randomized, controlled trials. The serotonin 1a receptor partial agonist **buspirone** has also been shown to be efficacious but appears to have a relatively smaller magnitude of effect. **Benzodiazepines** have appeared as effective as SSRIs in several randomized, controlled trials, but their use is limited by risks of abuse and dependence. Other medications with some evidence for efficacy include tricyclic antidepressants and antihistamines.

Cognitive-Behavioral Therapy

CBT for generalized anxiety disorder typically focuses on normalizing and controlling worry, reducing avoidant behavior, and increasing stress management. Treatment often includes relaxation training. Patients may also be trained in mindfulness techniques, such as observing worries and related feelings without trying to exert control over them or judging them. They are often told to schedule a specific time during the day when they must worry, and are told to prolong worrying until this prescribed time period. Patients learn to differentiate between productive and unproductive worry (e.g., "what if" questions), as well as how to tolerate and accept uncertainty (e.g., repeat a feared thought and focus on accepting it). Distorted thoughts (e.g., catastrophizing, fortune telling) are identified, challenged, and altered. Imaginal or in vivo exposure is often used to help patients confront avoided situations.

Finally, problem solving related to productive worries and interpersonal interventions (e.g., assertiveness training) are often also part of treatment. Some CBT therapists teach patients how to distract themselves from their worries, which may include mental exercises such as counting backward or scheduling pleasant activities (Leahy et al. 2012). One meta-analysis of 65 treatment studies for generalized anxiety disorder indicated that CBT was superior to control conditions, and "at least as" efficacious as benzodiazepines (Mitte 2005b).

Specific Phobias

Etiology

Specific phobias have been associated with fear circuitry that is hypersensitive to specific threat-related cues.

Pharmacotherapy

Pharmacotherapy of specific phobias has not been well studied, although there is anecdotal evidence for efficacy of benzodiazepines taken on an as-needed basis for anticipated phobic situations, such as a taking an airplane flight.

Cognitive-Behavioral Therapy

In CBT, patients are provided with psychoeducation regarding evolutionary, behavioral, and cognitive models of the relationship among fear, escape, and avoidance. Typically, CBT therapists will help the patient generate a fear hierarchy of potential imaginal and/or in vivo situations using the SUDS system outlined earlier. In vivo exposures are considered most preferable. Activities lower on the hierarchy may include viewing pictures of the feared stimulus or participant modeling, which entails watching the therapist engage in appropriate behavior with the feared stimulus or activity before the patient does (e.g., being in a room with a clown, holding a snake). Graduated exposure, or working up the patient's hierarchy, is better tolerated than flooding, which involves immediately engaging the patient in the most feared situation until the anxiety decreases (e.g., putting a patient with a dog phobia into a dog run until his or her anxiety is reduced). Patients are encouraged to eliminate safety behaviors, such as carrying anxiolytic medication or engaging in prayer. Cognitive restructuring may also be used (Leahy et al. 2012).

CBT for specific phobias is often effective in very few sessions, and studies have demonstrated that one-session exposure therapy for various specific phobias (e.g., airplane, spider) is as effective as five sessions. Conducting exposure tasks through virtual reality equipment (i.e., computerized, visual and auditory depictions and kinesthetic sensations of feared situations) is an innovative, effective method for treating specific phobias such as airplanes and heights (Krijn et al. 2004) and can be useful as part of graduated exposure or if initial in vivo exposure would be financially costly (e.g., plane tickets). Applied tension (tensing muscles to increase arousal) treatments are often effective for treating blood-injury phobias. One meta-analysis of 33 studies of treatment for specific phobia found that exposure-based treatment was superior to placebo or alternative psychotherapeutic treatments (Wolitsky-Taylor et al. 2008).

Substance/Medication-Induced Anxiety Disorder

Etiology

The concept that an addictive substance may induce an anxiety disorder is intriguing and controversial. Although it may seem illogical that an "anxiolytic" such as alcohol can, in the long run, actually create an anxiety disorder, **prolonged alcohol consumption** and repeated alcohol withdrawals may sensitize individuals via a **kindling** effect, in which each successive withdrawal decreases the threshold for anxiety (Racine 1979). Panic and other types of anxiety could conceivably be kindled by repeated, progressively more severe episodes of alcohol withdrawal. The possibility of such a development underscores the importance of adequately treating all episodes of alcohol withdrawal. It has been shown that the blunted responsiveness of the noradrenergic α_2-autoreceptors is correlated with the number of episodes of alcohol withdrawal; this lends support to the kindling hypothesis.

Although use of a substance or withdrawal from a substance may be a primary cause of anxiety, in other cases use of a substance may be a way to "self-medicate" and temporarily relieve feelings of nervousness and worry caused by an underlying anxiety disorder. Often treatment must be directed at both the substance use disorder and the anxiety disorder symptoms to maximize benefit.

REFERENCES CITED

Beck, J. *Cognitive Therapy: Basics and Beyond.* New York: Guilford Press, 1995.

Bisson, J. I., A. Ehlers, R. Matthews, S. Pilling, D. Richards, and S. Turner. Psychological treatments for chronic post-traumatic stress disorder. *British Journal of Psychiatry* 190:97–104, 2007.

Etkin, A., and T. D. Wager. Functional neuroimaging of anxiety: a meta-analysis of emotional processing in PTSD, social anxiety disorder, and specific phobia. *American Journal of Psychiatry* 164:1476–1488, 2007.

Hofmann, S. G., and A. J. Smits. Cognitive-behavioral therapy for adult anxiety disorders: a meta-analysis of randomized placebo-controlled trials. *Journal of Clinical Psychiatry* 69:621–632, 2008.

Klein, D. F. False suffocation alarms, spontaneous panics, and related conditions: an integrative hypothesis. *Archives of General Psychiatry* 50:306–317, 1993.

Krijn, M., P. M. G. Emmelkamp, R. P. Olafsson, and R. Biemond. Virtual reality exposure therapy of anxiety disorders: a review. *Clinical Psychology Review* 24:259–281, 2004.

Leahy, R. L., S. J. F. Holland, and L. K. McGinn. *Treatment Plans and Interventions for Depression and Anxiety Disorders*, 2nd ed. New York: Guilford Press, 2012.

LeDoux, J. E. Emotion circuits in the brain. *Annual Review of Neuroscience* 23:155–184, 2000.

Mitte, K. A meta-analysis of the efficacy of psycho- and pharmacotherapy in panic disorder with and without agoraphobia. *Journal of Affective Disorders* 88:7–45, 2005a.

Mitte, K. Meta-analysis of cognitive-behavioral treatments for generalized anxiety disorder: a comparison with psychotherapy. *Psychological Bulletin* 131:785–795, 2005b.

Racine, R. Kindling: the first decade. *Neurosurgery* 3:234–252, 1979.

Wolitsky-Taylor, K. B., J. D. Horowitz, M. B. Powers, and M. J. Telch. Psychological approaches in the treatment of specific phobias: a meta-analysis. *Clinical Psychology Review* 28:1021–1037, 2008.

SELECTED READINGS

Barlow, D.H., ed. *Clinical Handbook of Psychological Disorders, Fourth Edition: A Step-by-Step Treatment Manual*. New York: Guilford Press, 2008.

Herman, J. L. *Trauma and Recovery*. New York: Basic Books, 1992.

James, W. *The Principles of Psychology*. New York: Holt, 1890.

Kardiner, A., and H. Spiegel. *The Traumatic Neuroses of War*. New York: Paul Hoeber, 1947.

Leonardo, E., and R. Hen. Anxiety as a developmental disorder. *Neuropsychopharmacology* 33:134–140, 2008.

Milrod, B., A. C. Leon, F. Busch, M. Rudden, M. Schwalberg, J. Clarkin, A. Aronson, M. Singer, W. Turchin, E.T. Klass, E. Graf, J. J. Teres, and M. K. Shear. A randomized controlled clinical trial of psychoanalytic psychotherapy for panic disorder. *American Journal of Psychiatry* 164:265–272, 2007.

Poulton, R., G. Andrews, and J. Millichamp. Gene–environment interaction and the anxiety disorders. *European Archives of Psychiatry and Clinical Neuroscience* 258:65–68, 2008.

Simpson, H. B., Y. Neria, R. Lewis-Fernandez, and F. Schneier, eds. *Anxiety Disorders: Theory, Research and Clinical Perspectives*. Cambridge, UK: Cambridge University Press, 2010.

Stein, D. J., E. Hollander, and B. O. Rothbaum, eds. *Textbook of Anxiety Disorders*, 2nd ed. Washington, DC: American Psychiatric Publishing, 2010.

7

Substance-Related and Addictive Disorders

Benjamin R. Bryan and Frances R. Levin

Alcohol and illicit drug use are common in the United States, and alcohol and other substance use disorders are among the most common problems encountered in medical settings. These disorders are associated with extraordinary personal and societal costs. Health problems, decreased academic or job performance, crime and violence, and relationship difficulties are all associated with substance use disorders. Two large, face-to-face surveys employing structured interviews to estimate the prevalence and severity of substance use disorders within the adult population of the United States found that substance use disorders are common, disabling, and undertreated (Compton et al. 2007; Hasin et al. 2007; Kessler et al. 2005). The surveys estimated the lifetime prevalence of alcohol and drug use disorders at 30.3% and 10.3%, respectively. See Box 7.1 for additional details about the epidemiology of substance use in the United States.

The detection of substance use disorders is often complicated by patients' inability or unwillingness to acknowledge their problematic use of substances. Although these disorders often include significant physical and emotional complications, many patients tend to have limited insight about the impact that substance use has on their lives and may deny or underreport the extent of their use. Detecting alcohol and substance use disorders is made even more difficult by the insidious nature of addictive illness. Many people can drink alcohol or use other psychoactive drugs occasionally without any negative effects on their physical or emotional well-being. Only a minority of individuals who use alcohol or other substances will develop problematic use. Predicting who these individuals will be is difficult.

DIAGNOSTIC AND CLINICAL FEATURES

The *Diagnostic and Statistical Manual of Mental Disorders,* Fifth Edition (DSM-5) conceptual approach to psychiatric disorders associated with substance use, referred to as substance-related and addictive disorders, distinguishes substance use disorders from substance-induced disorders.

BOX 7.1

EPIDEMIOLOGY OF SUBSTANCE USE IN THE UNITED STATES

The following statistics were gathered in 2010 and 2011 and where applicable are based on DSM-IV diagnostic criteria for substance abuse (maladaptive pattern of substance use without substance dependence) and substance dependence diagnoses.

GENERAL TRENDS IN ALCOHOL USE

According to 2011 estimates, over half of Americans report being current drinkers of alcohol, meaning they consumed alcohol at least once in the past 30 days. Nearly one in four people age 12 or older report binge drinking (more than five drinks in a given day) in the past 30 days and about 6% of people age 12 or older report binge drinking on 5 or more out of the past 30 days. In 2011, 14.4 million Americans met DSM-IV criteria for alcohol abuse or dependence.

GENERAL TRENDS IN TOBACCO USE

Approximately 30% of Americans over age 12 are past-month users of tobacco. Approximately 13% of the U.S. population over age 12 is thought to be have a nicotine use disorder. The highest rate of current tobacco use is among adults age 18 to 25 (43.9%). Over 10% of young people age 12 to 17 are current users of tobacco, with equal numbers of male and female smokers. According to the Centers for Disease Control and Prevention, tobacco use remains the leading preventable cause of death in the United States. Approximately 440,000 premature deaths per year are attributable to tobacco use. An estimated $75 billion in direct medical costs are attributable to smoking. Use of illicit drugs and alcohol is much more prevalent among current cigarette smokers than among nonsmokers. The yearly number of alcohol- and tobacco-related deaths eclipses the number of deaths from all illicit drugs combined.

GENERAL TRENDS IN ILLICIT DRUG USE

Nearly half (45.4%) of Americans age 12 years or older have tried an illicit drug during their lifetime. Of those, nearly 90% have used marijuana or hashish, approximately 45% have used a prescription drug for a nonmedical reason, and approximately 30% have used cocaine. Approximately 8.3% of individuals aged 12 years or older have used illicit drugs within the past 30 days. Most people who have used illicit drugs do not continue to use regularly.

Marijuana

Nearly 75% of all current illicit drug users use marijuana. More than 1 in 10 marijuana users is a daily or almost daily user. An estimated 40% of past year marijuana users meet criteria for marijuana abuse or dependence (Compton et al. 2004).

Cocaine

Approximately 14% of Americans age 12 years or older have used cocaine at least once in their lifetime. In 2011, 0.5% of Americans age 12 years or older had used

(continued)

cocaine within the past month, and approximately 0.1% are current crack cocaine users. Approximately 8% of all substance use treatment admissions are for cocaine. The number of treatment admissions for cocaine declined from 1996 to 2006. During 2011, almost 40% of drug-related emergency room visits involved cocaine.

NONMEDICAL USE OF PRESCRIPTION MEDICATIONS

One in five Americans has used prescription medications (e.g., pain relievers, stimulants, and sedatives) nonmedically at least once in their lifetime, and nearly 3% are current nonmedical users of prescription medications, making it the most frequently used class of illicit drugs apart from marijuana.

Opioid Pain Relievers

Nearly 15% of Americans age 12 and older has used opioid pain relievers nonmedically at least once in their lifetime, and approximately 2% are current nonmedical users of prescription pain relievers. The 2007 Monitoring the Future study (Johnston et al. 2008) reported that approximately 1 in 10 twelfth graders had used hydrocodone without a doctor's prescription. Among persons who use pain relievers nonmedically, over half report obtaining the drug from a friend or relative for free.

Sedatives

Fewer than 1% of Americans age 12 and older are current nonmedical users of prescription CNS depressants (benzodiazepines and barbiturates).

Stimulants

Approximately 0.5% of the population age 12 and older are current nonmedical users of prescription stimulants (amphetamine preparations, methylphenidate). Misuse of these medications is prevalent and on the rise. In the past year, an estimated 5% to 9% of grade and high school–aged children have taken a stimulant medication not prescribed to them or taken a stimulant medication in a way it was not prescribed (higher dosage, combined with alcohol or illicit drug use). The 2012 Monitoring the Future study (Johnston et al. 2012) reported that approximately 1 in 10 twelfth graders used amphetamine without a doctor's prescription. This type of misuse of prescription stimulant preparations is even more common among college-aged individuals, ranging from 5% to 35%. Approximately 1 in 10 individuals with a diagnosis of ADHD and a prescription for a stimulant medication report selling their medication during the prior 4 years, and nearly 1 in 3 report selling their prescription at least once in their lifetime (Wilens et al. 2008).

METHAMPHETAMINE

An estimated 5.1% of the United States population aged 12 or older has used methamphetamine at least once in their lifetime for nonmedical purposes. Methamphetamine use is more common in western states in the United States. The 2012 Monitoring the Future survey indicated that 1.7% of twelfth graders

(continued)

had used methamphetamine at least once. Approximately 6% of all substance abuse treatment admissions were for methamphetamine in 2010. The number of treatment admissions for methamphetamine increased greatly over the 10 years from 1996 to 2006. During 2011, 8.2% of drug-related emergency room visits involved methamphetamine.

HEROIN

Approximately 1.6% of Americans age 12 or older has used heroin at least once during their lifetime, and 0.1% are current heroin users. Over 40% of past-year heroin users inject heroin intravenously. The average age at first use is 20.7 years. Approximately 14% of all substance abuse treatment admissions are for heroin. The number of treatment admissions for heroin increased over the 10 years from 1996 to 2006. During 2011, 20% of drug-related emergency room visits involved heroin.

HALLUCINOGENS

Approximately 14.1% of Americans age 12 or older has used hallucinogens at least once during their lifetime, and approximately 0.4% report past-month use of hallucinogens. In 2010, treatment admissions for hallucinogens accounted for only 0.1% of the total number of admissions.

INHALANTS

Approximately 8% of Americans age 12 and older has used inhalants at least once in their lifetime. Approximately 0.2% are current inhalant users. In 2010, treatment admissions for inhalants accounted for only 0.1% of the total number of admissions. Of these treatment admissions, most were male and nearly 30% were under the age of 18.

Source: *Office of Applied Studies (OAP). 2011 National Survey on Drug Use & Health: National Results. http://oas.samhsa.gov (accessed July 2013).*

Substance Use Disorders

A *substance use disorder* refers to a patient's problematic pattern of substance use that results in **significant impairment or distress**. To make a judgment about the problematic nature of a patient's behavior, the physician must view it within the context of the patient's individual circumstances and societal strictures (e.g., while it may be socially appropriate for a healthy young adult to drink two glasses of wine at dinner, it is generally not acceptable for a 6-year-old or an elderly individual with diabetes to drink in a similar manner). Tolerance and withdrawal are two signs of problematic use. **Tolerance** means that increasing amounts of a drug are needed to produce the same degree of intoxication, or, to put it another way, that the same amount of the drug produces less of the desired effect. **Withdrawal** symptoms are defined as symptoms that are judged by the physician to occur because the patient has stopped using or is using less of a particular drug. Not all substances of abuse have a defined withdrawal syndrome; therefore, this criterion does not apply to all substances. Patients have **physical dependence** if they demonstrate tolerance or suffer from, or must use a drug to avoid, symptoms of withdrawal. Although the term **addiction** is not used diagnostically in the DSM-5, the term is still commonly used to describe a patient's substance use. Addiction can be conceptualized as the behavioral problems associated with maladaptive substance use (see case example in Box 7.2).

Importantly, physiological dependence is not the same as addiction. For example, therapeutic use of opioid analgesics may lead to physiological dependence with tolerance and withdrawal, but this is not the same as addiction or the DSM-5 diagnosis of

---

BOX 7.2

EVOLUTION OF ADDICTION: A CASE OF METHAMPHETAMINE DEPENDENCE

A 26-year-old recent law school graduate relocated to Manhattan to start his first job as an attorney. Throughout college and law school he regularly binge-drank alcohol on weekends and occasionally used cocaine intranasally (less than monthly). Shortly after arriving in New York City, he began frequenting gay bars and nightclubs to meet men. He eventually befriended a group of men who frequently used cocaine and crystal methamphetamine during the course of a night out.

Over the course of 6 months he began occasionally using methamphetamine on Friday or Saturday nights. Over the following months his use became more frequent and in larger amounts. When high, he would have sex with anonymous partners who were also using. Occasionally, he would engage in unprotected sex. He began binging most weekends, starting Friday and ending on Sunday afternoon. He started having trouble paying his rent despite his adequate salary. As time passed, he began occasionally missing work on Mondays because of his weekend use, despite a weekly promise to himself that he would not use again. While he initially had only used methamphetamine intranasally, he began smoking and finally began using intravenously. With increasing frequency, he began using the Internet to find other anonymous sexual partners with whom he would get high. His use continued until his supervisor at his firm became alarmed by his increasing absenteeism and dramatic weight loss. After the confrontation by his supervisor, he sought treatment at an outpatient clinic. His initial evaluation found that he had contracted syphilis and hepatitis C but remained HIV negative.

This case demonstrates a typical progression of substance use from casual use without many negative consequences to a substance use disorder with significant difficulty controlling substance use and marked social impairment. Disinhibition and increased risk-taking with drug and alcohol use may increase the likelihood of high-risk sexual behaviors. Substance-using young adults have higher rates of sexually transmitted infections than their non-using counterparts. Stimulant use has been positively associated with an increased number of sexual partners. Intravenous drug use put the individual in this case at extraordinarily increased risk for contracting HIV and hepatitis C. Involvement with an employee assistance program may be key in getting a patient into formal addiction treatment.

opioid use disorder. Substance use disorders are classified according to the particular substance: alcohol; cannabis; phencyclidine; other hallucinogens; inhalants; opioids; sedatives, hypnotics, or anxiolytics; stimulants; tobacco; and caffeine (see DSM-5). These disorders are designated as mild, moderate, or severe depending on the number of criteria met during the past 12 months.

Substance-Induced Disorders

Intoxication occurs when a substance's effect on the central nervous system (CNS) produces **maladaptive behavioral or psychological changes**. Intoxication can be either **acute or chronic,** and it can occur in the absence of a substance use disorder. Withdrawal is frequently associated with more severe substance use but, as previously described, is neither necessary nor sufficient to make this diagnosis. Other substance-induced disorders tend to occur in the context of a substance use disorder. Although substance use and substance-induced disorders are separate entities, the two types of disorders frequently coexist in the same patient, making the physician's index of suspicion and detection of substance-induced disorders doubly important (see Differential Diagnosis, later in this chapter).

Psychiatric symptoms caused by the substance-induced states of intoxication or withdrawal can mimic symptoms of primary psychiatric disorders, particularly mood, psychotic, anxiety, and neurocognitive disorders, including delirium and dementia (see Chapter 3, Mood Disorders; Chapter 4, Schizophrenia and Other Psychotic Disorders; Chapter 5, Neurocognitive Disorders and Mental Disorders Due to Another Medical Condition; and Chapter 6, Anxiety, Obsessive-Compulsive, and Stress Disorders). They are distinguished from the primary disorders in these categories on the basis of their etiology, which is substance use.

To make an adequate diagnosis and distinguish substance-induced disorders from preexisting psychiatric conditions, it is necessary to know which psychiatric symptoms are produced by which classes of drugs at different stages of use. This is particularly true of the symptoms of acute and chronic intoxication and withdrawal. The most common signs and symptoms of the substance-induced disorders are presented according to the major classes of abused substances.

Alcohol and Other Sedatives

Alcohol and other CNS depressants (e.g., benzodiazepines, barbiturates, and many other drugs known as "downers" or by a plethora of other street names) are commonly abused. The **symptoms of acute intoxication** (see DSM-5) are the same for all of these substances (see Table 7.1). An individual's age, weight, sex, and level of tolerance and the setting in which the substance is used influence the effect that alcohol has on the individual's

TABLE 7.1 Symptoms of Acute Intoxication with Alcohol and Other Sedatives

- Slurred speech
- Impaired coordination
- Unsteady gait
- Nystagmus (horizontal)
- Impairment of attention or memory
- Stupor or coma

TABLE 7.2 Symptoms of Withdrawal from Alcohol and Other Sedatives

- Autonomic hyperactivity (increased heart rate, blood pressure, respiratory rate, body temperature, sweating)
- Anxiety
- Insomnia
- Psychomotor agitation
- Nausea or vomiting
- Tremor
- Transient visual, tactile, or auditory hallucinations or illusions
- Grand mal seizures

behavior. During heavy alcohol consumption, some drinkers will experience **blackouts** in which they forget or are unaware of what occurred while drinking. This phenomenon is due to high levels of alcohol impairing memory formation in the hippocampus and *is not the same* as "passing out" from drinking.

When chronic users of large amounts of alcohol or other sedatives abruptly discontinue their use, they can experience dramatic **symptoms of withdrawal** (see DSM-5) (see Table 7.2). Symptoms of alcohol withdrawal can be assessed with the **Clinical Institute Withdrawal of Alcohol Scale (CIWA)** (Table 7.3), a 10-item structured assessment of objective and subjective signs and symptoms of withdrawal. Symptoms of withdrawal can emerge as soon as 4 to 8 hours after cessation of drinking, usually reach **peak intensity by day 2**, and improve by day 5. Mild symptoms may persist for months. Severe withdrawal occurs in less than 5% of alcohol-dependent people and includes seizures or delirium. **Delirium tremens**, or DTs, is characterized by **severe autonomic hyperactivity**, **tremor**, **altered consciousness**, and **hallucinations**. Delirium tremens is associated with older age, large quantity of alcohol consumption, longer history of dependence, and concomitant medical problems. Because substance withdrawal delirium can be a life-threatening condition, it is imperative that physicians consider this diagnosis when evaluating delirious patients (see Chapter 5, Neurocognitive Disorders and Mental Disorders Due to Another Medical Condition). The failure to obtain a history of heavy drinking from a patient prior to surgery may result in the development of seizures or delirium due to withdrawal a few days postoperatively.

Depression is a less dramatic but nonetheless life-threatening complication associated with chronic sedative use and withdrawal. Depressive symptoms associated with sedative withdrawal usually diminish within a few weeks, but they may persist, requiring pharmacological intervention, inpatient hospitalization, or both. While intoxicated or distressed by withdrawal symptoms, patients may act on suicidal impulses.

Heavy chronic alcohol use over a period of years is associated with hallucinations and delusions. **Alcohol-induced psychotic disorder with hallucinations or delusions** usually occurs in the context of a **clear sensorium** and does not represent a medical emergency. Unlike the hallucinations associated with withdrawal, alcoholic hallucinations are primarily, but not exclusively, auditory. In contrast to delirium tremens, **alcoholic hallucinosis** and **paranoia** can persist for several weeks, rather than several days, after alcohol cessation. Alcohol-induced psychotic disorder usually remits after a period of abstinence. Chronic heavy alcohol use has also been associated with brain atrophy and degeneration leading to a number of **cognitive deficits**, including **dementia** and **encephalopathy**.

TABLE 7.3 Clinical Institute Withdrawal of Alcohol Scale

Clinical Institute Withdrawal Assessment of Alcohol Scale, Revised (CIWA-Ar)

Patient:_____   Date: _____

Time: _____ (24-hour clock, midnight = 00:00)

Pulse or heart rate, taken for 1 minute:_____

Blood pressure:_____

NAUSEA AND VOMITING—Ask "Do you feel sick to your stomach? Have you vomited?" Observation.

0 no nausea and no vomiting

1 mild nausea with no vomiting

2

3

4 intermittent nausea with dry heaves

5

6

7 constant nausea, frequent dry heaves and vomiting

TACTILE DISTURBANCES—Ask "Have you any itching, pins and needles sensations, any burning, any numbness, or do you feel bugs crawling on or under your skin?" Observation.

0 none

1 very mild itching, pins and needles, burning or numbness

2 mild itching, pins and needles, burning or numbness

3 moderate itching, pins and needles, burning or numbness

4 moderately severe hallucinations

5 severe hallucinations

6 extremely severe hallucinations

7 continuous hallucinations

TREMOR—Arms extended and fingers spread apart.

Observation.

0 no tremor

1 not visible, but can be felt fingertip to fingertip

2

3

4 moderate, with patient's arms extended

5

6

7 severe, even with arms not extended

AUDITORY DISTURBANCES—Ask "Are you more aware of sounds around you? Are they harsh? Do they frighten you? Are you hearing anything that is disturbing to you? Are you hearing things you know are not there?" Observation.

0 not present

1 very mild harshness or ability to frighten

2 mild harshness or ability to frighten

3 moderate harshness or ability to frighten

(continued)

TABLE 7.3 Continued

Clinical Institute Withdrawal Assessment of Alcohol Scale, Revised (CIWA-Ar)

4 moderately severe hallucinations

5 severe hallucinations

6 extremely severe hallucinations

7 continuous hallucinations

PAROXYSMAL SWEATS—Observation.

0 no sweat visible

1 barely perceptible sweating, palms moist

2

3

4 beads of sweat obvious on forehead

5

6

7 drenching sweats

VISUAL DISTURBANCES—Ask "Does the light appear to be too bright? Is its color different? Does it hurt your eyes? Are you seeing anything that is disturbing to you? Are you seeing things you know are not there?" Observation.

0 not present

1 very mild sensitivity

2 mild sensitivity

3 moderate sensitivity

4 moderately severe hallucinations

5 severe hallucinations

6 extremely severe hallucinations

7 continuous hallucinations

ANXIETY—Ask "Do you feel nervous?" Observation.

0 no anxiety, at ease

1 mild anxious

2

3

4 moderately anxious, or guarded, so anxiety is inferred

5

6

7 equivalent to acute panic states as seen in severe delirium or acute schizophrenic reactions

HEADACHE, FULLNESS IN HEAD—Ask "Does your head feel different? Does it feel like there is a band around your head?" Do not rate for dizziness or lightheadedness. Otherwise, rate severity.

0 not present

1 very mild

2 mild

3 moderate

(continued)

TABLE 7.3 Continued

Clinical Institute Withdrawal Assessment of Alcohol Scale, Revised (CIWA-Ar)

4 moderately severe

5 severe

6 very severe

7 extremely severe

AGITATION—Observation.

0 normal activity

1 somewhat more than normal activity

2

3

4 moderately fidgety and restless

5

6

7 paces back and forth during most of the interview, or constantly thrashes about

ORIENTATION AND CLOUDING OF SENSORIUM—Ask "What day is this? Where are you? Who am I?"

0 oriented and can do serial additions

1 cannot do serial additions or is uncertain about date

2 disoriented for date by no more than 2 calendar days

3 disoriented for date by more than 2 calendar days

4 disoriented for place/or person

Total CIWA-Ar Score _____

Rater's Initials _____

Maximum Possible Score 67

NOTE: The CIWA-Ar is not copyrighted and may be reproduced freely.

This assessment for monitoring withdrawal symptoms requires approximately 5 minutes to administer.

The maximum score is 67 (see instrument).

Patients scoring less than 10 do not usually need additional medication for withdrawal.

Sullivan, J. T., K. Sykora, J. Schneiderman, C. A. Naranjo, and E. M. Sellers. Assessment of alcohol withdrawal: The revised Clinical Institute Withdrawal Assessment for Alcohol scale (CIWA-Ar). *British Journal of Addiction* 84:1353–1357, 1989.

Nicotine

Nicotine is **highly addictive**. The **withdrawal** (see DSM-5) symptoms associated with dependence may be intense and are often accompanied by **craving** for the drug (see Table 7.4). Symptoms usually begin within a few hours of smoking cessation, increase over 3–4 days, and then gradually decrease over 1–3 weeks. Individuals with comorbid psychiatric illnesses have a much higher prevalence of smoking. Additionally, depressed individuals have a higher rate of relapse to smoking than their nondepressed counterparts.

Cannabis

The psychoactive component of cannabis, tetrahydrocannabinol (THC), can be found in several different preparations of the hemp plant (marijuana, hash, sinsemilla). The potency

TABLE 7.4 Symptoms of Withdrawal from Nicotine

- Depressed mood
- Insomnia
- Irritability, frustration, or anger
- Anxiety
- Difficulty concentrating
- Restlessness
- Decreased heart rate
- Increased appetite or weight gain

of marijuana varies with the THC concentration. Symptoms of acute **intoxication** (see DSM-5) include **conjunctival injection** and **increased appetite** (see Table 7.5). Users commonly describe an **altered sense of time and distance** as well as **intensified bodily perceptions**. Acute intoxication may result in **anxiety** and **paranoid ideation**. Rarely, auditory or visual hallucinations may be experienced. The high of smoked marijuana typically lasts between **1 and 2 hours**; the high from ingested THC typically is of longer duration. No deaths from marijuana overdose have ever been reported. A recent review of longitudinal, population-based studies suggests that cannabis use increases the risk of developing a psychotic disorder later in life (Moore et al. 2007). Chronic marijuana use has been correlated with pulmonary dysfunction associated with smoking (e.g., COPD), but not as clearly with pulmonary malignancies. Although marijuana withdrawal was not included in the DSM-4, mounting evidence supported a withdrawal syndrome experienced by chronic users and cannabis **withdrawal** (see DSM-5) is included in the DSM-5 (see Table 7.6).

Stimulants

Acute intoxications from **cocaine, amphetamines** ("speed"), and **methamphetamine** ("crystal," "meth," "tina") (see DSM-5) produce similar symptoms (see Table 7.7).

TABLE 7.5 Symptoms of Acute Intoxication with Cannabis

- Conjunctival injection
- Increased appetite
- Dry mouth
- Tachycardia

TABLE 7.6 Symptoms of Withdrawal from Cannabis

- Sleep disturbance
- Vivid dreams
- Depressed mood
- Decreased appetite or weight loss
- Irritability, anger, or aggression
- Increased anxiety
- Restlessness
- Flu-like symptoms

TABLE 7.7 Symptoms of Acute Intoxication with Stimulants

- Tachycardia or bradycardia
- Pupillary dilation
- Elevated or lowered blood pressure
- Perspiration or chills
- Nausea or vomiting
- Weight loss
- Decreased need for sleep
- Distractability
- Psychomotor agitation or retardation
- Anxiety
- Paranoid ideation and delusions
- Hallucinations
- Muscular weakness, respiratory depression, chest pain or cardiac arrhythmias
- Dyskinesias, and dystonias
- Confusion, seizures, or coma

Stimulant intoxication may induce **manic-like symptoms**, such as a **decreased need for sleep, rapid flow of speech and ideas, inflated self-esteem,** and **distractibility**. Acute stimulant intoxication can also induce **paranoid ideation** and **delusions**, as well as auditory and visual **hallucinations**. These symptoms usually subside within a few days. Upon the initial presentation of the patient, it may be extremely difficult to differentiate stimulant-induced psychosis from schizophrenia. Anxiety disorders are also common among stimulant users, particularly **panic disorder**. Drug screening, which includes a test for the cocaine metabolite benzoylecgonine, can be useful diagnostically, particularly with patients for whom adequate histories cannot be obtained. Physical examination of acutely intoxicated individuals may reveal dilated pupils (except in cases of multiple substance use that includes an opioid) or physical manifestations of **intranasal** use (e.g., nasal septum erosions), **intravenous** use (e.g., needle track marks), or **smoking** (e.g., burns on the fingers or lips). Repeated assessments over time are important because stimulant-induced psychosis usually improves without pharmacological intervention, whereas an acute exacerbation of schizophrenia or mania does not.

Stimulant withdrawal (see DSM-5) symptoms are often described as a "crash" (see Table 7.8). It is not uncommon for individuals to complain of **anhedonia** and **lack of energy** for weeks after their last use of cocaine. Symptoms of stimulant withdrawal

TABLE 7.8 Symptoms of Withdrawal from Stimulants

- Depressed or irritable mood
- Anhedonia
- Fatigue
- Vivid, unpleasant dreams
- Insomnia or hypersomnia
- Increased appetite
- Psychomotor retardation or agitation

usually **peak within 24 hours** of drug cessation and rapidly diminish over the course of a few days.

Stimulant **overdoses can be life-threatening**. Smoking stimulants ("crack" or "crystal meth") results in much higher blood levels than does intranasal "snorting" of these drugs. **Myocardial infarctions, arrhythmias, strokes**, and symptoms consistent with a **neuroleptic malignant syndrome** have been related to stimulant use. Medical interventions are usually the first line of treatment. Because **depression** is common in cocaine addicts, particularly during periods of withdrawal, the possibility that the patient has used the drug to attempt suicide must be considered and aggressively investigated. Depressed mood and suicidal ideation usually abate within a few days, but some individuals continue to experience these psychiatric symptoms and may require appropriate intervention.

Opioids

The term *opioid* refers to all naturally occurring, synthetic and semisynthetic analgesic compounds with morphine-like action. Possible symptoms of acute opioid **intoxication** (see DSM-5) are listed in Table 7.9. Opioid **overdoses can be life-threatening**. When patients are brought to the emergency room with an opioid overdose, the first goal is to ensure adequate respiratory function, which may require ventilatory support and opiate antagonists, such as naloxone. After patients have been medically stabilized, they should be assessed for suicidality. Depression is common among chronic opioid users, and suicide attempts are not uncommon.

In contrast to alcohol and other sedative withdrawal, the **withdrawal** (see DSM-5) from opioids is a very unpleasant but not life-threatening experience (see Table 7.10). Symptoms of opioid withdrawal can be assessed with the **Clinical Opiate Withdrawal Scale**, an 11-item structured assessment of objective and subjective signs and symptoms

TABLE 7.9 Symptoms of Acute Intoxication with Opioids

- Pupillary constriction
- Drowsiness
- Slurred speech
- Impairment in attention or memory
- Coma

TABLE 7.10 Symptoms of Withdrawal from Opioids

- Depressed or irritable mood
- Nausea or vomiting
- Muscle aches
- Lacrimation or rhinorrhea
- Pupillary dilation
- Piloerection (goose bumps)
- Sweating
- Diarrhea
- Yawning
- Fever
- Insomnia

of withdrawal (see Table 7.11). The time to onset of withdrawal symptoms and the duration of withdrawal symptoms are both dependent on the specific opioid used. Heroin withdrawal symptoms usually **peak within 36 to 72 hours** and subside significantly by day 5. However, it is common for mild disturbances of mood and sleep to persist for 6 or more months in a protracted withdrawal syndrome from any opioid.

Hallucinogens (LSD, PCP, Ecstasy, Mescaline)

The most commonly used hallucinogen in the United States is the stimulant hallucinogen, 3,4-methylenedioxymethamphetamine (MDMA, "ecstasy"). Other hallucinogens used include lysergic acid diethylamide (LSD), phencyclidine (PCP), psilocybin ("magic mushrooms"), mescaline, and dimethyl-tryptamine (DMT).

TABLE 7.11 Clinical Opiate Withdrawal Scale

Clinical Opiate Withdrawal Scale

For each item, circle the number that best describes the patient's signs or symptom. Rate on just the apparent relationship to opiate withdrawal. For example, if heart rate is increased because the patient was jogging just prior to assessment, the increase pulse rate would not add to the score.

Patient's Name:_____   Date and Time ____/_____/____:_____

Reason for this assessment:_____

Resting pulse rate: _____beats/minute	GI upset: over last ½ hour
Measured after patient is sitting or lying for 1 minute	0 no GI symptoms
0 pulse rate 80 or below	1 stomach cramps
1 pulse rate 81–100	2 nausea or loose stool
2 pulse rate 101–120	3 vomiting or diarrhea
4 pulse rate greater than 120	5 multiple episodes of diarrhea or vomiting
Sweating: over past ½ hour not accounted for by room temperature or patient activity.	Tremor observation of outstretched hands
0 no report of chills or flushing	0 no tremor
1 subjective report of chills or flushing	1 tremor can be felt, but not observed
2 flushed or observable moisture on face	2 slight tremor observable
3 beads of sweat on brow or face	4 gross tremor or muscle twitching
4 sweat streaming off face	
Restlessness observation during assessment	Yawning observation during assessment
0 able to sit still	0 no yawning
1 reports difficulty sitting still, but is able to do so	1 yawning once or twice during assessment
3 frequent shifting or extraneous movements of legs/ arms	2 yawning three or more times during assessment
5 unable to sit still for more than a few seconds	4 yawning several times/minute
Pupil size	Anxiety or irritability
0 pupils pinned or normal size for room light	0 none
1 pupils possibly larger than normal for room light	1 patient reports increasing irritability or anxiousness
2 pupils moderately dilated	2 patient obviously irritable anxious
5 pupils so dilated that only the rim of the iris is visible	4 patient so irritable or anxious that participation in the assessment is difficult

TABLE 7.11 Continued

Clinical Opiate Withdrawal Scale

Bone or joint aches. If patient was having pain previously, only the additional component attributed to opiates withdrawal is scored.	Gooseflesh skin
	0 skin is smooth
	3 piloerrection of skin can be felt or hairs standing up on arms
0 not present	5 prominent piloerrection
1 mild diffuse discomfort	
2 patient reports severe diffuse aching of joints/muscles	
4 patient is rubbing joints or muscles and is unable to sit still because of discomfort	
Runny nose or tearing not accounted for by cold symptoms or allergies	Total Score _____
	The total score is the sum of all 11 items
0 not present	Initials of person completing
1 nasal stuffiness or unusually moist eyes	assessment: _____
2 nose running or tearing	
4 nose constantly running or tears streaming down cheeks	

Score: 5–12 = mild; 13–24 = moderate; 25–36 = moderately severe; more than 36 = severe withdrawal.

Reprinted with permission of the California Society of Addiction Medicine.

Acute **intoxication** (see DSM-5) from hallucinogens leads to **perceptual changes** occurring in a **state of full wakefulness** and alertness (see Tables 7.12 and 7.13). These changes may include **intensification of perceptions, depersonalization, derealization, illusions, hallucinations** (visual, tactile, and auditory), or **synesthesia** (e.g., hearing a sound produces a sensation of color; seeing an object produces a sensation of sound). Some users may experience **anxiety** or **panic reactions** ("a bad trip") that are characterized by odd sensations of time slowing down or physical boundaries being lost. Drug-induced changes in mental status usually resolve within 8 hours.

TABLE 7.12 Symptoms of Acute Intoxication with Phencyclidine (PCP)

- Psychomotor agitation and belligerence
- Vertical or horizontal nystagmus
- Numbness or diminished responsiveness to pain
- Ataxia
- Hypertension or tachycardia
- Dysarthria
- Muscle rigidity
- Seizure
- Coma
- Hyperacusis

TABLE 7.13 Symptoms of Acute Intoxication with Other Hallucinogens

- Anxiety or depression
- Ideas of reference and paranoid ideation
- Pupillary dilation
- Tachycardia
- Pupillary dilation
- Sweating
- Palpitations
- Blurred vision
- Tremors
- Incoordination

Although there are no life-threatening medical complications associated with hallucinogen intoxication, deaths have resulted from psychiatric or physical stress. In a confused, psychotic state, individuals may run out into traffic or jump from a high building because they think they can fly. Psychosis, depression, and disorientation may require individuals to be hospitalized in order to protect them from harming themselves or others. MDMA in particular is popular among adolescents and young adults, and is frequently used in the context of dancing. The stimulant effects of MDMA may fuel all-night dancing. A number of deaths related to dehydration and cardiac effects have occurred following such use.

No clear-cut **withdrawal** symptoms are associated with chronic hallucinogen use. Some individuals experience **flashbacks** of prior drug-induced experiences after they have ceased using hallucinogens, which may cause severe anxiety and require psychiatric intervention. The flashbacks are usually of a limited duration and occur in patients who are under stress or are physically ill. Most patients respond positively to verbal reassurance, although some may require pharmacological intervention.

Unless physicians consider the possibility of hallucinogen use, patients may be diagnosed with schizophrenia. There are few physical manifestations that suggest hallucinogen use. One may observe dilated pupils with LSD use or pupillary constriction with PCP use. Many diagnostic laboratories do not routinely screen for hallucinogens. If hallucinogen intoxication is suspected, specific screening tests should be requested.

Anabolic-Androgenic Steroids

Testosterone and synthetic derivatives of testosterone are types of anabolic-androgenic steroids that are taken by body builders, athletes, and other individuals who wish to improve their physical appearance and increase their muscle mass. The **euphoria** caused by steroids can be another important reinforcer of their use. Unless physicians are aware that patients are misusing steroids, the psychiatric symptoms associated with their use can lead to a misdiagnosis of bipolar disorder (see Table 7.14). **Withdrawal** (see DSM-5) from steroids has also been associated with psychiatric symptoms, such as **irritability, anxiety, and depression**. Anabolic-androgenic steroids typically are not screened for during routine laboratory urine drug testing and screening must be ordered for specific agents. Given the large number of agents potentially being used and their presence in very small amounts, urine testing may be difficult.

TABLE 7.14 Psychiatric Symptoms Associated with Anabolic Steroid Use

- Aggression
- Anxiety
- Impulsivity
- Irritability
- Impaired judgment
- Paranoid delusions

Inhalants (Volatile Solvents, Propellants, Medical Anesthetics, Nitrites, "Poppers")
Inhalants are volatile substances that can produce a state of intoxication (see Table 7.15). Inhalant intoxication is generally of **short duration**. Chronic use of some inhalants produces a neurocognitive disorder (dementia) or irreversible **neurological damage**. Inhalants can cause renal, hepatic, hematological, or pulmonary damage or death from cardiac arrhythmias or other organ-system dysfunctions. A thorough physical examination and appropriate laboratory tests are, therefore, crucial for patients in whom solvent use is suspected. Presently, no clinically significant inhalant withdrawal syndrome has been definitively identified. As inhalant use is most common among adolescents and young adults, physicians must remember to keep inhalant use as part of the differential diagnosis when caring for young people.

COURSE OF ILLNESS

Patients with a long-standing pattern of heavy substance use are at high risk for developing a substance use disorder, which tends to have a **chronic progressive course**

TABLE 7.15 Symptoms of Acute Intoxication with Inhalants

- Dizziness
- Nystagmus
- Incoordination or unsteady gait
- Slurred speech
- Lethargy
- Depressed reflexes
- Psychomotor retardation
- Tremor
- Generalized muscle weakness
- Blurred vision or diplopia
- Stupor or coma
- Cardiac arrhythmias
- Euphoria
- Disinhibition
- Disorientation
- Aggression
- Hallucinations
- Delirium

characterized by waxing and waning use, with periods of particularly heavy use alternating with periods of lesser use or even complete abstinence. Individuals who develop a substance use disorder generally progress from escalating use to substance use disorder of increasing severity. Some users progress slowly through these stages, others quickly, while others never progress at all.

Alcohol

Perhaps the most well-known work regarding the usual course of alcohol use is that of George Vaillant (1983). He found that most individuals who develop problematic drinking progress from asymptomatic social drinking to alcohol use disorder over a span of 3–15 years, although some individuals drink alcohol for more than 20 years before their use can be defined as problematic. He observed the **death rate** among alcoholics age 40–70 years to be approximately three times that of age-matched controls. Other studies suggest that **women** become "sicker quicker" from alcohol. This tendency may be related to biological factors. For example, women have decreased amounts of the gastric enzyme that metabolizes alcohol before it enters the bloodstream. Consequently, the same amount of alcohol will produce higher blood levels in women than in men and, ultimately, greater organ damage.

Alcohol use disorder (see DSM-5) tends to have a progressive course with varying outcomes. Some individuals die early as a result of their heavy drinking; some continue to drink heavily into their senior years; and some diminish or discontinue their use spontaneously or through treatment. Individuals who develop alcohol use disorder in their later years (late-onset alcoholics) are often reacting to the losses associated with aging, such as the deaths of family members or friends, retirement, separation or divorce, or ill health (see case example in Box 7.3). **Early-onset** alcoholics are more likely to have a **family history** of alcoholism, commit crimes, and respond less well to treatment.

Recreational Drugs

The evolution of problematic **cocaine** and **marijuana** use also tends to follow a pattern, which may include **experimental, social-recreational, circumstantial-situational, intensified**, and **compulsive phases**. Individuals may skip one or more of these phases. Many users have episodes of decreased use or abstinence. Over time, many cocaine users progress from a lower to a higher level of use, but some do not progress at all. Hallucinogens and other abused substances tend to be used more intermittently. Some individuals may continue to use substances recreationally for years without developing a substance use disorder.

The evolution of a drug use pattern into a substance use disorder of increasing severity seems to be related to the rate of onset of each agent's effects and the rate at which the effects diminish or are lost. The **rate of onset of action** is related to both the pharmacokinetic and pharmacodynamic properties of the substance, as well as the route of administration. **Routes of administration** that bypass first-pass metabolism by the liver (smoking, injecting, sniffing) may increase bioavailability and effective dosage of the drug that reaches the brain. Smoking and intravenous drug administration generally produce much more rapid onset of euphoric effects than nasal insufflation (snorting) or oral administration. Snorted stimulants produce a high within 3 to 5 minutes, whereas the intravenous route causes a high within 15 to 30 seconds, and smoked stimulants

> **BOX 7.3**
>
> ## CASE EXAMPLE OF OLDER ADULT ALCOHOL USE DISORDER
>
> A 67-year-old retired schoolteacher moved to a warmer climate with her husband of 30 years, who had also retired. Shortly after relocating, her husband became terminally ill with cancer. During the year before his death she served as his sole caregiver. During that time she felt very isolated and developed depression and difficulty sleeping. Her primary care physician prescribed alprazolam, which she took nightly in gradually escalating doses. As her husband became sicker in the weeks before his death, her sleep became more disturbed and she started having "night caps" to help her get to sleep. After her husband's death, her feelings of depression and isolation increased. Additionally, the majority of their life savings had been spent on her husband's medical care. She asked her primary care physician to increase her dose of alprazolam and would frequently ask for early refills. While she had always been a social drinker, she began drinking throughout the day, starting in the early morning and drinking into the night. She started losing significant amounts of weight. One night, as she was on her way to bed, she tripped, fell, and broke her hip. After a number of hours her neighbors heard her cries and called EMS. After her hip replacement surgery she had a lengthy stay in the intensive care unit and then a physical rehabilitation facility. Upon discharge she moved to a senior living community and resumed drinking daily but at lesser amounts. Her physician prescribed daily mirtazapine and naltrexone, recommended multivitamin and vitamin B supplementation, and conducted weekly psychotherapy sessions focused on loss and building social supports as well as increasing her motivation to reduce her alcohol use. As her depressive symptoms abated and she began to deal with her grief, her alcohol consumption decreased to less dangerous levels.
>
> For individuals who develop substance use problems later in life, substance use is often in response to loss. In this case, escalating alcohol use was also an attempt to mask painful feelings and alleviate psychiatric symptoms such as insomnia. For some, but certainly not all, patients, treating an underlying psychiatric disorder may have positive effects on substance use. As body composition changes with age, the negative effects of substance use may increase even if there is no change in the amount of substance used. Older adults are generally much more sensitive to the motor and cognitive impairments caused by sedatives and alcohol. Nutritional and vitamin deficiencies may be more marked in individuals with chronic alcohol use disorder and in older individuals and increase morbidity and mortality in older substance users.

produce an almost immediate high. Intravenous heroin causes a rapid sense of euphoria that has been compared with sexual orgasm; the response gradually diminishes over several hours. Crack cocaine also causes a rapid, intensely pleasurable high followed by a rapid loss of the feeling over a period of minutes. This "roller coaster" effect of changing drug plasma levels seems to reinforce the drug-taking behavior. Epidemiological studies

TABLE 7.16 Relative Addictiveness (Decreasing Order from Most to Least Addictive)

- Nicotine
- Heroin
- Cocaine
- Alcohol
- Marijuana
- Benzodiazepines

indicate that the development of dependence happens much more quickly for cocaine than for alcohol or marijuana. Comparing the number of individuals who have ever used a substance to the number who develop dependence on that substance gives an indication of the relative addictiveness of different substances (see Table 7.16).

THE INTERVIEW

Substance Use History

Any patient who is suffering from psychiatric symptoms must be evaluated for drug use. As described earlier, each class of drugs can induce psychiatric symptoms. Depression, psychosis, anxiety, and delirium are all common symptoms associated with drug use. Before assuming that these symptoms are the result of an underlying psychiatric disorder, the physician needs to consider the possibility of a substance-induced disorder.

Whenever the possibility of a substance use or substance-induced disorder exists, a detailed, specific drug and alcohol use history should be obtained (see Box 7.4 for specific items to be covered during history-taking and Box 7.5 for evaluation guidelines). An opening question such as, "How much do you drink or use drugs?" does not usually provide fruitful information. Often, patients who have problems with alcohol or drugs respond in a vague manner or claim that they use substances only occasionally. Whenever possible, several approaches should be used in tandem in order to attain the proper diagnosis.

Many patients **underestimate** the amount of alcohol or drugs they use when asked by a physician. Often patients believe physicians hold harsh, negative, and punitive ideas regarding alcohol and drug users. These beliefs may grow from past experience with health care providers, as well as with other people in their lives. Aggressively confrontational or judgmental approaches to patients with substance use disorders are generally counterproductive. A **respectful, direct, and empathic approach** will generally elicit the most useful information. Asking questions assuming an affirmative answer is often helpful. For example, a physician might ask, "How many days a week do you drink alcohol (use marijuana)? When you drink (use) how much do you drink (smoke)? How often do you use cocaine?" These types of questions, asked in a nonjudgmental way, **convey permission** to the patient to answer in the affirmative.

Occasionally, physiologically dependent substance users who are afraid of experiencing withdrawal symptoms may exaggerate the amounts they use, thinking that by doing so they will receive greater amounts of the medication used in opioid or sedative detoxification. Unfortunately, this distortion can lead to difficulties in determining the appropriate dosage of medication for detoxification.

BOX 7.4
HISTORY OF SUBSTANCE USE

- **Age of first use** and **first regular use** of alcohol and each specific drug used
- **Pattern of current use**: frequency of use, amount used per use, route of administration, as well as the duration of this pattern
- **Last use of alcohol or drugs**
- **Periods of heaviest use**: frequency of use, amount used per use, route of administration, as well as the duration of this pattern
- **Periods of abstinence:** supports and obstacles to past abstinence
- **Previous substance abuse treatment:** pharmacological treatments, psychosocial treatments (group or individual therapy), participation in mutual self-help groups, formal inpatient or outpatient treatments (detoxification, rehabilitation, intensive outpatient treatments), and the usefulness of these interventions
- **Patient's perception of positive** and **negative consequences of use:** why substances are used, in what ways substance use is helpful or positive, as well as what problems have arisen from drug use (legal, relationships, employment)
- **Patient's perception of the need for change**

BOX 7.5
EVALUATION GUIDELINES

- Always ask about alcohol and drug use.
- Gather collateral substance use history from family, significant others, and friends.
- Perform urine drug screening tests (with patient's permission), if recent drug use is suspected. The urine test is most useful for determining whether drugs have been used in the past 48 hours.
- Perform a breathalyzer or blood alcohol test to screen for recent alcohol use, if current alcohol intoxication is suspected.
- Examine the patient for physical signs of drug use, including signs related to the route of administration.
- Monitor vital signs and the neurological status.
- Obtain laboratory tests. Abnormal liver, renal, or hematological screens may all indicate chronic use.
- Observe the patient for a period of time. The effects of drugs may diminish within a few hours, days, or weeks.

Screening Tests

A variety of screening instruments can be used to detect whether a patient has a problem with alcohol or drugs. The most commonly used screening tool for alcohol-related disorders is the **CAGE** (an acronym for the questions that the physician asks the patient) questionnaire (see Box 7.6). The CAGE is worded to minimize denial and allow for rapid screening.

The Alcohol Use Disorders Identification Test (**AUDIT**) is a brief, 10-item self-report instrument that can be administered and scored within 5 minutes (Babor et al. 1992). Eight of the items are scored on a 0–5 scale and two are scored as 0, 2, or 4. A score of 8 or more generally indicates a hazardous level of drinking and requires more specific evaluation.

The Michigan Alcoholism Screening Test (**MAST**) is a 25-item self-report or clinician-administered instrument that screens patients for problematic alcohol use (Selzer 1971). A Short Michigan Alcoholism Screening Test (**SMAST**), a 10-item version of the MAST, can also be used for screening purposes (Selzer et al. 1975).

The Drug Abuse Screening Test (**DAST**) is a 20-item self-report instrument used to screen for non–alcohol related substance abuse or dependence (Skinner 1982). Additionally, the CAGE questions can be easily and validly altered to screen for other drugs of abuse (e.g., marijuana, by changing drinking to "marijuana use" and changing the last question to "have you ever used marijuana first thing in the morning?").

These instruments merely screen for problematic use and do not provide enough information to accurately diagnose a substance use disorder or develop an appropriate treatment plan. They can also produce false-positive and false-negative results. Therefore, complete alcohol and drug assessments should be performed whenever problem substance use is suspected.

Family, Social, and Legal Histories

Obtaining thorough family, social, and legal histories during an alcohol and drug use assessment is of great importance. The patient's perception of what constitutes addictive behavior and whether treatment is necessary is influenced by familial and peer patterns of substance use. To obtain a **genetic history,** as well as to assess the **familial norms**, the physician should ask about the use of alcohol and other drugs by biological as well as any nonbiologically related family members (adoptive parents, step-parents, or step-siblings). Any substance use problems among parents, siblings, grandparents, or aunts and uncles should be noted. Additionally, any participation in substance abuse treatment (e.g., pharmacological treatment, individual or group therapy, mutual self-help groups) by family

---

BOX 7.6
CAGE SCREENING INSTRUMENT

- **C** Have you ever felt you should **cut down** on your drinking?
- **A** Have people **annoyed** you by criticizing your drinking?
- **G** Have you ever felt bad or **guilty** about your drinking?
- **E** Have you ever had a drink first thing in the morning to steady your nerves or get rid of a hangover (**eye-opener**)? An affirmative answer to two or more questions suggests problem drinking.

members should be assessed, as well as the perceived success of these interventions, as these experiences may largely inform the patient's beliefs about what may or may not be helpful about treatment.

The patient's social history can provide a wealth of information. The patient's physical and social environments can strongly affect his or her ability to achieve sobriety. Significant personal **losses** or physical or sexual **abuse** can influence a patient's pattern of use. More than half of women with substance use disorders and more than 40% of adolescent male drug users seeking treatment are estimated to have been sexually or physically abused. To obtain a complete assessment, the physician needs to sensitively explore the patient's experience of any current or past abuse (physical, sexual, or emotional, including domestic violence). Housing, the substance using and non-using individuals who are important in the patient's life, employment, and means of obtaining and paying for drugs are important factors in understanding a substance using patient's social situation.

Obtaining a patient's legal history is also crucial. Patients who have been **arrested** for driving while intoxicated, selling or carrying drugs, public intoxication, or disorderly conduct should be evaluated for problematic alcohol or drug use. Some individuals with substance use disorders will turn to petty crime (panhandling, shoplifting, etc.) or prostitution to support their drug use. Notably, patients who are court mandated to treatment may have a similar prognosis for recovery to that of patients who come of their own accord.

History Timeline

A timeline can be particularly helpful for integrating data from the patient's history. Indications are made on the timeline to mark when the patient first used psychoactive substances, the periods of heaviest use for each substance, the periods of abstinence, and significant losses or crises experienced by the patient. If a patient has a significant psychiatric history, another timeline can be drawn that indicates the first manifestations of psychiatric problems, periods of psychiatric symptoms, and hospitalizations. One timeline is then placed above the other, using the same demarcations (Figure 7.1). In complicated cases, the two timelines may reveal relationships between the timing of the psychiatric symptoms and of alcohol or drug use, which can have important treatment implications. If a patient has persistent psychiatric symptoms during a period of prolonged abstinence, the physician may prescribe a psychotropic agent. Conversely, if the patient becomes symptomatic only during periods of heavy use, pharmacological approaches may not be indicated. Varying levels of psychiatric symptoms despite chronic unvarying substance use may also indicate a primary psychiatric disorder meriting pharmacologicol treatment. Clearly, this method is limited by the patient's ability to recall past psychiatric episodes and periods of alcohol or drug use.

Assessment of Patient Reliability

Patients with addictive behaviors demonstrate varying degrees of **denial**. Clues to the presence of a substance use disorder include vague medical complaints, social isolation, or erratic and irresponsible behavior. Substance users can use hostility and evasiveness to distance themselves from the interviewer and avoid self-exploration or outside scrutiny of their alcohol or drug use. Cultural, gender, or socioeconomic differences between clinicians and patients may interfere with the patient's ability to trust the interviewer. Patients who feel guilty or ashamed may minimize the extent of their use and the negative impact it has had on their lives.

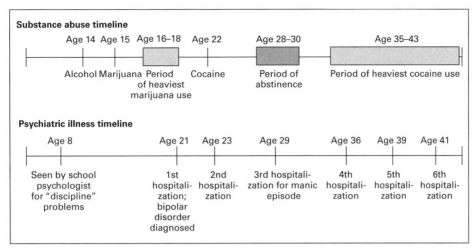

FIGURE 7.1 Timelines. The parallel timelines indicate the superimposed substance abuse history and psychiatric history.

When physicians ask questions regarding substance use, they may elicit an angry response. Patients who have experienced hostile reactions from friends or family regarding their substance use may expect the physician to treat them in the same way. Health professionals may be viewed as adversaries rather than allies. Women may be particularly reluctant to admit to alcohol or drug use because of the historically increased social stigma associated with problematic substance use by women. They may minimize alcohol or drug use and evade questions regarding addictive behavior.

The physician must assess the **validity** of the information provided by the patient in the interview. The patient's level of denial and ability to trust the physician can influence the accuracy of the data. On a more basic level, the patient's ability to remember past and present details of his or her life may be impaired by substance use or other psychiatric or medical conditions and must be evaluated in order to assess the reliability of the data obtained. Whenever possible, **collateral history** should be obtained from other persons, such as family members, health care workers, or friends. When patients resist having the physician contact a spouse or other significant persons, the physician's suspicions of a substance use problem should be heightened.

During the initial part of a substance use interview, it is essential that physicians demonstrate **sincerity** and **empathy**. Once the patient's **trust** is elicited, the information the patient provides will be more reliable. It is often useful for the physician to state specifically the confidential nature of the interview and the limits of that confidentiality. A physician might state, "Information obtained during this interview regarding your drug and alcohol use may be shared with other staff members, but no information will be released to anyone else without your explicit consent."

Often, once rapport is established, the physician may obtain a patient's permission to contact non–drug-using family members or significant others and engage them in the treatment. In most cases, family involvement is beneficial. Contacting an employer is not commonly done, as this might result in loss of employment. However, if there is any possibility that the patient might be endangering his or her life or the lives of others because of continued alcohol or drug use (e.g., the patient is a school bus driver who is continuing to use heroin), the patient's employee assistance program or an appropriate professional organization must be contacted.

The patient's hostility and minimization of substance use can engender powerful feelings in the physician. When interviewers seek to help patients and are met with belligerence and evasiveness, they may become angry and be tempted to adopt a more punitive stance. It is useful for physicians to be aware of and understand their own attitudes toward patients who abuse alcohol and drugs. Physicians' personal experiences with alcohol and drugs can significantly influence their approach. A physician who grew up in an alcoholic household and avoids all psychoactive substances may have little tolerance for substance users. Conversely, physicians who frequently binge on alcohol themselves may minimize the negative consequences of such behavior in their patients. Box 7.7 describes guidelines for safe drinking for adult men and women.

Patient Engagement

Relatively simple interventions can have a significant impact on patients with substance-related disorders. Even brief (e.g., 5- to 10-minute) interventions, in which the physician diagnoses a patient with a substance use disorder, presents the diagnosis to the patient, and offers a treatment referral, have been demonstrated to be effective in reducing or eliminating substance use.

If a substance problem is suspected by the physician but denied by the patient, the physician should attempt to bridge this gap and engage the patient rather than turn away and regard the patient as a liar. The physician could suggest that the patient attempt to abstain from alcohol or drugs for 2 weeks and then return to see the physician after that time to discuss the success or failure of the goal of **abstinence**. This approach works best for patients whose families do not have problematic substance use and with whom they have close

---

BOX 7.7
SAFE DRINKING GUIDELINES

The National Institute on Alcohol Abuse and Alcoholism (NIAAA) outlines safe levels of alcohol consumption as up to two standard drinks daily for men and up to one standard drink daily for women. The NIAAA has set forth guidelines for defining heavy drinking (levels of drinking shown to put individuals at risk for substance use disorders and negative health consequences). For men up to 65 years of age, NIAAA defines heavy drinking as 5 or more standard drinks on any drinking day and greater than 14 standard drinks in a week. For women up to age 65 years of age and healthy men over 65 years of age, NIAAA defines heavy drinking as four or more standard drinks on any drinking day and greater than seven standard drinks in a week. For comparison purposes, a standard drink is defined as a drink containing 14 gm of pure alcohol. By this standard:

- One 12 oz beer or wine cooler is one standard drink
- One 12 oz malt liquor is 1.5 standard drinks
- A 750 mL bottle of table wine contains five standard drinks
- One single shot mixed drink or 1.5 oz of hard liquor (80-proof spirits) is one standard drinkSource: National Institute on Alcohol Abuse and Alcoholism, 2008. http://www.niaaa.nih.gov

relationships. The physician can ask families to confirm the agreement that was made and to provide feedback about patients' progress. When a patient's alcohol or drug use continues despite an agreement to try to stop, the patient may accept a referral for substance abuse treatment. Identifying the medical sequelae associated with problematic alcohol or drug use can also be an extremely effective intervention aimed at engaging a patient.

If problematic substance use is suspected and the patient actively denies it, a substance use disorder specialist may be consulted (see case example in Box 7.8). A consultation from an addiction specialist, which is often requested in an inpatient setting by the treating

---

BOX 7.8

CASE EXAMPLE OF PATIENT ENGAGEMENT IN A PRIMARY CARE SETTING

A 42-year-old roofer came to his family physician, accompanied by his wife, with complaints of upset stomach and insomnia. His wife told the doctor that she was concerned that these symptoms were caused by his drinking. The patient became visibly irritated at this suggestion and stated, "I don't have a problem with alcohol! What? You think I'm an alcoholic?" Upon careful evaluation, the patient endorsed drinking four to six standard drinks most days of the week for the past 10 years. He denied ever having symptoms of physiological withdrawal when he didn't drink. He stated, "I can stop any time I want to." His physician recommended some blood tests, described the NIAAA guidelines for safe drinking for men his age, and suggested that the patient try to abstain from alcohol for the next 2 weeks. They agreed to meet in 2 weeks to discuss the laboratory test results and see how the patient had done abstaining. When they met again, the patient stated, "Doc, I didn't make it the whole 2 weeks, but I'm not sure I really wanted to stop." They reviewed the laboratory test results, including mildly elevated liver function tests (AST, ALT and GGT values), which the physician explained could be a result of hazardous levels of alcohol consumption. His doctor recommended he attend AA, which he refused outright. The physician then recommended a referral to a psychiatrist with whom he frequently collaborated for the patient to continue talking about his drinking. The patient agreed to meet with the psychiatrist and spent several weeks discussing his drinking and his motivation to decrease his use. Ultimately, the patient identified several negative consequences of his drinking and was agreeable to a trial of naltrexone, which he found helpful in reducing both the number of days he drank and the amount he drank on each drinking day.

As demonstrated in this example, patients with drug and alcohol use problems often present to a primary care physician with vague complaints. Asking a patient to try and abstain can be a helpful exercise for patients to better understand their motivation or perhaps the compulsive nature of their use. Importantly, the primary care physician provided specific individualized feedback to this patient regarding his drinking, identified an alcohol problem, and recommended that he reduce his drinking. Physicians should convey that they are allies and are willing to address problems over time. When a patient remains ambivalent about change, a referral to an addiction specialist can be very helpful.

physician, may not be welcomed by the patient, who may regard the interview as an intrusion. The patient may wish to focus only on the medical sequelae of the addiction rather than the underlying addictive behavior. In these situations, physicians should inform patients that a specialist will be meeting with them. By initially focusing on, and demonstrating their concern for, the patient's medical problems, the specialist may be able to facilitate rapport.

In a psychiatric setting, patients are more accustomed to being asked about personal issues. However, these patients frequently view their psychiatric problems as being of primary importance and their substance use as a secondary issue. Again, the physician should empathize with the patient's psychiatric problems but also make it clear that an understanding of the alcohol or drug use is necessary to provide effective treatment.

Special Considerations in Children and Adolescents

Generally, the best indication of psychoactive substance use in children and adolescents is **pronounced behavioral changes in their lives** (see Table 7.17). Any of these changes may indicate that a child or adolescent is having trouble with alcohol or drugs and, therefore, deserves careful evaluation. However, such changes can be related to other factors (e.g., depression, parental conflict). Some potential risk factors for adolescents are listed in Table 7.18. The greater the number of risk factors, the more likely it is that an adolescent will use drugs. Substance-using adolescents are at a much higher risk for suicide attempts than are their non–substance-using peers. A depressed adolescent who is a using drugs or alcohol should be thoroughly evaluated (see case example in Box 7.9).

TABLE 7.17 Indicators of Psychoactive Substance Use in Children and Adolescents

- Deteriorating academic performance
- Breaking off relationships with old friends and acquiring new friends
- Personality changes
- Behavioral changes
- Changes in sleep patterns
- Changes in appetite

TABLE 7.18 Risk Factors Associated with Adolescent Alcohol and Drug Use

- Early alcohol intoxication
- Observed adult drug use
- Perceived peer approval of drug use
- Perceived parental approval of drug use
- Frequent absences from school, truancy
- Poor academic achievement, low grade-point average
- Distrust of teachers
- Distrust of parents
- Low educational aspirations
- Little religious commitment
- Emotional distress
- Dissatisfaction with life

CASE EXAMPLE OF ADOLESCENT POLYSUBSTANCE USE

A 17-year-old high school junior was arrested for selling prescription medications to his classmates. Previously a straight-A student and member of the swim team, in the year before the arrest his family had noticed several alarming changes. He had left a group of friends that he had known for several years, abruptly quit the swim team, started sleeping erratically, and began missing school frequently.

At the end of the first semester of his sophomore year of school, a friend gave him dextroamphetamine to help him pull an all-nighter while studying for finals. First he began buying dextroamphetamine from friends at school for studying and alertness, but later he began crushing and snorting dextroamphetamine at parties with friends to get high. These parties usually involved binge drinking and smoking marijuana as well. He would frequently drink to the point of vomiting or blacking out on Friday or Saturday evenings. During his summer break he began taking oxycodone from his grandmother's medicine cabinet.

The family took their son to his pediatrician, who did an office-based urine test that was positive for amphetamines and marijuana and negative for cocaine, benzodiazepines, and opiates. When confronted with the results of the urine test he stated, "It's not a big deal. I take some dextroamphetamine to help me study. Everyone does it. Marijuana is *not a drug*." The family took the boy to a psychotherapist recommended by the pediatrician, who tried to engage him around his substance use and to increase his motivation to stop this behavior. He remained resistant to openly discussing his substance use and continued sneaking out of the house and using with friends. The therapist referred the family to a therapist specializing in contingency reinforcement and family training (CRAFT). This therapist was able to help the family develop positive and negative contingencies that encouraged their son's participation in treatment and discouraged his continued substance use.

Adolescent substance use is often marked by behavior changes demonstrated in this case, including a drastic change in social circle, abandoning previously enjoyed extracurricular activities, truancy, weight change, and changes in sleeping pattern. With increasing regularity, adolescents misuse prescriptions medications that they get from friends or family members, either paying for them, stealing them, or being given them freely. Importantly, common urine drug screens used in doctors' offices or at home often test for opiates, but, unless the individual uses very high doses of opioids, the tests will not detect opioids such as oxycodone, leaving a problem undetected. When an individual with a substance use problems is in a social circle of other users, their own substance use may appear normal and decrease their motivation to make any changes in their behavior. Some groups of adolescents have very permissive, minimizing views of drug and alcohol use. A patient's motivation to decrease his or her substance use may be much less than that of concerned adults. Parents may need assistance in finding ways to set positive and negative contingencies that encourage the behavior changes they are hoping their child will make.

Special Considerations in the Elderly

Normal human aging causes physiological changes (e.g., in body mass composition) leading to **greater susceptibility** to the effects of alcohol and other drugs. Without increasing substance use, the physiological effects of drugs and alcohol may increase dramatically as a person ages. Because elderly persons often suffer neurological impairment from other causes, the physician may overlook substance-induced **cognitive changes** in these patients. **Social problems** related to substance use often are not as obvious in older adults. Because older individuals' responsibilities have often diminished (e.g., they no longer have to care for children or are retired), a substance use problem may go unrecognized for a longer period of time. New-onset substance use disorders in the geriatric population are not uncommon and are often associated with personal loss, including retirement, death of friends, death of a spouse or partner, or failing health or disability. A psychiatric and substance use assessment is indicated when an elderly individual shows diminished interest in social activities or becomes more isolated.

Historically, adults over 50 years of age have represented a relatively small percentage of all individuals with substance use disorders in the United States. Evidence suggests that substance use disorders, which generally start in late adolescence or early adulthood, tend to persist as a patient ages. As Americans live longer and relatively healthier lives, the number of older adults with substance use disorders is expected to increase. The aging of the baby boomer generation (born 1946–1964) is greatly increasing the percentage of Americans over 50, likely leading to a substantial rise in the percentage of substance use disorders represented by older adults.

DIFFERENTIAL DIAGNOSIS

The differential diagnosis of substance-related disorders can be complicated. More than one substance-related disorder frequently coexists in the same patient, making the physician's detection of substance-induced disorders doubly important. Substance-induced disorders not only require treatment themselves but also serve as clues to a maladaptive pattern of substance use that could benefit from medical attention once the patient acknowledges the self-destructive process.

In addition, primary psychiatric disorders often coexist in patients with substance-related disorder. They are referred to as **co-occurring disorders**. In most cases, a patient's alcohol or drug use must be treated simultaneously with any coexisting psychiatric disorder, such as a primary mood disorder. Often, the coexisting psychiatric condition may require medication. Determining with certainty whether the two disorders are completely unrelated can be difficult. The National Epidemiologic Survey on Alcohol and Related Conditions found that drug use disorders were positively associated with mood, anxiety, and personality disorders. Individuals with co-occurring substance use disorders and other psychiatric disorders tend to have a **greater severity** of illness, **higher rates of relapse** of substance use and psychiatric symptoms, and a **poorer prognosis** for both illnesses. These patients tend to more frequently use emergency and inpatient services and have more medical problems. Among these patients, treatment retention and medication adherence are both lower. Importantly, they tend to have increased levels of psychological distress with increased rates of violence, suicide, and legal difficulties (Ross, 2008).

Large epidemiological studies have found the rates of comorbid substance use disorders to be high among several specific psychiatric illnesses. Nearly 50% of individuals with **schizophrenia** have a substance use disorder; nicotine use disorders are the most common, followed by alcohol, cocaine, and cannabis use disorders. Over 50% of patients with **bipolar disorder** have a lifetime history of a substance use disorder. Among **depressed** patients, nearly 20% have a history of a lifetime diagnosis of an alcohol use disorder, and a similar number have a history of a drug use disorder. Thirty percent of individuals with a history of an anxiety disorder have a comorbid drug use disorder compared with 16% of individuals without a mental illness. Posttraumatic stress disorder, panic disorder, and obsessive-compulsive disorder all have particularly high rates of comorbidity with substance use disorders. Between 20% and 40% of patients with attention-deficit hyperactivity disorder have a lifetime history of a substance use disorder (Ross, 2008).

When patients are open about their substance use, physicians can work with them to try to sort out the patterns of causality, such as whether the substance use or the psychiatric syndrome developed first and how much one disorder contributed to the development of the other. When a patient is not honest about substance use, the differential diagnosis process becomes even more complicated.

The physician's approach to the differential diagnosis will vary depending on whether substance use is revealed. For example, a patient who presents to the emergency room in a jittery, suspicious state and admits that he has been binging on crack cocaine for the past 2 days will most likely receive the diagnosis of cocaine intoxication, while the diagnoses of primary anxiety and psychotic disorders will be much less likely. The same clinical presentation in a patient who adamantly denies recent drug use would prompt the physician to consider a different diagnostic hierarchy, with primary anxiety and psychotic disorders placed at the top of a list of possible causes.

The differential diagnosis of substance-related disorders should be approached from the following perspectives. When a patient with psychiatric signs and symptoms gives a recent history of substance use, the physician should consider how likely it is that all of the psychiatric findings are substance-induced. Alternatively, when a patient presents with psychiatric signs and symptoms but denies substance use, the physician must decide whether the clinical picture suggests that a substance-induced disorder be included in the differential diagnosis. For example, a 25-year-old patient with a recent onset of psychosis who denies substance use may have schizophrenia but may also be suffering from a cocaine- or amphetamine-induced psychosis.

Although it is essential that substance-related disorders not be overlooked, it is equally important that other medical conditions not be mistaken for substance-related disorders. Many medical conditions cause syndromes that resemble alcohol intoxication. Some of these are quite common (e.g., hyperglycemia; hypoglycemia; postictal syndrome, which occurs after a generalized seizure; and other neurological disorders, such as multiple sclerosis). Any medical condition that can cause delirium can mimic alcohol or sedative intoxication (see Chapter 5, Neurocognitive Disorders and Mental Disorders Due to Another Medical Condition). The other medical conditions to be considered in the differential diagnosis of alcohol and sedative withdrawal are essentially the same as those for anxiety disorders (see Chapter 6, Anxiety, Obsessive-Compulsive, and Stress Disorders).

MEDICAL EVALUATION

A comprehensive medical history and physical examination can provide evidence of a substance use disorder. A host of medical symptoms and physical signs are associated with chronic alcohol or other substance use (see Table 7.19). Laboratory testing may also reveal findings consistent with problematic substance use. Patients often present to physicians complaining of physical symptoms rather than concerns regarding substance use. Physicians

TABLE 7.19 Complaints, Findings, and Conditions Related to Substance Use

Substance	Symptoms/Physical Complaints	Physical Findings	Related Conditions
Alcohol	Frequent injuries	Smell of alcohol	Gastritis
	Abdominal pain	Elevated blood pressure	Alcoholic hepatitis
	Nausea/vomiting	Bruising	Fatty liver
	Diarrhea	Enlarged liver	Cirrhosis
	Headache	Signs of liver failure	Hypertension
	Insomnia	• Spider angiomas	Peripheral neuropathy
	Erectile dysfunction	• Palmar erythema	Anemia
	Palpitations	• Jaundice	Congestive heart failure
	Gait disturbance		Cardiomyopathy
			Cerebellar atrophy
			Wernicke-Korsokoff syndrome
Cannabis	Cough	Smell of marijuana	Chronic obstructive pulmonary
	Weight gain	Injected conjunctiva	disease
	Memory complaints	Tachycardia	
	Sleep disturbance	Dilated, sluggishly reactive pupils	
Cocaine	Insomnia	Rhinitis	Myocardial infarction
	Fatigue	Irritation of nares	Stroke
	Chest pain	Perforation of nasal septum	HIV
	Weight loss	Burns on fingers and lips	Viral hepatitis (especially HCV
	Headache	Elevated blood pressure	in IV users)
	Seizure	Tachycardia	
	Arrhythmias	Hoarseness	
		Track marks (IV users)	
Stimulants	Insomnia	Tachycardia	HIV
	Weight loss	Elevated blood pressure	Viral hepatitis (especially HCV
		Worn down teeth (meth mouth)	in IV users)
		Excoriations of skin	
		Burns on fingers and lips	
		Track marks	
Opioids	Pain complaints	Track marks	HIV
	Constipation	Skin lesions	Viral hepatitis (especially HBV
	Diarrhea	• Cellulitis	and HCV)
	Rhinitis	• Abscess	Tuberculosis
		Constricted pupils	
		Thrombosis	
		Rhinorrhea	
		Lacrimation	
		Goose bumps	

(continued)

TABLE 7.19 Continued

Substance	Symptoms/Physical Complaints	Physical Findings	Related Conditions
Sedatives	Insomnia	Slurred speech	
	Restlessness	Unsteady gait	
	Seizures		
	Pneumonia		
	Falls		
Hallucinogens	Palpitations	Muscle weakness	Myopathy
	Chest pains		Renal failure
	Seizure (PCP)		
	Muscular pain or weakness		
	Urinary symptoms		
Inhalants	Weight loss	Halitosis	Cognitive impairment
	Respiratory complaints	Rash	
	Fatigue	Paint around mouth / nose	
	Epistaxis		
	Stomach upset		
	Cognitive changes		

HBV, hepatitis B virus; HCV, hepatitis C virus; HIV, human immunodeficiency virus; IV, intravenous.

Adapted from Wartenberg, A., C. E. Dubé, D. C. Lewis, and M. G. Cyr. Diagnosing chronic substance use problems in the primary care setting: related physical problems, psychological problems, physical findings and relevant labs. In Dubé, C. E., M. G. Goldstein, D. C. Lewis, E. R. Myers, and W. R. Zwick, eds. *Project ADEPT Curriculum for Primary Care Physician Training. Vol. 1: Core Modules.* Providence, RI: Brown University Press, 1989. Reprinted by permission of the publisher.

must be aware of substance use as a possible etiology of these symptoms, to appropriately identify and treat both the substance use disorder and the presenting symptoms.

Individuals with substance use disorders are at increased risk for serious medical comorbidity. Some substances can potentially cause medical sequelae as a direct effect of acute or chronic use (e.g., cocaine causing myocardial infarction or seizure, alcohol causing cirrhosis or cardiomyopathy). Other medical sequelae are more indirect. Alcohol and drug use is associated with increased risk for **sexually transmitted diseases**. Intravenous (IV) drug use puts individuals at increased risk of **infectious disease** (e.g., abscess, endocarditis, HIV, hepatitis C). Individuals with a history of opioid dependence or of any IV drug use should be screened for HIV and viral hepatitis and vaccinated for hepatitis A and B, as these infections are exceedingly common among IV drug users. Individuals with chronic alcohol use disorder tend to have multiple **vitamin B deficiencies** that can lead to serious complications, including **peripheral neuropathy** and **anemia**.

As patients age, the amounts of drugs and alcohol that they tolerated without problems in the past may cause problems due to decreased plasma clearance and increased volume of distribution. Chronic alcohol and drug use can be associated with temporary or more long-lasting cognitive dysfunction, and a thorough mental status examination is a crucial component of the assessment of substance use disorders (see Chapter 5, Neurocognitive Disorders and Mental Disorders Due to Another Medical Condition). For example, chronically alcohol-dependent individuals may develop **Korsakoff syndrome**, a consequence of chronic **thiamine deficiency**, which leads to damage of the mamillary bodies and results in prominent short-term memory loss with confabulation.

Laboratory Tests for Alcohol-Related Disorders

Chronic alcohol use in hazardous amounts can lead to end-organ damage, which may be revealed in laboratory abnormalities. Such ingestion of alcohol can cause elevated levels of γ-**glutamyl transpeptidase** (GGT/GGTP). Serum GGT is a sensitive but not specific measure of alcohol-induced liver damage and enzyme induction. Alcohol-induced GGT levels quickly return to normal in the first weeks of abstinence. The **mean corpuscular volume** (MCV) may also be elevated in heavy drinkers (via direct toxicity to bone marrow or interruption of folate metabolism). Elevated MCV is a relatively late manifestation of chronic heavy alcohol use but increases the specificity of elevated GGT in diagnosing alcohol-induced liver damage.

Carbohydrate-deficient transferrin (CDT) is a relatively sensitive and specific marker of heavy alcohol consumption. Elevated CDT levels decrease by approximately 50% with every 2 weeks of abstinence from alcohol. Unfortunately, this test usually must be sent to a specialty lab and is not a practical measure clinically. **Alanine aminotransferase** (ALT) and **aspartate aminotransferase** (AST) are elevated in about 50% of chronic heavy drinkers. These elevations are nonspecific markers of liver damage. Chronic heavy alcohol consumption can also lead to **vitamin B_{12}**, **folate**, and **thiamine** (B_1) deficiencies with resultant evidence of megaloblastic anemia.

Other laboratory abnormalities found in a minority of alcohol-dependent individuals include elevated serum **urate**, **triglycerides**, **bilirubin**, or **alkaline phosphatase**. Alcohol use is not the only cause of these abnormalities. A wide range of medical conditions may produce similar laboratory findings as well.

Recent alcohol use is most accurately detected by **breathalyzer** test or blood test, although urine testing is possible. These test abnormalities suggest problematic alcohol use, but only information obtained in a clinical interview can confirm an alcohol use disorder.

Laboratory Tests for Drug-Related Disorders

An array of blood, urine, and hair sample tests can reveal the use of a wide variety of drugs. Urine toxicology is the most commonly used detection method for screening purposes (see Table 7.20). Each test has a different sensitivity, specificity, and cost. Generally, screening tests such as thin-layer chromatography (TLC) or radioimmunoassay (RIA) are used initially because they are simple, rapid, and inexpensive. If the result is positive, drug use can be confirmed by tests such as gas chromatography or high-performance liquid chromatography, which are more expensive and should be used judiciously. When submitting samples to a laboratory, physicians must specify which drugs should be tested for, rather than merely sending a sample to a diagnostic laboratory and asking whether any drugs can be detected.

Physicians should be aware that the sensitivity of the laboratory test is not the only factor that affects drug detection. Other factors include the half-life of the substance, the patient's ability to metabolize or excrete the substance, the extent of substance use,

TABLE 7.20 Urine Toxicology Screening

Substance (Metabolite Detected)	Window for Detection	False Positives
Cannabis (cannabinoids)	Occasional user: 1–3 days or longer Chronic heavy user: 1 month or longer	Dronabinol Efavirenz NSAIDs Proton pump inhibitors Tolmetin
Cocaine (benzoylecogonine)	Up to 3 days	Virtually no false positives
Amphetamine/ methamphetamine/MDMA (amphetamine)	Up to 5 days	Bupropion Desipramine Ephedrine Methylphenidate Phenylephrine Pseudoephedrine Ranitidine Selegiline Trazodone Vick's inhaler
Opioids: Morphine Oxycodone Hydrocodone Methadone	48 hours 2–4 days 2–4 days 3 days	Dextromethorphan Diphenhydramine Poppy seeds Quinine Quinolones Rifampin Verapamil
Benzodiazepines	Short-acting (e.g., lorazepam): 3 days Long-acting (e.g., diazepam): 30 days	Sertraline Oxaprozin
Barbiturates	Short-acting (e.g., pentobarbital): 24 hours Long-acting (e.g., phenobarbital): 3 weeks	
Phencyclidine	8 days	Dextromethorphan Diphenhydramine Doxylamine Ibuprofen Imipramine Ketamine Meperidine Mesoridazine Thioridazine Tramadol Venlafaxine

Source: Moeller, K. E., K. C. Lee, and J. C. Kissack. Urine drug screening: practical guide for clinicians. *Mayo Clinic Proceedings* 83(1):66–76, 2008.

the method of collecting the sample, intentional or inadvertent tampering with the sample, and the method used to store the sample. Positive drug test results or abnormal lab findings may suggest problematic substance use but are not diagnostic. Only information obtained in a clinical interview can confirm a substance-related disorder.

Specific lab abnormalities sometimes seen in users of PCP include myoglobinuria, and elevated creatine phosphokinase (CPK), blood urea nitrogen (BUN), and creatinine. Users of inhalants may show changes in complete blood count (CBC), elevated BUN and creatinine, or elevated liver enzymes.

ETIOLOGY

For individuals with alcohol or drug problems, a complex, unique set of **biological, psychological**, and **social** variables influence their addictive behavior. Individual vulnerability to developing a drug addiction results from a complex interaction of genetic and environmental factors. Importantly, these factors do not predestine an individual to a substance use disorder but only confer vulnerability.

Neurobiological Factors

The past decade has seen an explosion in molecular biology, human genetics, and neuroscience research leading to a richer understanding of the biological underpinnings of addiction. Multiple lines of evidence have emerged for individual genetic variation resulting in an increased vulnerability to developing a substance use disorder. Neurobiological mechanisms underlying the evolution and maintenance of substance use disorders have also been hypothesized.

Genetic Factors

Epidemiological studies of twins and families have demonstrated a genetic contribution of **30–60%** in developing addiction. Adoption studies have also supported the model of genetic transmission of problematic alcohol and drug use. Even if their adoptive parents are not alcoholics, adopted men with one biological parent who is an alcoholic are four times as likely to become alcoholics themselves, compared with their counterparts whose biological parents are not alcohol dependent. In contrast, epidemiological studies also provide strong evidence that developing a substance use disorder has important nongenetic, experiential determinants.

Twin and family studies have helped differentiate genes that influence initiation of drug use and genes influencing the evolution of problematic substance use. These studies have identified genetic variations that are common across all addictions and others that are common to a particular addiction. Genes have been identified that influence personality traits as well as physiological traits that are associated with increased vulnerability to developing substance dependence. Genetic variations in genes coding neurotransmitter receptors and transporters have been identified that influence drug pharmacodynamics (drug effects at receptors and effect of receptor binding). Genetic variations in genes influencing pharmacokinetics (drug absorption, distribution, metabolism, and excretion) have also been identified.

The heritability of problematic substance use was first demonstrated for alcohol. **Genetic polymorphisms influencing alcohol metabolism** (alcohol dehydrogenase and aldehyde dehydrogenase) were identified and are directly correlated to differential rates of alcohol consumption and alcohol dependence. Approximately 50% of northeast

Asians, including Chinese, Japanese, and Koreans, carry a dominant mutation of a gene, rare among non-Asians, involved in the production of aldehyde dehydrogenase and resulting in deficient enzyme activity. Individuals with this genetic variation experience a "flushing reaction" that causes visible redness, increased heart rate, and feelings of warmth when they consume alcohol. Individuals with this genetic variation drink less and have lower rates of alcohol use disorder than their counterparts with normal aldehyde dehydrogenase activity. Some small groups of Native Americans have been found to have an increased frequency of a variant of gene involved in the production of alcohol dehydrogenase with a similar protective effect. Nonetheless, high rates of alcohol use disorders are seen generally in the Native American population.

Recently, a specific variation in the *OPRM1* gene that encodes the opioid receptor has been shown to cause altered receptor-binding affinity. Individuals with this variant allele experience differences in subjective effects of alcohol compared with individuals without this variant. Individuals with this variant appear to have an increased response to naltrexone and may have a better response to naltrexone treatment for alcohol use disorders. This is likely the first example of **addiction pharmacogenetics**—pharmacotherapy guided by genotype.

Neurotransmitter Factors

A commonly held hypothesis borne out by animal studies holds that most substances of abuse exert their initial reinforcing effect via a large, rapid rise in **dopamine** in the **nucleus accumbens**, which is innervated by the **ventral tegmental area** and has wide-ranging projections. Dopamine pathways have a central role in **reward** and **reinforcement** in the brain. However, dopaminergic neurons are modulated by a wide array of other neurotransmitter systems (γ-aminobutyric acid [**GABA**], **glutamate, opioid, cholinergic, serotonin, and neuropeptide y**) that also are thought to be involved in important ways in establishing and maintaining substance use disorders. Cocaine, amphetamine, methamphetamine, and MDMA directly activate the dopamine system by facilitating dopamine release or inhibiting its uptake. Other drugs, including alcohol, nicotine, opioids, and marijuana, increase dopamine indirectly through GABAergic and glutamatergic neurons that are stimulated by **GABA, nicotine, μ-opioid**, or **cannabinoid CB_1 receptors** (Baler and Volkow 2006). Stimuli that have been repeatedly paired with drug use through classical conditioning are hypothesized to generate increased dopamine activity in the nucleus accumbens without use and cause **drug craving** even during periods of abstinence.

Neuroendocrine Factors

Both biological sex and sex hormone milieu may have an as yet undefined impact on the development of substance use disorders. Defining the differences between male and female substance users is an active area of research. Stress response and activation of the hypothalamic–pituitary–adrenal (HPA) axis are under genetic control and are influenced by exposure to drugs of abuse. The role of variation in stress response in substance use disorders is currently being investigated.

Psychological Factors

Personality traits that are genetically influenced can contribute to a vulnerability to the development of a substance use disorder. Individuals with high **impulsivity**, the tendency to act without planning or considering consequences; **novelty seeking**, the tendency to seek new behaviors or sensations; and **risk taking**, the tendency to act in a planned way despite knowing possible negative consequences, have an increased vulnerability to addiction. Related to impulsivity is the concept of **delayed discounting**—the longer the delay to a reward, the less the reward is valued. Individuals with substance use disorders tend to choose smaller immediate rewards over larger delayed rewards.

A cognitive-behavioral framework can be used to understand the development of problematic substance use. Substance use can be seen as a **learned behavior** initially modeled from others and rehearsed over time, often over the course of years. Drug taking and associated behaviors can receive **positive reinforcement** from the pleasurable effects of substance use and **negative reinforcement** from using substances to remove the aversive effects of abstinence. After repeated pairing of previously neutral stimuli with substance use, many previously neutral stimuli such as people (e.g., using friends), places (e.g., liquor store), and things (e.g., drug paraphernalia) become strongly associated with substance use. Even during periods of abstinence, these stimuli can serve as **triggers** for substance **craving** and use. Substance use can also be conceptualized as a learned, inappropriate means of dealing with life stressors when ineffective coping skills are overwhelmed.

The **self-medication hypothesis** proposes that psychoactive substances are used by individuals to treat distressing psychiatric symptoms. For example, a person starts drinking in an attempt to alleviate panic attacks. Although this hypothesis is appealing in many ways, studies have been mixed as to whether substance use or psychiatric disorders manifest first. Once a substance use disorder has developed, the addiction will likely require specific treatment regardless of the reason why the substance use began. Additionally, this hypothesis does not take into account that these substances are appetitive stimuli (positively reinforcing). This is in contrast to taking an antibiotic for infection, in which the antibiotic is likely only to have a negative reinforcing effect (alleviates aversive stimuli without being pleasurable in and of itself).

Cognitive deficits hypothesized to be important in self-control have been studied using neurocognitive testing in individuals with substance use disorders. Changes in the brain areas thought to be important in **self-control** have been investigated using neuro-imaging studies (functional magnetic resonance imaging [fMRI] and positron emission tomography [PET]). Imaging studies have suggested altered functioning in the orbito-frontal cortex (involved in motivation, drive, and shifting the relative value of reinforcers) and the anterior cingulate gyrus (involved in inhibitory control), as well as in the amygdala and hippocampus (central for memory and learning).

Social Factors

An individual's **culture** is an important factor influencing alcohol and drug use. For example, in the Mormon religion, strong prohibitions exist against alcohol and other substance use. Alcohol and drug use and substance use disorders are much less common among Mormons in the United States than in the general population. Among other cultural groups, substance use is common, and heavy drinking or regular drug use may be culturally sanctioned. Historically, bars and nightclubs have been the predominant venue for socialization for the gay, lesbian, bisexual, and transgendered communities. Epidemiological studies of gay and bisexual men have consistently shown greater prevalence rates of alcohol and drug use but not necessarily substance use disorders compared with matched heterosexual controls. The **peer group** or culture to which an individual belongs models what is considered normative substance use.

Context of use can have a powerful influence on substance use. Approximately 20% of American military men who served in Vietnam became dependent on heroin during their tour of duty. Heroin was widely available in Vietnam at that time. Interestingly, upon return to the United States less than 5% remained dependent, demonstrating the importance of culture and the context of substance use in both developing and maintaining a substance use disorder.

Societal factors can also influence the prevalence of addictive behavior. If a psychoactive substance is **illegal**, it is less widely available and more expensive. As a result, generally fewer people have the opportunity to begin using the substance, resulting in lower rates of problematic use. Society has attempted to curtail the use of legal psychoactive substances (alcohol and tobacco) by adolescents by prohibiting purchase or consumption by minors. Drugs are readily available in many communities on the black market despite illegality, and adolescents can easily obtain and use alcohol and cigarettes despite minimum ages for purchase and consumption.

The rates of problematic alcohol and drug use are lower in women than in **men**. The reason for this differential is likely multifactorial and includes genetic and social factors. Generally, there have been stronger cultural and societal prohibitions against substance use by women than those for men, and these prohibitions may be suppressing the expression of addictive behavior. More recently, this gender gap has been shrinking with changing social mores.

Marital conflict may cause children to seek out peers who use drugs or drink alcohol. Peer associations are a major influence in the initiation and maintenance of adolescent substance use. Parental and familial attitudes toward substance use, as well as parents' own substance use, significantly affect adolescent substance use.

Some specific factors that may lead to substance use disorders in midlife are job loss or dissatisfaction, divorce, separation, children leaving home, emotional distress, and medical illness. Most people who encounter these stressors do not develop a substance use disorder. Those who do may have never learned effective stress management or coping skills.

TREATMENT

Recovery from Substance-Related Disorders

Only a minority of people with a substance use disorder seek treatment. According to the 2011 National Survey on Drug Use and Health, of the 21.1 million Americans estimated to be in need of substance use treatment, 95% felt they did not need treatment. Diagnosing patients with a substance use disorder, alerting them to the diagnosis, and referring them to appropriate treatment are critical.

Recovery from a substance use disorder is the process by which an individual learns effective coping strategies for regaining control over compulsive substance use. Recovery requires making a commitment to change substance use behaviors and to maintain these changes. For many individuals, a return to controlled substance use is their initial treatment goal, a goal that often proves difficult or impossible. Most patients find that recovery requires total abstinence from the substance they were using in a problematic way. Treatment programs in the United States have traditionally been based on an **abstinence model**, viewing total abstinence from all psychoactive substances as the only acceptable goal of addiction treatment. In recent years, a **harm reduction model** has been gaining favor. This model conceptualizes reduction of negative consequences (e.g., health, social, psychological, legal) of substance use as a meaningful treatment goal. Needle exchange programs are an example of an intervention based on a harm reduction model. Less frequent, less risky, and lower-dose substance use are acceptable goals to be encouraged in this model. Complete abstinence can be conceptualized as the greatest degree of harm reduction. In some abstinence-based treatment programs patients are asked to leave if they continue to use or repeatedly relapse to use. In treatment programs based on harm reduction, some patients may continue to use substances while in active treatment.

The **transtheoretical model** describes five stages that patients pass through when making intentional behavior change (see Box 7.10). Patients normally experience a varying degree of ambivalence regarding changing their substance use behavior. The physician's task is to help patients understand this ambivalence and foster increased motivation for change. Readiness to change substance use behavior may vary among the multiple substances a patient is using. For example, a patient may feel ready to decrease his or her alcohol consumption but not ready to consider quitting smoking cigarettes. Physicians should strive to match treatment interventions to patients' needs as well as to their readiness for change and acceptance of different treatment modalities.

BOX 7.10
THE TRANSTHEORETICAL MODEL

The transtheoretical model (TTM) provides a framework to understand how people make **intentional health behavior changes**. The model describes **five stages** of change that individuals move through when making changes in behavior including substance use. In the **precontemplation** stage, the individual has no thoughts of or is uninterested in changing his or her behavior in the near future. During the **contemplation** stage, the individual is considering behavior change in the near future, and marked ambivalence is a hallmark of this stage of change. At the **preparation** stage, the individual has decided to make change and is planning to start implementing that change. In the **action** stage, the individual is implementing changes in the targeted behavior. Not uncommonly, individuals move rather quickly from the preparation to action stage once they have decided to make change. At the **maintenance** stage of change, the individual has made significant behavior changes and is working on maintaining those changes. These stages are relatively fluid, and it is common for individuals to progress to a next level of change and then fall back to an earlier stage of change as they move toward long-lasting behavior change. Once the maintenance phase has been established (usually defined as 6 months of consistent behavior), this new behavior can be considered the baseline behavior and the individual can be considered precontemplational in terms of the original behavior that was changed.

Motivational interviewing (MI) and **motivational enhancement therapy** (MET) are built upon the TTM. A large empirical database supports the usefulness of these interventions for substance users. Initially developed for smoking cessation, MI has been found to be useful for treatment across problematically used substance classes. Doctors can learn to use MI and other brief interventions and make a big impact on patient behavior.

Addiction treatment is designed to help patients become abstinent, maintain abstinence, and avoid relapse to use. A major goal of treatment is to help individuals recognize the warning signs of relapse in time to prevent it. In the past, any return to alcohol or drug use was usually viewed as a treatment failure. Currently, distinctions are often made between a lapse and a relapse. A **lapse** is a brief return to substance use. In contrast, a **relapse** is a return to excessive or uncontrolled use. When patients experience a lapse, the physician can help them to cognitively restructure the situation. Instead of perceiving the loss of sobriety as a personal failure, patients can see it as a chance to understand what prompted them to return to substance use and can learn improved methods of coping so that it will not happen in the future.

Recovery can occur spontaneously or with treatment. Formal substance abuse treatment is associated with improved outcomes in substance use. Regardless of the substance used, recovery must be seen as a long-term process that is measured in years rather than weeks.

Successful maintenance of recovery is usually positively associated with the length of prior periods of abstinence and the involvement of supportive significant others in the patient's treatment. Although it is not clear whether demographic variables such as income, race, gender, or marital status can predict the outcome of treatment, income and marital status often reflect social supports that are correlated with a higher probability of a good outcome. The amount or frequency of alcohol or drug use does not seem to be predictive of outcome. A chronic course of problematic substance use and many previous addiction treatment episodes are both predictive of poorer treatment outcome. As in other areas of medicine, individuals with more severe and more chronic illness are often harder to treat, but this does not mean that treatment will not be helpful or should be withheld.

Individuals who have long histories of problematic substance use are often difficult to treat. Some chronic users, particularly alcoholics, manage to avoid the treatment system altogether. Alcohol use disorder is often first detected when the patient has work-related difficulties and is forced to enter an **employee assistance program** (EAP). Some alcoholics are initially diagnosed when they require medical treatment for pancreatitis or liver disease. It may be extremely difficult for these individuals to identify themselves as addicts requiring substance abuse treatment.

Other habitual users admit they have a problem with their substance use and repeatedly seek help, but despite the efforts of a myriad of treatment programs, they continue to have difficulties related to their chemical use. Because of their long string of perceived failures, they lose faith that they can be helped. It is the physician's role to remain optimistic and refer these patients to addiction specialists who may be able to offer additional treatment strategies.

Treatment for patients who suffer from drug use disorders involves various approaches and takes place in different settings. The patient's needs should dictate the treatment strategy, but the availability of community resources or the patient's insurance or financial means often dictate the mode of therapy.

Therapeutic Settings

As physicians have gained a better understanding of addicted patients, they have recognized the importance of matching each patient to the appropriate treatment. The needs of the patient and the patient's conceptual understanding of the addictive behavior must be explored before a treatment plan is designed and implemented. Treatment is effective only if it is appropriate to the needs of the patient and if the patient and the physician have a working alliance. Most patients with substance use disorders have a variety of problems related to life functioning. They may lack job skills, have family or marital difficulties, suffer from a variety of medical ailments caused by neglect or poor nutrition, or experience significant emotional distress. Although it may be beyond the scope of any one treatment program to address all of these areas, it is crucial that the areas of greatest difficulty or of greatest concern to the patient be addressed.

An essential part of understanding the individual needs of the patient is recognizing the patient's level of motivation for change, conceptualization of the addictive behavior, and individual treatment goals. Individuals enter treatment for a multitude of reasons. Some are forced to do so by the legal system or their families and may not accept that they have a problem with psychoactive substances; therefore, they will be resistant to any form of treatment. These patients often benefit from substance use education and nonjudgmental presentation of specific individualized feedback about the consequences that substance use has had in their lives or on their bodies (e.g., laboratory abnormalities, loss of job). Individuals who freely choose to enter treatment may recognize their problems with alcohol or drugs but may believe that they can use chemicals in a controlled manner.

Because patients with severe psychiatric problems tend to do poorly in standard substance use disorder programs, they must be identified and provided appropriate pharmacological and psychosocial treatments. If the chemical treatment program does not have an adequate psychiatric staff or consultants for these patients, the patients should be referred to a more appropriate program. Patients with co-occurring substance use disorders and other psychiatric illness are best served at programs designed to treat both issues simultaneously. These programs have adequate psychiatric staff or consultants to appropriately address the needs of these patients. Individuals with current severe psychiatric problems tend to have a poorer prognosis than those with less severe psychiatric symptoms.

Patients with substance use disorder often assume that their addictive behavior is due to moral weakness or a lack of will power. These assumptions cause them to feel enormous guilt and to view treatment as punitive. Unless they are coerced into entering treatment, they may avoid it altogether. For these individuals, a dialogue with an addiction specialist who takes a different view (i.e., that addictive behavior can be due to a variety of biological, psychological, and environmental factors) may be extremely productive. If such patients can accept the view that they are not morally reprehensible for having an addiction but *are* responsible for changing their behavior, they may be willing to embrace treatment.

Even for individuals who have had frequent relapses, drug treatment can eventually be successful. Ideally, with each treatment attempt patients gain new insights and learn more strategies for living a drug-free lifestyle. Treatment can also be effective for individuals who are reluctant to seek treatment or are forced into it. In fact, substance-using individuals who are pressured into treatment by their families, their employers, or the criminal justice system often do just as well as patients who enter treatment voluntarily.

After physicians and patients agree that treatment is necessary, they must decide what level or intensity of care will be most appropriate. Inpatient treatment including medically managed detoxification or rehabilitation provides the highest level of monitoring, structure, and intervention. Other patients will do well in outpatient treatment, which can range from day programming and intensive outpatient programs, to groups (professionally lead or mutual self-help), to individual treatment with an addiction specialist. Understanding the benefits and drawbacks of each setting is important for making appropriate treatment referrals.

Much of American substance use disorder treatment has been based on 12-step treatment models. In many treatment settings, patients are encouraged to attend Alcoholics Anonymous (AA) or Narcotics Anonymous (NA) meetings. In inpatient settings, these meetings are often one component of the treatment. In outpatient settings, these meetings may be the patient's only form of support, or they may be used in conjunction with other therapies. AA and NA meetings are run by lay members of the groups. Using a self-help supportive model, individuals are encouraged to admit their powerlessness over alcohol or other drugs and accept their need for help from a higher power. In AA, the **12-step program** helps the individual to begin a process toward recovery (see Table 7.21). Meetings may be closed (i.e., only members or potential members of the group can attend) or open (i.e., any interested person can attend). All physicians should attend at least one open meeting so that they can adequately answer patients' questions regarding these groups. Referral to a 12-step group is not effective for all patients and does not necessarily replace the need for substance abuse disorder treatment.

Inpatient and Residential Chemical Dependence Programs

Medically managed inpatient **detoxification units** are the highest level of medical intervention for substance use disorders. Patients are most often admitted to detoxification units for management of withdrawal from alcohol, sedative-hypnotics (benzodiazepines, barbiturates), or opioids. Detoxification itself does not generally require an inpatient admission, but severity of illness and comorbidity may necessitate inpatient treatment. Detoxification admissions vary in length depending on the substance the patient is withdrawing from but generally last 3–7 days. This treatment is generally focused on safe detoxification management and arranging appropriate aftercare treatment. Detoxification may be a necessary first step but is rarely adequate treatment of substance use disorders.

Inpatient rehabilitation programs are often based in freestanding treatment units (i.e., other than hospitals) or in psychiatric hospitals. Psychiatric hospitals often treat adolescents and patients with co-occurring disorders, including patients who require close monitoring because of suicidal ideation or other psychiatric symptoms. Patients usually stay for 2–4 weeks. Treatment usually includes individual, group, and family therapy;

TABLE 7.21 The 12 Steps of Alcoholics Anonymous

1. We admitted we were powerless over alcohol and that our lives had become unmanageable.
2. Came to believe that a Power greater than ourselves could restore us to sanity.
3. Made a decision to turn our will and our lives over to the care of God as we understood Him.
4. Made a searching and fearless moral inventory of ourselves.
5. Admitted to God, to ourselves, and to another human being the exact nature of our wrongs.
6. Were entirely ready to have God remove all these defects of character.
7. Humbly asked Him to remove our shortcomings.
8. Made a list of all persons we had harmed, and became willing to make amends to them all.
9. Made direct amends to such people wherever possible, except when to do so would injure them or others.
10. Continued to take personal inventory and when we were wrong promptly admitted it.
11. Sought through prayer and meditation to improve our conscious contact with God as we understood Him, praying only for knowledge of His will for us and the power to carry that out.
12. Having had a spiritual awakening as the result of these steps, we tried to carry this message to alcoholics, and to practice these principles in all our affairs.

education; exercise; relaxation techniques; and attendance at AA or NA meetings. Some inpatient rehabilitation programs are able to identify and treat individuals with coexisting psychiatric disorders, but many of these programs have no such capability.

Freestanding rehabilitation units usually utilize the AA 12-step model of treatment. The focus of these intensive programs is to comprehensively evaluate each patient from a psychosocial approach, develop a treatment plan, and implement the 12-step program. In the past, these programs were often the first treatment option, but with the advent of managed care, they now most commonly treat individuals who have repeatedly relapsed in outpatient settings, have required removal from drug-plagued environments to achieve abstinence, or have been referred by their employers because of occupational difficulties related to substance use. Patients are usually admitted for 2–4 weeks and then are referred to further outpatient treatment and encouraged to attend AA or NA meetings. Patients often enter freestanding programs after they have been detoxified in a medical facility. Units with full-time physicians may provide pharmacological treatment for uncomplicated detoxification or helping maintain abstinence. Physicians at these facilities may also perform physical examinations and provide medical treatment as needed. In many instances, therapy is provided by counselors who are themselves in recovery.

Outpatient Programs

Outpatient treatment programs offer a wide range of addiction treatment services including individual, group, and family therapy. Patients entering outpatient programs may be new to treatment, referred from other treatment settings, or forced to enter treatment (e.g., by the legal system or an EAP). Certain elements are essential. The program should carry out a **comprehensive initial psychosocial evaluation** of the patient to detect major complicating psychiatric, social, or medical problems that may require additional psychotherapy, family therapy, psychiatric medication, or referral to an inpatient program. This evaluation may allow for tailoring of the outpatient services selected to the specific needs of the patient. Additionally, **urine testing** must be done frequently during outpatient treatment to ensure that treating clinicians are aware of the extent of the patient's substance use and to document treatment efficacy and patient progress.

Outpatient clinics often provide individual and group therapy and education groups that teach patients about the negative social, psychiatric, and medical consequences of substance use. Comprehensive outpatient treatment clinics may also include pharmacological treatment. To better meet the needs of their patients, many outpatient treatment clinics also offer a variety of specialty groups for women; gay, lesbian, or bisexual individuals; HIV-positive individuals; and adolescents. Other groups may teach parenting skills or help patients learn how to find a job or write a resumé.

Twelve-step groups are not the only type of mutual-self help groups available in the community. Individuals who are uncomfortable with the spiritual aspects of traditional 12-step groups or those who do not have complete abstinence from psychoactive substances as a goal may do well in alternative mutual self-help groups such as Rational Recovery or Self-Management and Recovery Training (**SMART**). Groups that do not embrace the 12-step approach are much less widespread and therefore may be hard to use. Nonetheless, they may serve as alternative adjuncts to formal substance abuse treatment.

Residential Therapeutic Community Programs

Residential programs, also known as **therapeutic communities**, stress the importance of having fellow addicts and ex-addicts provide nonprofessional treatment to individuals recovering from substance use disorders within a residential setting. These communities are often staffed by ex-addicts. Rewards and penalties are used to shape the residents' behaviors, and confrontation by their peers regarding the consequences of their behaviors is virtually constant. These programs are highly structured, and residents are required to work. The jobs are allocated according to the patient's length of stay in the community, competence, and ability to behave responsibly.

Most residential community programs recommend that residents stay a number of months. Many individuals with substance use disorders are unwilling to make a commitment to a highly structured treatment program and may resist the strict regulation of their behavior. Because these programs rely heavily on confrontation, they are not recommended for patients with comorbid psychiatric disorders or for emotionally fragile individuals. Residential programs have been criticized because their dropout rate is high. However, even individuals who leave precipitously benefit from the treatment because the longer they remain in the facility the more likely they are to reduce their drug use or illegal activities after they leave.

Treatment programs in general have a wide range of strategies for engaging and maintaining patients in therapy, including behavioral or psychotherapeutic techniques, religious beliefs, and pharmacological interventions. These methods are commonly used in combination.

Psychotherapy

Evidence-based psychotherapeutic interventions for the treatment of substance use disorders include motivational interviewing (MI), motivational enhancement therapy, cognitive behavior therapy, relapse prevention therapy, skills training, community reinforcement approach, community reinforcement approach family training, and 12-step facilitation (Anton et al. 2006). Psychotherapy may be used in individual, group, and family therapy settings. The evidence shows that all of these therapy approaches are effective in helping patients reduce their substance use.

The goal of early recovery is cessation of substance use. Therapies utilized in early treatment are designed to help patients stop substance use and remain abstinent. Uncovering core conflicts and confronting maladaptive defenses can produce a significant degree of anxiety, and exploratory, uncovering type therapies have not been shown to be helpful in early recovery. Not until the patient has had an extended period of recovery should a more traditional psychodynamic psychotherapy be applied. Only then is a patient more likely to tolerate anxiety without returning to self-destructive drug use.

The initial psychotherapeutic treatment of substance use disorders usually begins with motivational work (**motivational interviewing** and **motivational enhancement therapy**), with the goals of increasing patient motivation and readiness to change or helping patients design an action plan for treatment. This type of intervention uses specific techniques to help patients navigate the normal ambivalence toward their substance use and abstinence. Underpinning this model of treatment is the idea that patients will successfully make changes in their behavior when they reach an appropriate stage of readiness. As patients often continue to experience ambivalence during treatment, these techniques can be helpful in later stages of treatment, when other psychotherapy modalities may be employed.

Cognitive-behavioral therapy (CBT) is a time-limited intervention directed at understanding the learning processes that have been integral to the development and continuation of the substance use disorder (see Chapter 17, Psychotherapy). **Functional analysis** (the identification of thoughts, feelings, and circumstances preceding and following substance use) and **skills training** (teaching specific effective coping strategies other than substance use to deal with life's challenges and maintain abstinence) help the patient learn to recognize and manage high-risk situations and feelings that might cause them to use drugs, as well as the early warning signs of an impending relapse.

Behavior therapy techniques are based on the psychological theories of operant or respondent conditioning. In **operant conditioning**, a behavior is shaped by the environmental consequences of that behavior. If a behavior is rewarded, it is more likely to be repeated, and if it is punished, it will eventually diminish. When operant techniques are applied successfully to problematic substance users, salient reinforcers or punishers effectively compete with the rewarding aspects of drug use. In **respondent conditioning**, aversive stimuli serve to eliminate or reduce the pleasant effects of drugs or drug stimuli. **Disulfiram** is an example of such an aversive behavioral technique (see Pharmacotherapy, later in this chapter). The difficulty with all aversive behavioral techniques is finding stimuli that are negative enough to suppress drug use, acceptable to the patient, and ethically and medically responsible.

The underpinning of the **community reinforcement approach** is that social, vocational, familial, and recreational reinforcers or contingencies play a pivotal role in encouraging or discouraging substance use. Positive and negative contingencies are put in place to help patients maintain abstinence. For example, patients may receive vouchers redeemable for non–substance-related goods or activities that promote a healthy lifestyle as a contingent reward for a negative urine test, or patients may contract to let therapists inform their families, colleagues, or bosses if they break their abstinence and resume using drugs. Community reinforcement approach family training (CRAFT) engages family members or significant others and helps them impose positive and negative contingences on the impaired individual to encourage him or her to seek treatment. CRAFT also can help family and significant others effectively deal with their loved one whether the addict seeks treatment or not.

Supportive psychotherapy can be modified to meet the treatment needs of patients with substance use disorders. An empathetic and nonjudgmental therapist can help patients replace drug-seeking behaviors with new behaviors that are compatible with a healthier, drug-free lifestyle. Patients learn to avoid relapse by developing new areas of interest and activities as substitutes for their former drug behaviors. Finding new, rewarding, healthy activities to replace substance use is an essential goal of substance abuse treatment that maintains long-term abstinence, as stopping substance use often initially leaves a sense of emptiness in the former user's life.

At times, issues of loss, past physical or sexual abuse, or other traumatic events impede the patient's ability to achieve prolonged abstinence. For such patients, the therapeutic focus on the present situation may require some modification. These patients have often used substance use to avoid painful feelings associated with disturbing past events. These events may need to be addressed early in treatment, but the purpose of such exploration should be to teach the patient new strategies for coping with distressing memories and help the patient build self-esteem.

Pharmacotherapy

Various pharmacological strategies may be employed in the treatment of substance use disorders. Antagonist agents are given to block the pleasant effects of drugs of abuse or emergently in cases of overdose. Other medications produce aversive effects if an abused substance is taken concomitantly. Agonist or partial-agonist medications produce the same effects as the substance being used but with less euphoric effect and fewer physical or psychosocial consequences. Other medications are used to treat withdrawal symptoms or to decrease cravings for alcohol or drugs.

Pharmacotherapy is most effective when combined with other forms of treatment. To assess which pharmacological approach may be appropriate, a patient's **psychological and physical status**, as well as his or her **motivation** for treatment should be assessed. The symbolic aspect of administering drugs (medications) to individuals with substance use disorders should not be overlooked. Some patients may be seeking a "magic bullet" in the form of a medication that will solve their problems. Patients need instruction from physicians to understand that medications are being prescribed to help reduce harmful substance use but will not take the place of work toward change on their part.

Alcohol Use Disorder

Three medications are U.S. Food and Drug Administration (FDA) approved for the treatment of alcohol use disorder. **Disulfiram** is an **aversive** treatment that acts via the inhibition of aldehyde dehydrogenase. If patients drink alcohol or ingest substances containing alcohol after taking disulfiram, acetaldehyde levels rise, resulting in **flushing**, decreased blood pressure, **nausea and vomiting, and pounding in the chest**. More serious but rare consequences include seizures, myocardial infarction, cerebrovascular hemorrhage, and cardiovascular collapse. Despite the use of this medication for over 50 years, deaths have rarely occurred. Disulfiram is generally indicated for highly motivated patients or for those who have had success with the medication in the past. Adherence to disulfiram is poor, and individuals can quickly return to drinking (within a week) after discontinuing disulfiram.

Naltrexone is an opioid antagonist that **diminishes the reinforcing effects** of alcohol. Naltrexone has been demonstrated to reduce the number of drinks consumed per drinking day and to increase the number of days of abstinence in individuals striving for abstinence. Naltrexone is available in both daily oral dosing and monthly depot injections. **Acamprosate**, which is thought to modulate GABA and glutamate neurotransmitter pathways, has been demonstrated to increase the time to relapse to drinking in patients who have already achieved abstinence. Both naltrexone and acamprosate therapy have been shown to be more successful in conjunction with psychosocial treatment targeting alcohol dependence. Neither naltrexone nor acamprosate is an aversive therapy, and combining these medications with alcohol does not produce unpleasant symptoms. Neither medication blocks the intoxicating effects of alcohol.

The anticonvulsant **topiramate** has also shown utility in reducing relapse to heavy drinking (five or more standard drinks per drinking day) in multiple double-blind, randomized controlled trials. It does not currently have FDA approval for this indication.

Detoxification from Alcohol and Other Sedatives

If a patient wishes to be detoxified or is experiencing withdrawal symptoms associated with alcohol or other classes of sedatives (e.g., barbiturates and benzodiazepines), a number of pharmacological approaches can be used. The agent for detoxification is chosen on the basis of medical status of the patient, intended route of administration, and desired half-life. **Benzodiazepines** are the most commonly used agents for alcohol or sedative detoxification, although barbiturates (e.g., phenobarbital) can also be used. Some studies suggest that anticonvulsants (e.g., carbamazepine or valproic acid) may be useful detoxifying agents, especially if there is a prior history of withdrawal seizures, but neither is commonly used for alcohol detoxification. The basic principle of pharmacological detoxification is to rapidly substitute a sufficient amount of the detoxifying agent to prevent withdrawal symptoms and then gradually decrease the dose of the detoxifying agent over several days. Adequate substitution can be estimated using conversion tables.

Flumazenil, a benzodiazepine receptor antagonist, can be administered intravenously in emergency situations to reverse benzodiazepine overdose. This agent must be used cautiously, as it may precipitate withdrawal symptoms (including seizures) in chronic benzodiazepine users.

Opioid Use Disorder

In emergency settings, physicians may administer **naloxone**, an opioid antagonist, to reverse the effects of opioid overdoses. Naloxone can be administered intravenously, intramuscularly, subcutaneously, or via endotracheal tube if necessary. As the action of naloxone may be shorter than the duration of action of the administered opioid, naloxone may need to be administered repeatedly, and patients should be monitored closely.

Medication strategies for long-term maintenance treatment of opioid dependence include agents that are μ-opioid receptor agonists, antagonists, or partial agonists. **Naltrexone**, a long-acting, orally active opioid antagonist, is used to help maintain abstinence by competitively binding at μ-opioid receptors and blocking the effects of opioids. For maintenance purposes, patients must first be detoxified, as naltrexone can quickly precipitate withdrawal in physiologically dependent individuals who have recently used. Patient adherence to oral naltrexone is generally poor. Opioid-dependent individuals treated with naltrexone often continue to experience significant cravings for drug use. Naltrexone treatment can be abruptly stopped without adverse effects, leading to rapid removal of the opioid receptor blockade and allowing patients to easily and quickly return to use. Adherence may be improved with depot naltrexone injections. Naltrexone treatment has been most successful for patients who have much to lose because of their use or who are highly motivated for treatment (e.g., physicians or individuals under the control of the criminal justice system, see case example in Box 7.11).

Methadone maintenance is the most established form of substitution pharmacotherapy for opioid dependence, and it has been used successfully for nearly 50 years. Methadone is a long-acting (i.e., it can be dosed once daily) full **opioid agonist** with good oral availability. In contrast to heroin and other short-acting opioids, it does not produce significant fluctuations in mood or alertness throughout the day. Methadone is titrated to a dose that blocks opioid withdrawal, halts non-methadone opioid use, and quells cravings. Patients can be directly transitioned from heroin or other opioids to methadone without prior detoxification.

Federal and state laws closely regulate the requirements for patient eligibility for methadone maintenance therapy, medication dispensing, and program structure. Methadone maintenance for opioid dependence can only be prescribed through a licensed methadone clinic. To qualify for maintenance therapy, patients must be opioid dependent and demonstrate observable signs of physical withdrawal. Physical signs of withdrawal may be spontaneous or precipitated by administering a test dose of an opioid antagonist such as naloxone (known as a **naloxone challenge**). Patients entering methadone maintenance must be 18 years of age or older with at least a 1-year history of opioid dependence (exceptions include pregnant women, previously treated patients, and individuals being released from prison). Alternative criteria apply to individuals under the age of 18. During the first year of treatment, patients generally must come daily to a methadone clinic to obtain their medication. Depending on response to treatment and adherence, patients can receive a limited number of take-home doses, again regulated by state and federal law. The tight **regulation** of methadone maintenance is an attempt to ensure appropriate

CASE EXAMPLE OF OPIOID USE DISORDER AND TREATMENT IN AN IMPAIRED PHYSICIAN

A 30-year-old anesthesiology resident received a hydrocodone prescription for a shoulder injury and noticed that he enjoyed both the euphoric and calming effects of the medication. He got two additional prescriptions for hydrocodone from coworkers, despite achieving adequate pain control with NSAIDs. He then began using fentanyl, a potent opioid available to him at work, in order to "cope with the stress and anxiety of work" and "trouble" with his marriage. As his drug use began to escalate, he began missing days of work and the operating room staff noticed that he had become more argumentative than usual. He began inconsistently responding to pages. Frustrated with his behavior at home, his wife was staying at her parents' home in a neighboring city with their young son. None of his colleagues suspected substance use as the cause of these behavior changes, until an overdose brought him into the emergency room. After emergency stabilization, the resident was transferred to a hospital at which he did not work, for opioid detoxification. The consulted addiction psychiatrist was required by the laws of his state to report the resident as an impaired physician. As a contingency of returning to work as a physician, the state agency devised a plan for addiction treatment and monitoring including a 1-month participation at an inpatient rehabilitation geared toward impaired physicians, followed by 12 months of mandatory outpatient treatment. Additionally, ongoing random urine drug screening and monitoring by a psychiatrist was stipulated. The resident also opted for antagonist treatment with naltrexone. On his own, the resident began attending Caduceus meetings (12-step–based meetings for health care professionals). The resident did exceptionally well, maintaining long-term abstinence from illicit opioid use and adhering to his treatment and monitoring plan. He was ultimately able to finish a residency in family medicine and get a job in the community.

As illustrated in this case, opioid use disorder commonly begins with a legitimate prescription for pain. Physicians, nurses, and pharmacists tend to have increased access to opioids and other abusable prescription medications. This case highlights several red flags for a substance use disorder in physicians: personality changes, absenteeism, and inconsistent responding to pages or phone calls. Often coworkers are slow to suspect substance use problems among professional colleagues. Some impaired physicians are able to maintain their professional lives as their substance use escalates and other areas of their life are falling apart.

Each state has its own requirements for reporting impaired physicians and other medical professionals. State impaired-physician programs and contact information for these programs can be found at the website for the Federation of State Physician Health Programs: www.fsphp.org. Impaired physicians are often able to keep or regain their medical license and continue in their profession if they comply with treatment and monitoring regulations that are in place. Physicians as a group tend to have exceptionally high success rates of recovery from substance use disorders, exceeding 90% in some samples.

use of this treatment strategy, maximize treatment outcomes, and minimize diversion of methadone. Methadone does not prevent the euphoric or other psychological effects associated with other classes of drugs and thus would not be expected to directly reduce other substance use. Methadone-maintained individuals often continue other problematic substance use (especially cocaine, alcohol, or benzodiazepines).

Buprenorphine is another agent used for maintenance treatment. It is a **partial opioid agonist**. It **blocks opioid withdrawal**, causes **limited euphoria**, and **eliminates craving**. Because it is a partial agonist, buprenorphine has a ceiling effect, thus making overdose less likely and attenuating the effects of additional full opioid agonists with lower receptor affinity (e.g., heroin). Patients can be directly transitioned from heroin or other opioids to buprenorphine without detoxification. Because buprenorphine can precipitate opioid withdrawal, patients must be in moderate withdrawal before being inducted into buprenorphine treatment. Buprenorphine is often formulated in combination with naloxone to reduce abuse potential. If the combination tablet is crushed and injected intravenously, the naloxone, which has low oral availability, will act to block the effects of buprenorphine. Unlike methadone, buprenorphine can be prescribed by physicians with special training and Drug Enforcement Agency (DEA) license exemptions in their offices and does not require daily visits by patients.

Methadone and buprenorphine maintenance have been demonstrated to be clearly effective in treating opioid use disorder. Both agents have been shown to decrease mortality and morbidity, as well as to improve social and vocational functioning. Maintained patients are less likely to contract HIV and hepatitis or commit crimes than nonmaintained opioid-dependent individuals. Because of the opioid effect, patients are more willing to adhere to treatment with methadone or buprenorphine than with naltrexone. Up to 75% of patients relapse to use after stopping agonist maintenance treatment. The mortality rates for individuals leaving agonist treatment are markedly increased.

Opioid Detoxification

Detoxification from opioids is usually accomplished with **methadone or buprenorphine** substitution and gradual withdrawal. The α-adrenergic agonist **clonidine** can reduce many of the autonomic components of the opioid withdrawal syndrome and can be used alone or adjunctively for management of opioid withdrawal. Rapid detoxification strategies involving an opioid antagonist given under heavy sedation or general anesthesia are effective, but no more so than other detoxification strategies, and are usually much more expensive and involve the risks associated with anesthesia. Symptomatic treatment of opioid withdrawal can be used adjunctively or by itself and includes nonopioid analgesics, antispasmodics, antidiarrheals, antiemetics, and benzodiazepines.

Cocaine Use Disorder

There are currently no FDA-approved pharmacotherapies for cocaine use disorder. Over 50 medications have been tested, but none have been found to be generally effective. Researchers have attempted to find medications that might attenuate intoxication, promote abstinence, prevent relapse, ameliorate withdrawal, or reduce craving. Agents that modulate neurotransmitters (direct or indirect agonists, antagonists) thought to be involved in cocaine dependence (dopamine, GABA, glutamate, serotonin, norepinephrine) have generally been targeted for investigation. Recently, small, double-blind placebo-controlled trials have shown limited promise for **disulfiram** and **modafinil**. Clinical trials of a cocaine vaccine are underway.

Cannabis Use Disorder

Although cannabis use disorder is the most common reason that substance users enter treatment, there has been little investigation of pharmacological agents targeting cannabis use. The previously held mistaken belief that marijuana use does not produce a withdrawal syndrome may explain why little investigation of medications that may ameliorate withdrawal symptoms has been undertaken. Since the medical and social sequelae of marijuana use are generally less than those of the heavy use of cocaine or heroin, the negative impact of marijuana use on work, interpersonal relations, and psychological functioning has been underappreciated. More recently, laboratory and treatment studies have investigated several medications to reduce withdrawal symptoms and self-medication. To date, the medication that appears most promising is **dronabinol**, oral δ-9-tetrahydrocannabinol, which is the primary psychoactive component of marijuana. However, cannabinoid antagonists, partial agonists, or combined pharmacotherapies might have clinical utility.

Nicotine Use Disorder

The optimal treatment of nicotine use disorder is comprised of both pharmacological and behavioral interventions provided simultaneously (see Box 7.12). **Nicotine replacement therapy** (NRT) works via the principle of drug substitution. NRT is available in several formulations, including gum, transdermal patch, inhaler, lozenge, and nasal spray. NRT works by reducing symptoms of withdrawal and craving as a patient stops smoking. Although most patients who use NRT resume their cigarette use, enough individuals succeed in stopping smoking that the use is justified. Combining NRT with behavioral treatment increases the success rate significantly. NRT is not recommended for patients who have acute cardiovascular disease, are pregnant, or have an allergic reaction.

The antidepressant **bupropion** is also FDA approved for smoking cessation. Bupropion has been demonstrated to be superior to placebo and NRT in smoking cessation. The partial agonist selective for $\alpha_4\beta_2$ nicotinic acetylcholine receptor subtypes, **varenicline**, is the most recently FDA-approved treatment for smoking cessation. Varenicline acts via its agonist activity while simultaneously blocking nicotine binding, thereby **attenuating symptoms of nicotine withdrawal** while patients are attempting to quit smoking. Varenicline has been demonstrated to be three times more effective than bupropion for smoking cessation. Varenicline and bupropion are intended for use during early smoking cessation. The starting dose of either medication should be gradually titrated to full dose during the first week of treatment. Patients are instructed to set a quit date during the second week of treatment. Treatment should be continued for 12 weeks even if patients are not initially successful in achieving complete abstinence. Patients successful in smoking cessation can be maintained for an additional 12 weeks of treatment.

Both bupropion and varenicline have been associated with **neuropsychiatric symptoms,** including suicidal thinking and changes in mood, and are contraindicated for individuals with bipolar disorder. Patients initiated on bupropion or varenicline should be closely monitored for emerging suicidal thinking or behavior, agitation, and depression. These medications should be used cautiously in individuals with preexisting depression or schizophrenia. Because of the extremely detrimental effects of chronic cigarette smoking, pharmacological strategies that are even partially successful or have some limitations are useful.

BOX 7.12
SMOKING CESSATION

Tobacco smoking is the leading preventable cause of mortality and morbidity in the United States. Quitting smoking is the single most important health behavior change that most smokers can make. Unlike individuals dependent on other substances, most smokers say they want to quit. Brief interventions (those lasting less than 3 minutes) by physicians such as simply advising patients to quit have been shown to increase the rate of smoking cessation. Physicians should use the "Five A's" to guide these brief interventions with all patients: **A**sk patients if they smoke; **A**dvise patients to quit; **A**ssess patients' motivation level for quitting; **A**ssist with quit attempts; **A**rrange follow-up contacts.

Given the higher prevalence of smoking among patients with other substance use disorders (75–98%) and other mental illnesses, screening and intervention are imperative in these populations. Depression is more prevalent among smokers, and depressed smokers have more difficulty quitting. Individuals with schizophrenia are more likely to be smokers (75–90%) and smoke more heavily than the general population. Nicotinic acetylcholine receptor dysfunction is thought to be important in the cognitive deficits seen with schizophrenia. Smoking by individuals with schizophrenia may ameliorate some of this cognitive dysfunction. Smoking may also reverse some side effects from commonly used antipsychotic medications.

Debate exists about the sequencing of smoking cessation and the cessation of other substance use. Individuals may have differing levels of motivation to reduce or quit smoking cigarettes compared with their motivation to change their alcohol intake or substance use behavior. Controlled studies have demonstrated that alcohol and other drug use tends to increase cigarette smoking. Smoking cessation in the context of ongoing drug or alcohol use may prove especially difficult for many patients.

Group, individual, and telephone counseling have all been shown to be effective in increasing rates of abstinence. Therapeutic interventions shown to be effective in smoking cessation include motivational interviewing, cognitive behavior therapy, and relapse prevention therapy.

REFERENCES CITED

Anton, R. F., S. S. O'Malley, D. A. Ciraulo, et al.; COMBINE Study Research Group. Combined pharmacotherapies and behavior interventions for alcohol dependence. The COMBINE study: a randomized controlled trial. *JAMA: Journal of the American Medical Association* 295:2003–2017, 2006.

Babor, T. F., J. R. de la Fuente, J. Saunders, and M. Grant. *AUDIT: The Alcohol Use Disorders Identification Test. Guidelines for Use in Primary Health Care.* Geneva: World Health Organization, 1992.

Baler, R. D., and N. D. Volkow. Drug addiction: the neurobiology of disrupted self-control. *Trends in Molecular Medicine* 12:559–566, 2006.

Compton, W. M., B. F. Grant, J. D. Colliver, M. D. Glantz, and F. S. Stinson. Prevalence of marijuana use disorders in the United States: 1991–1992 and 2001–2002. *JAMA: Journal of the American Medical Association* 291:2114–2121, 2004.

Compton, W. M., Y. F. Thomas, F. S. Stinson, and B. F. Grant. Prevalence, correlates, disability, and comorbidity of DSM-IV drug abuse and dependence in the United States: results from the national epidemiologic survey on alcohol and related conditions. *Archives of General Psychiatry* 64:566–576, 2007.

Hasin, D. S., F. S. Stinson, E. Ogburn, and B. F. Grant. Prevalence, correlates, disability, and comorbidity of DSM-IV alcohol abuse and dependence in the United States: results from the national epidemiologic survey on alcohol and related conditions. *Archives of General Psychiatry* 64:830–842, 2007.

Johnston, L. D., P. M. O'Malley, J. G Bachman, and J. E. Schulenberg. *Monitoring the Future national results on adolescent drug use: Overview of key findings*, 2007 (NIH Publication No. 08-6418). Bethesda, MD: National Institute on Drug Abuse, 2008.

Johnston, L. D., P. M. O'Malley, J. G Bachman, and J. E. Schulenberg. *Monitoring the Future national results on adolescent drug use: Overview of key findings, 2011.* Ann Arbor: Institute for Social Research, The University of Michigan, 2012.

Kessler, R. C., W. T. Chiu, O. Demler, and E. E. Walters. Prevalence, severity and comorbidity of 12-month DSM-IV disorders in the National Comorbidity Survey replication. *Archives of General Psychiatry* 62:617–627, 2005.

Moore, T. H., S. Zammit, A. Lingford-Hughes, T. R. Barnes, P. B. Jones, M. Burke, and G. Lewis. Cannabis use and risk of psychotic or affective mental health outcomes: a systematic review. *Lancet* 370:319–328, 2007.

Ross, S. The mentally ill substance abuser. In M. Galanter and H. D. Kleber, eds. *The American Psychiatric Publishing Textbook of Substance Abuse Treatment.* Arlington, VA: American Psychiatric Publishing, 2008.

Selzer, M. L. The Michigan Alcoholism Screening Test: the quest for a new diagnostic instrument. *American Journal of Psychiatry* 127:1653–1658, 1971.

Selzer, M. L., A. Vinokur, and L. Van Rooijen. A self-administered short Michigan Alcoholism Screening Test. *Journal of Studies on Alcohol* 36:117–126, 1975.

Skinner H. A. The drug abuse screening test. *Addictive Behavior* 7:363–371, 1982.

Vaillant, G. E. *Natural History of Alcoholism*, Cambridge, MA: Harvard University Press, 1983.

Wilens T. E., L. A. Adler, J. Adams, et al. Misuse and diversion of stimulants prescribed for ADHD: a systematic review of the literature. *Journal of the American Academy of Child and Adolescent Psychiatry* 47:21–31, 2008.

SELECTED READINGS

American Psychiatric Association. *APA Practice Guideline for the Treatment of Patients with Substance Use Disorders*, 2nd ed. Arlington, VA: American Psychiatric Publishing, 2006.

Galanter, M., and H. D. Kleber, eds. *Textbook of Substance Abuse Treatment*, 4th ed. Arlington, VA: American Psychiatric Publishing, 2008.

Kalivas, P. W., and C. O'Brien. Drug addiction as a pathology of staged neuroplasticity. *Neuropsychopharmacology* 33:166–180, 2008.

Miller, W. R., and S. Rollnick. *Motivational Interviewing: Helping People Change*, 3rd ed. New York: Guilford Press, 2013.

Ruiz, P., and E. Strain, eds. *Lowinson and Ruiz's Substance Abuse: A Comprehensive Textbook*, 5th ed. Philadelphia: Lippincott Williams and Wilkins, 2011.

Web Resources

Motivational Interviewing

Substance Abuse and Mental Health Services Administration (SAMHSA) and Center for Substance Abuse Treatment (CSAT) Treatment Improvement Protocols (TIP) at: http://www.ncbi.nlm.nih.gov/books/NBK64967/?term=motivational interview

TIP 34—Brief Interventions and Brief Therapies for Substance Abuse

TIP 35—Enhancing Motivation for Change in Substance Abuse Treatment

Smoking Cessation

The U.S. Department of Health and Human Services maintains a website (updated annually) providing evidence-based practice guidelines for the treatment of tobacco use and dependence at: http://www.ahrq.gov/path/tobacco.htm

Patients interested in quitting smoking can be referred to http://www.smokefree.gov or can call 1-800-QUIT NOW to gain free access to up-to-date information about smoking cessation, strategies for quitting, and real-time access to counselors.

Other Useful Alcohol and Substance Abuse Websites

Substance Abuse and Mental Health Services Administration: http://www.samhsa.gov

National Institute on Drug Abuse: http://www.nida.nih.gov

National Institute on Alcohol Abuse and Alcoholism: http://www.niaaa.nih.gov

Alcoholics Anonymous: http://www.alcoholics-anonymous.org

Narcotics Anonymous: http://www.na.org

Cocaine Anonymous: http://www.ca.org

Marijuana Anonymous: http://www.marijuana-anonymous.org

Self-Management and Recovery Training—an alternative to 12-step based self-help: http://www.smart-recovery.org

National Alliance of Advocates for Buprenorphine Treatment (matching opioid-dependent patients with physicians able to prescribe buprenorphine): http://www.naabt.org

American Academy of Addiction Psychiatry: http://www.aaap.org

American Society of Addiction Medicine: http://www.asam.org

/// 8 /// Personality Disorders

EVE CALIGOR, FRANK YEOMANS, AND ZE'EV LEVIN

A 22-year-old female graduate student with a prior history of 15 emergency room visits and 3 psychiatric hospitalizations is brought by EMS to her local emergency room, having ingested a bottle of pills when her boyfriend announced that he was breaking up with her. A socially isolated 50-year-old male postal worker with crescendo angina admitted to the cardiac unit is adamantly refusing all diagnostic testing, hatefully accusing his caretakers of incompetence while insinuating that they actually may be out to do him harm. A 40-year-old administrative secretary seen in the ambulatory clinic with a broken arm acknowledges that her chronically abusive husband pushed her down the stairs, yet she insists on going home with him because, "I love him too much to live without him."

While it is not difficult to appreciate that there is something terribly wrong with the ways in which the three individuals described above are experiencing and relating to the world around them, it is not so easy to describe exactly what it is that is wrong. Neither is it manifestly clear that these three individuals have much in common. Yet they do:all three have personality disorders that can account for their apparently irrational and self-destructive behavior. The graduate student has borderline personality disorder, the postal worker paranoid personality disorder, and the administrative secretary dependent personality disorder.

Physicians frequently encounter patients with personality disorders, both in psychiatric and other medical settings. In fact, it has been estimated that among patients seeking psychiatric services, roughly 50% of patients have personality disorders. Personality disorders are common in the general population, with an estimated lifetime prevalence of 12%. Patients with personality disorders often seek treatment for comorbid depression and anxiety, as well as for difficulties coping with acute stressors. They sometimes seek treatment because they become aware of repetitive, unsatisfying patterns in their work or personal lives.

The presence of a personality disorder will typically complicate management of surgical and other medical conditions. These patients may be poorly adherent to treatment recommendations, and the presence of personality pathology will often adversely impact the therapeutic relationship between physician and patient. Patients with personality disorders typically require longer and more intensive treatment for other psychiatric disorders than do patients without personality disorders, and the presence of a personality disorder is a negative prognostic indicator with regard to treatment response and rate of relapse for many general psychiatric disorders, including anxiety and mood disorders, eating disorders, and substance abuse. For all of these reasons, it is important that personality disorders be identified when present, regardless of the patient's manifest complaints.

PERSONALITY AND PERSONALITY PATHOLOGY

Personality refers to the **enduring and habitual patterns of behavior, cognition, emotion, motivation, and ways of relating to others** that are characteristic of the individual. Personality is manifested in the individual's characteristic reactions to the environment and to his or her own feelings, desires, urges, and fears. An individual's personality can be observed and will be expressed as a particular *personality style*. For example, an individual with an obsessive style is highly attentive to detail, perfectionistic, risk-averse, and constricted in emotional expression and may seem distant or controlling when interacting with others. In contrast, someone with a histrionic style is impressionistic rather than detail-oriented, "colorful" in speech and presentation, extroverted and emotional, but superficial. Each of these descriptors is viewed as a *personality trait*. Thus, the integration of a person's personality traits in a fashion characteristic of that individual constitutes his or her personality. Everyone has a personality and a personality style. One's personality is part of "who I am" or "the kind of person I am" and need not imply psychopathology.

In contrast with personality, the term *personality disorder* does imply psychopathology. Personality traits become more rigid and more extreme as one moves from normal to pathological personality functioning. A person with **rigid** personality traits is unable to change his or her behavior, even when the individual would like to and when it would be highly maladaptive not to do so. Rather than learning from experience and modifying maladaptive patterns, these individuals will activate the same behaviors, emotional responses, and ways of relating time and time again and across a broad array of circumstances, regardless of whether or not they are appropriate to the setting. **Extreme** personality traits refer to an increasingly wide deviation from commonly encountered and culturally normative behaviors, reactions, and ways of functioning.

In the normal personality, traits are not extreme, and they are flexibly and adaptively activated in different settings. For example, an individual with a normal personality and an obsessive style might be perfectionistic and attentive to detail but is able to be less fastidious if need be when working under a deadline; is risk-averse but is able to take a chance when it seems the best solution to a problem; and though emotionally distant in general, is able to establish a few deep and long-lasting friendships. In contrast, for the individual with obsessive-compulsive personality disorder, these same traits are sufficiently rigid and extreme as to interfere with daily functioning. The individual with obsessive personality pathology might be so rigidly perfectionistic and bogged down in detail that nothing is ever finished and deadlines are never met; so cautious and risk-averse that he or she cannot make a decision even when making no decision causes obvious and immediate problems; and emotionally unavailable even with the person's spouse and children.

Personality pathology exists on a **spectrum**, with traits becoming more rigid and more extreme, and interfering with the individual's functioning more profoundly and more broadly, as personality pathology becomes more severe. When personality rigidity reaches a point where it significantly, consistently, and chronically **interferes with daily functioning** or causes **significant distress** to the individual and those around him or her, a personality disorder may be diagnosed. Personality disorders typically adversely affect psychological and social functioning in many different domains. In particular, **interpersonal relationships** tend to be profoundly affected by personality pathology. Relationships may be unstable, stormy, superficial, excessively clinging, exploitative, devaluing, avoidant, distant, or simply absent, depending on the particular personality disorder in question. People with personality disorders also typically experience profound disturbances in their **sense of self**, harboring views of themselves that are unrealistic and poorly integrated. Such views may be unstable, contradictory, and, in some instances, grossly distorted, for example, extremely self-aggrandizing or self-denigrating.

Other common features often associated with personality disorders include erratic or contradictory behavior patterns and personality traits, failure to achieve professional success commensurate with level of education or to pursue long-term goals, and chronic unhappiness or dysphoria over many years, often associated with anxiety and depression. Individuals with personality disorders typically have low frustration tolerance, difficulty coping with stress, and a tendency to respond to adverse life events in ways that only exacerbate their difficulties. These individuals often blame others, rather than taking responsibility for their problems. They may be entirely oblivious to the degree to which they contribute to or even cause their own difficulties, or, alternatively, they may deny that they have problems whatsoever, experiencing themselves simply as the unfortunate victims of circumstance or mistreatment.

There are many different personality disorders, each with a characteristic presentation and course. However, in the clinical setting, it may be less important to identify exactly which personality disorder(s) a patient has than it is to recognize in a more general sense that the patient has clinically significant personality pathology. This recognition on the part of the physician can lend coherence to presenting complaints that may be vague, confusing, and seemingly contradictory. Such insight can begin to provide explanation for life difficulties, typically chronic and severe, that may be otherwise difficult to explain and will enable the physician to better identify and manage the challenges and frustrations that frequently emerge in the doctor–patient relationship when treating patients with personality disorders.

DIAGNOSTIC AND CLINICAL FEATURES

The DSM-5 provides two different classification systems for the personality disorders: the current standard, and an alternative approach requiring further study. In both systems, diagnosis is organized in relation to identifying first, the general criteria for a personality disorder and second, the presence of specific maladaptive personality traits.

According to the current system, the general criteria for the diagnosis of all personality disorders are the presence of an **enduring pattern of experience and behavior that is maladaptive, inflexible, and pervasive,** affecting the individual across a **broad range of personal and social situations** and **deviating markedly from the expectations of an individual's culture.** To make the diagnosis of a personality disorder, these rigid and maladaptive patterns must lead to **clinically significant distress or impairment in social, occupational, or other important areas of functioning.** By definition, personality disorders **begin by adolescence or young adulthood** and are persistent across time. However, adults with personality disorders can often identify maladaptive personality traits dating back to preadolescence. The DSM-5 specifies that to meet diagnostic criteria for a personality disorder, personality rigidity must be manifest in at least two of the following areas of psychological functioning: (1) **cognition** (including ways of perceiving and interpreting the self and other people, as well as events) (2) **affectivity** (including the range, intensity, lability, and appropriateness of emotional response), (3) **interpersonal functioning**, and (4) **impulse control** (see DSM-5).

TABLE 8.1 Prototypical Traits of DSM-5 Personality Disorders

Cluster A: Odd or Eccentric
Paranoid: guarded, touchy
Schizoid: aloof, isolative
Schizotypal: eccentric, idiosyncratic in cognition and perceptions
Cluster B: Dramatic, Emotional, or Erratic
Antisocial: disregards the rights of others, lacks remorse
Borderline: unstable, impulsive
Histrionic: dramatic, attention-seeking
Narcissistic: grandiose, feeling entitled
Cluster C: Anxious or Fearful
Avoidant: fearful, self-denigrating
Dependent: clinging, fears autonomy
Obsessive-compulsive: emotionally constricted, detail-oriented

The current standard system of classifying personality disorders describes criteria for **10 specific personality disorders** (see Table 8.1) plus two additional categories: (1) personality change due to another medical condition and (2) other specified personality disorder and unspecified personality disorder. The latter diagnostic category is used when the general criteria for a personality disorder are met and traits of several different personality disorders are present but the individual fails to meet the criteria for any particular personality disorder, or when the general criteria for a personality disorder are met but the individual is considered to have a personality disorder that is not included in the DSM-5 classification.

As indicated in Table 8.1, the DSM-5 divides the 10 specific personality disorders into **three clusters**, based on similarities in their presentation. Each personality disorder can be seen to have its own prototypical traits or personality style. In addition, there is a wide spectrum of severity, with regard to degree of impairment of functioning and long-term prognosis among the different personality disorders. Nonetheless, all share the general criteria for a personality disorder, as well as pathology in three **core domains of personality functioning**: (1) disturbance or distortion in the **sense of self**, (2) pathology of **interpersonal relationships**, and (3) faulty **affect regulation** with a predominance of negative emotions.

In this current system, diagnoses are made categorically (*categorical* diagnostic systems can be contrasted with *dimensional* or spectrum approaches to classification), in keeping with a long tradition within descriptive psychiatry. In a **categorical diagnostic system**, a patient will either meet criteria for a given disorder or will fail to do so; the answer to whether or not a given patient has a particular DSM-5 personality disorder is "yes" or "no." Each personality disorder has between seven and nine individual criteria, and an individual must endorse a particular number of these criteria to make the diagnostic threshold. This approach to diagnosis is **polythetic**, referring to a system in which a particular number of listed criteria, but not all criteria and not any single criterion, must be present to diagnose a particular disorder. One consequence of this system is that there are many different ways to meet criteria for any given personality disorder. As a result, there is a fair amount of **heterogeneity** among patients meeting criteria for a specific DSM-5 personality disorder and often a wide spectrum of severity of pathology among patients meeting criteria for the same diagnosis. This is problematic for clinicians, as it means that making the diagnosis of a particular personality disorder may not be especially helpful in predicting prognosis or selecting a particular treatment approach. Another outcome of this diagnostic approach is that many if not most patients who meet criteria for one personality disorder also meet criteria for another one, and not infrequently for several personality disorders, especially in the setting of more severe personality pathology. In other words, there is a high degree of **comorbidity** among the personality disorders.

In part in response to these concerns about the current diagnostic system, the DSM-5 provides an alternative approach to the classification of personality disorders, with the aim of generating further research. This approach is different from the current approach in several important ways and reflects a growing consensus about the nature of personality pathology. The alternative classification of personality disorders is (1) dimensional rather than categorical; (2) organized in relation to personality *functioning* in addition to personality traits, identifying core psychological capacities that define personality health and disorder across the different personality disorders; and (3) focuses on the dimension of severity of personality pathology, which has proven to be a robust predictor of prognosis and response to treatment.

The alternative approach redefines the general criteria for a personality disorder in terms of disruption of personality *functioning* in the *core domains* of **self** and **interpersonal** *functioning* (see DSM-5, Section III: Emerging Measures and Models, Alternative DSM-5 Model for Personality Disorders). Psychological functions related to the self are defined in terms of **identity** and **self-direction**. Interpersonal functioning is defined in terms of the individual's capacity for **empathy** and for **intimacy**. Self and interpersonal functioning, and pathology in these domains, exist across a spectrum of severity, from healthy functioning to severe impairment. This spectrum is described in a **Level of Personality Functioning Scale (LPFS)** (see DSM-5). The LPFS rates severity of personality pathology on a five-point scale ranging from 0 to 4, where 0 is "no impairment" and 2 is "moderate impairment," the threshold for diagnosing a personality disorder. The LPFS provides clinically useful descriptions of personality functioning at different levels of pathology, and reading it provides a valuable introduction to personality functioning and pathology across the spectrum of severity.

In the alternative diagnostic system, all personality disorders are described in terms of characteristic impairment in self and interpersonal functioning, in conjunction with the presence of specific maladaptive or pathological personality traits. Pathological traits are selected from five broad domains (see Definitions of DSM-5 personality disorder trait domains and facets): negative affectivity, detachment, antagonism, disinhibition, and psychoticism. The alternative approach also includes criteria for six specific personality disorders (see DSM-5): antisocial, avoidant, borderline, narcissistic, obsessive-compulsive, and schizotypal. Four personality disorders included in the standard approach, as well as in the DSM-IV, have been excluded from the new approach: paranoid, schizoid, histrionic, and dependent. This decision was made because these disorders have a limited research base. Individuals falling into these diagnostic groups are classified on the basis of impairment in self and interpersonal functioning in association with the presence of specific maladaptive personality traits characteristic of the disorder.

Cluster A—The Odd or Eccentric Cluster

Core clinical features of the cluster A disorders are 1) profound problems in interpersonal relationships, characterized by **severe mistrust or lack of interest in others**, and 2) a tendency toward **paranoid or idiosyncratic thinking** in the absence of frank psychosis. Individuals with cluster A personality disorders **rarely seek psychiatric treatment**. When they are seen by psychiatrists it is generally for treatment of an associated axis I disorder such as depression or anxiety or because they were sent by concerned or frustrated family members.

Paranoid Personality Disorder

Prevalence estimates for paranoid personality disorder suggest a prevalence of 2.3% to 4.4% of the general population, and it is more common in **men** than women. There is evidence for an increased prevalence in relatives of probands with schizophrenia and for a more specific familial relationship with delusional disorder, persecutory type. The hallmark of paranoid personality disorder is an **angry mistrust** of others that is pervasive, persistent, and inappropriate (see DSM-5). These individuals incorrectly interpret the motives of others to be malevolent, suspecting that others are exploiting, deceiving, or harming them. They endlessly question the loyalty and trustworthiness of friends and romantic partners. Interpersonally, individuals with paranoid personality disorder are suspicious, irritable, easily angered, and exquisitely sensitive to slights. They do not confide in others, and they tend to read demeaning and threatening meanings into benign remarks or events (see case example in Box 8.1).

Schizoid Personality Disorder

Schizoid personality disorder is rare in clinical settings. There is an estimated prevalence of 3.1–4.9% in the general population, and there may be an increased prevalence among relatives of people with schizophrenia or schizotypal personality disorder. It is more common among **men** than women. The hallmark of schizoid personality disorder is a **lack of interest** inand an **inability to establish meaningful relationships** with others (see DSM-5). These individuals tend to lead isolated lives, engage in solitary activities, and choose professions that enable them to avoid interactions with others. They typically do not marry and are not interested in sexual activity with another person. People with schizoid personality disorder tend to pursue cerebral or mechanical activities, such as Web-based games, and they often develop elaborate fantasy lives that substitute for engagement in the world. Their affective experience is flattened, with a general lack of pleasure resulting in chronic anhedonia. Interpersonally, they typically appear aloof and detached (see case example in Box 8.2).

BOX 8.1

CASE EXAMPLE OF PARANOID PERSONALITY DISORDER

A 45-year-old shopkeeper was known throughout her small town to be bizarrely irritable and suspicious. She constantly and unpredictably snapped at customers for being rude or ignorant, often while angrily mumbling to herself. It seemed that even the most innocuous question or gesture on the part of a customer could set her off, causing her to be suspicious, accusatory, and even verbally assaultive. She had been married briefly, but became convinced that her husband was having an affair, and divorced him.

BOX 8.2

CASE EXAMPLE OF SCHIZOID PERSONALITY DISORDER

A 36-year-old man presented to his internist complaining of fatigue and weight loss. Interacting with his doctor, the patient was cool and aloof. The patient lived an isolated life, working from home editing text for online instruction manuals. He spent at least 6 hours daily playing interactive games on the Web, and many additional hours lost in a fantasy world in which he was one of the characters in the game. He had no complaints beyond those that brought him to treatment, and he made it clear that he had no interest in sharing information about himself with his physician.

Schizotypal Personality Disorder

In community settings, reported rates of schizotypal personality disorder range from 0.6% to 4.6%, while the prevalence in clinical populations seems to be quite low (0–1.9%). It is equally common among men and women. Schizotypal personality disorder appears to aggregate familially and is more prevalent among the first-degree biological relatives of people with schizophrenia than among the general population. There may also be a modest increase in the rate of schizophrenia and other psychotic disorders in the relatives of probands with schizotypal personality disorder. The hallmark of schizotypal personality disorder is the presence of **cognitive or perceptual distortions** in a person who is not frankly psychotic (see DSM-5). The other anchor point for this diagnosis is a lack of desire for relationships with others, often stemming from social anxiety. Cognitive distortions include ideas of reference, odd beliefs, or magical thinking not consistent with cultural norms, such as belief in clairvoyance or telepathy. Interpersonally these individuals appear eccentric or odd and emotionally constricted. Their speech may be circumstantial, overinclusive, or difficult to follow (see case example in Box 8.3). Schizotypal personality disorder is not associated with gradual deterioration of social and cognitive functioning, though some of these individuals may be subject to brief psychotic decompensation.

Cluster B—The Dramatic, Emotional, or Erratic Cluster

Features shared by the cluster B disorders include (1) **emotional reactivity**, (2) **poor impulse control**, and (3) an **unclear sense of identity**. In addition, patients with

---

BOX 8.3

CASE EXAMPLE OF SCHIZOTYPAL PERSONALITY DISORDER

A 62-year-old schoolteacher lived alone and had never married. She had no close friends. In the teacher's lounge she would talk at length and in ways sometimes difficult to follow about her belief in faith healing and about various "crystals" that could be used to predict the future. Her colleagues and students viewed her as "weird but harmless."

borderline, narcissistic, and antisocial personality disorders are also often characterized by (4) high levels of **aggression**. In contrast to individuals with cluster A disorders, individuals in cluster B are generally more extroverted, although their relationships tend to be highly charged, stormy, and problematic. Patients with cluster B personality disorders are often seen by psychiatrists, typically for treatment of depression as well as for anxiety, substance use, and eating disorders, along with problems with relationships, impulsivity, and affective dysregulation. These patients are often seen in emergency settings when in crisis. At these times they may be at risk for self-destructive behavior.

Borderline Personality Disorder

The median population prevalence of borderline personality disorder has been estimated at 1.6%, but it may be as high as 5.9%. The prevalence is about 6% in primary care settings, about 10% among patients seen in outpatient mental health clinics, and about 20% of psychiatric inpatients. Borderline personality disorder is five times more common among first-degree biological relatives of those with the disorder than in the general population. There is also an increased familial risk for substance use disorders, antisocial personality disorder, and depressive or bipolar disorder. Though borderline personality disorder is more commonly diagnosed in **women** in clinical populations, this likely reflects a greater propensity to seek treatment on the part of women. In community-based samples, no difference in prevalence has been found between men and women. As a group, patients with borderline personality disorder tend to be **treatment seeking**, and they make disproportionate use of psychiatric services in both inpatient and outpatient psychiatric settings.

The key features of borderline personality disorder are emotional dysregulation, pathology of interpersonal relationships, and poor impulse control, often associated with recurrent self-destructive behavior and a poorly integrated and unstable sense of self (see DSM-5). These individuals are severely compromised in their ability to form secure attachments with others, and their relationships are typically quickly formed and unstable, often associated with frantic efforts to avoid perceived abandonment. They may engage in self-destructive behavior in the setting of disruption or threat of disruption of a relationship ("If you leave me I'll kill myself") or as a means of dealing with intense emotion or to punish themselves.

Faulty affect regulation (referred to as "affective instability") leads to rapid and wide swings of emotion in individuals with borderline personality disorder. These individuals can easily and seemingly instantaneously alternate between intense feelings of gratification and pleasure, and equally intense feelings of deprivation, rage, and/or anxiety. Their relationships are stormy, highly affectively charged, and unstable, often marked by idealization of the other person that is associated with clinging behavior, alternating with hatred and devaluation. This switch, which is typically very rapid and may happen many times in the course of a relationship, reflects defensive "**splitting**" of the image of the other person into an idealized, positive image and a negative, hated and devalued image. There is a corresponding split in the sense of self, which in a moment can shift from feeling special to feeling worthless. Given their lack of a solid sense of self, the way in which these patients view themselves depends to a large extent on outside cues. Individuals with borderline personality disorder are prone to a host of chronic self-destructive behaviors, such as superficially cutting or burning themselves, and many patients with borderline personality disorder make **frequent suicide attempts** or gestures. Drug and alcohol abuse, eating disorders, and sexual promiscuity are other forms of self-destructive behavior commonly encountered in this population. Sometimes self-destructive behaviors and superficial cutting are premeditated, designed to relieve internal pain and emptiness,

---

BOX 8.4

CASE EXAMPLE OF BORDERLINE PERSONALITY DISORDER

An undergraduate seeing a counselor at Student Health Services filled her therapy session with rapturous praise of her new "boyfriend," a young man she had met at a bar the previous evening while drunk whom she had taken home to her apartment. The next afternoon, the therapist received a call from the emergency room. When the emergency room physician put the patient on the phone, the patient unleashed a tirade about how the man she had met the previous day had not wanted to see her again; he was cold and heartless and her entire life situation was hopeless. She saw nothing to live for and had taken a Tylenol overdose while on the phone with him, at which point he had called 911 and she had been brought to the emergency room.

---

chronic dysphoria, and free-floating anxiety. At other times, self-destructive behaviors, including suicidal gestures and attempts, may be more impulsive, typically triggered by interpersonal frustration or disappointment. Whether premeditated or impulsive, self-destructive behaviors often are used interpersonally as a way to communicate distress and to control or strike out at others (see case example in Box 8.4).

Histrionic Personality Disorder

Histrionic personality disorder has been estimated to occur in approximately 1.8% of the general population and is more common among **women** than men. The key features of histrionic personality disorder are a need to be the **center of attention** along with **rapidly shifting, dramatic, and superficial expression of emotion** (see DSM-5). These individuals characteristically use their physical appearance to gain attention, often in a sexually provocative or seductive fashion. People with histrionic personality disorder are impressionistic in their speech and cognition, self-dramatizing, and emotional; they often consider relationships to be more intimate than they are. Interpersonally these individuals tend to be engaging initially, but over time they often come to seem superficial and excessively demanding of attention. Individuals with histrionic personality disorder **often seek treatment** and generally have a **positive prognosis**. Severe impairment in functioning may be largely limited to the realm of romance and sexual intimacy. Compared with the other cluster B personality disorders, histrionic personality disorder is associated with a greater capacity to establish stable and meaningful relationships and with better work functioning (see case example in Box 8.5).

Narcissistic Personality Disorder

Narcissistic personality disorder (see DSM-5) has an estimated prevalence of 0% to 6.2% in community samples. In addition, many individuals with other personality disorders have clinically significant narcissistic pathology, without meeting full criteria for narcissistic personality disorder. Narcissistic personality disorder is diagnosed more commonly in **men (50%–75%)**, but it is unclear if this reflects a higher prevalence in men or diagnostic bias. The core features of narcissistic personality disorder are a **grandiose sense of self, fantasies of unlimited success and power, and excessive need for admiration from others**. Underneath their grandiosity, individuals with

---

BOX 8.5
CASE EXAMPLE OF HISTRIONIC PERSONALITY DISORDER

A young woman consulted a psychiatrist because of a crisis in her romantic and professional life. She arrived to the first meeting wearing an attractive, tight-fitting outfit and heavy makeup. In the interview, she alternated between weeping dramatically and then behaving seductively with the male psychiatrist who was evaluating her. She explained that the reason she was so upset was that her live-in boyfriend was pushing for marriage. She was very fond of him, and happy living with him, but she often treated him unkindly and had no sexual feelings for him. Meanwhile, she had been maintaining a flirtation with her married boss for several years, and had spent a handful of drunken evenings in bed with him while traveling together on business. She found her boss sexually exciting and loved the attention he secretly gave her in the office. She had been quite happy maintaining the two relationships, but now felt that her situation had been destabilized by the boyfriend's insistence that they either move ahead or move on.

---

narcissistic personality disorder are often plagued by painful feelings of **inferiority and envy**. These latter feelings are more evident in a type of narcissist that is not included in the DSM criteria, the covert or masochistic narcissist (Cooper 1998). These individuals usually present with chronic, treatment-refractory depression. Exploration in therapy reveals that these individuals harbor a sense of superiority in the degree of their suffering, a "moral superiority," and thus need their suffering to bolster their self-esteem in a somewhat perverse way.

Interpersonally, individuals with narcissistic personality disorder appear self-centered, arrogant, and haughty, and they can be exploitative and strikingly lacking in empathy in their relationships with others. Because their sense of self depends on feeling superior to others, setbacks, slights, and criticism are poorly tolerated, often leading to emotional collapse and depression or, alternatively, rage and devaluation of others. It is during these **depressive crises** that narcissistic patients tend to seek treatment. In general, these individuals have no tolerance for needing help from or relying on others; seeking help stimulates painful feelings of envy and inferiority (see case example in Box 8.6).

Antisocial Personality Disorder
Antisocial personality disorder occurs in about 1.7% of the population and is much more common among **men** than among women. The highest prevalence (greater than 70%) is among the most severe samples of men with alcohol use disorders and from substance abuse clinics, prisons, or other forensic settings. Prevalence is higher in individuals affected by adverse socioeconomic factors, like poverty, or sociocultural factors, like migration.

Antisocial personality disorder is more common among the first-degree biological relatives of those with the disorder than in the general population. Biological relatives of people with this disorder are also at increased risk for somatic symptom disorder and substance use disorders. Adoption studies indicate that both genetic and environmental

> ### BOX 8.6
> ### CASE EXAMPLE OF NARCISSISTIC PERSONALITY DISORDER
>
> A 45-year-old businessman was preoccupied with accruing massive wealth; he spent all of his time thinking about his business plans, about how much money he had, and about how much money he would have someday. He chose to associate only with people who were extremely wealthy or well connected. He was chronically angry at his wife, an attractive and well-educated woman who had put him through graduate school, feeling that she should be doing more to help him climb socially and resenting that she did not have better social connections. Although he had insisted she leave her career as a lawyer to devote herself to decorating their home and maintaining their lifestyle, he was contemptuous of her for not working, and he spoke openly with her of his admiration for and sexual interest in the female bankers he came into contact with.

factors contribute to the risk of developing antisocial personality disorder. The core feature of antisocial personality disorder is a pervasive pattern of behavior reflecting **disregard for and violation of the rights of others**. Diagnostic criteria include engaging in repeated illegal acts, lying, conning or the use of aliases, reckless disregard for the safety of self and/or others, and a **lack of remorse** for unlawful, dishonest, destructive, or exploitative acts (see DSM-5). These individuals live in a "dog-eat-dog" world and, from their perspective, anyone who believes otherwise is by definition a fool. Many, but not all, individuals with antisocial personality disorder show evidence of impulsivity, irritability, aggressiveness, and lack of concern for the consequences of their actions. However, there is a group of con men, embezzlers, imposters, and white-collar criminals with antisocial personality who present as charming, seductive, and clever (see case example in Box 8.7).

> ### BOX 8.7
> ### CASE EXAMPLE OF ANTISOCIAL PERSONALITY DISORDER
>
> A respected trial lawyer came under scrutiny for tax evasion. As the government began to look into his background, it emerged that he was not a member of the bar and, in fact, had been expelled from law school 20 years earlier and never received a diploma. Yet he had built a career over the course of 10 years, posing as a graduate of an Ivy League school. He had assumed an alias, gotten jobs, gone to court, represented clients, and built a reputation for being a clever litigator, always cool under fire. To sustain his deception and generate sympathy, he had told everyone that he had no family, that both of his parents had been murdered when he was a teenager. In fact, his parents were alive and well but had not heard from him for over 20 years.

Cluster C—The Anxious or Fearful Cluster

The key feature shared by the cluster C disorders is a **propensity toward anxiety**. Avoidant patients are fearful of other people in general, and of criticism and derision in particular. Dependent patients are fearful of losing others or having to function autonomously. Obsessive-compulsive individuals fear loss of control. Along with histrionic personality disorder, cluster C personality disorders tend to be the **least severe** of the personality disorders. Individuals with obsessive-compulsive personality disorder tend to be the highest functioning, followed by avoidant and dependent personality disorders. Patients in the cluster C group **often seek treatment**, and they have a relatively **positive prognosis**.

Avoidant Personality Disorder

Avoidant personality disorder is estimated to have a prevalence of about 2.4% in the general population. The disorder appears to be more common in certain cultures and in **women**. The avoidant behavior often starts in infancy or childhood with shyness, isolation, and fear of strangers or new situations. Shyness in childhood is a common precursor of avoidant personality disorder, but in most people it tends to remit gradually as they get older. In contrast, people who go on to develop avoidant personality disorder may become increasingly shy during adolescence and early adulthood. The key features of avoidant personality disorder are a pervasive pattern of **social inhibition, feelings of inadequacy, and hypersensitivity to criticism** (see DSM-5). These individuals are fearful and uncomfortable in social situations and in intimate relations. They have strong wishes to have relationships with others, yet anticipate being ridiculed, rejected, or humiliated. As a result, they tend to avoid social or intimate settings, are unwilling to become involved with others unless they are certain of being liked, and will avoid occupational activities that involve significant interpersonal contact, for fear of humiliating themselves or being criticized. These individuals are risk-averse and are plagued by feelings of inferiority and shame. Interpersonally, individuals with avoidant personality disorder tend to be anxious, awkward, and timid, and they often display an attitude of self-derision. There is a high co-occurrence of avoidant personality disorder with social phobia, as well as with a broad spectrum of other anxiety disorders (see case example in Box 8.8).

Dependent Personality Disorder

Dependent personality disorder is estimated to have a prevalence of between 0.49% and 0.6% in the general population. In clinical settings, dependent personality disorder

---

BOX 8.8

CASE EXAMPLE OF AVOIDANT PERSONALITY DISORDER

A 20-year-old college student presented for treatment of anxiety. Though an attractive and intellectually accomplished individual, he quickly communicated his painful feelings of inferiority and self-criticism. He never spoke in class, for fear of making a fool of himself, and often would skip classes and spend the day in his room, anticipating that if he were to go out people would ridicule his appearance, manner, and insecurity.

has been diagnosed more frequently in **women, but some studies report similar prevalence rates among men and women. T**he key feature of dependent personality disorder is an **excessive need to be taken care** of that leads to **submissive and clinging behavior and fears of separation** (see DSM-5). These individuals have exaggerated and unrealistic fears of being unable to take care of themselves; they tend to devalue their own abilities and decision-making, while viewing others as much more powerful and able. As a result, they not only look to others to make decisions and take care of them but will also go to excessive lengths to seek out and maintain dependent relationships with partners they feel can provide nurturance and guidance. They feel panicked at the prospect of being left to care for themselves, and if a relationship ends, they will quickly initiate a new one. Interpersonally, people with dependent personality disorder often seem ingratiating and appealing. In the setting of a dependent relationship they often become submissive and childlike, while experiencing a desperate need to maintain the relationship in the face of fear of losing their partner (see case example in Box 8.9).

Obsessive-Compulsive Personality Disorder

Obsessive-compulsive personality disorder is one of the most **common** personality disorders, with estimated prevalence ranging from 2.1% to 7.9%. It is diagnosed about twice as often among **men**. The key features of this disorder are **a preoccupation with orderliness, perfectionism, and control**, in the setting of **severe emotional constriction** (see DSM-5). These individuals are excessively devoted to work, to the exclusion of friendships and leisure activity, so much so that they may avoid taking vacations. They are overly conscientious in their morals, and they are miserly with regard to spending money. People with obsessive-compulsive personality disorder often experience themselves as "living machines" or robots; their emotional lives are constricted and flattened, and they value self-control above all else. They also tend to be controlling of others, and they have difficulty delegating tasks, feeling that no one can do the task the way they want it done. Interpersonally, obsessive-compulsive individuals appear stiff, excessively controlled, and emotionally distant and constricted. Some individuals with obsessive-compulsive personality disorder are able to functioning relatively well, especially in their professional lives, while others suffer significant impairment in all domains of functioning (see case example in Box 8.10).

BOX 8.9

CASE EXAMPLE OF DEPENDENT PERSONALITY DISORDER

A young woman was dating a man who treated her poorly, devaluing her in front of others and frequently threatening to leave her. Though her friends were outraged to witness her boyfriend's behavior, the young woman's response was to appease and cajole him. Her friends told her she would be much better off without the boyfriend, but the young woman was preoccupied with the possibility that he might leave her, believing that she could not make it on her own, and that she loved him too much to live without him.

BOX 8.10

CASE EXAMPLE OF OBSESSIVE-COMPULSIVE PERSONALITY DISORDER

A partner in a law firm was meticulous and detail-oriented to a fault; it took him twice the expected time to prepare a document. He described himself as losing sight of the big picture at these times, getting lost in detail. He micromanaged and would not delegate to his associates, feeling that their work was sloppy and inadequate. To compensate for his inefficiency and perfectionism, he consistently worked 14-hour days. Though a faithful husband and a responsible father, he rarely showed any warmth toward his family. He experienced himself as cut-off and remote, and when at home often felt that he just wanted to be left alone.

COURSE OF ILLNESS

Personality disorders are characterized by an **early onset**, and the patterns of inner experience and observable behavior that constitute a personality disorder are enduring across the life cycle. By definition, personality disorders lead to distress and impairment in social, occupational, or other important areas of functioning. However, there is a great degree of variability in severity of illness among the different personality disorders, and within each personality disorder there is a **spectrum of severity** as well. The degree of severity of an individual's personality pathology will have a great impact on the degree of impairment in any given domain of functioning, the number of domains affected, the course of illness, and the responsiveness to treatment. All of these must be taken into account when considering course of illness.

A cornerstone of understanding personality and of personality disorder is the expectation that an individual's personality traits, or personality style, will be **stable across time**. This is to say that an avoidant person is unlikely to become extroverted, a histrionic individual is unlikely to become emotionally constricted and detail-oriented, and an antisocial individual is even less likely to become empathic and respectful of the rights and needs of others. However, even though personality traits are from a dimensional perspective stable, they can become less extreme and less rigid across time, resulting in significant overall improvement in functioning and decrease in subjective distress.

In fact, empirical studies have to some degree challenged the assumption that personality pathology is enduring (Lenzenweger et al. 2004; Zanarini et al. 2003, 2006). Rather, it may be a more accurate perspective to view personality pathology as persistent, but waxing and waning across time, affected by life circumstances, phase of life, social supports, and psychosocial stressors. As a result, there is currently greater optimism regarding the overall prognosis of many individuals diagnosed with personality disorders. It now appears that severity of personality pathology, as reflected in impairment in functioning and level of subjective distress, often improves over time and may diminish across the life cycle for at least some of the personality disorders. In particular, personality traits such as impulsivity, aggressiveness, and chaotic interpersonal relationships often "mellow" as individuals move from early adulthood into their 30s and 40s (Stone 1990, 1993). In addition, the normal process of maturation can benefit some individuals with personality disorders, leading to maturation of defensive strategies for coping with adversity and an evolution toward increasingly flexible and adaptive personality traits. In particular, it seems that the personality pathology of individuals who are able to establish meaningful relationships often improves over time in the setting of attachments with others, and those who enjoy professional success may benefit as well. Thus, despite the long-standing assumption that personality disorders are stable and lifelong, there is a body of evidence to suggest that for many of the personality disorders there may be more variability in the course of personality pathology than had previously been assumed.

Odd or Eccentric Cluster

The cluster A personality disorders are among the more severe of the personality disorders, associated with **profound compromise of functioning** across many domains and across the lifespan. Interpersonal functioning is always severely and often permanently compromised, and these individuals tend to lead isolated lives. Work functioning is typically also impaired, though often to a lesser extent if the individual is able to find work that involves minimal contact with others. Individuals with schizotypal personality disorder are vulnerable to psychotic decompensation when under stress, and some patients with paranoid personality disorder will develop transient psychotic symptoms as well. It is important to identify and treat **psychotic symptoms** in cluster A patients, recognizing that frank psychosis cannot be attributed to underlying personality pathology. However, because of their tendency to avoid interpersonal contact, individuals in this group rarely come for psychiatric treatment. When they do, it is most commonly for treatment of depression or anxiety. They are sometimes brought for treatment by concerned family members. Because cluster A patients are suspicious of others and isolative, it is difficult to establish a therapeutic relationship.

Dramatic, Emotional, or Erratic Cluster

Even though individuals with cluster B personality disorders often present with impulsive and self-destructive behaviors, some of these patients can have a relatively favorable prognosis. The degree to which individuals with a cluster B personality disorder are able to establish and sustain meaningful relationships, the degree to which their moral functioning is intact, and the extent to which their behavior and subjective experience are not flooded with rage and hatred are positive prognostic factors. Using these criteria, antisocial individuals have the poorest prognosis and individuals with histrionic personality disorder are most likely to do well. Individuals with borderline personality disorder fall in between; while there is a fair amount of heterogeneity among patients in the borderline group, it appears that many improve over time, at least in terms of a decrease in symptoms. Many individual scan achieve an adequate degree of satisfaction in love relations and work achievement. In contrast, individuals meeting full criteria for DSM-5 narcissistic personality disorder generally have a more guarded prognosis.

Histrionic Personality Disorder

Individuals with histrionic personality disorder have a favorable prognosis. The healthiest patients in this group may function adequately in all areas except intimate relations. For those at the more severe end of the spectrum, chaotic and inappropriate interpersonal behaviors disrupt professional functioning as well as interpersonal relations. Comorbid anxiety, depression, and substance abuse are common, affecting prognosis and requiring treatment. Patients with histrionic personality disorder often seek treatment, can benefit from psychotherapy, and may do especially well with long-term psychodynamic psychotherapy.

Borderline Personality Disorder

Patients with borderline personality disorder tend to present for treatment and to experience the most disruption in adolescence and early adulthood, often complicated by substance abuse and eating disorders. Not uncommonly, during these years patients' lives may come to be dominated by cycles of destructive and self-destructive behavior. However, though 8–10% of patients may die from suicide, those who survive early adulthood typically will improve over time. Most of these individuals will at some point no longer meet DSM-V criteria for borderline personality disorder (Zanarini et al. 2003, 2006), although they still tend to experience dissatisfaction in life. Positive long-term prognosis in this population is associated with high intelligence, physical attractiveness, and self-discipline. Poorer outcome is associated with increased severity of symptoms, multiple hospitalizations, history of childhood physical and sexual abuse, antisocial behavior, high levels of aggression and rage, and chaotic impulsivity (Stone 1990). Patients with borderline personality disorder can benefit from both psychodynamic and cognitive behavioral therapies, typically supplemented with medication management.

Narcissistic Personality Disorder

Patients with narcissistic personality disorder have a variable course. At the healthiest end of the spectrum, patients with prominent narcissistic traits who do not meet full criteria for the personality disorder may do relatively well. Patients in this group are characterized by relatively intact ethical functioning, the absence of overtly aggressive behavior, the capacity to achieve professional success, and the ability to sustain superficial relations (even while demonstrating extreme, and sometimes shocking, impoverishment of intimate relationships). As narcissistic pathology becomes more severe, maladaptive traits tend to interfere profoundly with all domains of functioning, and antisocial features become more common. Narcissistic patients are vulnerable to **depression**, especially as they age. Narcissistic patients generally tolerate treatment poorly since they have difficulty acknowledging flaws. However, as individuals with narcissistic personality disorder reach middle age they may become more highly motivated to seek treatment, as it becomes increasingly clear that the reality of their lives does not match their exaggerated view and expectations of themselves. Positive prognostic factors are some capacity to establish and sustain nonexploitative relationships, relatively intact moral functioning, and the absence of extreme aggression.

Antisocial Personality Disorder

Arguably, antisocial personality disorder is the most severe of the personality disorders, and this diagnosis generally carries a **bleak prognosis**. Among individuals with antisocial personality disorder, those who are overtly aggressive and violent do poorest of all. Less aggressive individuals may superficially function better, and those who are especially intelligent and socially skilled may attain professional success. However, by and large most antisocial individuals tend to function very poorly overall, and **comorbid substance abuse** is common. The typical life course of the individual with antisocial personality disorder is marked by multiple disruptions of relationships and work, often with recurrent encounters with the penal system. With age, antisocial individuals may become less overtly aggressive, destructive, and impulsive. These patients rarely seek treatment and are generally considered to be untreatable in conventional therapeutic settings.

Anxious or Fearful Cluster

Along with histrionic personality disorder, the cluster C disorders carry the most favorable prognosis among the personality disorders, and individuals with cluster C personality disorders often function adequately in some and occasionally several domains.

Avoidant Personality Disorder

Avoidant personality disorder affects social and intimate relations most profoundly. Some of these individuals may function adequately professionally and even in nonintimate interpersonal situations. Avoidant patients may self-medicate social anxiety with alcohol or anxiolytics. Patients with avoidant personality disorder often seek treatment, most typically for anxiety, depression, or problems with self-esteem. They can benefit from various forms of psychotherapy and social skills training, often supplemented with medication management to target symptoms of anxiety and depression.

Dependent Personality Disorder

Dependent personality disorder also carries a relatively favorable prognosis. Those individuals able to sustain long-term relationships that gratify their dependency needs can do well over time. People with dependent personality disorder will often seek treatment in the setting of depression or anxiety triggered by the ending of an important relationship. These individuals do well in psychotherapies that focus on promoting independence.

Obsessive-Compulsive Personality Disorder

Obsessive-compulsive personality disorder is arguably the least severe of the personality disorders. These individuals often function adequately and even well in some areas. Emotional life is chronically constricted, and the enjoyment of leisure activities is typically profoundly compromised; people with obsessive-compulsive personality disorder often come to be overly dependent on work as a source of pleasure and as a way to maintain self-esteem and avoid anxiety. Though they can benefit greatly from psychodynamic psychotherapy, these individuals often do not seek treatment, as their personality traits are often both egosyntonic and culturally sanctioned. When they do come to treatment, it is often at the bequest of a spouse, who complains of the patient's emotional distance and/or controlling behavior.

THE INTERVIEW

The interview is the central evaluative tool for diagnosing personality disorders. Assessment and diagnosis of personality pathology is typically more challenging than assessment of other psychiatric disorders. It is helpful to keep in mind that diagnosis of a personality disorder requires that rigid and maladaptive personality traits are not only present but also responsible for chronic problems across several domains of functioning. Further, to diagnose a personality disorder, it must be established that the patient's difficulties cannot be attributed to another mental disorder. As a result, when evaluating personality pathology, the interview needs to include a thorough general psychiatric assessment coupled with a careful evaluation of personality functioning.

The psychiatric interview begins with evaluation of the patient's presenting complaints and history. The patient's general level of functioning is assessed next, focusing on the degree to which personality traits are rigid and maladaptive and interfere with functioning across various domains. Finally, if there is evidence of significant personality pathology, specific maladaptive personality traits are identified and evaluated in order to make the diagnosis of a particular personality disorder.

Evaluation of a patient's personality functioning requires inquiring specifically about the nature of the individual's functioning in the following areas: (1) relationships and capacity to maintain a view of significant others that is stable, realistic, and nuanced; (2) performance and degree of satisfaction at work or school along with the capacity to invest in and pursue long-term goals; (3) capacity to pursue and enjoy interests and leisure time; and (4) self-concept. This overall line of inquiry is best approached from the perspective of getting to know the patient as an individual, with the explicit goal of developing a clear impression of how the patient experiences and moves through the world.

Typically, much information that pertains to evaluation of personality functioning and personality pathology will emerge naturally in the course of taking a standard history. As a result, even before beginning a formal evaluation of the patient's personality, the interviewer may have a general sense of the patient's overall level of functioning. While taking the general psychiatric history, the interviewer should be attentive to information regarding personality functioning, such as the nature of the patient's relationships and work situation. In addition, it is important to consider whether the patient seems to be someone who has enjoyed life for significant periods or has been chronically unhappy. Are there aspects of the history that point to impulsive or self-destructive behavior? Does the patient seem to be suspicious or critical of others or of the interviewer? Does the patient constantly put himself or herself down, or assume a general attitude of superiority in the telling of his or her story? When trying to identify personality traits, it can be helpful to try to listen for **patterns of behavior** (for example, ignoring problems until they reach a crisis) or attitudes (for example, feeling inadequate or suspicious of others) that repeat themselves in the patient's narrative in different settings. Finally, it is helpful to make note of the patient's **style of communicating** and interacting during the interview. For example, is the patient withholding of information and hostile, dramatic, and impressionistic? Or is the patient emotionally constricted and providing excessive amount of detail?

After the physician has elicited presenting difficulties, current symptoms, and psychiatric and medical history, the interview will focus explicitly on the patient's personality and general level of functioning. It can be helpful to introduce this portion of the interview with a statement such as, "I have gotten a pretty clear sense of the symptoms and difficulties that bring you here. I want to shift gears a bit now and learn more about you as a person. Can you tell me a bit about yourself, about what your daily life is like, and about the ways in which your difficulties have and have not interfered with your functioning?" It is often fruitful to begin with this sort of **open-ended inquiry** and see where the patient takes things; ultimately, most patients will benefit from a more structured approach. It is the task of the interviewer to ensure that by the time the evaluation is completed, all central domains of functioning have been evaluated.

When evaluating the nature of the patient's **relationships**, one must first determine whether the patient has any significant relationships and, if so, whether he or she has been able to sustain them over time. What are these relationships like for the patient? Are they stable and characterized by mutual concern and affection, or are they stormy and marked by hostility? How does the patient describe significant others—in detail or superficially? Are they sources of support or of pain? Are they criticized or idealized, or are they viewed in a seemingly realistic fashion? It can be helpful to ask the patient, "Who is the person you are closest to? Can you tell me a bit about this person and your relationship with him or her? How often do you see this person or talk to him or her?" The goal of this portion of the interview is to reach a point at which the people the patient is describing and the nature of the patient's relationships with them can be imagined in the interviewer's own mind. Because people often minimize the degree of pathology in their interpersonal functioning, clarification and detail in the setting of specific examples should always be requested when a patient is vague.

The interview in Box 8.11 illustrates the process of clarification. The patient gives brief and superficial answers that minimize his own pathology and place blame on his wife. The interviewer is persistent, following up on vague responses, asking for further

---

BOX 8.11

CLARIFICATION IN AN INTERVIEW WITH A "COMPLAINING HUSBAND"

Interviewer: Who is the person you are closest to?

  Patient: My wife.

  I: How long have you been married?

  P: For 22 years.

  I: Do you have children?

  P: No

  I: Can you tell me a bit about the marriage and about what your wife is like?

  P: Well, my wife is lazy.

  I: What do you mean?

  P: She never cleans up the house, is a lousy cook.

  I: How do the two of you get along?

  P: OK.

  I: Do you sometimes lose your temper with her about these things?

  P: Sometimes, but I never lay a hand on her.

  I: What happens when you lose your temper?

  P: Well I tell it like it is, that she's a no good piece of crap and she's lucky I put up with her.

  I: Do you ever lose your temper to the point where you want to hit her?

  P: Sure, sometimes I want to beat the livin' daylights out of her. She sure deserves it, but like I said, I never touch her. She'd just start calling around to her family and I'd never hear the end of it.

  I: What does she do to "deserve it"?

  P: Well, she complains about my not working and her having to work nights to pay the bills.

  I: Can you tell me more?

  P: Well, she always throws in my face that she has to ask her hotshot brother for help. I know he gives her money just because he wants to show off. Just because

(continued)

> he's a lawyer, doesn't mean he's any better than me or has more going for him. He just got lucky—right place, right time. But she's always singing his praises.
>
> **I:** You know, you seem to have a lot of pretty negative things to say about your wife, yet you describe her as the person you are closest to. Is it true that this is your closest relationship? Is there anyone else you are close to?
>
> **P:** No. I don't think most people are worth getting to know.
>
> **I:** Well, given that your wife is the person you describe as the person closest to you, I wonder if there are things about her that you value, aspects of your relationship that involve intimacy or friendship.
>
> **P:** Well, she gives me sex. And since we got married, I haven't had to work.

information, greater level of detail, and specific examples. As the patient begins to speak more freely, he reveals that he is in fact not working, while his "lazy" wife is supporting him. His feelings for her are hostile and critical, and his attitude toward her is devaluing, yet he has indicated that this is his closest relationship. The basis of the relationship, from the patient's perspective, seems to depend on what his wife does for him and provides him with, with little sense of reciprocity or interest in or concern for her needs.

Patients who do not have significant personality pathology tend to see relationships in terms of give and take; they are able to rely on and value others in a mutual fashion and to attain a significant level of intimacy with another person. As personality pathology becomes more severe, relationships typically become unstable, infused with hostility, or, alternatively, superficial or even entirely absent. While many individuals with personality pathology lack a capacity for intimacy, patients at the more severe end of the spectrum come to view relationships purely and simply in terms of need fulfillment. As illustrated by the husband in Box 8.11, these individuals may have little or no sense of give and take between two people (see assessment of this patient in Box 8.12). Rather, relationships are viewed solely in terms of "What can this person do for me?"

In addition to evaluating the nature of a patient's relationships, evaluation of personality should include exploration of the patient's **vocational functioning**. One can

---

BOX 8.12

ASSESSMENT OF THE "COMPLAINING HUSBAND"

On the basis of the severe pathology in the patient's view of relationships, particularly in his relationship with and attitude toward his wife, in conjunction with chronic unemployment, high levels of hostility, and externalization of the source of his difficulties, the "complaining husband" appears to have clinically significant personality pathology. Maladaptive personality traits include exploitation of others, sense of entitlement, a superior and devaluing attitude toward others, feelings of envy, and egosyntonic aggression, all pointing to the diagnosis of narcissistic personality disorder.

begin by asking about employment or school attendance, duration of the patient's present position, and his or her attitude toward it. Has the patient pursued a career path or jumped about from job to job or from career to career? Has the patient ever been fired or laid off? If so, under what circumstances? Has the patient had the same sort of difficulties more than once and in different settings? How does the patient get along with bosses and with coworkers? The clinician should inquire about the patient's level of education and determine whether the patient's professional performance is compatible with the level of education and training. While making these inquiries, it is important to consider ways in which the patient's personality traits might interfere with work performance or success.

The presence of a personality disorder can interfere with an individual's capacity to function at work in a number of ways. Some personality disorders, in particular borderline personality disorder, antisocial personality disorder, and, to a somewhat lesser degree, narcissistic personality disorder, may be associated with pronounced limitations in the capacity to stick with a particular pursuit or to obtain satisfaction from work. These individuals often find that they easily become bored or lose interest in a task when it loses its novelty. The impulsivity and erratic behavior that is often associated with borderline, antisocial, and, at times, histrionic and paranoid personality disorders can interfere with an individual's ability to hold down a job or succeed in the workplace. The interpersonal problems frequently associated with personality disorders are another common cause of problems in the workplace; suspiciousness of others, social anxiety, fears of being exploited or told what to do (or fear of telling others what to do), intolerance of being in a subordinate position, grandiosity, a sense of entitlement, irritability, and interpersonal hostility all make it difficult to succeed in an environment that involves working with others. As a result, many individuals with personality disorders gravitate toward jobs where they can function relatively independently. For example, the patient in Box 8.13 chose a solitary work setting with a lower wage to avoid having to interact with others. This is a choice commonly made by patients with schizoid personality disorder who present, like the patient described, with little interest in relationships, an emotional detachment and flatness, and a general lack of concern for how they are perceived by others.

In addition to evaluating interpersonal and work functioning, it is also useful to inquire about how patients use **leisure** time. Often patients with personality disorders do not have developed interests or hobbies, easily becoming bored or losing interest. Individuals with narcissistic, antisocial, and, to some degree, histrionic and dependent personality disorders may describe feeling restless, empty, or at loose ends when confronted with unstructured time. Individuals with obsessive-compulsive personality disorder present a somewhat different picture; though able to invest and engage fully in work-related pursuits, they typically have little interest in leisure activities, preferring to work at times that others might spend socializing or engaging in recreational activities.

During the course of obtaining the history, the interviewer should consider whether a clear sense of how the patient views him- or herself has developed. Patients with severe personality pathology may provide information about themselves and their lives that is inconsistent and even frankly contradictory, reflecting a poorly integrated and unstable **self-concept** and a poorly developed capacity to think about themselves. This may become apparent if the information provided by the patient is discrepant with data obtained from other sources, or if a particular comment made by the patient contradicts something he or she said only moments earlier. For example, a patient who has spent more time than not collecting unemployment might describe herself as hard-working and industrious, or a patient whose wife has an order of protection against him might describe himself as a very caring person. Other patients with personality disorders will present with distorted

---

BOX 8.13

INTERVIEW WITH A NIGHT-SHIFT WORKER

Interviewer: Are you employed?

Patient: Yup.

I: What kind of work do you do?

P: Been working as a nurse for 40 years.

I: At the same hospital?

P: I work the night shift in a nursing home.

I: Do you enjoy your work?

P: Pretty much.

I: Do you enjoy helping the patients?

P: Doesn't really mean much to me.

I: What is it that you like or find satisfying about your work?

P: Pays the bills, steady income, good benefits.

I: It's unusual for someone with your seniority to be working nights. What's that about?

P: Oh, I like nights.

I: Why?

P: Things are quiet and then I can get things done when other people are at work during the day.

I: How have you done in your job? What kind of reviews do you get from your supervisors?

P: Oh, they like me, but that doesn't mean much to me. In fact, they're always wanting me to be charge nurse or move to days. But I have no interest. I like the quiet. Don't like working when there's a lot of staff around, doctors rounding. You know what it's like. And I certainly wouldn't want to be in the position of managing other people.

I: So you prefer working on your own.

P: Sure thing.

I: Would it be fair to say that you're pretty much of a loner?

P: Yup.

I: And have I gotten this right, that because you prefer to work on your own you have chosen to turn down offers that would involve taking on a busier and higher paying position?

P: Yes. I like what I do and I like not having to deal with anyone.

---

views of themselves predominantly in the area of self-esteem. Many patients with narcissistic personality disorder, for example, tend to feel greatly superior to others, even though they may be objectively highly unsuccessful, while others may be grandiose and feel entitled while at the same time struggling with feelings of envy and inferiority. Patients with avoidant personality disorder tend to see themselves as inferior and damaged, even though they may be successful in particular domains of functioning, while patients with obsessive-compulsive personality disorder strive for perfection and can become highly self-critical when failing to live up to their lofty self-imposed standards.

Finally, the process, as well as the content, of the psychiatric interview can provide useful data. The interview with the physician is an **interpersonal interaction** that patients often experience as stressful. It is common for patients' personality traits and, in particular, their customary ways of relating to others and of coping with anxiety to be expressed in their behavior during the interview and in their interactions with the physician. In essence, patients will "show" the interviewer aspects of their personality functioning that they do not necessarily describe in their narrative. When personality pathology is absent or relatively mild, the interviewer can attend to and make use of, but generally will not be troubled by, this aspect of the interview process. However, as personality pathology becomes more severe, the interaction between the patient and the interviewer often becomes not only a source of valuable diagnostic information but also by necessity a focus of clinical attention.

In the setting of a diagnostic evaluation, patients with personality disorders will often powerfully call upon their customary and generally maladaptive patterns of coping with anxiety and of interacting with others. Observing the patient's behavior in the interview and attending to his or her nonverbal communication serve as an invaluable source of information with regard to the nature of the patient's pathological personality traits. However, managing this aspect of the diagnostic interview can be challenging. At best, the interviewer may be left feeling frustrated and overwhelmed. At worst, the entire interview process may be derailed (see Table 8.2).

As personality pathology becomes more severe, the patient's interactions with the interviewer may prove to be one of the most useful ways to gain information about the nature and severity of the patient's problems. Patients with personality disorders characteristically evoke unusually strong and often uncomfortable emotional reactions in

TABLE 8.2 Typical Interview Behavior in Patients with Personality Disorders

Personality Disorder	Interview Behavior
Paranoid	Hostile, guarded, and unrevealing
Schizotypal	Circumstantial and difficult to follow
Schizoid	Patient provides detailed descriptions that fail to provide a coherent sense of the patient's history or life story
Antisocial	Manipulative, bullying, or glib, often concealing much of the relevant history
Narcissistic	Demanding or devaluing; patients present views of themselves and their life experience so profoundly colored by idealization and devaluation that it may be difficult to obtain a realistic impression of a patient's current and past life experience
Borderline	Affectively labile, easily and visibly angered, and unable to provide a clear history or explanation of why the patient is seeking treatment
Histrionic	Alternating between flirtation and uncontrollable weeping while leaving the interviewer with very little understanding of the difficulties that bring the patient to treatment
Avoidant	Self-denigrating and reluctant to reveal vulnerabilities
Dependent	Clinging and overly ingratiating
Obsessional	Patient tells a story seemingly stripped of emotion, or interacts in a controlling or subtly critical manner

others, including in their physicians. In moving through the diagnostic interview, interviewers should attend to their **own emotional responses**, be they positive or negative, and reflect on whether or not their feelings in relation to a particular patient fall within their customary range of emotional reactions to patients, or if they are responding to this individual in a fashion that is in some way more extreme than is typical. It is important for physicians to keep in mind that there is nothing incorrect about having strong emotional reactions to patients, even if the emotions involved are hostile, critical, or even expressions of sexual interest. The goal is not to eradicate these feelings but rather to be aware of the feelings without necessarily acting on them. This skill can only be developed with time and experience. The capacity of physicians to make use of their internal responses as they interact with patients is a hallmark of an expert clinician.

Guidelines for addressing particular challenges in the evaluation of patients with personality disorders are described in Box 8.14.

BOX 8.14
CHALLENGES IN THE EVALUATION OF PERSONALITY DISORDERS

CHALLENGE 1: PRESENTING COMPLAINTS

Patients with personality disorders may present in many different ways and with a broad spectrum of possible complaints. For example, they may present with complaints of depression, anxiety, social or interpersonal problems, substance abuse, or eating disorders or in an acute crisis that may involve self-destructive or impulsive behavior or paranoid thinking. Patients may endorse many of these complaints, or they may focus entirely on external circumstances, with no reference to internal difficulties. As a result, at the beginning of the interview it may not be obvious that the presence of a personality disorder plays an important role in the presenting picture.

GUIDELINES

Always consider the possibility of a personality disorder when evaluating a psychiatric or medical patient, regardless of the patient's complaints or presentation. In particular, the following situations should increase the interviewer's suspicions about the presence of a personality disorder:

- The patient's complaints are vague.
- The patient has multiple complaints and problems that do not seem to hang together.
- The patient's complaints are chronic, either beginning early in life or without a clear time of onset.
- The patient consistently blames others people and external circumstances for his or her difficulties in life.
- The patient describes a pattern of maladaptive behavior.
- The patient conveys a sense of chronic dissatisfaction.

(continued)

CHALLENGE 2: EGOSYNTONICITY

Problem

Many personality traits are "egosyntonic"—that is, individuals with personality disorders may be unaware of their maladaptive personality traits or, if aware of them, may not view them as a problem.

Advice

Ask if others have commented on particular aspects of the patient's behavior.

Example

Rather than asking patients with borderline personality disorder if their behavior is erratic, one might say, "Have the people close to you ever told you that they have difficulty anticipating how you are going to behave?"

Advice

Obtain information from other informants in addition to the patient whenever possible. The perspective of people close to the patient can be an essential component of the evaluation of personality pathology. Consultation with significant others will often reveal information the patient has not disclosed and can introduce a different perspective on the patient's story.

Problem

Patients minimize the presence or impact of maladaptive personality traits, especially when the traits are socially undesirable.

Examples

Even though envy is central to the subjective experience of individuals with narcissistic personality disorder, many such patients will deny that they suffer from painful feelings of envy when asked directly. Similarly, paranoid patients who are sensitive to slights and suspicious of others will often deny these traits when asked about them in so many words.

Advice

Normalize the trait that is being evaluated, and avoid reviewing a laundry list of diagnostic criteria.

Example

One might say to a patient with unstable self-esteem characteristic of narcissistic personality disorder, "Many people find that they tend to compare themselves to others. Sometimes people who do this feel superior, while at other times they may find themselves feeling envious. Does anything like this ever happen to you?"

Advice

Allow patients to externalize their difficulties.

(continued)

Example

Rather than inquiring as to whether a patient is sensitive to slights, one might ask,"Do you find that the people around you tend to be tactless or critical, frequently saying things that offend you?"

CHALLENGE 3: HETEROGENEITY AMONG THE PERSONALITY DISORDERS

The individual personality disorders are very different from one another. In addition, the criteria used to diagnose personality disorders span many different domains of psychological functioning, subjective experience, and maladaptive behavior. As a result, it is not easy to ask about the many different traits that form the core features of the various personality disorders as part of a routine clinical interview.

GUIDELINES

- Begin with a general evaluation of personality functioning before focusing on particular maladaptive traits or trying to assess the presence of a particular personality disorder. This approach puts personality pathology in perspective and sheds light on the degree to which personality pathology is clearly maladaptive and compatible with the diagnosis of some sort of personality disorder or just represents a particular personality "style."
- Be familiar with the general criteria for the various personality disorders, so that if it appears that the patient does have chronic ways of functioning that are clearly maladaptive and cause distress to the patient and those around him or her, the particular personality disorder(s) present can be honed in on.
- Keep in mind that approximately 50% of patients meeting criteria for one personality disorder will meet criteria for at least two.

DIFFERENTIAL DIAGNOSIS

Each of the following differential diagnostic decisions can have a profound effect on treatment planning.

Distinguishing Between Personality Pathology and Another Psychiatric Disorder

Many of the features of personality disorders are also associated with a variety of other psychiatric disorders. It is important to distinguish between a patient who is presenting with symptoms associated with another psychiatric disorder and a patient presenting with a personality disorder (Kernberg and Yeomans 2013). For example, suspiciousness is commonly associated with psychotic disorders, avoidant behavior with anxiety disorders, grandiosity with mania or hypomania, affective instability with rapidly cycling bipolar illness, and self-criticism with depressive disorders. When making the differential diagnosis, it should be kept in mind that personality disorders by definition have an onset before early adulthood, are chronic, and are relatively stable. As a result, a careful history and evaluation of symptoms, complemented if possible by history from a family member, is an essential diagnostic tool when it comes to ruling out or ruling in a personality disorder. A personality disorder should not be diagnosed if the relevant symptoms are present only during an episode of another psychiatric disorder or can be attributed to another psychiatric condition. Having said this, it can at times be difficult to distinguish between psychiatric disorders that are chronic and often of early onset, such as dysthymia or social phobia, and a personality disorder.

Distinguishing Between Personality Pathology and Physiological Manifestations of Another Medical Condition

Medical disorders that affect the central nervous system can cause personality changes on a physiological basis and may appear to present as personality pathology. As a result, a complete medical history and evaluation should always be part of the clinical assessment of patients being evaluated for personality pathology. Strokes, brain tumors, demyelinating diseases, and Alzheimer's disease can at times present with personality changes that may mimic a personality disorder. Suspicion of an underlying medical cause for personality changes should be elevated in patients already carrying a diagnosis of a central nervous system disorder or a chronic systemic medical condition, as well as in older patients, who are at elevated risk for medical illness. When enduring changes in personality arise as a result of the direct physiological effects of a medical condition, personality change due to another medical condition should be diagnosed rather than a personality disorder (see Chapter 5, Neurocognitive Disorders and Mental Disorders Due to Another Medical Condition).

Evaluating the Patient with Other Psychiatric Disorders and Comorbid Personality Pathology

Because other psychiatric disorders can mimic and complicate the presentation of personality disorders, it can be difficult to make a reliable personality disorder diagnosis in a patient presenting with acute symptomatology. For example, hypomania can mimic the grandiosity of narcissistic personality disorder, agoraphobia can present with socially avoidant behavior suggestive of avoidant personality disorder, and panic disorder can be associated with clinging behavior that resembles that seen in dependent personality disorder. In addition, symptoms of other psychiatric disorders may impact and distort the manner in which patients characterize their baseline functioning. For example, a patient in the midst of a depressive episode will often exaggerate professional disappointments or personal failures, while a patient who is hypomanic may minimize chronic interpersonal or professional difficulties. At the same time, the presence of a comorbid personality disorder diagnosis will inform treatment planning for many other psychiatric disorders. As a result, even though it is customary to defer diagnosing personality disorders until acute symptoms resolve, it is clinically useful to attempt to evaluate premorbid personality functioning if at all possible, especially if the physician is able to obtain a clear, detailed, and accurate description of the patient's baseline functioning from others. When evaluating patients with a history of substance use disorders, it is necessary to distinguish between baseline personality pathology and behaviors that are sequelae of substance use or efforts to obtain drugs (most commonly, antisocial behavior). If personality pathology appears to have emerged or have been exacerbated after an individual has been exposed to extreme stress, a diagnosis of posttraumatic stress disorder should be considered.

Patients with personality disorders have an elevated risk of many other psychiatric conditions, including mood, anxiety, eating, and substance use disorders. In patients with comorbid diagnoses, it is important to comprehensively evaluate and identify all active disorders. Other psychiatric disorders can cause personality traits to become even more extreme and maladaptive in the patient with a personality disorder and, similarly, the presence of a personality disorder will predict poorer prognosis and complicate management in the patient being treated for an acute psychiatric disorder. Often the physician will make a presumptive diagnosis of a personality disorder in a patient with an active acute disorder and then reevaluate the nature of personality pathology and functioning as those symptoms remit.

Evaluating the Patient for Comorbid Personality Disorders

There is a high rate of comorbidity among the personality disorders. The presence of comorbid personality disorders will often profoundly affect prognosis and treatment planning. For example, a patient with only a diagnosis of borderline personality disorder has a vastly more favorable prognosis than does a patient with both borderline personality disorder and antisocial personality disorder. As a result, in the same way that it is important to do a complete review of systems in every medical patient, it is important to do a complete evaluation of personality functioning and personality traits in every psychiatric patient. This remains true even after a patient has met the diagnostic criteria for a particular personality disorder.

MEDICAL EVALUATION

When evaluating a patient presenting with what appears to be a psychiatric disorder, it is always necessary to rule out the possibility that some or all of the patient's presenting difficulties can be attributed to the physiological manifestations of another medical condition. In the case of personality disorders, this entails, at the very least, obtaining a complete medical history, performing a thorough cognitive evaluation, and obtaining routine blood work to rule out metabolic and endocrine abnormalities. If this screening suggests the presence of medical illness, medical and neurological evaluation, including CT or MRI of the brain, may be indicated.

ETIOLOGY

Current understanding of the etiology of personality disorders points to a complex interaction between **temperament**, that is, constitutional factors determined by genetic and other biological factors, and **environment**, or developmental experience as it impacts individuals and their psychological development. It appears that the relative degree to which constitutional and environmental factors play a role in the etiology of personality pathology is variable among the different personality disorders. Because developmental and environmental experiences affect gene expression, while temperamental factors help to shape environmental experience, it can be difficult to sort out the relative contribution of temperament and environment in the etiology of any particular disorder. As a result, in working with an individual patient, it is important to appreciate that the reason why some patients develop personality pathology and others do not is most often unknown. For example, extreme environmental stressors, such as growing up during wartime or being physically or sexually abused in childhood, do not affect all individuals equally.

More **resilient** individuals may suffer severe trauma and environmental stressors without developing clinically significant personality pathology, while others may be scarred for life. Similarly, some individuals do not develop personality disorders despite a heavy genetic loading for personality pathology and maladaptive personality traits.

Neurobiology

There has been a recent explosion in the understanding of the genetics and neurobiology of many of the personality disorders. On the basis of twin and adoption studies, it appears that **genetic** factors play at least some role in the etiology all of the personality disorders. In addition, studies looking at individual personality traits such as introversion, extroversion, submissiveness, and neuroticism suggest that approximately half the variance seen in these personality traits can be attributed to genetic factors. The genetics of schizotypal, borderline, and antisocial personality disorders have been studied extensively, and there is strong support for an important role for genetic factors in the etiology of these disorders. Schizotypal personality has been found to be genetically associated with schizophrenia, while traits such as impulsivity, affective instability, stimulus seeking, hostility, and callousness, many of which are associated with the cluster B personality disorders, appear to be highly heritable. In addition, harm avoidance, physiological arousal, trait anxiety, and social anxiety are seen in family members of individuals with avoidant personality disorder.

The neurobiology underlying maladaptive personality functioning is a current area of research. For example, structural abnormalities in brain anatomy characteristic of schizophrenia are also found in individuals with schizotypal personality disorder. The brains of individuals with antisocial personality disorder have reductions in whole brain volume, particularly in the temporal lobe, and antisocial personality disorder has been associated with deficient brain activation in response to fear conditioning in forensic populations.

Structural neuroimaging studies have found borderline personality disorder to be associated with reduction in frontal and orbitofrontal volume, areas of the brain that serve an inhibitory function and are involved in affect regulation. Findings of functional neuroimaging studies of patients with borderline personality disorder are also compatible with salient clinical features of the disorder, in particular poor impulse control and affective instability. Studies that present individuals with borderline personality disorder with stressful conditions while measuring brain activity using fMRI show decreased levels of activation of frontal and orbitofrontal areas and heightened levels of activation in the amygdala in the patients relative to controls.

Studies point to the role of abnormal dopamine activity in schizotypal personality disorder, and impulsive and aggressive personality traits have been linked to abnormalities in serotonin activity in patients with antisocial and borderline personality disorders. In general, serotonin appears to play a role in behavioral inhibition such that low serotonin activity is linked to impulsivity and aggressive behavior, while high levels of serotonin activity have been linked to behavioral inhibition and the personality traits of compulsiveness and conscientiousness associated most prominently with obsessive-compulsive personality disorder.

Environment

Environmental factors have long been understood to play a role in the etiology of personality pathology. The role of environmental factors in the etiology of personality pathology has been most systematically studied in relation to borderline and antisocial personality disorders. Because these disorders carry a disproportionately high cost with regard to utilization of psychiatric and forensic services, there is great interest in identifying environmental risk factors for the development of these disorders that could be targeted for early intervention.

Psychodynamic theories emphasize the role of excessive frustration, parental unresponsiveness, and inappropriate parental responsiveness—lack of emotional attunement—in the etiology of borderline personality disorder, and psychodynamic approaches consider similar factors to play a role in the origins of narcissistic personality disorder as well. These **pathogenic experiences early in life** are thought to amplify an inborn propensity toward aggression, leading to chronic rage and the development of pathological or "primitive" defense mechanisms that attempt to diminish anxieties in ways that are very maladaptive in life (see Box 17.3, Chapter 17, Psychotherapy), pathological attachment patterns, and a failure to form stable and realistic experiences of oneself and others.

Consistent with these theories, empirical studies have found a high frequency of physical and sexual abuse as well as abandonment and traumatic neglect in the early lives of adults with borderline personality disorder. However, in an analysis of the data, Paris (2009) cautions that the percent of borderline patients reporting a history of severe abuse (25%) is not that much greater than that in general-community samples, and that 30% of patients with bipolar disorder report no history of abuse. Family dysfunction, emotional neglect, and parental psychopathology are cited as risk factors that may interact with a history of abuse in the etiology of the condition. Studies of antisocial personality disorder also point to a high frequency of early trauma and abuse, often at the hands of caretakers who themselves may have impulsive and antisocial traits as well as high rates of substance abuse.

The predominant cognitive-behavioral view of the development of borderline personality disorder emphasizes an early environment that consistently invalidates the subjective experience of children who have inborn difficulties with emotional regulation.

TREATMENT

Treatment of the patient with a personality disorder must be tailored to the needs, goals, and capabilities of the individual patient. While in the past personality disorders were viewed as relatively intractable conditions, recent empirical studies have provided a more optimistic perspective on the responsiveness of many of the personality disorders to a relatively broad menu of therapeutic approaches. Treatment typically combines multiple therapeutic modalities, focusing on psychoeducation, individual and group psychotherapies, and medication management. Psychotherapy, provided in an individual or group setting, remains the backbone of treatment (Oldham et al. 2001). Psychopharmacology is used to target the various symptoms frequently associated with many of the personality disorders, as well as to treat other comorbid psychiatric disorders, but it is generally agreed that medications do not lead to personality change.

Psychodynamic Psychotherapy

Contemporary psychodynamic therapies for personality disorders seek to improve overall functioning by modifying the way in which patients experience themselves and the world around them. Psychodynamic treatments for personality disorders tend to be relatively

long term, typically lasting at least a year and often several years. Psychodynamic treatment approaches emphasize the clinical challenge of modifying personality traits that are egosyntonic, either invisible or of no concern to the patient. The first step is to help patients become more aware of their maladaptive ways of behaving, thinking, and feeling and of interacting with others. Over time, as attention is focused on maladaptive traits, they become more visible to the patient, and ultimately they come to be experienced as a problem. At this point it is possible to explore the motivations and cognitive distortions underlying maladaptive traits and to begin to modify them. Many psychodynamic approaches make a link between maladaptive personality traits and pathological defensive operations, with the expectation that, as the treatment progresses, the patient will come to use healthier and more adaptive defenses (see Chapter 17, Psychotherapy).

Different personality disorders are more or less amenable to a psychodynamic approach, depending to a large extent on the patient's level of **motivation** for long-term treatment and the degree to which personality pathology interferes with the patient's **capacity to form a therapeutic alliance**. Motivated patients presenting with histrionic, obsessive-compulsive, dependent, and avoidant personality disorders tend to do well in psychodynamic therapy. In contrast, individuals with cluster A personality disorders rarely seek long-term treatment because of their fundamental mistrust of others and their difficulty tolerating anything but superficial relationships.

Specialized forms of psychodynamic psychotherapy, such as transference-focused psychotherapy (TFP) (Clarkin et al. 2006) and mentalization-based treatment (MBT) (Bateman and Fonagy 2012), have been developed, manualized, and found to be effective for treatment of patients with more severe personality pathology, particularly those with borderline personality disorder. These treatments share a structured treatment approach, limit-setting, development of the patient's capacity to be aware of his or her emotional states and those of others, and maintenance of a stable and consistent "holding" relationship with the therapist, that is, a relationship that welcomes and can deal with the intense emotions at the root of the disorder. TFP focuses more than MBT on contracting around destructive behaviors that interfere with exploring thoughts and feelings, and on resolving conflicts within the patient's mind that underlie symptoms and subjective distress (see Chapter 17, Psychotherapy). Individuals with antisocial personality disorder should not be treated in psychodynamic psychotherapy, as they are unlikely to benefit from that treatment approach.

Cognitive-Behavioral Therapy

Cognitive-behavioral therapy (CBT) can be helpful to many patients with personality disorders. It is generally more **structured** and **focused** on specific goals than dynamic therapies. CBT also tends to be of **shorter duration**, typically lasting less than a year and sometimes maybe as brief as several sessions. Cognitive-behavioral therapists actively help patients to identify maladaptive behavior patterns and ways of thinking, focusing on the core beliefs that color and distort patients' experiences of themselves and of the world around them. Cognitive-behavioral therapists provide the patient with specific strategies and skills to modify these patterns, making use of techniques such as practicing and homework assignments. For example, for patients with avoidant personality disorder, CBT will address avoidant behavior patterns by gradually increasing the patient's exposure to anxiety-provoking social situations they typically would avoid, while also working to challenge and modify self-deprecating cognitive patterns such as "I'm a loser and no one will want to talk to me."

In addition to more conventional forms of CBT, a number of long-term versions of this treatment approach have been developed to treat specific personality disorders. **Dialectical behavior therapy** (DBT) (Linehan 1993) integrates elements of CBT and is widely used to treat individuals with borderline personality disorder. DBT combines weekly group **skills training** with weekly individual therapy. It has been found to be effective for patients who are chronically self-destructive and impulsive (see Chapter 17, Psychotherapy). **Schema-based therapy** (Young et al. 2003) focuses on modifying patients' cognitive schemata underlying many maladaptive personality traits and offering "**limited reparenting**" to make up for perceived flaws in the original parenting experience.

Supportive Psychotherapy

Supportive psychotherapy (Winston et al. 2012) is another form of individual psychotherapy frequently used to treat personality disorders. Supportive psychotherapies are highly flexible in their approach. Their duration and frequency are variable, depending on the needs of the patient and his or her current life and psychological situation. The goal of supportive psychotherapy is to help patients mobilize the most adaptive ways of coping they have available to them while eschewing more destructive responses to external and internal stressors. In supportive therapy, the therapist plays an active role, often making use of psychodynamic and cognitive-behavioral strategies, while providing advice, guidance, and psychoeducation and mobilizing social supports. Supportive psychotherapy is often combined with a variety of other treatments and interventions, including social skills training, family therapy, 12-step programs, and vocational counseling and rehabilitation, tailored to the needs of the individual patient over time.

Good psychiatric management (GPM) is a recent addition to the evidence-based treatments for borderline personality disorder. It combines psychoeducation about genetics, flexible integration of medications, and group and family options, to focus the patient on the tasks required to gain a good life outside of the therapy. GPM is seen as a basic approach to be used by general clinicians. It is suitable for most borderline patients, leaving those who prove unresponsive to seek psychotherapies provided by experts in borderline personality disorder.

Group Psychotherapy

Group psychotherapy supports self-esteem by helping patients appreciate that others struggle with difficulties similar to their own. In this setting, members of the group can challenge one another, calling attention to maladaptive behaviors and ways of thinking and interacting with others. Group treatments carry the benefit of being especially cost-effective. They are commonly used in inpatient settings and in day hospitals as well as in more conventional outpatient settings.

Pharmacotherapy

While the psychotherapies are the backbone of treatment for the personality disorders, treatment will often involve combining pharmacotherapy as well. Medications are prescribed to treat specific symptom complexes;this can be helpful even when the patient does not meet full criteria for another psychiatric disorder. In particular, impulsivity and aggression may respond to selective serotonin reuptake inhibitors (SSRIs). Instability of mood may also respond to SSRIs, as well as to other antidepressants and mood stabilizers. Psychotic-like experiences may respond to low-dose antipsychotics, as may symptoms of anxiety in patients with schizotypal personality disorder.

As emphasized, patients with personality disorders frequently have other comorbid psychiatric disorders. It is important to carefully evaluate, diagnose, and aggressively treat these disorders in this population. Mood, anxiety, substance use, and eating disorders should be treated using standard approaches. However, patients with personality disorders tend to be more refractory to conventional treatments for these disorders than patients without personality disorders, and special attention should be paid to maintenance of the treatment alliance and adherence when working with this population. When comorbid psychopathology is successfully treated, personality pathology may become less severe or disabling, and treatment for underlying personality pathology may become more effective.

REFERENCES CITED

Bateman, A. W., and P. Fonagy, eds. *Handbook of Mentalizing in Mental Health Practice*. Washington, DC: American Psychiatric Publishing, 2012.

Clarkin, J. F., F. E. Yeomans, and O. F. Kernberg. *Psychotherapy for Borderline Personality: Focusing on Object Relations*. Washington, DC: American Psychiatric Press, 2006.

Cooper, A. M. Further developments in the clinical diagnosis of narcissistic personality disorder. In E. F. Ronningstam, ed. *Disorders of Narcissism: Diagnostic, Clinical and Empirical Implications*. Washington DC: American Psychiatric Press, 1998.

Kernberg, O. F., and F. E. Yeomans. Borderline personality disorder, bipolar disorder, depression, attention deficit/hyperactivity disorder, and narcissistic personality disorder: practical differential diagnosis. *Bulletin of the Menninger Clinic* 77(1):1–22, 2013.

Lenzenweger, M. F., M. D. Johnson, and J. B. Willett. Individual growth curve analysis illuminates stability and change in personality disorder features. *Archives of General Psychiatry* 61:1015–1024, 2004.

Linehan, M. M. *Cognitive-Behavioral Treatment of Borderline Personality Disorder*. New York, Guilford Press, 1993.

Oldham, J. M., G. O. Gabbard, M. K. Goin, J. Gunderson, P. Soloff, D. Spiegel, M. Stone, and K. A. Phillips. Practice guideline for the treatment of patients with border line personality disorder. *American Journal of Psychiatry* 58:1–52, 2001.

Paris, J. Borderline personality disorder. In T. Millon, P. H. Blaney, and R. D. Davis, eds. *Oxford Textbook of Psychopathology*. New York: Oxford University Press, 2009, pp. 625–652.

Stone, M. H. *The Fate of Borderline Patients: Successful Outcome and Psychiatric Practice*. New York: Guilford Press, 1990.

Stone, M. H. Long-term outcome in personality disorders. In P. Tyrer and G. Stein, eds. *Personality Disorder Reviewed*. London: Gaskell, 1993, pp. 321–345.

Winston, A., R. N. Rosenthal, and H. Pinsker. *Learning Supportive Psychotherapy, An Illustrated Guide*. Washington, DC: American Psychiatric Publishing, 2012.

Young, J. E., J. S. Klosko, and M. E. Weishaar. *Schema Therapy: A Practitioner's Guide*. New York: Guilford Press, 2003.

SELECTED READINGS

Bateman, A. W., and P. Fonagy P, eds. *Handbook of Mentalizing in Mental Health Practice*. Washington, DC: American Psychiatric Publishing, 2012.

Beck, A. T., A. Freeman, D. D. Davis, et al. *Cognitive Therapy of Personality Disorders*, 2nd ed. New York: Guilford Press, 2004.

Clarkin, J. F., F. E. Yeomans, and O. F. Kernberg. *Psychotherapy for Borderline Personality: Focusing on Object Relations*. Washington, DC: American Psychiatric Press, 2006.

Gabbard, G. O. Dynamic approaches to axis II disorders. In *Psychodynamic Psychiatry in Clinical Practice*, 4th ed. Washington, DC: American Psychiatric Publishing, 2005, pp. 401–599.

Gunderson, J. G., and G. O. Gabbard, Eds. *Psychotherapy for Personality Disorders. Review of Psychiatry*, Vol, 19. Washington, DC: American Psychiatric Publishing, 2000.

Linehan, M. M. *Cognitive-Behavioral Treatment of Borderline Personality Disorder*. New York: Guilford Press, 1993.

MacKinnon, R. A., R. Michels, and P. J. Buckley. *The Psychiatric Interview in Clinical Practice*, 2nd ed. Washington, DC: American Psychiatric Publishing, 2007.

Oldham, J. M., A. E. Skodol, and D. S. Bender, eds. *The American Psychiatric Publishing Textbook of Personality Disorders*, 2nd ed. Washington, DC: American Psychiatric Publishing, 2014.

Zimmerman, M., L. Rothchild, and I. Chelminski. The prevalence of DSM-IV personality disorders in psychiatric outpatients. *American Journal of Psychiatry* 162:1911–1918, 2005.

/// 9 /// Feeding and Eating Disorders

MICHAEL J. DEVLIN AND
JOANNA E. STEINGLASS

The majority of patients with anorexia nervosa or bulimia ner-
vosa are young women who, as a result of their disorders, face serious psychosocial and
health consequences. In contrast, binge-eating disorder, newly classified in DSM-5 as a
feeding and eating disorder, affects a broader demographic. Additional disorders, which
occur primarily in children and adolescents, have been reclassified as feeding and eating
disorders; these include rumination disorder, pica, and avoidant/restrictive food intake
disorder (ARFID) (see Chapter 15, Child and Adolescent Psychiatry).

Eating disorders highlight the distinctions that need to be made between the spectrum of normal behavior and frank psychopathology. A large percentage of Americans
diet. Furthermore, significant body image *concern*, particularly among women, is common. But fewer than 5% of women and even fewer men develop a frank eating disorder.
This discrepancy between the number of individuals engaging in at-risk behavior and the
much smaller number developing full clinical syndromes suggests, among other things,
the presence of a preexisting biological vulnerability. Yet, as with much of psychopathology, there are also important cultural and social influences. The eating disorders present
particularly clear examples of the challenge to physicians to understand their patients'
illnesses not only on a psychological level but also on biological, social, and cultural levels. All of these factors must be taken into account as physicians evaluate the onset and
maintenance of eating disorders and devise appropriate treatment strategies.

DIAGNOSTIC AND CLINICAL FEATURES

Core Shared Features

The eating disorders share a core behavioral feature, which is a disturbance of eating habits. Most share a core psychological feature, which is a preoccupation with or disturbance
in the perception of body image. In anorexia nervosa, the **eating disturbance** takes the
form of undereating, while in bulimia nervosa or anorexia nervosa binge-eating/purging
type it takes the form of severely restrained eating alternating with loss of control and
consumption of large amounts of food. Binge-eating disorder is also characterized by
episodic uncontrolled eating, frequently in a lifetime context of intermittent attempts at
dieting, but without fasting, vigorous exercise, purging, or other attempts to compensate

for the binge-eating episodes. Patients with binge-eating disorder consider themselves "compulsive eaters" and often gain large amounts of weight during periods of extreme binge eating.

The second feature shared by the eating disorders is a preoccupation with or **disturbance in the perception of body image**. Most evident in anorexia nervosa, this excessive concern about body weight and shape is also a major component in bulimia nervosa and binge-eating disorder. This feature was added to the diagnostic criteria for bulimia nervosa in the DSM-III-R and has been retained. Some consider it to be the central characteristic of these illnesses and the source of the behavioral disturbances. Many patients with eating disorders consider body weight and shape to be the most important factors in determining how they feel about themselves at a given moment. These factors are more significant to these patients than their performance at work or school; their relationships with friends, spouses, or children; or any other aspect of their lives that might contribute to a sense of well-being. It is not unusual for a patient to find that her weight intrudes constantly into her thoughts to the point that she cannot focus on her work or even on a conversation.

Anorexia Nervosa

Anorexia nervosa is characterized by **severe restriction** of food intake, leading to weight loss and the medical sequelae of starvation. Patients with anorexia nervosa, unlike those who lose weight for other reasons, are unable to acknowledge their emaciated state and are continually afraid of becoming fat. Patients are not always able to express this fear verbally, but it drives their behavior.

The first criterion (see DSM-5) for diagnosing anorexia nervosa is **weight loss** or absence of expected weight gain in a person who does not maintain a minimum healthy weight. Of note is that the phrase "refusal to maintain body weight," from DSM-IV, has been altered in DSM-5 to focus on behavior and to eliminate possibly misleading implications regarding conscious intent. The minimum healthy weight is usually defined in terms of body mass index, with 18.5 kg/m^2 as the lower limit of normal and 17.0 kg/m^2 as moderate to severe thinness. The diagnosis cannot be based on this criterion alone, however, because it is not unusual for women especially to weigh less than the minimum healthy weight. Amenorrhea as a physiological indicator of starvation has been removed as a diagnostic criterion for anorexia nervosa in DSM-5. In addition to these behavioral and biological features, the diagnosis of anorexia nervosa requires two psychological features: an **intense fear of gaining weight,** and a **body image disturbance.** The latter is especially difficult to manage because patients with anorexia nervosa usually see themselves or parts of their bodies as fat, even though they appear emaciated to others. Some patients, often older or chronic patients, will admit that they are thin, but are unduly invested in maintaining this degree of emaciation or seem not to appreciate the consequences of maintaining such a low weight. These patients should receive the diagnosis of anorexia nervosa if they meet the other DSM criteria.

The DSM-5 recognizes **two subtypes** of anorexia nervosa. Anorexia nervosa **restricting** type is seen in underweight patients who have engaged in dieting, fasting, or excessive exercise but do not engage in binge eating or purging. Anorexia nervosa **binge-eating/purging** type is seen in underweight patients who engage in a cycle of binge eating and purging. Several studies have shown that patients with the binge-purge subtype have more impulsive behaviors (e.g., stealing, abusing drugs, mutilating themselves, and attempting suicide) and more maladaptive personality traits than anorectic-restrictors.

In addition, they more commonly have a personal and family history of obesity and more frequently report psychiatric illness in their parents. Severity of anorexia nervosa is rated according to body mass index.

Patients with anorexia nervosa display a number of characteristic behaviors. Initially, they may be enthusiastic about the discipline involved in dieting, exercising, and continuing to lose weight. As starvation progresses, a depressed mood may develop, which is accompanied by lethargy, irritability, social isolation, and decreased interest in sex.

Patients with anorexia nervosa tend to have high levels of baseline **anxiety** and high levels of baseline **obsessionality**, in some ways similar to obsessive-compulsive disorder (see case example in Box 9.1). The personality trait of perfectionism is often found among patients with anorexia nervosa before the onset of the illness. Similarly, these patients

---

BOX 9.1
CASE EXAMPLE OF ANOREXIA NERVOSA

Anna is a 20-year-old single woman who had to take a medical leave from college after 2½ years. When she was in high school, she was always on the thinner side compared to her peers. She participated in school sports and activities, while maintaining an excellent academic record. She was accepted to the college of her choice and set off for school, looking forward to living on her own and getting out of a difficult household. She had heard that women tend to gain weight in college and was mindful of her eating. When she got to college, she discovered that it was harder than she expected to keep up with her classes and to make friends. She found that she was able to keep herself from feeling anxious if she focused on very specific tasks for the day. At meals, she could prevent herself from worrying about who to sit with by focusing instead on exactly the right thing to eat. She discovered that she could feel good about the day if she did not eat any dessert. She liked the effect this was having on her shape and weight, and decided to add a regular exercise routine to her day.

With this new routine, she lost a few pounds. As she saw the numbers go down on the scale, she discovered that she really liked that feeling, and that she felt less and less anxiety about her life at college. She decided to select her meals carefully, cutting out all "fat" in her diet. She then found that she felt better at the gym than she did in class, and began to spend several hours there a day—sometimes missing plans with friends, or even skipping classes to complete her exercise routine. She felt that she had to complete 330 sit-ups in order to get on with her day. Her weight continued to go down.

As she became underweight for her height, she found that she was thinking about food all day. In class in the morning, she would be carefully adding up the caloric content of what she ate for breakfast and using that information to determine what she would allow herself for dinner. She would plan to skip lunch and go to the

(continued)

gym. It quickly became important to eat her meals in a very precise way. She would select her salad from the salad bar. Dressing was too many calories, so she added mustard for flavor. Some days she put Equal on her lettuce instead. If she ate a yogurt, she would put a small amount on the spoon, lick the back of the spoon, then take small bites from the front of the spoon. It could take an hour to eat a yogurt, and she was always careful to leave a small amount behind. She weighed herself each morning at the same time, wearing the same thing each day. Periodically, during the day, she would check to be sure that her thighs were not touching when she stood up.

Her weight began to drop to new lows and Anna went from enjoying seeing the number on the scale to being afraid of seeing any increases on the scale. The number dictated what she had to do at the gym that day. She was increasingly tired and worried about what the scale would tell her. She was too tired to do any of the extracurricular activities she used to enjoy. Her friends noticed that she lost her sense of humor and didn't come out with them anymore. Over time, her friends' concerns about her made an impression and Anna sought out treatment. Her weight had dropped to 75% of what would be considered her "ideal body weight" and her eating was sufficiently poor that Anna agreed to begin treatment with an inpatient program that aimed to restore normal weight. Her inpatient treatment was followed by outpatient cognitive-behavioral therapy that helped her to maintain her weight and to challenge some of the rigidity in her thinking about eating, shape, and weight.

commonly have high levels of rigidity and "harm avoidance." The illness includes intrusive thoughts about food, shape, and weight that can be preoccupations, obsessions, or even on the spectrum of delusional beliefs (i.e., an emaciated patient believes that she is "fat"). The patient develops a series of behaviors that are extremely ritualized. The rituals may be related to procedures around eating, or body-checking, or exercise. The rituals and obsessions are worse in the underweight state and tend to improve somewhat with weight normalization.

These seemingly compulsive behaviors and obsessions about "counting calories" and following weight have led to speculation that there may be a relationship between anorexia nervosa and obsessive-compulsive disorder. Although most patients with anorexia nervosa do not suffer from a clinically defined obsessive-compulsive disorder that can be distinguished from their preoccupations with weight and food, the prevalence of an obsessive-compulsive disorder that appears to be separate and distinct from the eating disorder is higher than would be expected among these patients.

Bulimia Nervosa

Bulimia nervosa, which is usually diagnosed in patients of **normal weight**, is also characterized by attempts to restrict food intake, but the eating behavior is somewhat different from that found in anorexia nervosa. The attempts at restriction are interspersed with **binge eating,** periods of consumption of **objectively large amounts of food** accompanied by a feeling of **loss of control** followed most frequently by the compensatory behavior of vomiting. The use of syrup of ipecac, which is an emetic that is available without prescription, can result in a potentially lethal cardiomyopathy. Because patients may not volunteer such information, the physician should specifically ask about the use of syrup of ipecac.

Other **methods of compensation** include laxatives and over-the-counter or prescription diuretics. Stimulant laxatives may be taken in amounts that far exceed the recommended dosage. Some patients use vigorous exercise and fasting to prevent weight gain. Patients with comorbid diabetes mellitus may restrict or withhold insulin following a binge to facilitate elimination of glucose, in effect, purging. This may, of course, lead to worsening of diabetic symptoms and complications.

The diagnosis of bulimia nervosa is no longer divided into purging and nonpurging subtypes as it was in the DSM-IV because this did not prove to be a useful distinction (see DSM-5). Severity of bulimia nervosa is rated according to the frequency of compensatory behaviors.

Many patients with bulimia nervosa experience an **escalation** of their behavior (see case example in Box 9.2). Many patients describe a euphoric feeling (a "high") associated with binge-eating or purging, or both. Over time the pattern of binge eating and purging

---

BOX 9.2
CASE EXAMPLE OF BULIMIA NERVOSA

Brittany is a 24-year-old female college graduate working full time in an exciting and demanding job in the performing arts. She is not an actress, but derives great enjoyment from being surrounding by artists. She has always been very aware of beauty in the world, and has applied her tasteful eye to her own appearance. She dresses with flair. Her shape has always bothered her, as it doesn't quite fit with her own standard for beauty. Though not an athlete, she played enough sports in high school to keep her weight at about normal for her height. When she got to college, she found a group of friends who were very social. They went to parties, and enjoyed late-night meals. She began to gain some weight and became very concerned. One night, after a few beers and a few slices of pizza, she felt very concerned about what might happen to her weight and decided to throw up to get rid of it. She thought she had found the perfect solution. She could fully enjoy the social activities with her friends, and then get rid of all the extra calories right afterward.

After a few months of throwing up late at night once a week, she found herself looking forward to binge eating and thinking more and more about how good she felt after purging. She started to go out of her way to schedule in a time to binge and purge. In order to prepare, she would purchase all of her favorite foods—a large bag of chips, a couple of slices of pizza, some ice cream. Over time, she found that she was buying larger quantities of food—a whole pizza, a pint of ice cream, a bag of chips, and a bag of cookies—to achieve the same effect, and she began to feel more out of control during the episodes. Binge eating and purging was starting to take more time in her day, and she was not able to go out with her friends because

(continued)

she would take the time to be alone in her room for a full binge–purge episode. She began to do this every night.

In the morning, she felt terrible. She was exhausted from the effort, and felt guilty about how much food she had eaten. She felt disgusting and vowed to skip breakfast and lunch to make up for it. This became a daily pattern. She noticed that some months her weight went up, and she would become more vigilant in her routine. She could lose 20 pounds in a month, get back to her regular weight, and then the binge eating would increase and her weight would drift up again.

After college, she found a demanding job in a theater company. She had a diet shake every morning for breakfast before rushing to work. At work, there simply wasn't time for lunch. At the end of the day, her friends from work would head out to a bar or a restaurant and she would relish eating everything that was ordered. She would continue to buy food at each deli on her way home at night, and arrive home late at night to spend an hour vomiting. The effort was exhausting. At times, following the purge, Brittany would start to nibble, with the intent of keeping down the food. But if she ate more than she set out to, even a little, she would decide to keep eating and then purge. On nights when she had more than one binge–vomit episode, she would finish by taking six laxatives just to reassure herself that she had gotten rid of everything. After a year of this escalating behavior, Brittany was so depressed by her lack of control that she sought treatment. She worked with a cognitive behavioral therapist for 6 months to develop new strategies around eating and to challenge some of her automatic thoughts about herself.

can change with increasing size of the binge or increasing time spent binge eating and purging. This pattern can be likened to the phenomenon of tolerance seen with substance abuse, in which increased amounts of drug are required to achieve the same effect over time. Patients with bulimia nervosa also commonly describe impulsivity in their behavior. Sometimes even a normal meal impulsively turns into a binge when an invisible line is crossed. For example, the patient described in Box 9.2 begins each day with a plan to "be good" but finds that she nonetheless ends the day with a binge/purge episode. Many patients with bulimia nervosa have other mental health problems related to **impulse control** as well, such as **substance use disorders**. Eating binges are sometimes **triggered by unpleasant feelings or circumstances** (e.g., a disappointing personal relationship, stress at work or school) or by an experience that affects the patient's perception of her body (e.g., trying on clothes that no longer fit). The binge eating and purging cycle may relieve or neutralize these feelings for a short period of time but later often results in an overall decline in self-esteem.

Most patients with bulimia nervosa express significant concern with body shape and weight when they are asked to evaluate their appearance and overall self-worth. Individuals with bulimia nervosa are usually of normal weight, although occasionally they may be obese or somewhat underweight. It is normal in the United States for physical appearance to influence a person's overall self-esteem, but patients with bulimia nervosa often consider body weight and shape to be *the* most important factors in determining how they feel about themselves. They derive less satisfaction from other areas of life, such as personal relationships or achievements at work or school.

Binge-Eating Disorder

Binge-eating disorder, which was included in the DSM-IV as a provisional diagnosis, has been granted full diagnostic status in DSM-5. Binge-eating disorder is characterized first and foremost by recurrent **uncontrolled eating binges.** The binges are similar to those in bulimia nervosa but cannot be broken down into discrete episodes, as they often occur continuously over several hours and are not punctuated by purges. In order to be diagnosed with this disorder (see DSM-5), patients must experience a **loss of control** as well as exhibit the behavioral indicators of loss of control. Loss of control differentiates these episodes from "normal" overeating. They must have significant distress related to eating. Patients with binge-eating disorder often feel that their lives are dominated by eating and have significant impairment in their abilities to work and relate to others. Severity of binge-eating disorder is rated according to the frequency of binge episodes.

Because binge-eating disorder is a relatively new entity, little is known about its descriptive features and psychopathology. There is an association between binge-eating disorder and **obesity**, but binge-eating disorder is not synonymous with obesity. Obesity is considered to be a medical rather than a psychiatric disorder, although some obese individuals probably do have an eating disorder, and recent efforts have been made to study, diagnose, and treat such individuals. It is not yet known what proportion of obese individuals suffers from the disorder or what proportion of individuals with the disorder is obese. Preliminary studies demonstrate that persons of normal weight as well as overweight persons may meet the criteria for binge-eating disorder and that most obese patients in weight loss clinics do not fulfill the criteria. There is some evidence that obese patients who engage in binge eating, many of whom probably meet the criteria for binge-eating disorder, have increased psychopathology, particularly depressive symptoms, compared with obese persons who do not engage in binge eating.

It is not certain whether binge-eating disorder will become a permanent diagnostic category in the psychiatric classification system. New approaches to the classification and treatment of obese patients are needed, however, as it becomes increasingly clear that long-term weight loss programs are largely ineffective.

Other Specified Feeding or Eating Disorder/Unspecified Feeding or Eating Disorder

This category is used for patients who have clinically significant symptom constellations that do not meet the threshold for full diagnosis. For example, patients with atypical anorexia nervosa meet all criteria for the diagnosis of anorexia nervosa except that they are not in an abnormally low-weight range. This may occur when patients lose a large amount of weight from an overweight baseline. Patients with bulimia-like or binge-eating disorder–like syndromes include those who do not meet frequency criteria, as well as those who chew and spit out large amounts of food. The regular occurrence of purging in the absence of objective binge eating has come to be known as **purging disorder** and is posited to have distinct biological and clinical features.

Another eating pattern currently classified in this category is **night eating syndrome**. Classically defined by the triad of morning anorexia, evening hyperphagia, and insomnia, it is now seen is as a disorder of circadian sleep and eating rhythms, such that an unusually large proportion of daily eating takes place at night, after the evening meal. Similarly, sleep-related eating disorders are characterized by the consumption of food following awakenings from sleep during the night, often with partial or complete amnesia regarding this eating.

EPIDEMIOLOGY AND COURSE OF ILLNESS

One of the practical reasons for studying epidemiology is to better understand the ways in which an illness is contracted and dispersed. Although this model may be more easily applied to infectious diseases, it is nonetheless applicable to eating disorders, which may be considered, in some ways, "communicable." Many patients with bulimia nervosa report that they first got the idea of binge eating and purging from friends or from television programs designed to discourage eating disorders. Although it is overly simplistic to view such influences as being entirely responsible for the development of these disorders, they may be significant contributing causes. Another significant influence may be the pervasive societal promotion of thinness, which may lead to a preoccupation with dieting, a core feature of anorexia nervosa and bulimia nervosa, and to the development of eating disorders at least in some individuals predisposed to the disorders.

Incidence and Prevalence

Anorexia nervosa has an overall incidence of 4.2–8.1 new cases per 100,000 persons per year (Miller and Golden 2010). The figures increase by an order of magnitude when the population base is restricted to young women. Among young women, the point prevalence is reported at 0.28%, and lifetime prevalence for women is about 1%. Anorexia nervosa occurs in men as well, but at one-tenth the rate of females.

Bulimia nervosa is more common than anorexia nervosa, with an incidence of approximately 11.4–13.5 per 100,000 individuals per year (Miller and Golden 2010). Its point prevalence is estimated at 1% among young women, with lifetime prevalence reported as 1–4.2%. It is likely that these figures underestimate the true incidence and prevalence of bulimia nervosa, as many cases may be unreported. The most recent studies suggest that the prevalence of bulimia nervosa reached its peak in the early 1990s and has begun to decrease since that time (Keski-Rakhonen et al. 2008). As is the case for anorexia nervosa, 90–95% of individuals with bulimia nervosa are **female**.

Although available research is limited, the prevalence in community samples of binge-eating disorder appears to be greater than that for anorexia nervosa and bulimia nervosa, with the most reliable current estimates being 0.7–4%. Binge-eating disorder also differs from anorexia nervosa and bulimia nervosa in its gender ratio of approximately 60% women to 40% men.

Age of Onset

The mean age of onset for anorexia nervosa is 16–17 years, with a **bimodal** distribution that peaks at age 14 and 18 years. Bulimia nervosa also usually has its onset in adolescence or early adulthood. Little reliable information is yet available regarding the age of onset of binge-eating disorders. Although it is relatively uncommon for preteenage children to present with clinical eating disorders, it is not uncommon for them to begin dieting and, perhaps, unwittingly lay the groundwork for future eating disorders. Dieting seems to be a risk factor for these disorders; in the vast majority of cases, onset occurs during or following a period of dieting or non-dieting weight loss. Persons who are under pressure to diet (e.g., ballet dancers, models, and actresses) are at a particularly high risk of developing bulimia nervosa as well as anorexia nervosa. For both disorders, there is a relatively high prevalence of subthreshold or transitory cases in high-risk populations (i.e., women of high school or college age, especially those who are dieting).

The age at which patients first present for treatment is often very different from the age of onset. Patients with anorexia nervosa and bulimia nervosa commonly present between the early teenage years up through early adulthood, and patients with binge-eating disorder may present at any age. There is also some suggestion that prevalence of anorexia nervosa among older women has increased in the past decade. The presentation may be different in the different age-groups. Family issues tend to be more of a concern in younger patients who are living at home, and these patients are more likely to be brought in by family members, sometimes unwillingly. Patients who are older at the time of presentation are more likely to have experienced adverse effects from the disorder and may have a somewhat higher motivation to take part in treatment.

Morbidity and Mortality

Anorexia nervosa is one of the most lethal psychiatric illnesses. Long-term studies have reported alarmingly high mortality rates of 5% per decade of illness. Half of these deaths are due to **suicide**, and half are related to **complications of starvation**. More recent shorter-term studies have suggested that these figures may be somewhat lower in patients who receive adequate treatment. Bulimia nervosa is less frequently lethal, but catastrophic complications of vomiting, such as gastric rupture or esophageal tears, cardiac arrhythmia secondary to severe electrolyte imbalance, and cardiomyopathy resulting from abuse of syrup of ipecac can lead to death (see Table 9.1 for medical and dental complications of anorexia nervosa and bulimia nervosa). In the case of binge-eating disorder, medical morbidity is generally thought to be related to obesity, which may result in part from binge eating. The severely disruptive effects of an eating disorder on personal development (i.e., on the tasks of young adulthood, such as forming intimate relationships, obtaining an education, and setting career goals) should not be underestimated.

There is substantial **comorbidity** of anorexia nervosa and bulimia nervosa. About 50% of patients with anorexia nervosa develop bulimia nervosa within 7 years of onset, and about one-half of patients with bulimia nervosa who are of normal weight report a history of anorexia nervosa. Crossover between diagnoses can occur repeatedly over time (see case example in Box 9.3). In other words, patients with either subtype of anorexia nervosa can go on to develop bulimia nervosa, and then over time can return to a diagnosis of anorexia nervosa. Crossover may also occur between bulimia nervosa and binge-eating disorder.

Patients with anorexia nervosa, bulimia nervosa, and binge-eating disorder are at increased risk for certain other psychiatric disorders. Studies over the past decade have revealed that roughly one-third to one-half of patients with eating disorders suffer from concurrent **major depression,** and about one-half to three-quarters have a lifetime history of depression. Similarly, **obsessive-compulsive disorder** and **social phobia are common comorbid diagnoses**. Patients with bulimia nervosa and with anorexia nervosa binge-eating/purging type have a higher than expected prevalence of **substance use disorders,** especially alcohol and stimulant abuse or dependence. Stimulants are often used in an attempt to lose weight. Some physicians view bulimia nervosa as a form of substance abuse, with the substance being food, and point to common features (see

TABLE 9.1 Associated Physical Symptoms and Signs of Anorexia Nervosa and Bulimia Nervosa

Physical Symptoms

Anorexia Nervosa	Bulimia Nervosa
• Constipation	• Emesis with flecks of blood
• Abdominal discomfort	• Menstrual irregularities
• Cold intolerance	• Large bowel abnormalities (laxative abuse)

Physical Exam

Anorexia Nervosa	Bulimia Nervosa
• Bradycardia	• Teeth enamel erosion
• Hypotension	• Salivary gland enlargement
• Hypothermia	• Russell's sign: ulcerations and calluses on
• Dryness/yellow skin	the dorsum of the hand
• Lanugo (fine body hair)	
• Peripheral edema	

Laboratory Findings

Anorexia Nervosa	Bulimia Nervosa
• Leukopenia	• Hypokalemia
• Elevated blood urea nitrogen (BUN)	• Hyponatremia
• Elevated liver function tests (AST, ALT)	• Hypochloremia
• Hyponatremia	• Hypomagnesemia
• Hypokalemia	• Elevated serum amylase
• Low estradiol	• Metabolic alkalosis
• Low LH and FSH	• Metabolic acidosis (laxative abuse)
• High cortisol	
• High growth hormone	
• Low triiodothyronine, high reverse triiodothryonine	
• Head CT: mild atrophy and increased ventricular–brain ratio	
• ECG: sinus bradycardia, rarely prolonged QT interval	
• Bone scan: osteoporosis	

ALT, alanine transaminase; AST, aspartate aminotransferase; CT, computed tomography; ECG, electrocardiogram; FSH, follicle-stimulating hormone; LH, luteinizing hormone.

Box 9.4). However, the analogy is limited in that abstinence from alcohol or drugs leads to better health, whereas abstinence from food leads to another eating disorder, namely, anorexia nervosa.

Researchers have also been interested in the comorbidity of eating disorders and **personality disorders**. Most studies agree that patients with eating disorders have elevated rates of personality disorders in cluster B (antisocial, borderline, histrionic, narcissistic) and cluster C (avoidant, dependent, obsessive-compulsive). The cluster B disorders, including borderline personality disorder, are especially common in patients who engage in binge eating and purging. The reported rates of personality disorders vary widely, depending on the methods of assessment used. Sexual abuse has been reported in

> **BOX 9.3**
> ## CASE EXAMPLE OF COMORBID ANOREXIA NERVOSA AND BULIMIA NERVOSA
>
> Cora, a 21-year-old single college student, presented for treatment of binge eating and vomiting that had been occurring since she was 16 years old and that, as she put it, "had taken over my life." When asked about the onset of her eating disorder, she stated, "I have never eaten normal meals. . . . I've always been a dieter." She initially got the idea to purge after seeing a television program about eating disorders. Although the program was intended to discourage eating disorders, it seemed at the time to be describing to Cora the ideal method of "eating whatever [she] wanted and not having to pay the consequences." However, once she started to induce vomiting after normal meals, she soon found herself eating large quantities of food and vomiting on a daily basis. During the current semester, she had broken up with her boyfriend and was taking a particularly heavy course load. Her binge eating and vomiting went from once per day to four or five times per day. Much of her day was spent planning her next binge and making sure that she would have the opportunity to vomit without being detected. She was ashamed to relate that, at times, she had taken her roommates' food during a binge and was not always able to replace it. Although she had always taken pride in being a good student, she was beginning to miss her morning classes after she stayed up eating and vomiting. She had initially lost weight when she started vomiting, with a body mass index nadir of 17.4 kg/m². At that time, she lost her menstrual cycling for 5 months. Her weight had now returned to the low-normal range. Despite her apparent thinness, she was distressed by what she perceived as her "fat thighs," so much so that she avoided seeing herself in the mirror and had gone from weighing herself several times per day to completely avoiding the scale. In her words, "I hate myself and I hate what my life has become. I can't find my way out of this trap."

a substantial proportion of patients with bulimia nervosa, but the rate does not appear to exceed that in other psychiatric patients. Personality traits of harm avoidance and perfectionism are high among patients with anorexia nervosa and have been shown to precede the onset of illness (see Box 9.5).

Long-Term Course of Illness

Eating disorders commonly lead to a downward spiral in functioning, and diagnostic migration across eating disorder categories commonly occurs (as illustrated in the case example in Box 9.3).

Anorexia Nervosa

Although the number of published longitudinal follow-up studies of patients with anorexia nervosa is relatively small, certain findings have emerged fairly consistently. The following characteristics predict a **poorer prognosis**: older age of onset, binge-purge

BOX 9.4
BINGE EATING AND THE BIOLOGY OF REWARD

As is underscored by the experience of the patient described in Box 9.2, patients with bulimia nervosa and binge-eating disorder bear a certain resemblance to patients with substance use disorders. Similar features include (1) the initial casual use of a substance, followed by escalating use and progressive loss of control; (2) craving for and preoccupation with the substance; (3) the phenomenon of tolerance, in this case, the need for increasing amounts of food to achieve the same effect; (4) impairment in social or occupational activities (in the case of Brittany, described in Box 9.2, spending less time with her friends at college); (5) continued use despite increasing awareness of harmful effects—for example weakness and exhaustion after binge eating and purging. Individuals who have suffered both from substance use disorders and binge eating often report that the experiences are quite similar. Self-help programs based on the idea of binge eating as an addiction, such as Overeaters Anonymous, a 12-step approach based on Alcoholics Anonymous, and other similar programs are widespread. An obvious difficulty is in defining abstinence, since a complete abstinence from food is not compatible with life. As such, the concept of abstinence is often based on a pattern of eating or a subset of foods that seem to relate most to the individual's experience of addiction.

Underlying this phenomenological similarity may be an underlying similarity in the biology of reward systems and the ways in which this is disrupted by both substance use and binge-eating disorders. Pertinent genetic studies are in a relatively early stage. While it is clear that genes account for a significant proportion of the vulnerability or resistance to various addictions, and it is likely that genes contribute at least somewhat to eating behaviors, such as binge eating, the overlap in genetic risk factors has yet to be established. However, the brain's central reward system, consisting of dopaminergic neuronal projections from the ventral tegmental area of the midbrain to the striatal nucleus accumbens, known as the mesolimbic pathway, is clearly activated during the consumption of palatable foods, giving rise to the "natural high" familiar to all. Inputs to this system mediated by other neurotransmitters, such as serotonin, which increases the sensation of satiety and endogenous opioids that promote the consumption of palatable foods, may account for the interface between the consumption of food and the activation of the reward system. In rats, the feeding of palatable foods on an intermittent schedule, mimicking binge eating, gives rise to a cyclic activation of the dopaminergic reward system and upregulation of endogenous mu-opioid receptors, thereby reinforcing this pattern of eating. This form of intermittent feeding appears to heighten the rewarding effects of multiple substances of abuse, suggesting that at least some of the pathways mediating binge-related and substance-related reward are overlapping.

(continued)

Neuroimaging studies in humans provide further evidence of a link between addictive disorders and binge eating. Using positron emission tomography (PET), investigators demonstrated that the quantity of dopamine receptors in the striatum of obese individuals correlated negatively with body mass index, which is in turn known to be associated with the frequency of binge eating. The interpretation was that very obese individuals, or perhaps those with frequent binge eating, may suffer from a dopaminergic reward deficit, thereby causing them to seek out repeated food-mediated stimulation of the reward system. Other studies have focused on other components of the reward system, such as the amygdala, that may account for the powerful conditioned learning of rewarding behaviors in response to particular cues—in Brittany's case, particular foods or sets of circumstances. Just as cocaine addicts, on a PET scan, show activation of the amygdala in response to thin white lines of powder, the amygdala of a hungry individual will activate in response to food, but will not activate once the hunger has been satiated. An additional brain circuit that has an impact on reward-seeking behavior is the "top-down" corticostriatal system, which involves projections from the orbitofrontal and prefrontal cortex to the striatum. This circuit appears to perform regulatory function, permitting or inhibiting reward-seeking behavior. Another study using PET demonstrated that the orbitofrontal cortex is highly reactive to rewarding foods such as chocolate. A dysfunction of this regulatory system could conceivably account for the impulsivity that individuals like Brittany experience around highly stimulating foods.

While the evidence at this point is limited and indirect, the idea that the brain's reward circuitry that functions to maintain essential appetitive behaviors might somehow be "hijacked" in the service of substance use and perhaps binge-eating disorders remains a compelling one. This will undoubtedly be the focus of further investigation in the years to come.

symptoms, longer duration of illness before presentation for treatment, lower weight, personality disturbance, social and family difficulties, and failure to respond to previous treatments. Patients who are ill for 5–7 years or longer are likely to have a chronic course and are at increased risk of death. It is important to note that it is possible for patients to recover even after many years of illness. Recent research suggests that as many as 75% of patients may experience partial recovery, though the rate of full recovery is much lower, closer to 25%.

Most patients in inpatient refeeding programs attain a weight within the normal range by the time of discharge. At long-term follow-up (4–12 years), about half of these patients continue to maintain a normal weight and are menstruating, while 10–20% are still markedly underweight. About two-thirds of patients continue to be preoccupied with weight and body shape and do not have a regular pattern of eating. As noted earlier, a substantial proportion of patients with anorexia nervosa develop bulimic behaviors at some point in their illnesses. The longest-term follow-up studies suggest that, over the course of time, most patients either recover to a significant degree or die from their illnesses.

BOX 9.5

ANOREXIA NERVOSA AND THE BIOLOGY OF PERFECTIONISM

Many patients with anorexia nervosa, though by no means all, are high achievers, with perfectionist personality traits. The patient described in Box 9.1 maintained good grades and had a very active life in multiple arenas. Her anxieties became more manifest at college, and she found that anxiety was relieved through ritualized behaviors (eating the "right" food; her exercise routine included a specific number). As she lost weight, her rituals became more pronounced. In addition, she became "obsessed" with food, finding herself thinking about her meals all day and unable to think about other things. She found that focusing on the rules around eating relieved her social discomfort. Many patients with anorexia nervosa describe anxiety around meals, avoidance of eating-related situations, and rituals to manage their food-related anxiety. These rituals can include exercise. This clinical picture bears a striking resemblance to obsessive-compulsive disorder and other anxiety disorders.

Patients with anorexia nervosa more commonly have a comorbid anxiety disorder or obsessive-compulsive disorder than would be expected in the general population. Some twin studies have suggested shared genetic influence in the development of these disorders and eating disorders.

The obsessive/perfectionist nature of anorexia nervosa is particularly noticeable when patients are in the underweight state. In addition to impaired concentration and attention, which have been repeatedly demonstrated in underweight patients, more recent cognitive neuroscience findings have suggested that patients with anorexia nervosa may have specific difficulty with "set shifting" or "task switching." In tasks where the rules change during the course of the task, patients are unable to absorb the change—even if they understand it—and they make perseverative errors. Collectively, these neuropsychological findings, seen at low weight in recovered patients, suggest that patients with anorexia nervosa may have impaired cognitive flexibility, and this impairment may be related to the illness.

Neuroimaging findings, though new, are suggestive. One consistent finding among patients with anorexia nervosa has been that in the underweight state, brain volume is diminished. This may return to normal with weight restoration. More recently, functional neuroimaging studies have led to speculation that patients with anorexia nervosa have excessive activity in the amygdala when presented with food images. In addition, some volumetric studies and some PET studies have pointed toward abnormalities in the basal ganglia (caudate, putamen, and thalamus).

These findings suggest that there may be overlap in the neural mechanisms that subserve eating disorders and obsessive-compulsive disorder as well as anxiety disorders. As seen in obsessive-compulsive disorder, there may be abnormalities in the neural circuits connecting the basal ganglia and the prefrontal cortex (frontostriatal circuits). Or, as seen in many anxiety disorders, there may be irregularities in the amygdala or in cortical control of the amygdala. Probing of these circuits through cognitive neuroscience and neuroimaging is a very active area of research in eating disorders.

Bulimia Nervosa

While much of the available evidence on course of illness and prognosis in bulimia nervosa is derived from treatment studies that have followed patients over the short term, a few long-term, naturalistic follow-up studies have been conducted, and meaningful patterns are beginning to emerge. In the most successful outpatient studies, particularly psychotherapy studies, approximately half of patients are in remission following treatment; most of the remaining patients have improved significantly from their baseline status. Full remission is a significant predictor of ongoing success. Patients who fail to fully remit by the end of treatment, even if they have only mild symptoms, are more likely to relapse. A small number of patients lose a significant amount of weight during or following treatment. It is also becoming clear that patients who fail to respond to one treatment approach may respond more favorably to a different approach. Therefore, patients who are persistent and motivated to accept treatment are more likely to do well. Bulimic patients who are treated as inpatients are, for the most part, a more severely ill group. A follow-up study (Fallon et al. 1991) done on the authors' inpatient unit found that of patients contacted 2–9 years following hospitalization, about 40% had recovered, 40% still met the full criteria for bulimia nervosa, and 20% had an intermediate outcome.

The experience that significant proportions of patients fail to fully recover or relapse following full recovery has led to the conceptualization of bulimia nervosa as a chronic vulnerability. Patients often do well with treatment and may recover fully, but they should be prepared to detect early warning signs of clinical slippage and have a plan in place to respond to lapses quickly and effectively.

As more becomes known about the effective treatment of bulimia nervosa and the patient factors that predict success with a particular form of treatment, it makes increasing sense to regard most cases of bulimia nervosa as treatable rather than chronic. A few patients may have a more chronic course and require long-term treatment, however. More chronically ill patients tend to have impaired functioning in maintaining interpersonal relationships and performing occupational activities, in part because of the length of their illness. A small number of patients are able to accommodate the eating disorder and maintain a relatively high level of functioning. Some older patients with bulimia nervosa report that their level of concern with body shape and weight has decreased over the years but that they have become so accustomed to binge eating and purging that it is hard to imagine living any other way.

Binge-Eating Disorder

There is little firm information on the course of binge-eating disorder. Preliminary studies show that these patients, like those with bulimia nervosa, usually begin binge eating in late adolescence or early adulthood, but often do not present for treatment until much later. The course of binge eating appears to be fluctuating, with a great deal of diagnostic migration in and out of the disorder. Interestingly, while binge eating at a given time point is not a very strong predictor of binge eating at a particular later time point, some studies suggest that binge eating is associated with weight gain over time.

THE INTERVIEW

Once an eating disorder is suspected, the physician should obtain a thorough history, including lifetime patterns of weight fluctuation and dieting, menstrual history, personal and family attitudes toward eating and weight, and the onset and progression of binge eating. The patient should be questioned carefully about methods of attempted compensation, including fasting, laxative abuse, purging, vigorous exercise, and the use of syrup of ipecac or over-the-counter, prescription, or illicit drugs to control weight. The physician should determine whether symptoms of depression, anxiety, or alcohol and drug use disorders are present, and whether the patient is engaging in behaviors such as impulsivity, self-mutilation, or the stealing of food. It is often useful for family members to be interviewed, especially if the patient is young. Common presenting complaints of patients with eating disorders are listed in Box 9.6. Each patient should have a thorough medical evaluation (discussed later in this chapter).

During the interview of a patient with an eating disorder, the first priority is for the physician to **establish an alliance** with the patient. The physician must try to understand the patient's view of herself and determine what caused the patient to seek treatment at this time (see Box 9.7). While this determination must always be made in psychiatry, eating disorders can present particular challenges because of the egosyntonic nature of the symptoms. That is, many patients feel that they value their thinness or drive for thinness.

Anorexia Nervosa

Fully developed anorexia nervosa is more easily diagnosed than bulimia nervosa because of the objective measure of low weight. Nonetheless, patients and families sometimes **deny** the presence of the illness for a surprisingly long time. Patients who are thought to be at risk should be asked about the methods they use to lose weight and should be encouraged to discuss their attitudes toward food, body weight, and body shape. Patients whose weight loss has been entirely voluntary are at the highest risk for anorexia nervosa. Patients who initially lose weight because of an illness or some other external factor but then decide to "keep going" and lose more weight have a somewhat lower risk. Patients who deny their

---

BOX 9.6

PRESENTING COMPLAINTS OF PATIENTS WITH EATING DISORDERS

- Obsession with dieting or thinness, or both
- Fatigue, inability to exercise, or other sequelae of malnutrition
- Uncontrolled binge eating or purging, or both
- Depressed mood or other symptoms of depression
- Functional impairment (e.g., inability to concentrate at school or work due to one or more of the above factors)
- Family or marital discord related to eating disorder
- Dental erosion or salivary gland enlargement (particularly seen in patients presenting to dentists)
- Weakness, light-headedness, amenorrhea, bloating, abdominal discomfort, blood in vomitus, or other symptoms resulting from malnutrition, binge eating, or purging (particularly seen in patients presenting to nonpsychiatric physicians)
- Desire to lose weight despite, in many cases, being of normal or low weight (particularly seen in patients presenting to weight loss centers)

> ## BOX 9.7
> ### INTERVIEWING GUIDELINES
>
> - A thorough history should include the following items:
>   - Eating patterns and fluctuations in weight
>   - Important life events and transitions
>   - Attitudes toward the body and overall self-esteem
>   - Depression, substance use disorders, and other psychiatric symptoms
>   - Other medical disorders
>   - Previous treatments and responses
>   - Reason for the patient presenting for treatment at this particular time
>   - Family context of the eating disorder
> - Convey an attitude of understanding and expertise.
> - Avoid statements that evoke shame or guilt.
> - Identification of the following information can be particularly helpful in forming a treatment alliance:
>   - What the patient desires from treatment
>   - How the eating disorder has been interfering with her life
>   - How the eating disorder is preventing her from attaining her goals
> - Inform the patient fully about the structure of, rationale for, and expected outcome of treatment.
> - Provide reassurance that treatment will take place one step at a time and that the patient will be assisted in maintaining control.
> - Recognize the patient's anxiety about sudden drastic changes (e.g., rapidly gaining a large amount of weight).
> - It may be helpful to interview family members or other informants, especially in the case of adolescents and extremely undernourished patients who are cognitively impaired.
> - Emphasize (empathically) the medical sequelae of remaining underweight to strengthen motivation for treatment.

weight loss or are not appropriately concerned about its medical sequelae, such as amenorrhea, should be evaluated carefully for the other symptoms of anorexia nervosa.

Patients with anorexia nervosa are frequently motivated by the physical manifestations of their low weight to ask for professional help. For example, a patient may be so malnourished that she can no longer carry out activities that are important to her, such as exercise or work. Occasionally, a patient will ask for help because she wants to have children and is seeking treatment for amenorrhea. On some level, a patient with anorexia nervosa knows that she needs to gain weight, and the physician must ally himself or herself with this goal. The physician must be aware, however, that the patient is extremely **ambivalent** and tremendously fearful about giving up what has become the central focus of her life. Although the physician needs to understand the patient's resistance to eating and fear of uncontrolled weight gain, he or she must tell the patient that treatment cannot be successful without weight gain and must not collude with the patient in her attempts to defer it. Once the patient feels that she can trust the physician, she will be able to risk gaining weight and may realize that this is not as unmanageable as she may have thought. The patient's malnourished state is likely to affect her ability to think. Extremely cachectic patients tend to have concrete, rigid thought patterns. Initially, therefore, much of the focus is on weight gain, and only later is it possible to shift the focus to other important issues in the patient's life that may underlie the eating disorder.

There are some common themes in the responses that patients suffering from anorexia nervosa have to their physicians. The patient often sees the physician as an authority figure who is acting as a dictator by telling her how much weight she is expected to gain. Depending on the patient's psychological makeup, she usually reacts with covert or open rebellion. The physician may become frustrated by the rigidity of the patient's thinking and her resistance to efforts to help.

Bulimia Nervosa and Binge-Eating Disorder

Patients with bulimia nervosa and binge-eating disorder tend to have surprisingly few medical sequelae of their behavior. These disorders are often more subtle in their presentation than anorexia nervosa because most patients are not underweight. Patients tend to be extraordinarily **ashamed** of their behavior, and even if they have reached the point where they want help, they will often not come forward with their concerns unless the physician conveys a sense of understanding and familiarity with the disorder.

Occasionally, patients with bulimia nervosa will admit to recurrent vomiting but not to the voluntary induction of vomiting and will be subjected to extensive gastrointestinal workups. In order to diagnose bulimia nervosa as quickly as possible in patients who do not complain of binge eating or purging, the physician should bear in mind the risk factors for this illness. Women of high school or college age, particularly those who have had significant weight fluctuations, are known to be dieting strictly, have a rigorous exercise regimen, or suffer from depression or substance abuse, should be considered to be at risk. Unanticipated dental problems or unexplained electrolyte disturbances, particularly hypokalemia, should raise the index of suspicion.

Patients often present for treatment when they have become aware of the destructive effects of binge eating and purging on their lives and their inability to control this behavior. They are often extremely ashamed of their binge-eating and purging episodes and associated behavior (e.g., stealing food) and expect others to be repulsed by it. Not uncommonly, the physician is the first person they have told about the problem. When asked to describe their binge-eating behavior in detail, however, some patients describe episodes that do not fit the usual classification of binge eating. A patient may say that she had eaten a large amount of food, particularly if she thinks of the food as fattening or forbidden, and felt that purging was necessary, even though she had eaten only a small amount, such as three cookies or a candy bar. The physician must ask for **specific details** about the amount and type of food consumed. Patients often find this difficult to discuss because they are afraid that the physician will be shocked by the details of their eating. Therefore, it is important for the physician to assume an empathic but matter-of-fact attitude when questioning patients and to let them know that he or she is familiar with and not disgusted by the amount of food that may be consumed during a binge-eating episode, is experienced in working with the disorder, and wants to find out more about the particular difficulties.

Like patients with anorexia nervosa, patients with bulimia nervosa are usually terrified of gaining weight. A surprisingly large number of patients state, at least initially, that even though they are truly distressed about their bulimic behaviors, they would not be willing to accept a 10-pound weight gain in exchange for remission of the disorder. The physician must create a bond of trust with patients so that they are willing to change their eating habits and take the risk of gaining weight (although most patients do not gain a significant amount of weight as they recover from bulimia nervosa).

Patients with eating disorders often provoke intense reactions in the physician. Patients with anorexia nervosa and bulimia nervosa are often young adults who are functioning at a reasonably high level in other areas of their lives. Younger physicians tend to identify strongly with them. Bulimic patients of normal weight may have an appearance and style of interaction that is quite appropriate, which may cause the physician to **underrate** the severity of the illness. This may be a serious problem if the physician discharges a patient from an inpatient unit on the assumption that the patient will continue to do well but has not given the patient enough education on how to prevent relapse and how important it is to do so. Physicians sometimes view the illness as self-inflicted and may become angry and **frustrated** when patients refuse to give up their self-destructive behavior. (Patients are likely to provoke these feelings in their family and friends as well.) In the case of binge-eating disorder, particularly when it is accompanied by obesity, physicians may similarly be inclined to view the illness as a deficit in character or lack of will power. When the physician becomes aware of these feelings, he or she should remember that patients' perceptions of their bodies are seriously impaired, that their behavior is deeply entrenched, and that this behavior makes a certain amount of sense when seen from their point of view.

DIFFERENTIAL DIAGNOSIS

Anorexia Nervosa

The differential diagnosis for anorexia nervosa includes medical causes of wasting, such as occult **malignant tumors** or, rarely, lateral hypothalamic tumors or trauma. Psychiatric syndromes, such as major depression, may also be associated with weight loss. Patients with these diagnoses may feel unable to eat enough to maintain their weight but rarely display the psychological features of anorexia nervosa. The differential diagnosis between anorexia nervosa and **depression** can at times be difficult because patients with anorexia nervosa not uncommonly suffer from major depression. Patients who are depressed may say that they realize they are thin and need to gain weight, but if they are also suffering from anorexia nervosa, their unexpressed fears of becoming fat usually become evident as they begin to gain weight, and they will exhibit a resistance to gaining more weight. Patients with anorexia nervosa may have a body image disturbance so severe that it seems psychotic (i.e., a patient may claim that she is fat when she is actually extremely emaciated). However, a psychotic disorder should not be considered in these patients unless the distorted thinking extends into other areas of their lives. For example, one underweight patient with a fear of gaining weight believed that God would not be able to lift her into heaven if she weighed more than 88 pounds. Because her body image disturbance existed in the context of a larger delusion, she was diagnosed as having a psychotic disorder rather than an eating disorder.

Bulimia Nervosa and Binge-Eating Disorder

The differential diagnosis of binge eating in bulimia nervosa or binge-eating disorder includes rare medical causes, such as genetic disorders (e.g., Prader-Willi syndrome) and ventromedial hypothalamic tumors, or trauma. Atypical depression can present with overeating and weight gain. In all of these cases, patients usually do not meet the criteria for bulimia nervosa, either because their overeating does not take the form of discrete eating binges or because they do not attempt to compensate for binge eating by purging, fasting, or vigorous exercising. Similarly, such patients often fail to meet criteria for binge-eating disorder because they may not exhibit the requisite level of distress regarding binge eating.

MEDICAL EVALUATION

Patients should have a complete physical examination, including height, weight, and vital signs. Laboratory tests should include serum **electrolytes**, **magnesium**, and **phosphate**; **blood urea nitrogen**, **creatinine**, and **liver enzymes**; and a **complete blood count** (see Table 9.1). Given the coexistence of eating disorders and substance abuse, urine toxicological screening is often useful. An **ECG** should be part of the baseline workup for patients who are seriously underweight, have significant electrolyte disturbances, or have a history of ipecac abuse. Other laboratory tests may be suggested by the history or physical examination (e.g., a chest x-ray is indicated in patients with evidence of pulmonary congestion or pleural effusion on physical examination). Patients who purge regularly should be referred for **dental examination**. **Bone density scans** to evaluate for osteoporosis are recommended for patients who have been amenorrheic for 6 months. Patients who are obese should be evaluated for known medical comorbidities of obesity, including hypertension, diabetes mellitus, and hyperlipidemia.

ETIOLOGY

The factors that predispose an individual to developing an eating disorder, trigger the onset of the illness, and sustain the disorder once it is established are as yet incompletely understood. Biological factors may predispose certain individuals, but they are not sufficient to explain these disorders completely. As with many psychiatric syndromes, interaction among biological, psychological, and cultural factors clearly contributes to the onset and continuance of eating disorders. In addition, any coherent theory of causation must attempt to explain why the eating disorders are much more common in women than in men.

In considering the factors that lead a given individual to develop an eating disorder, it is useful to distinguish among predisposing factors, precipitating factors, and amplifying and maintaining factors (see Figure 9.1). It is also useful to consider, at each stage, the factors or interventions that propel the individual in the opposite direction, that is, toward health.

Predisposing factors are relatively static factors that may include, for example, female gender, genetic endowment, or cultural environment. Such factors contribute to risk but by no means ensure that an affected individual will develop an eating disorder. Primary prevention programs (e.g., public awareness programs promoting body acceptance) strive to mitigate the effects of a culture that promotes unrealistic body ideals; they are aimed at reducing the overall population risk and mitigating the effects of predisposing factors.

Precipitating factors are events that propel a vulnerable individual further along the road to an eating disorder. For example, the onset of adolescence may be associated with both body changes and environmental changes (e.g., the social environment of junior high and high school) that could lead to the onset of unhealthy dietary practices. Secondary prevention programs target at-risk individuals, for example, high school

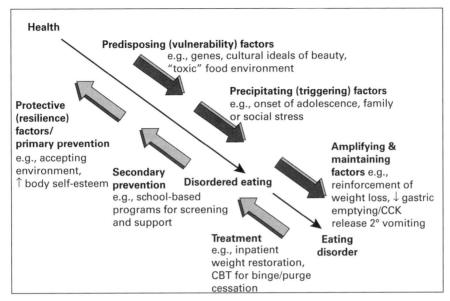

Health

Predisposing (vulnerability) factors
e.g., genes, cultural ideals of beauty, "toxic" food environment

Precipitating (triggering) factors
e.g., onset of adolescence, family or social stress

Protective (resilience) factors/ primary prevention
e.g., accepting environment, ↑ body self-esteem

Secondary prevention
e.g., school-based programs for screening and support

Disordered eating

Amplifying & maintaining factors e.g., reinforcement of weight loss, ↓ gastric emptying/CCK release 2° vomiting

Treatment
e.g., inpatient weight restoration, CBT for binge/purge cessation

Eating disorder

FIGURE 9.1 Etiological factors in the development of eating disorders: bidirectional movement between health and illness.

girls, and provide both screening for early detection and support for those vulnerable to becoming ill.

Amplifying or maintaining factors provide positive feedback whereby disordered eating creates changes that reinforce disturbed eating and compensatory behavior patterns and lead to further spiraling down into full-syndrome eating disorders. For example, weight loss in the early stages of anorexia nervosa may elicit praise that motivates the individual to increase her commitment to dieting and weight loss. As detailed later in the chapter, binge eating and/or vomiting may lead to gastrointestinal changes that interfere with the development of normal satiety following a meal and that promote further binge eating. Once an individual has reached this stage, some form of acute treatment is usually required to reach a level of wellness at which less intensive preventive or maintenance strategies can help her to continue moving toward robust physiological and psychological health.

The etiology of the eating disorders can be considered from two different perspectives. One perspective focuses on the disturbed biological states found in patients with these disorders and the degree to which these states give rise to the characteristic abnormal behaviors. From another perspective, these disorders can be seen as attempts by individuals to solve problems in their lives by developing, either consciously or unconsciously, disturbed behaviors that ultimately have physiological consequences.

Biological Theories

Patients with anorexia nervosa are suffering from, among other things, starvation, and they have most of the expected biological (and psychological) sequelae. Patients with bulimia nervosa, although usually of normal weight, also have some of the physiological signs of starvation, probably because of the pattern of dieting and undereating on which their intermittent binges are superimposed. It is important to distinguish between biological factors that *give rise to* eating disorders and biological abnormalities that *result from* the illness. The latter do not contribute to the onset of the eating disorder, but in some case they may contribute to its continuance (see Boxes 9-6 and 9-7).

Genetic Factors

Family and twin studies suggest that there is a genetic diathesis for both anorexia nervosa and bulimia nervosa. In anorexia nervosa, there is a 50% concordance in monozygotic twins and 7% in dizygotic twins; in bulimia nervosa, there is a 23% concordance in monozygotic twins and 9% in dizygotic twins. For both disorders, first-degree relatives of probands are at increased risk for eating disorders, affective disorders, and substance abuse. Patients with anorexia nervosa binge-eating/purging are more likely to have relatives with bulimia nervosa and substance abuse disorders. Although these studies suggest that certain individuals may be genetically **predisposed** to eating disorders, the mechanism is not yet understood. A genetic predisposition does not mean that a person is predestined to develop an eating disorder, but rather that a person is at increased risk if the right cultural and psychological milieu is present. Given what is known about the different rates of the eating disorders in different cultures and historical periods, it is unlikely that a person is destined from birth to suffer from these disorders. It is more likely that a predisposition is inherited, which may or may not be expressed in the course of a person's lifetime. A person with a predisposition to obesity who is living in a culture that overvalues thinness might restrict her eating, which would put her at increased risk of developing a full-blown eating disorder. A person with a genetic predisposition to dysphoria and low self-esteem might react to cultural influences by manipulating her body shape and weight in an attempt to feel better about herself. The biological changes resulting from an eating disorder might also in some way counter the dysphoria. Further sophisticated genetic epidemiological studies will be needed in order to discriminate between competing hypotheses concerning the nature of genetic risk.

Research is now focused less on the magnitude of the genetic contribution to risk and more on the nature and mechanisms of genetic risk. Candidate genes have been identified that may confer risk to the development of an eating disorder. Some studies have focused on genes related to the serotonin system, for example, the serotonin 1D receptor and the serotonin transporter (5-HTTLPR), as serotonin is known to be dysregulated in eating disorders. Attention has also focused on genes known to be involved in regulation of body weight, such as the *BDNF* gene.

Neurotransmitters and Neuropeptides

Neurotransmitters such as norepinephrine and serotonin regulate the appetite, feelings of satiety, and emotional moods. It is tempting to speculate on the influence of abnormal levels or imbalances of neurotransmitters on the behavior of patients with eating disorders. Abnormal levels of neurotransmitters and their metabolites have been found in the central nervous system and the peripheral circulation in patients with eating disorders and in some patients who have recovered from these disorders. Longitudinal data that would definitively distinguish preexisting abnormalities (that might have triggered the disorder) from abnormalities resulting from behavior related to the disorder (and that may also play a role in maintaining the disorder) are as yet lacking. Some interesting patterns have emerged, however.

Serotonergic systems, which are involved in regulating feelings of satiety (and are also implicated in the production of depressive and obsessive symptoms), appear to be underactive in patients with eating disorders. This abnormality may reverse in patients who have recovered from eating disorders, and serotonergic activity may actually be increased in long-term recovered patients. Abnormalities in the serotonin system may reflect a biological vulnerability to the development of eating disorders, and changes in serotonergic function that accompany the progression of illness may function as amplifying or maintaining factors. In addition, altered striatal **dopamine** function may contribute to altered reward and affect regulation, stereotypic motor behavior, and abnormal eating in eating disorders.

Neuropeptides involved in appetite regulation have been implicated in eating disorders as well. Peptide YY, an appetite stimulant, may be related to the maintenance of binge eating. Leptin levels have been shown to be low in patients with bulimia nervosa and are thought to contribute to binge eating and reduced metabolic rate. Low leptin levels in patients with anorexia nervosa may contribute to some of the behavioral symptoms seen at low weight, such as increased exercise.

Neuroendocrine Factors

The neuroendocrine system (i.e., the hypothalamus, pituitary gland, and endocrine glands) has been regarded for many years as a "window" through which the functioning of the brain can be observed. The many neuroendocrine abnormalities that have been described in anorexia nervosa were at one time thought to be potential causes of the illness. It is now clear that, for the most part, they are **consequences of starvation** rather than preexisting trait markers. The existence of some of these abnormalities in women with bulimia nervosa who are of normal weight or in normal-weight or overweight individuals with binge-eating disorder suggests that intermittent dieting and binge eating can have biological consequences similar to those of semistarvation.

In some cases, the neuroendocrine abnormalities may reinforce the illness, setting up a positive-feedback cycle that is difficult to interrupt. **Corticotropin-releasing hormone** is elevated in patients with anorexia nervosa, probably as a result of malnutrition. When this hormone is injected into the cerebral ventricles of laboratory animals, it may produce an anorexia nervosa–like syndrome characterized by decreased feeding, diminished sexual activity, and increased physical activity. Thus, elevated levels of this hormone result from and may contribute to the behavior of patients with anorexia nervosa. Treatments based on normalizing hypothalamic–pituitary–adrenal function are theoretically possible, but have not yet been investigated.

Another example of bidirectional feedback between illness-related behavior and neuroendocrine abnormalities involves the hypothalamic–pituitary–gonadal axis. In patients with anorexia nervosa, the abnormal secretion of **luteinizing hormone** is the underlying cause of amenorrhea. This abnormality in luteinizing hormone secretion is related to low levels of leptin, in turn reflecting the reduction in fat mass that occurs in starvation. As weight is lost, the pattern of luteinizing hormone secretion regresses to a prepubertal state. Recovery from starvation is associated with the recurrence of mature patterns of secretion of luteinizing hormone and the resumption of menstruation. This physiological regression, which also occurs in patients who are undernourished for other reasons, is often reinforcing in patients with anorexia nervosa who have a fear of sexual maturity.

Gastrointestinal Factors

Studies of eating behavior suggest that patients with bulimia nervosa have a deficit in the satiety response to eating (i.e., after eating a normal amount of food, they do not feel "full" or wish to stop eating). Although this may reflect abnormalities in the way the brain processes signals of hunger and satiety, it may also reflect abnormalities in the signals themselves. Preliminary evidence suggests that gastrointestinal abnormalities mediate this deficit. Following a test meal, patients with bulimia nervosa secrete subnormal amounts of the hormone **cholecystokinin,** which, among other functions, acts as a mediator of satiety. This abnormality in peripheral satiety signals is thought to result from repeated binge eating and purging and to reflect, at least in part, abnormal gastric motility. Once the blunted release of cholecystokinin has become established, it leads to further blunting of the satiety response after meals. In this way, a positive-feedback cycle develops in which the illness causes a biological abnormality that becomes a factor in sustaining the binge eating. Further research is needed to clarify the role of this and other gastrointestinal mechanisms in the pathophysiology of eating disorders. Patients with anorexia nervosa also display abnormalities in gastric motility and appetitive sensations, but their reports of hunger and fullness are difficult to disentangle from affects and cognitions related to the feared consequences of eating.

Psychosocial Theories

Cognitive Model
According to the cognitive model, patients with bulimia nervosa and binge-eating disorder are driven to binge and purge by strict dietary rules that periodically break down. This dieting is in turn driven by an excessive concern with body shape and weight that has its basis in **poor self-esteem**. The system is **self-reinforcing** at many levels. Binge eating and purging further damage self-esteem, which increases the concern with body weight and shape, leading to further dieting, binge eating, and purging. The cognitive model of anorexia nervosa is similar, except that uncontrolled starvation rather than binge eating and purging is the behavioral component of the vicious circle.

Behavioral Model
The behavioral model views binge eating and vomiting as being **positively reinforced** by the sensations associated with the consumption of highly palatable "forbidden foods" and, for some patients, by the **reduction of anxiety** they experience after vomiting. In patients with anorexia nervosa, reinforcement may be derived from the physiological responses to starvation and, in the early stages of the illness, from praise received for their thinness. For patients with binge-eating disorder, the alternating behaviors of binge eating and strict dietary control may occur for days or weeks at a time, that is binge days or weeks versus dieting days or weeks.

Interpersonal Perspective
Viewed from an interpersonal perspective, eating disorders are maintained by disturbances in relationships (e.g., difficulty in negotiating major role transitions, such as leaving the family and taking on an adult role). Other disturbances include interpersonal disputes, unresolved grief reactions, and pervasive interpersonal deficits.

Cultural Factors

Only a modern-day Rip van Winkle could fail to notice and be affected by the cultural preoccupation with body image in the United States (see Box 9.8). Young women at risk for developing eating disorders are assailed daily by images of perfect bodies, with the implication that it is this and only this which guarantees happiness and fulfillment.

BOX 9.8
HISTORICAL PERSPECTIVE ON EATING DISORDERS

Descriptions of syndromes that resemble anorexia nervosa date back to medieval times, when the psychological context of the illness had more to do with spiritual beliefs than with the aesthetic aspects of emaciation. Narratives of self-starvation can be found in accounts and writings of several saints. The "fasting girls" of the 19th century attracted the attention of both religious admirers and skeptical physicians. One of the earliest medical descriptions of an anorexia-like syndrome is that of Mr. Duke's daughter, written by Richard Morton in 1689:

In the month of July, she fell into a total suppression of her monthly Courses from a multitude of Cares and Passions of her Mind, but without any symptoms of the Green-Sickness following upon it. From which time her Appetite began to abate, and her Digestion to be bad; her flesh also began to be flaccid and loose, and her looks pale . . . she was wont by her studying at Night and continual poring upon Books to expose herself both Day and Night to the Injuries of the Air. . . . I do not remember that I did ever in all my practice see one that was conversant with the Living so much wasted with the greatest degree of Consumption (like a Skeleton only clad with Skin).

The term *anorexia nervosa* was coined in the 19th century by Sir William Gull. Anorexia, meaning "lack of appetite," is now thought to be a misnomer, because patients with anorexia nervosa are often quite preoccupied with food but deny, to a greater or lesser extent, the experience of hunger and refuse to act upon it.

In contrast to anorexia nervosa, which has been discussed in the medical literature for more than a century, bulimia nervosa did not appear in the literature until quite recently. Although the practice of occasional excessive eating followed by purging has precedents extending as far back as ancient Rome, the first recognition of bulimia nervosa as a psychiatric syndrome occurred in the 1970s, in the United States, Japan, and Great Britain, where the term *bulimia nervosa* was coined. It is not clear whether the syndrome has truly originated in our current cultural climate or whether it has existed as an unrecognized entity for decades or even centuries. Certainly, there has been a rapid escalation in research and popular interest in eating disorders. During the past decade, they have been the subject of television movies, feature films, medical journals, and many books.

The most recent chapter in the history of eating disorders has been the recognition of binge-eating disorder. First described in the 1950s, binge eating in the absence of compensatory behavior received little systematic study until the last decades of the 20th century and is first included in the classification of eating disorders in DSM-5.

For women, the ideal image has changed in recent decades. This shift has been documented by studies of women who have posed for the centerfold in *Playboy* magazine or won the Miss America title. On average, these women have become substantially thinner over the past 30 years, while the percentage of American women who are overweight has increased. Therefore, the gap between actual weight and the culturally ideal weight has progressively widened. The perception that one is 20 pounds overweight compared with the culturally sanctioned body type is more likely to lead to drastic attempts at weight control, such as vomiting or laxative abuse, than is the perception that one is 5 pounds overweight. As these cultural factors have promoted greater degrees of food restriction, the risk of eating disorders may have increased.

An important epidemiological feature of the eating disorders is that they appear to be bound to certain cultures, occurring primarily in the developed countries of North America and Europe, as well as Australia, New Zealand, South Africa, and Japan. The risk of illness may be related to the degree of assimilation of a person into the dominant culture within a country. Although eating disorders are commonly thought of as illnesses of middle- and upper-class white women, studies have increasingly documented their occurrence among minority women and women from various social classes.

Interestingly, anorectic-like syndromes in different cultures may present somewhat differently. In Hong Kong, patients usually do not display a fear of obesity and distorted body image but rather tend to attribute undereating to a somatic disturbance, such as abdominal bloating. It is debatable whether this syndrome, which occurs in young women and has physiological features similar to those of anorexia nervosa but a different psychological context, should be excluded from the diagnosis of anorexia nervosa or whether the criteria for anorexia nervosa should be broadened to accommodate it.

Anorexia Nervosa

The classic patient with anorexia nervosa (particularly the restricting subtype) is described by Hilde Bruch in *The Golden Cage* (1978) as a "sparrow in a cage." She is an adolescent growing up in a privileged family that responds to her material needs but not her emotional needs. Her parents place excessive demands on her to conform to their expectations, and, as a result, she feels that none of her achievements are good enough. She seizes upon food restriction and excessive exercise as ways to feel successful and alter an intolerable family situation.

Individual psychodynamic factors related to anorexia nervosa can vary greatly. **Family characteristics** that have been observed include enmeshment and overintrusiveness of family members, overprotectiveness of parents toward children, rigid adherence to roles within the family, and avoidance of overt conflict. The eating disorder can serve in some way to keep family conflict at bay. The self-induced starvation can represent, among other things, **compliance** and **rebellion**, since the patient is engaging in the "healthy" behaviors of dieting and exercising but to a degree that brings her into conflict with the family. In addition, the patient may have an unconscious conflict between dependence and separation or individuation. By refusing food, which would nurture her physical body, the patient undercuts her ability to become an independent adult woman. Starvation also causes the cessation of menstruation and retards the development of secondary sexual characteristics, which may serve to alleviate anxiety in an adolescent who finds the prospect of womanhood threatening. This formulation is simplistic, but it applies, to a greater or lesser degree, to many patients with anorexia nervosa.

Bulimia Nervosa and Binge-Eating Disorder

The psychological factors involved in binge eating vary greatly from individual to individual. Binge eating is often experienced as a temporary escape from rigid control both in the realm of eating and in other areas of life. For patients with bulimia nervosa, purging becomes the means of undoing this lapse and regaining a sense of control. Many patients use binge eating and/or vomiting to **divert feelings** that they are unable to express because they are unacceptable to themselves or to others. Episodes of binge eating and/or purging are often triggered by situations in which the patient's self-esteem, which is often closely tied to body image, has been threatened (e.g., if a perceived slight from a boyfriend causes the patient to think she is fat and unattractive and to feel angry, despondent, and empty). Paradoxically, although patients who use compensatory behaviors often feel at first that they have found the ideal way of controlling their intake, they eventually feel that they have lost control and have little idea of how much they are eating and how much they are keeping down. As the patient becomes more involved in the eating disorder, she tends to become increasingly isolated, often refusing social opportunities because she feels fat and instead staying home to engage in binge eating and purging. From a psychodynamic perspective, a patient's conflicted need for and fear of greater independence may give rise to binge eating and purging episodes that simultaneously express her needs to assert herself and to maintain her dependent position.

For patients with chronic forms of eating disorders, the illness may be a way of avoiding difficult interpersonal or career issues. Patients recovering from severe eating disorders face the challenge of rebuilding a life in which important decisions and pursuits have been deferred, sometimes for several years.

TREATMENT

Anorexia Nervosa

The fundamental principle of treatment for anorexia nervosa is that it cannot proceed in a meaningful way in the absence of **weight gain**. The first order of business is to evaluate the patient's nutritional status and medical stability. Patients with severe electrolyte disturbances, abnormal findings on ECG, or other abnormalities may require medical hospitalization. When patients are medically stable, they may be treated on a psychiatric inpatient unit or in outpatient treatment. Some patients, especially those with solid support systems, do well with outpatient treatment, but many others, especially those who are extremely underweight, require **inpatient** treatment.

Behavior Treatment

Treatment for anorexia nervosa is usually multimodal. Inpatient treatment is most often based on **behavior modification**, with contingencies constructed to promote weight gain. A minimum acceptable weight is set by the physician (usually 85–90% of the ideal body weight). The physician prescribes a diet (consisting of variable amounts of food and a calorically dense liquid nutritional supplement) that will enable the patient to gain weight at the desired rate. The patient's weight is monitored on a regular basis (e.g., at least once per week) so that the physician and patient can detect any upward or downward trends and decide how to manage them. As the patient's weight increases, she is given more privileges and has more freedom to leave the hospital.

The **caloric requirements** increase as the patient gains weight. It is not unusual for a patient to require as many as 4,000 calories per day during the later phases of refeeding in order to continue to gain weight. This requirement decreases when the patient has achieved her target weight and needs only to maintain it. Most patients are able to achieve their minimum weight during hospitalization, but it is often difficult for them to maintain this weight and expand their food choices. After achieving normal weight, caloric requirements to maintain this weight can remain high (as compared to their peers) for some time. Patients in inpatient behavior weight control programs are especially likely to engage in **power struggles** with the treatment team over exactly how much weight must be gained, how much food must be consumed, and how many concessions will be made to accommodate patients' idiosyncratic needs and preferences. Patients often wish to ingest all of their calories in only one or two "safe foods" and will struggle mightily if a meal deviates even slightly from their set plan.

Patients who are superficially compliant should be encouraged to discuss their **ambivalence** about gaining weight. Some resolve to gain weight only so they can leave the hospital and lose it again. The physician must walk a tightrope with these patients while gently but firmly setting limits on the one hand, and, on the other hand, letting patients know that the treatment is ultimately in their control and cannot take place without their cooperation. Some patients may decide to end the treatment but will later reenter treatment when their motivation is stronger. Though longer duration of illness is generally a predictor of poor prognosis, physicians are limited in predicting the course of treatment for any individual patient. It is also common for a patient to require multiple hospitalizations to achieve health. Overall, patients should always be encouraged that they have a good chance of improvement with commitment to treatment.

Occasionally, a patient will have deteriorated so much that she must be fed **against her will**. This situation is difficult to manage on a psychotherapeutic level. Unless the patient comes to realize that she needs ongoing treatment, the gains made may be only temporary. However, some patients, even those who have had repeated and/or involuntary hospitalizations, eventually find the motivation to achieve and maintain recovery.

While this behavioral protocol is being followed, patients are involved in individual and group psychotherapy and family therapy, when appropriate. They also receive nutritional, vocational, and leisure counseling.

Patients who are treated on an **outpatient** basis cannot be supervised to the same degree as those in an inpatient setting. The physician often sets a minimum weight that patients must maintain and tells them that if they cannot maintain this weight, they will be hospitalized.

Psychotherapy

There is relatively little systematic information concerning the efficacy of different forms of psychotherapy in treating patients with anorexia nervosa. Psychodynamic, interpersonal, and, especially, cognitive-behavioral psychotherapies are often used (see Bulimia Nervosa, later in this chapter). There are compelling data to support the Maudsley method, or family-based treatment, a form of family therapy for younger patients who are living at home in which their parents take a very involved role in refeeding.

Pharmacotherapy

Drug treatment with antipsychotics, cyproheptadine (an antihistaminic and antiserotonergic drug that is used to treat allergies and tends to promote weight gain), or antidepressants has not significantly improved the outcome of anorexia nervosa. Recent trials examining the utility of the second-generation antipsychotics, particularly olanzapine, during the acute phase of treatment have yielded preliminary evidence of efficacy for some patients, but their use still lacks definitive empirical support. Overall, medications have been disappointing in the weight gain phase of treatment. The evidence concerning the utility of fluoxetine in the prevention of relapse following weight gain is mixed. Despite initial reports that fluoxetine may have been beneficial in patients who had been successfully restored to normal weight, more definitive study suggested that this was not the case, at least for patients receiving fluoxetine in combination with cognitive-behavioral therapy. Fluoxetine did not prevent relapse and did not appear to confer any benefit in associated mood symptoms when compared with placebo. Patients with symptoms of depression or anxiety that do not resolve with refeeding and weight gain may benefit from appropriate psychopharmacological interventions (see Chapter 3, Mood Disorders; and Chapter 6, Anxiety, Obsessive-Compulsive, and Stress Disorders).

Bulimia Nervosa

Treatments that appear to have little in common with one another, such as antidepressant medication, cognitive-behavioral therapy, and interpersonal therapy, are all effective in bulimia nervosa. This fact underscores the difficulty of making inferences about the etiology or pathophysiology of the disorder on the basis of treatment response. Carefully designed treatment studies may shed some light on the processes by which the illness arises and is maintained and may ultimately allow physicians to make better-informed decisions when they recommend particular forms of treatment.

Patients with bulimia nervosa are most often treated on an **outpatient** basis. Indications for inpatient treatment include medical instability (usually, extreme electrolyte imbalance), severe bulimic symptoms (i.e., binge eating and vomiting a number of times per day), significant coexisting disorders, or insufficient response to adequate trials of outpatient treatment. Hospital treatment is usually multimodal and similar to that for anorexia nervosa. Antidepressant medications and structured psychotherapy have been effective for this disorder. As with patients with anorexia nervosa, the physician should monitor the patient's weight on a regular basis (e.g., once per week) so that any upward or downward trends can be managed.

Psychotherapy

Although psychotherapy for bulimia nervosa usually takes place in an outpatient setting, in which the therapist has less control over what and how the patient eats, power struggles sometimes ensue. It is useful to create a collaboration with the patient in which both parties agree that the patient will make certain provisional changes in her eating (e.g., trying particular new foods in the coming week) and that the patient and therapist together will monitor the results and decide on further changes. The patient may consciously or unconsciously use binge eating and purging as a way to gain the physician's approval (i.e., may decrease or stop bulimic behaviors), ensure the physician's ongoing presence and concern, or divert the physician's attention from other anxiety-provoking issues. Decisions about whether, when, and how to address such patterns must be made on an individual basis. For example, one patient who had stopped binge eating and vomiting early in treatment enthusiastically praised the physician's skill in "curing" her. On closer examination, the physician realized that the patient was eating only salads and fruit. It was imperative for the physician to support the patient's efforts but also to reinforce the importance of developing a more normal eating pattern and dealing with the anxiety and discomfort involved in doing so.

The physician must acknowledge the patient's subjective experience and gradually begin to challenge it. The physician should then help the patient to modify her coping strategies, be more flexible in evaluating her body, and develop a more complete, better integrated view of herself. For example, the patient who was obsessed with her "fat thighs" (see Box 9.3) made little progress in altering this perception but was more successful in identifying and challenging the assumptions that stemmed from the perception (e.g., the idea that others were looking at her thighs disapprovingly and the thought that her overall appearance was ruined by this one feature).

Cognitive-behavioral therapy emphasizes patients' **self-monitoring** of eating and of thoughts, feelings, and circumstances surrounding eating binges in an attempt to identify patterns and triggering factors of binge eating and vomiting. In sessions with the physician and at home, the patient begins to identify dysfunctional thought patterns, such as all-or-nothing thinking ("I've blown my diet by eating this cookie, so I might as well go ahead and binge") or jumping to conclusions ("My boyfriend isn't paying attention to me because he thinks I'm too fat"). The next step is to develop rational responses to these thoughts. In situations likely to trigger binge eating, the patient systematically identifies dysfunctional thoughts and responds to them in ways other than binge eating and purging. The patient who feels that eating an extra cookie has "blown" her diet is encouraged to challenge this thought, marshal the arguments for and against it, and come up with a more reasonable, balanced response to the situation. Behavioral techniques such as systematically delaying binge eating and vomiting or using behavioral alternatives to binge eating and purging are also introduced and practiced. Alternative behaviors may be calling a friend, going for a walk, or reading a magazine. They must be appropriate to the specific situation, rewarding, and easy to execute. Finally, the patient is encouraged to develop her own ongoing treatment plan, including strategies for preventing relapse.

Controlled studies of this therapy in individual and group formats have revealed rates of improvement that are somewhat higher than those reported for drug treatment. Studies comparing psychotherapy with antidepressant treatment for bulimia nervosa have found psychotherapy to be more effective. Antidepressant treatment is clearly helpful for some patients, however, either alone or in combination with psychotherapy.

Other forms of psychotherapy have also been useful in the treatment of outpatients with bulimia nervosa. **Interpersonal therapy** focuses on the interpersonal disturbances that may underlie and reinforce bulimic behaviors. **Exposure with response prevention** is a behavioral technique also used in obsessive-compulsive disorder. During the therapy session, the patient consumes the foods that she would normally eat when binge eating and discusses the ensuing feelings of anxiety with the physician. **Psychodynamic psychotherapy** has not been well studied but may be particularly useful for patients presenting with coexisting personality disorders. **Dialectical behavioral therapy**, originally developed as a treatment to help patients with borderline personality disorder to more successfully control their impulses, regulate their emotions, and manage their relationships, has been adapted for patients with bulimia nervosa and binge-eating disorder.

Pharmacotherapy

Cyclic antidepressants, selective serotonin reuptake inhibitors (SSRIs), monoamine oxidase inhibitors (MAOIs), and atypical antidepressants have been effective in more than a dozen randomized controlled clinical trials. Only a few patients attain full remission when treated with drugs alone, however. There is little information concerning the long-term efficacy of these drugs, but they may be useful for many patients. Information about the interaction of drugs and psychotherapy and about factors that predict a successful response to a particular intervention is needed.

The usefulness of antidepressant drugs is not limited to patients with bulimia nervosa who are depressed. Trials of these drugs were originally stimulated by theories about the relationship between eating disorders and affective disorders. It is now known that the neurotransmitter systems targeted by these drugs also mediate feelings of hunger and satiety. Therefore, the mechanism of action of the drugs in bulimia nervosa may be largely **independent of their antidepressant effects**. In spite of the similarities between bulimia nervosa and anorexia nervosa, antidepressant medications are effective for the former but not the latter, suggesting that starvation may in some way interfere with their actions.

Binge-Eating Disorder

Preliminary studies of patients with symptoms similar to those of binge-eating disorder suggest that both antidepressant medication and cognitive-behavioral psychotherapy may be beneficial. For obese patients who suffer from binge eating, standard behavioral treatment for eating and weight control is usually effective both in controlling binge eating and promoting weight loss, at least in the short term. However, for patients who continue to binge eat, alternative treatment for binge eating may be a useful prerequisite to weight loss treatment.

Another approach to the treatment of binge eating and overeating is the **12-step method,** which is widely practiced but little studied. This approach is based on the method used at Alcoholics Anonymous and grounded in the **addiction model** of eating disorders (i.e., the patient is viewed as a food addict whose experience and behavior parallel that of alcohol- or drug-addicted individuals). One limitation of this approach is that abstinence from food is neither possible nor desirable, and many physicians believe that patients' attempts to severely restrict eating actually contribute to the maintenance of the illness. However, the concept of abstinence may be broadened to include avoidance of particular types of eating (e.g., eating in response to stress, eating large amounts of a particular food) or even avoidance of particular thinking patterns that have been recognized as deleterious. Systematic study is needed to assess the effectiveness of this approach, its possible risks, and the characteristics of patients who might benefit from it.

REFERENCES CITED

Fallon B. A., B. T. Walsh, C. Sadik, J. B. Saoud, V. Lukasik. Outcome and clinical course in inpatient bulimic women: a 2- to 9-year follow-up study. *Journal of Clinical Psychiatry* 52:272–278, 1991.

Keski-Rakhonen A., A. Raevuori, and H. Hoek. Epidemiology of eating disorders: an update). *Annual Review of Eating Disorders Part 2*, ed. Oxford: Radcliffe Publishing, 2008, pp. 58–68.

Miller C. A. and N. H. Golden. An introduction to eating disorders: clinical presentation, epidemiology, and prognosis. *Nutrition in Clinical Practice* 25:110–115, 2010.

SELECTED READINGS

American Psychiatric Association. Practice guidelines for eating disorders. *American Journal of Psychiatry* 163:S1–S54, 2006.

Birmingham, C. L., and P. Beumont. *Medical Management of Eating Disorders*. Cambridge, UK: Cambridge University Press, 2004.

Bruch, H. *Eating Disorders: Obesity, Anorexia Nervosa, and the Person Within.* New York: Basic Books, 1973.

Bruch, H. *The Golden Cage: The Enigma of Anorexia Nervosa.* Cambridge, MA: Harvard University Press, 1978.

Brumberg, J. J. *Fasting Girls: The Emergence of Anorexia Nervosa as a Modern Disease.* Cambridge, MA: Harvard University Press, 1988.

Franklin, J. C, B. C. Scheile, et al. Observations on human behavior in experimental semistarvation and rehabilitation. *Journal of Clinical Psychology* 4:28–45, 1948.

Garner, D. M., and P. E. Garfinkel, eds. *Handbook of Treatment for Eating Disorders,* 2nd ed. New York: Guilford Press, 1997.

Kaye, W. Neurobiology of anorexia and bulimia nervosa. *Physiology and Behavior* 94:121–135, 2008.

Lock, J., D. Le Grange, W. S. Agras, and C. Dare. *Treatment Manual for Anorexia Nervosa: A Family-Based Approach.* New York: Guildford Press, 2001.

Mitchell, J. E., M. J. Devlin, M. De Zwaan, S. J. Crow, and C. B. Peterson. *Binge-Eating Disorder: Clinical Foundations and Treatment.* New York: Guilford Press, 2008.

Nogami, Y., and F. Yabana. On kibarashi-gui (binge-eating). *Folia Psychiatrica et Neurologica Japonica* 31:159–166, 1977.

Russell, G. Bulimia nervosa: an ominous variant of anorexia nervosa. *Psychology and Medicine* 9:429–448, 1979.

Walsh, B. T. The enigmatic persistence of anorexia nervosa. *American Journal of Psychiatry* 170:477–484, 2013.

Walsh, B. T., A. S. Kaplan, E. Attia, M. Olmsted, M. Parides, J. C. Carter, K. M. Pike, M. J. Devlin, B. Woodside, C. A. Roberto, and W. Rockert. Fluoxetine after weight restoration for anorexia nervosa: a randomized controlled trial. *JAMA: Journal of the American Medical Association* 295:2605–2612, 2006.

/// **10** /// Somatic Symptom and Related Disorders

KELLI JANE K. HARDING AND BRIAN A. FALLON

Patients go to physicians with symptoms suggestive of an illness. The physician takes a careful history, performs a physical examination, orders diagnostic tests, and determines a diagnosis that explains the symptoms and dictates a particular prognosis and treatment plan. If the diagnosis remains undetermined after the physician has performed a careful medical workup, or if the symptoms seem in excess of an existing condition, either a physical illness of undetermined etiology is present, or the symptoms are related at least in part to psychological factors. Such bothersome physical symptoms are common, disabling, and costly, and they cause both patients and physicians distress.

Patients with **somatic symptom disorders** suffer from physical symptoms and related fears that seem disproportionate to objective medical findings. The physical symptoms are genuine; they are not intentionally produced. These debilitating conditions can cause functional impairments and a significant decline in a patient's quality of life. The **somatic symptom disorders** as a group are an enormous public health problem, estimated to account for 1 in 10 primary care patient visits and costing the U.S. health care system more than the annual estimated cost of diabetes care.

Patients with **factitious disorder** intentionally simulate or produce symptoms of illnesses in themselves or others for the purpose of appearing ill, impaired, or injured. Their primary motivation is to achieve the "sick role" of a patient. These perplexing disorders fall midway between somatic symptom disorder, in which symptom production is not intentional, and **malingering**, in which symptom production is motivated by external rewards, such as financial gain, obtaining controlled substances, or avoidance of incarceration or military service. Patients with factitious disorder consciously simulate illness for psychological purposes; pragmatic incentives are either absent or secondary. The relationship of psychological factors to medical symptoms lies on a spectrum of conscious awareness (see Table 10.1 and Figure 10.1).

DIAGNOSTIC AND CLINICAL FEATURES

The somatic symptom disorders were previously classified under the umbrella term "somatoform disorders." Reclassification is nothing new for these perplexing conditions,

TABLE 10.1 Differential Diagnosis of Distressing Somatic Symptoms

---

Unrecognized Disease (see Table 10.5)

Somatic Symptom Disorders (psychological factors contributing to symptoms)

Somatic Subtype

- Somatic symptom disorder
- Other specified somatic symptom and related disorder

Dissociative Subtype

- Conversion disorder

Obsessive/Cognitive Subtype

- Illness anxiety disorder
- Body dysmorphic disorder*

Factitious Disorders (symptoms intentionally produced without external gain)

Malingering (symptoms intentionally produced for external gain)

---

*Reclassified in DSM-5 as an obsessive-compulsive and related disorder.

which in the past have been called hysteria, neurasthenia, and psychogenic and psycho-somatic disorders. With expert consensus, the DSM-5 classification is more consistent with observed clinical similarities and emerging epidemiological and treatment data. For instance, the DSM-IV diagnosis of somatization disorder was so narrowly defined that only a small subgroup of patients with somatization symptoms met the criteria. Emphasis has been shifted in the DSM-5 from medically unexplained symptoms to **disproportionate concern or reaction to symptoms regardless of etiology**. Because studies specific for the new DSM-5 diagnoses have not yet been done, the evidence presented is extrapolated from the prior classification system.

It is important to note that the presence of ambiguous physical symptoms is not sufficient to classify someone as having a psychiatric disorder. As more is learned about

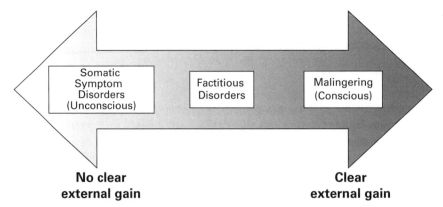

FIGURE 10.1 The relationship of psychological factors to medical symptom production is on a spectrum from the unconscious/involuntary to conscious/voluntary or intentional. Additionally, the symptoms range from no clear external gain to clear external gain or benefits (financial, medication seeking, avoidance of jail). Symptoms are consciously produced in patients with factitious disorder, while there is no clear external gain other than to play the sick role. Malingering is not considered a psychiatric disorder.

physical symptoms without a known etiology, classification can be further fine-tuned. For instance, many patients with functional somatic syndromes such as fibromyalgia, chronic fatigue syndrome, and irritable bowel syndrome would have been diagnosed as having a somatoform disorder according to the DSM-IV, but they are now only diagnosed with a somatic symptom disorder if their symptoms are accompanied by excessive concerns, distress, or behaviors.

Somatic Symptom Disorders

The somatic symptom disorders are a heterogeneous group unified by physical symptoms or concerns that are associated with prominent distress or impairment (see Table 10.2). Clinically it is useful to consider three subtypes: somatic/sensory, dissociative, and obsessional/cognitive.

Somatic/Sensory Subtype

Patients with **somatic symptom disorder (SSD)** (see DSM-5) experience **prominent somatic symptoms** that are disruptive to social, occupational, or other important areas of daily functioning. Somatic symptoms alone, however, are not sufficient for this diagnosis. Patients must also have excessive thoughts, feelings, or behaviors related to the somatic symptoms. If they have another medical condition, the thoughts, feelings, and behaviors associated with the medical condition are excessive. Patients with SSD may have persistently high levels of anxiety about health or symptoms, persistent thoughts about the seriousness of their symptoms, or spend excessive time and energy devoted to these symptoms or health concerns. Often the symptoms start before the age of 30 and may include a constellation of **pain**, gastrointestinal disturbances, sexual or reproductive symptoms, or neurological problems (e.g., weakness, swallowing difficulties, or sensation changes).

Patients with SSD usually present to internists, general practitioners, neurologists, or gynecologists. In general, pronounced physical symptoms associated with marked distress or functional impairment, as would be typical of SSD, are found in 4–12% of the general population with a median of 16.6% of primary care samples. Often, individuals with SSD have seen many different physicians and have received a variety of medical

TABLE 10.2 Key Features of Individual Somatic Symptom and Related Disorders

Somatic symptom disorder	Prominent somatic symptoms with distressing thoughts, feelings, and behaviors about illness lasting >6 months
Other specified somatic symptom and related disorder	Persistent somatic symptoms with distressing thoughts, feelings, and behaviors lasting <6 months and/or not fully meeting criteria for related disorders
Conversion disorder (functional neurological symptom disorder)	Impairing symptoms affecting voluntary motor system or sensory functions that are incompatible with recognized neurological or other medical conditions
Illness anxiety disorder	Fear of having or of acquiring a serious illness; somatic symptoms if present are mild in intensity
Body dysmorphic disorder*	Preoccupation with an imagined or slight defect in physical appearance

*Reclassified in DSM-5 as an obsessive-compulsive and related disorder.

diagnoses and treatments. The prototypical patient spends several hours a week at doctors' appointments and is treated symptomatically with a variety of over-the-counter and prescribed medications, which provide only temporary relief. Typically, none of the illnesses diagnosed are serious, nor does there seem to be a clear physiologically based connection between the various organ systems apparently affected. Also, despite having many symptoms, the afflicted patient often does not seem to be overly concerned about any specific diagnosis. Symptoms and treatments become central in these patients' lives, and they are often not aware of having any psychological, emotional, or interpersonal difficulties. The symptoms and extraordinary amount of time spent seeing physicians often interferes with employment or the enjoyment of a full social and family life. For a diagnosis of SSD, symptoms typically persist 6 months or longer, although they may wax and wane during that interval. Patients with a duration of symptoms less than 6 months or whose symptoms do not meet the full criteria for any of the disorders in the somatic symptom and related disorders class are diagnosed with other specified somatic symptom and related disorder (see DSM-5).

A common presentation of SSD is a localized painful symptom associated with a disproportionately high level of psychological distress or dysfunction. In as many as 4 out of 10 patients who present with pain, the pain appears related to psychological factors. Among patients with SSD manifesting as pain, there may be no clear pathophysiological mechanism that sufficiently accounts for the degree or location of pain. Even when there is a known cause, the pain the patient presents with is in significant excess of what the physical findings would suggest. Psychological contributants may include psychosocial stressors or conflict in the patient's life and the subsequent occurrence of pain symptoms. For example, a woman who was having problems at her job with a particular supervisor found that her back pain returned after each time she was criticized by that supervisor. When the supervisor was away on vacation, she did not have back pain. Even though the pain is not intentionally produced, it may result in secondary gain, such as increased attention and sympathy from others, time off from work, and financial compensation for the disability (see Box 11.10 in Chapter 11, Psychological Factors Affecting Medical Conditions).

Patients with SSD with predominant pain may present with a wide range of symptoms, including musculoskeletal (back), arthritic (joint), and cardiovascular (anginal) pain. Patients often visit a large number of physicians seeking relief. Analgesics of all sorts are prescribed to them and may be temporarily effective; however, the pain inevitably returns over time. Patients may undergo potentially dangerous invasive procedures or surgeries, which grant them little lasting relief. They generally do not recognize the contribution of psychological factors to the pain.

Dissociative Subtype

Patients with **conversion disorder** (functional neurological symptom disorder) (see DSM-5) present with neurological symptoms affecting their **voluntary motor** or **sensory function** that cannot be fully explained physiologically. Patients may experience sudden blindness, deafness, paralysis, inability to speak, seizures, or an inability to walk or stand. Although the symptoms or deficits suggest a physical condition, clinical findings are inconsistent with recognized neurological and medical disorders. Historically, conversion disorder was known as "hysteria" or "hysterical neurosis"; the origin of the term *conversion* is from Freud's theory that anxiety is "converted" into physical symptoms. The symptoms typically are considered symbolic representations that relieve an underlying emotional conflict (see case example in Box 10.1). Occasionally, more than

---

BOX 10.1

CASE EXAMPLE OF CONVERSION DISORDER RELIEVING AN UNDERLYING EMOTIONAL CONFLICT

A man who discovered his wife was unfaithful became enraged and developed a conversion paralysis of his right arm, preventing him from acting out murderous impulses toward his wife. On interview the patient appeared relatively unconcerned about the severity of his symptoms and resultant disability (**"la belle indifférence"**), stating, "I guess I can't move my arm." Although seemingly outside of his conscious awareness, the patient experienced both primary and secondary gain. The prevention of acting on his murderous impulses was the primary gain of his symptom. The secondary gain was the disability benefits the patient received because his paralysis prevented him from being able to work.

---

one person develops conversion symptoms, as reported in groups of school children and factory workers. This is called "mass psychogenic illness" or "mass hysteria."

Conversion symptoms often reflect patients' conceptions of what neurological disorders should be rather than what is neurologically possible, for example, sudden-onset "glove and stocking" paresthesia, stuttering, or "tunnel vision" (see case example in Box 10.2). While the diagnosis of conversion disorder is generally considered only after the results obtained from appropriate examination and testing have been used to rule out other underlying conditions, conversion symptoms may also coexist with documented

---

BOX 10.2

CASE EXAMPLE OF CONVERSION DISORDER WITH INCONSISTENT SENSORY NERVE DISTRIBUTION

A 42-year-old man complained to his physician about facial numbness, demonstrating the complaint by pinching his own cheeks and pushing his face very close to the physician's face. According to the patient, the distribution of the numbness was circular, running around the circumference of his face, along the hairline and under the jaw and chin. Because the sensory nerve distribution of the face does not follow such a pattern and instead is segmental and overlapping, the physician concluded that psychological factors contributed to the patient's symptoms. In taking the psychosocial history, the physician discovered that the patient was in a public fight with a boss at work who the patient experienced as excoriating and humiliating. When talking about the boss, the patient became agitated and said, "He is constantly in my face." Discussing his feelings of public humiliation enabled the patient to feel better and to request and receive a change in job assignment. The remainder of the "shamefaced" numbness symptom faded away.

---

medical illness. For example, an individual with epilepsy may also have coexisting conversion seizures or nonepileptic seizures.

A related condition that illustrates the profound relationship between the mind and body is **pseudocyesis**, in which a woman believes she is pregnant. Pseudocyesis is associated with symptoms and signs of pregnancy, such as cessation of menstruation, nausea, abdominal enlargement, breast enlargement, and hormonal changes. Despite these signs, there is no fetus. This phenomenon appears to be influenced by psychological factors, such as the wish for a child. It has been observed in animals, and reportedly the English Queen Mary Tudor, better known as "Bloody Mary," was believed to have suffered from the condition.

Obsessional/Cognitive Subtype

Patients who suffer with **illness anxiety disorder (IAD)** (see DSM-5) are preoccupied for 6 months or longer with the **fear or belief that they have or might acquire a serious disease**, to the point that their concerns interfere with social or occupational functioning. Although seen in all age groups, IAD is most likely to occur in people who are in their 30s or 40s; it is equally common in men and women. Minor bodily symptoms, which may be present, are catastrophically misinterpreted as signs of serious illness, causing anxiety to escalate out of control. For example, an individual with mild constipation and IAD may become convinced that he or she has an intestinal cancer. For those who suffer with severe health anxiety, just hearing about an illness can cause individuals to worry that they have it even in the absence of a somatic symptom. For example, media coverage about HIV/AIDS caused one individual with IAD to become convinced that he had the infection, even though he had no symptoms of the illness, had multiple negative tests, and had not engaged in any risky behaviors. Despite temporary reassurance from doctors, the fears would return. He sought repeated testing, missing so much work that he put his job in jeopardy. He avoided dating and socializing for concern that he might spread the illness to others.

Patients with IAD have behaviors associated with their anxiety. Either they are care seeking and frequently checking or they exhibit maladaptive avoidance of situations that might trigger their health anxiety. These individuals are often only temporarily relieved by much sought-after reassurance. They may spend inordinate amounts of time researching medical symptoms online, also known as "cyberchondria." Despite thorough physical examinations and reassurances that they are not ill, the worries often return, and so they seek out new physicians who they hope will discover the cause of their problem.

The essential difference between the diagnoses of IAD and SSD lies in the prominence of somatic symptoms. In both IAD and SSD, there is distress about illness or symptoms. However, in IAD, the somatic symptoms are either absent or only mild in intensity, but the preoccupation with illness and catastrophic thinking predominates. The presenting feature is more anxiety focused than symptom focused, as the case example in Box 10.3 illustrates. Some patients with IAD are so anxious that doctors may uncover a serious illness that they avoid medical care altogether, which can lead to poor health outcomes. **Care-avoidant** patients with IAD may get into conflicts with family members and friends over avoiding events that make them anxious about their health, including visiting sick relatives in hospitals or attending funerals.

Patients with the DSM-IV diagnosis of hypochondriasis are now diagnosed as having either illness anxiety disorder (approximately 25%) or somatic symptom disorder (approximately 75%). The previous term was eliminated as it was considered pejorative.

BOX 10.3

CASE EXAMPLE OF ILLNESS ANXIETY DISORDER

A 38-year-old physician engrossed in a very competitive grant-seeking phase of his academic career tripped on the street while running to catch a bus. He worried that he tripped because his foot dropped, which meant that he had a nerve palsy in his right leg. Over a period of weeks his worry progressed to a fear of multiple sclerosis. His physician took a careful history, performed a complete neurological examination, which indicated that all of his reflexes and strength testing were normal in the right lower extremity, and attempted to reassure him. He felt better immediately, experienced great relief, and rushed back into his busy academic life, only to find that his fear of multiple sclerosis returned within several days and increased over the next several weeks. He began to repeatedly test his Achilles tendon reflex throughout the day and found, as is typical in testing one's reflexes, that sometimes he elicited a brisk response and sometimes no response at all. He returned to see his doctor, who repeated the exam and again found no evidence of multiple sclerosis. At the patient's request, an MRI was ordered to definitively rule out any white matter changes. Waiting for the results, the patient stopped working on his grant because he was so anxious that he was unable to concentrate. He also turned down several social events he had been looking forward to because he felt he was "not any fun to be around." He started to anticipate life with a disability. When the results came back normal, the man felt tremendous relief. Again this lasted only a few days before the worries came creeping back. He returned to see his doctor, explaining, "I know this sounds crazy, but I can't stop worrying that I have undiagnosed multiple sclerosis, even though all of the evidence says I don't." On further history, the patient reported two previous episodes of health anxiety that interfered with his functioning, one in college after his grandfather had a heart attack and another during the second year of medical school. He recognized that his illness worries seemed related to the stress of his career concerns. He and his physician set up regularly scheduled "check-in" appointments.

Body Dysmorphic Disorder

The essential feature of body dysmorphic disorder (BDD) (see DSM-5) is a **preoccupation with a perceived defect in physical appearance.** Even if a slight physical defect exists, the person's complaints are markedly out of proportion to the objective findings. Perceived defects often concern the skin, hair, nose, eyes, and legs, although any part of the body, including breasts, muscles, or genitals, may be included. While many people may have concerns about certain aspects of their appearance, the preoccupation in patients with body dysmorphic disorder causes significant distress and impairment. Patients may spend hours a day in time-consuming checking behaviors and isolate themselves because they believe others are mocking their appearance; the latter belief would be considered an idea or delusion of reference. Insight about the irrational preoccupation can range from good to absent or delusional. Dermatological or surgical treatments are

---

BOX 10.4

CASE EXAMPLE OF BODY DYSMORPHIC DISORDER

A 22-year-old woman who had had a 3-mm precancerous growth on her forehead removed 6 months ago returned to her doctor concerned that the incision was not healing correctly and requested a corrective procedure. Repeated examinations showed good wound closure and no unanticipated swelling. Despite reassurance, the patient became so self-conscious about the scar that she would not leave home without wearing a hat. She felt people at work were treating her differently because of the scar, and she stopped joining her coworkers for their usual post-work socializing. She was reluctant to date because she didn't want to have to show the scar to a potential partner. The patient returned to her doctor again, requesting corrective surgery. Her doctor explained that it seemed she had been under a great deal of stress and it might be helpful to discuss it. She agreed.

---

commonly sought, but little satisfaction is obtained after the intervention. Many with BDD have suicidal thoughts. A case example is presented in Box 10.4.

Body dysmorphic disorder has been moved from the DSM-IV category of the somatoform disorders to the DSM-5 category of obsessive-compulsive and related disorders to reflect a growing consensus that it shares a similar etiology with the latter category of disorders.

Factitious Disorder

Why someone would fake being ill, without obvious gain, is mysterious, yet episodes of patients forging illness are not uncommon within the hospital setting. The only obvious motivation for the deception is to assume the sick role. Patients with factitious disorder (see DSM-5) may have physical symptoms, psychological symptoms, or a mixture of the two (see Table 10.3). They often present with signs and symptoms of illnesses that suggest rare medical conditions in order to interest physicians sufficiently to be admitted.

It is estimated that 1 in 10 patients with factitious disorder have the most severe form, popularly known as **Munchausen's syndrome**. Munchausen's is characterized by multiple hospitalizations with repeated invasive testing and surgical procedures. The condition is named for an 18th-century German baron who had a reputation for telling fantastic tales about his wartime adventures to impress his listeners. These patients may **wander** from city to city, state to state, or country to country in search of treatment for their symptoms. For example, one patient had over 200 documented hospitalizations over a 7-year span, from the coast of Maine to Boston, then to Albany, NY, and New York City, Philadelphia, and then Pittsburgh. His last documented hospitalization occurred in West Virginia. Another patient reported prolonged admissions at numerous prestigious hospitals around the country with a litany of diagnoses that were not verifiable. The flamboyant style and intriguing histories of these patients sometimes results in a single patient appearing as the subject of many case reports in a number of medical journals representing a variety of specialties. In this most severe and chronic form of factitious

TABLE 10.3 Clinical Features Associated with Factitious Disorders

Clinical Features Associated with Patients with Factitious Disorder

Symptoms are absent when patient does not think he or she is being watched

Multiple admissions in a variety of cities and states

Patient presents with very dramatic symptoms or rare disorders

No visitors

Patient relays "textbook" symptoms of an illness

Sophisticated medical knowledge and vocabulary

Patient works or studied in a medical field

Very accepting of discomfort and risk of invasive procedures and operations

Patient disputes test results

As soon as one set of symptoms is under control, new physical problems related to different organ systems or complications emerge

Extensive evidence of prior treatment (e.g., a gridiron abdomen, burr holes)

Pseudologia fantastica: pathological and fantastical lying about personal history or background

Patient predicts his or her disease will worsen

Patient left against medical advice from prior hospitalizations

Patient quickly leaves the hospital when confronted with evidence of his or her fabrication

Clinical Features Associated with Factitious Disorder Imposed on Another

A history of multiple emergency room visits and long hospitalizations

Child is under 4 years of age, or elderly homebound individual

History of infant death in family or children with failure to thrive

Family member in the medical field

disorder, patients spend the majority of their time in a self-destructive pattern of being either in the hospital or seeking admission to a hospital.

Men are more likely to present with Munchausen's syndrome, although factitious disorder with predominantly physical signs and symptoms is otherwise more common among women. Factitious disorder with predominantly psychological signs and symptoms occurs more commonly among men. While it is no longer specified in DSM-5, it can be clinically useful to consider factitious disorder with predominantly physical signs and symptoms versus those with psychological symptoms.

The symptoms of patients with factitious disorder with **predominantly physical signs and symptoms** are suggestive of a physical disorder that is intentionally produced. Simulation of almost every medical illness is possible, only limited by the patient's imagination, medical sophistication, and daring. Impressive physical signs can be fabricated. For instance, restricting blood flow with a ligature can produce significant edema. Falsified physical signs and symptoms are often supported by false histories and reported test results. Additionally, in a pattern akin to self-harm, medical signs can be induced through surreptitious means, such as inducing actual illness by infecting one's wounds or through ingestion of chemicals or other substances or by aggravating existing medical conditions (see Box 10.5 for a case example). Frequently seen factitious conditions include bleeding caused by the surreptitious ingestion of anticoagulant medication, endocrine abnormalities caused by the ingestion of thyroid hormone or insulin, abscesses caused by subcutaneous injection of saliva or feces, hyperthermia caused by manipulating the thermometer, and voluntary limb dislocation.

BOX 10.5

CASE EXAMPLE OF FACTITIOUS DISORDER WITH PREDOMINANTLY PHYSICAL SIGNS AND SYMPTOMS

A 37-year-old man who presented with hypoglycemia produced signs and symptoms of hypoglycemia by surreptitiously injecting himself with insulin with syringes that he had taken with him to the hospital. His doctor became suspicious of surreptitious insulin administration and on laboratory evaluation found an elevated insulin level with a low serum C-peptide, suggestive of exogenous insulin. (Serum C-peptide levels normally increase when pancreatic secretion of insulin increases; however, it is removed during the purification of commercial insulin preparations of recombinant human insulin.) A search of the patient's belongings found insulin and syringes. Following a confrontation by his physician, the patient became indignant that the doctors were wrong in their analysis and abruptly left the hospital. It seemed clear from the patient's behavior that he knew he was causing the symptoms. Later that evening, he was admitted via the emergency room to another hospital less than a mile away from the first hospital for hypoglycemic delirium. Because the computer systems at the two hospitals were not connected, the patient again was admitted for a medical workup. There was no obvious goal for the behavior other than to assume the psychological role of "patient."

Certain behavioral features are associated with patients with factitious disorder. **Pathological lying** about various aspects of history and background sometimes occurs. Patients may claim to be associated with rich, famous, and powerful individuals. The hospital staff treated one patient royally after he led them to believe that he was a prince from a central African country. Another patient claimed that he was related to the senator of an adjoining state. In addition, patients with factitious disorder may complain of **new physical problems** related to different organ systems as soon as one set of symptoms is under control. When hospitalized, many of these patients have **no visitors**, although some patients have **collaborators** who bring paraphernalia (e.g., syringes, medications) when they visit, to support the patients in their charades. Patients with factitious disorder often have an extensive **knowledge of medical terminology and procedures** and may have worked in the medical field. They **do not object to potentially dangerous procedures and operations** and may have received invasive and ultimately unnecessary treatments, such as catheterization, exploratory laparotomy, feeding tube placement, and even pacemakers. When these patients are confronted with evidence of their fabrication, they typically claim the medical team is incorrect and quickly **flee the hospital**, usually against medical advice. One patient with factitious illness in the medical intensive care unit suddenly stood up from his bed, tore off his monitoring leads, and walked out the door. Physicians encountering patients who have a **bewildering array of shifting complaints**, which are dramatic and not verifiable, should consider factitious disorder in the differential diagnosis.

People with factitious disorder **with psychological symptoms** simulate mental rather than physical illnesses. They either falsify their history or feign symptoms of mental illness. The presenting symptoms often reflect the individual's conception of mental illness rather than any recognized disorder. Such patients may present with a combination of psychotic, affective, and cognitive findings, as the case example in Box 10.6 illustrates. They may tell compelling tales of tragedy. For instance, one patient told his doctors about losing his wife and young daughter in a car accident and the severe depression that followed; collateral history revealed the patient had never been married. Factitious symptoms may arise in patients who have preexisting genuine mental disorders, but the new symptoms are not consistent with the previous diagnoses (see case examples in Box 10.7). Patients who are known to the staff at a hospital may present with factitious psychological symptoms to gain admission to an inpatient unit when their usual symptoms would not warrant admission. Such patients may report auditory hallucinations commanding them to kill themselves even though their chronic suicidal ideation has never previously included the presence of any hallucinations.

Variants of Factitious Disorder

Factitious disorder **imposed on another** (previously, factitious disorder by proxy), also known as Munchausen's syndrome by proxy, is a variant in which one individual (usually a parent) **fabricates illness in another person, often a child**, who then receives unnecessary medical interventions and hospitalizations. These individuals may be trying either to ensure that the person who is the victim receives appropriate medical attention or to gain attention or admiration for themselves by playing the role of the concerned or grieving caregiver. When a minor is involved, factitious disorder imposed on another is a form of **child abuse**. The average age of the child victim is under the age of 4 years, although it often takes over a year for the diagnosis to be made. Over half of victims have siblings that present with the same mysterious symptoms, and approximately a fourth of such

---

BOX 10.6

CASE EXAMPLE OF FACTITIOUS DISORDER WITH PREDOMINANTLY PSYCHOLOGICAL SIGNS AND SYMPTOMS CHARACTERIZED BY MULTIPLE SYMPTOMS

A man presented alone to the emergency room. He was able to provide only limited medical history and no contacts for collateral history. After a negative medical workup, he was admitted to a psychiatric inpatient unit for treatment of psychosis. On admission, he appeared to be responding to internal stimuli, often shouting out in a threatening voice to people who were not there. Despite increasing levels of antipsychotic medications he remained severely disorganized in his behavior and began to report frightening visual hallucinations of knights on white horses attacking him. Brain imaging was negative. On the second week of his hospital admission the patient suddenly developed stiff slowed movements and began drooling excessively. The night nurse, after hearing the report, became very concerned about him and decided to stop by the patient's room to check in on him. Much to the nurse's surprise, the patient was comfortably doing push-ups on the floor. A room search later revealed a stash of apparently "cheeked" medications hidden in the mattress. Additional history uncovered that the patient had an older brother with schizophrenia, whom he felt never got the care he deserved.

BOX 10.7

CASE EXAMPLES OF FACTITIOUS DISORDER WITH PREDOMINANTLY PSYCHOLOGICAL SIGNS AND SYMPTOMS IN PATIENTS WITH PREEXISTING PSYCHIATRIC DISORDERS

A patient with a known history of borderline personality disorder went to an emergency room complaining of hearing voices and seeing visions. Psychiatric examination revealed symptoms of mania, depression, and dementia, as well as panic attacks, conversion symptoms, and dissociative experiences. Since it is highly unlikely that any patient would have simultaneous presentation of all of these disorders, the physician extended the examination. Upon doing so, it became evident that the patient wanted to ensure her hospitalization.

A second patient had been previously diagnosed with major depressive disorder and dependent personality disorder. He had never claimed to experience hallucinations. He described seeing and hearing "spirits" just before he was to be transferred to a day hospital. As with factitious disorder with physical symptoms, no obvious recognizable goal explained the psychological findings. His physicians concluded that the patient was "dependent" on his present facility and was frightened about leaving a familiar environment and of adjusting to new surroundings. These psychological explanations indicated that the new, feigned symptoms were factitious rather than malingering. The man's original diagnosis remained the same, and the newly feigned symptoms supported an additional diagnosis of factitious disorder with psychological symptoms.

---

children have deceased siblings. The perpetrator is the mother in about three-fourths of cases. Of note, there are reports of factitious disorder in children and adolescents (mean age of 13.9, range 8–18 years) without known parental involvement. Another variant involves elder abuse.

There are case reports of virtual factitious disorders, or **Munchausen's syndrome by Internet**, in which individuals, sometimes referred to as cyberspace "trolls," exploit the Web's anonymity and assume the sick role in Internet groups and chat rooms to elicit sympathy and attention. The deception typically creates anger and frustration if discovered.

COURSE OF ILLNESS

Table 10.4 provides epidemiological information for each of the somatic symptom and related disorders as well as body dysmorphic disorder, in comparison with factitious disorder and malingering, and a summary of the age of onset and usual course of illness.

Somatic Symptom and Related Disorders

Patients with somatic symptom and related disorders often suffer tremendously, with difficulty functioning at work and in interpersonal relationships. Somatic symptom

TABLE 10.4 Epidemiological and Other Characteristics of Somatic Symptom Disorders, Factitious Disorders, and Malingering

Somatic Symptom and Related Disorders (Previously Somatoform Disorders and Factitious Disorder)

	Somatic Symptom Disorder (Previously Somatization Disorder and Pain Disorder)	Conversion Disorder	Illness Anxiety Disorder (Previously Hypochondriasis)	Body Dysmorphic Disorder*	Factitious Disorder	Malingering (not Considered a Psychiatric Disorder)
Prevalence	5–7% of the general population and 16.6% of primary care samples	0.01–0.3% of the general population 5% of referrals to neurology clinics 5–10% of general hospital psychiatric consultations	2–5% of patients seen by primary care physicians	1–2% of the general population 6–15% of plastic surgery or dermatological patients, including subclinical variants	1% of general hospital inpatients Higher incidence in health care workers 3.5–9.3% of patients with prolonged fevers of unknown origin	1% in civilian mental health clinical practice 5% in military mental health services
Age of Onset	<30 years old, often in adolescence	Majority of cases occur ages 10–35	Adulthood	Adolescence or early adulthood	Likely begins in adolescence, majority of cases ages 20–45	Can be seen starting in childhood
Gender	Females > males	Females > males	Females = males	Females = males	Varies by subtype	Males > females
Course	Chronic, with exacerbations	May be transient or persistent	Chronic or intermittent	Chronic, 25% attempt suicide	Chronic, patients often seek care elsewhere	"Symptoms" disappear after secondary gain is achieved
Familial Patterns and	Observed in 10–20% of female first-degree biological relatives of female patients	Occurs more frequently in relatives of afflicted patients Increased risk in monozygotic twins	Higher frequency in patients with OCD and their first-degree family members	Higher frequency in family members of patients with OCD	Patients often report a history of child abuse and neglect.	History of antisocial behavior. Homelessness. Psychosocial stress
Related Conditions	When pain predominates, depressive disorders and alcohol dependence are more common in first-degree relatives.		Possible greater frequency of SSD among relatives		Patients often have comorbid borderline personality disorder.	More likely in a setting in which there is an advantage to being ill

*Reclassified in DSM-5 as an obsessive-compulsive and related disorder.

disorder and body dysmorphic disorder are generally **chronic** conditions with a **fluctuating** course of exacerbations and temporary remissions.

Somatic symptom disorder, which often begins in adolescence, causes significant disability: patients with SSD spend more days in bed per month than patients with other major medical disorders and have twice the annual medical care costs of non-somatizing patients, even after adjusting for the presence of psychiatric and medical comorbidity. SSD typically presents during the most productive years of employment and is associated with significant disability, lower quality of life, and higher health care utilization.

Body dysmorphic disorder generally persists for years. In some instances, the symptoms worsen and become delusional in intensity. In other instances, the perceived defect may shift from one area of the body to another. Spontaneous remissions are rare. BDD has significant morbidity: patients with BDD report a poorer quality of life than those with a recent myocardial infarction or type II diabetes. In addition, one in four patients with BDD attempts suicide.

Illness anxiety disorder symptoms can present acutely, especially following the illness of a loved one. The typical course is chronic, interspersed with **remissions** and **relapses**. Ironically, patients with IAD may worry so much about having an undiagnosed illness that they may neglect attending to their known health risks. For example, a patient with tremendous fear about developing colon cancer felt too anxious to contemplate quitting smoking, a known risk factor, and actually increased her cigarette use when she felt anxious.

Conversion disorder is generally characterized by a **short duration with full resolution, although conversion symptoms may also persist**. Good premorbid functioning, abrupt onset of symptoms, and the presence of recognizable environmental stressors are all good prognostic indicators. For example, a 30-year-old woman with no prior psychiatric history was in a serious car accident in which a close friend was killed. Seeing her friend's body, she passed out and upon awakening had lost her vision. Her physical exam, brain imaging, and laboratories did not suggest an injury. Within 24 hours, this conversion disorder resolved. Patients with conversion symptoms occurring in the context of other physical disorders (e.g., conversion seizures in a patient with a preexisting seizure disorder) generally have a poorer prognosis. Any patient with recurrent conversion disorder or symptom-contingent secondary gain is also at risk for a poorer outcome. For example, a single mother with a history of abuse as a teenager suffered from chronic back pain. When she developed recurrent right arm and leg weakness that prevented her from going to work, she found that these additional symptoms provided her with attention and help from her siblings.

Patients with somatic symptom disorders frequently have **comorbid depression** and **anxiety**, as well as increased risk of **suicide**. Concomitant **abuse of prescribed medications** is not uncommon, nor is the risk of **unnecessary surgery or procedures**. Additionally, borderline, narcissistic, obsessive-compulsive, and histrionic personality traits may both predispose and perpetuate the somatic symptom disorders.

Factious Disorders

Factious disorders tend to have a poor prognosis with a **chronic** course associated with **iatrogenic morbidity**. These patients have a poor prognosis in part because they are disinclined to seek psychiatric care, flee from continuous care altogether, and are frequently lost to follow-up. It seems likely that some patients succumb either to the medical complications of their self-induced illnesses or to adverse effects of various invasive procedures. Patients with factious illnesses are at an increased rate of suicide as well.

THE INTERVIEW

Persistent somatic symptoms and unrelenting concerns can frustrate both patients and doctors. Patients may feel dissatisfaction with physicians and their situation, leading to nonadherence to medical recommendations and a disappointing quest for someone who can "cure" them or find the "correct" diagnosis. At the same time, persistent somatic symptoms serve as a humble reminder of medicine's current limitations, prompting physicians to maintain an open mind diagnostically and to respect patients' suffering regardless of etiology. Approaching somatic symptom disorders in this way provides an opportunity to treat patients holistically and refocus on the importance of the doctor–patient relationship.

Somatic Symptom and Related Disorders

Working effectively with patients with somatic symptom and related disorders requires health professionals to actively develop a good rapport (see Box 10.8). Good listening and detective skills are needed to sort out the information provided by patients and decide whether additional workup is required. Because patients' somatic complaints may mask depressive or anxiety disorders, physicians should explore those diagnoses. Additionally, the diagnosis of somatic symptom disorder does not preclude the development of another underlying medical disorder. It is essential that physicians guard against attributing any and all symptoms that patients experience to somatic symptom disorder, lest they miss the presence of other treatable medical conditions. In one dramatic case, a man who frequently complained of nonspecific pain and other physical symptoms died of a pulmonary embolism secondary to an undiagnosed deep vein thrombosis. Record review indicated that the patient had complained of lower extremity swelling on multiple occasions in the weeks prior to his death.

BOX 10.8

INTERVIEWING GUIDELINES FOR PATIENTS WITH SOMATIC SYMPTOM DISORDERS

- Approach the patient with empathy and acceptance.
- Recognize the difficulty the patient's symptoms are causing.
- Reassure the patient that the symptoms are being taken seriously.
- Be cautious in using medical jargon for normal variations in functioning.
- Focus on symptom management rather than "cure."
- Note whether the patient has insight into psychological functioning.
- Take a parallel psychosocial history.
- Search for depression and anxiety symptoms.
- Discourage "doctor shopping."
- Schedule appointments in a time-contingent rather than symptom-contingent manner.
- Try to ascertain whether the patient is receiving secondary gain from the symptoms.

Approaching patients with somatic symptom disorders with **empathy** and acceptance that the symptoms they are experiencing are real is helpful, as is acknowledgement of the patient's suffering and recognition of medicine's limitations in understanding somatic symptoms. Some patients with somatic symptom and related disorders are not in touch with their emotions and do not openly display them. They use their physical complaints as a form of communication. Unable to communicate directly about stress or conflict, they may express themselves through their somatic complaints. Such patients often show little psychological understanding of the relationship between their onset of symptoms and any environmental stressors that might have brought them about. The physician can emphasize the frequency with which **stress** can generate physical symptoms without the patient's awareness. By taking a **parallel psychosocial history**, the physician can usually make such stressors readily apparent. The corresponding affect, of which the patient may be unaware, is often clear from the manifest content of the story. It is sometimes useful to point out the affect that would be expected, as the case example in Box 10.9 illustrates.

Health professionals should be aware of their potentially negative emotional reactions to patients with persistent somatic symptoms and concerns. Otherwise, there is a risk of overprescribing, overordering unnecessary diagnostic tests and surgical procedures, or even ignoring patients (i.e., "running out of time" on morning rounds to see the patient, or focusing so much on the somatic complaints that the severe emotional distress and perhaps suicidality of the patient aren't ever uncovered). Finding the clinical balance between diagnostic and treatment factors while maintaining self-awareness of thoughts and feelings toward patients is an important professional skill to develop.

Factitious Disorder

The physician interacting with a patient with factitious disorder will do best if equipped with the wisdom of Solomon, the patience of Job, and the detective work of Sherlock Holmes. The history may be presented with great dramatic flair in a manner designed to intrigue caregivers. These patients may stir up feelings of helplessness, righteousness,

---

BOX 10.9

CASE EXAMPLE ILLUSTRATING THE UTILITY OF A PARALLEL PSYCHOSOCIAL HISTORY

The physician empathically observed that "many people would be quite sad for a number of weeks after their mother died." The patient to whom this was said was startled because he knew that the physician was pointing out the obvious, and yet he did not feel sad. Instead, he had numbness in a non-neurological distribution over his abdomen and thighs. He first noticed this when told of his mother's death. The symptom became much worse during the funeral and persisted for several weeks, at which point he saw his physician. The physician elicited the history of the patient's mother's death. The symptom of numbness displaced the expected emotional response of anxiety and sadness. The patient's conscious emotional reaction was to his physical symptoms, rather than to the traumatic event.

and rage in their physicians. The physician's awareness of these feelings will avoid unconsciously punishing the patient by ordering a host of painful and potentially dangerous diagnostic or therapeutic procedures. The prudent clinician will document historical inconsistencies without defaming the patient's character. Additionally, clinicians can increase their empathy toward patients with factitious illness when considering that hospitals and doctors are likely the only supportive source in the patient's life and that patients are often desperate to maintain this relationship.

When asked to discuss previous physicians or hospitalizations, these patients may report that they have forgotten the names of the physicians or hospitals. They may decline consenting to contact them because they had significant disagreements about the care that they received. It is important to obtain confirmatory collateral evidence whenever possible to find the facts within the fiction (see Box 10.10 for additional suggestions).

During a mental status examination, the patient may present with "**Vorbeireden,**" that is, inexact answers or talking past the point. A patient who is asked the name of the current president may reply "Lincoln." This response indicates that the patient has understood the nature of the task and is providing inexact answers to the questions. Whereas a single instance may be merely a mistake, such repeated answers may indicate deliberate intent. Reports from staff on other shifts who may observe inconsistencies in the patient's symptoms and behavior can be helpful.

Confrontation is a controversial intervention. Many patients will flee the hospital once confronted, negating any possible treatment intervention. Studies indicate that confrontation does not always lead to acknowledgement and is not necessary for management. If the treating team decides on confrontation, hospital security should be notified in advance, as patients sometimes become violent.

BOX 10.10
ASSESSMENT AND MANAGEMENT GUIDELINES FOR HOSPITALIZED PATIENTS WITH FACTITIOUS DISORDERS

- Note whether the patient uses medical jargon.
- Maintain a high level of suspicion if the patient's symptoms and signs seem to be a "textbook" description.
- Try to obtain corroborative information about the patient's history from family or other providers.
- Observe whether family or friends visit the patient.
- Look for temporal relationships between visitors and symptoms.
- Exclude visitors and observe for improvement.
- Consider borderline personality disorder and other comorbid psychiatric conditions.
- Assign one team member as the primary contact person.
- Place the patient on security watch for monitoring of unusual behavior.
- Consider a room search for substances.
- Confrontation should be done in a supportive and nonpunitive manner.

DIFFERENTIAL DIAGNOSIS

Somatic Symptom and Related Disorders

Somatic symptom and related disorders are diagnosed when patients present with subjective distress in excess of objective findings. Patients may have unrecognized, comorbid, and new illnesses. **Unrecognized illness** should always be placed first in the hierarchy of differential diagnosis. For instance, follow-up studies of patients diagnosed with conversion disorder suggest that about a fourth are diagnosed with neurological illness within 10 years that could account for their original presenting symptoms. Consideration should be given to the possibility that the symptoms represent an early stage of a difficult-to-diagnose syndrome that has an intermittent course or variable findings (see Table 10.5). Additionally, somatic symptom and related disorders may **coexist with other diseases.** For example, a patient can have both epileptic and nonepileptic seizures. Certain findings can suggest nonphysiological symptoms, such as collapsing weakness, distractible tremor, ictal stuttering, and Hoover's sign (contralateral hip extension with leg flexion in patients reporting hip weakness). However, these signs are not highly sensitive and can coexist with underlying physiological disease. Additionally, clinicians should monitor for the emergence of a **new physical disorder.** Even people with nonspecific somatic symptoms develop other medical problems. For example, a patient who was suspected to have a somatic symptom disorder presented with dysphasia. An MRI of her brain confirmed a recent cerebrovascular accident.

Psychiatric disorders such as **mood disorders, anxiety disorders,** and **substance abuse** are also part of the differential for somatic symptom and related disorders, as are psychotic disorders, including **major depression with psychotic features,**

TABLE 10.5 Commonly Unrecognized Diseases in Patients Diagnosed with Somatic Symptom and Related Disorders

Disorder	Example
Autoimmune disorders	Systemic lupus erythematosus, celiac disease, Sjogren's syndrome
Cardiovascular disorders	Abdominal angina, aortic aneurysm
Endocrine disorders	Thyroid dysfunction, Paget's disease
Gastrointestinal disorders	Biliary disease, intestinal motility disorders, chronic pancreatitis, gastroesophageal reflux disease
Gynecological disorders	Endometriosis, pelvic inflammatory disease
Infectious diseases	HIV, Lyme disease, babesiosis, hepatitis C, tuberculosis
Neurological conditions	Multiple sclerosis, abdominal migraine, encephalitis (i.e., anti-NMDA, herpes simplex virus), seizure disorders
Malignancies	Carcinoid tumors, pheochromocytoma, pancreatic cancer, brain tumors, paraneoplastic syndromes
Muscular abnormalities	Muscular dystrophy, mitochondrial disorders
Psychiatric conditions	Depression, delusional disorders, schizophrenia
Sleep disorders	Obstructive sleep apnea, narcolepsy
Toxic/metabolic disturbances	Porphyria, substance-related, vitamin B_{12}, folate, vitamin D, iron-deficiency anemia, Wilson's disease, hemochromatosis, lead toxicity, chronic arsenic exposure

schizophrenia with prominent somatic delusions, and **delusional disorder**. For instance, one patient who repeatedly presented for HIV testing was never reassured that the test was in fact negative. She felt that the way the doctor looked at her indicated that the test was positive, even requesting antiretroviral therapy. Her symptoms resolved with antipsychotic medication. **Panic disorder** can mimic cardiovascular symptoms (e.g., chest pain, dyspnea, palpitations); however, the symptoms occur in the context of the panic attacks.

While overconcern about perceived defects in appearance may occur during the course of **normal adolescence,** it may also be part of a more pervasive disorder, such as **anorexia nervosa**. One described phenomenon that should not be confused with body dysmorphic disorder is body integrity identity disorder, which is not included in the DSM-5, in which individuals are driven to have a healthy body part amputated because they feel the limb is somehow not a part of them. These individuals do not report believing that the limb is defective and do not feel ashamed or embarrassed by its appearance.

Factitious Disorder

Because of the nature of their illness, many patients with factitious disorder do, in fact, need treatment for **genuine physical illnesses**. For example, a patient who surreptitiously injected fecal material into his skin did have genuine infections, fevers, and septicemia that were life threatening and required medical intervention in the form of intravenous antibiotics. However, until the factitious etiology of the symptoms is uncovered, treatment is problematic.

People who **malinger** usually have an obvious, recognizable environmental goal, such as drug seeking, financial compensation, or avoidance of legal responsibility (e.g., outstanding warrants), accounting for the simulation of illness. Factitious disorder should be considered when no such goal explains the symptom production. Unlike the other disorders described in this chapter, malingering is not considered a psychiatric disorder. Treatment is rarely indicated because patients who engage in malingering are not usually motivated to change their behavior (see Box 10.11).

The major differential diagnosis for factitious disorder with predominantly psychological symptoms is a true **mental disorder**. A diagnosis of factitious disorder with psychological symptoms is even more difficult to establish with certainty in the absence of clear secondary gain than is factitious disorder with physical symptoms because, in most cases, no confirmatory laboratory or imaging findings exist. In most instances, physicians use their experience and intuition to determine whether patients have intentionally produced symptoms in an attempt to cope with stressors that they cannot communicate directly to their physicians.

Some patients with factitious disorders are diagnosed with schizophrenia because of their unusual lifestyle and strange affect (e.g., flat or inappropriate). However, psychiatric examination generally reveals the absence of symptoms of schizophrenia, particularly psychosis. Major depression with psychotic features should be considered in the differential, especially if the feigning of symptoms occurs only within the context of a mood disorder. Patients with factious disorders may have comorbid mood, substance, and/or personality disorders. Patients with significant character pathology such as borderline personality disorder or antisocial personality disorder may feign symptoms of mental illness for psychological reasons of attention, dependency, or indirect expression of anger. In these instances, both diagnoses should be made.

BOX 10.11

INTERVIEWING GUIDELINES FOR INDIVIDUALS SUSPECTED OF MALINGERING

- Listen carefully for inconsistencies in the history.
- Monitor for atypical or exaggerated symptoms and signs that are not consistent with what is known about usual disease presentation.
- Assess if symptom production is motivated by external incentives.
- Listen for pending litigation.
- Examine for evidence of antisocial personality disorder.
- Document inconsistencies in the medical chart without defaming the person's character.
- Remain open to the possibility that the patient is telling the truth.

MEDICAL EVALUATION

Somatic Symptom and Related Disorders

A thorough medical evaluation is vital for patients with somatic symptoms and related disorders. A careful history should include a detailed family history of medical illness. The physician is likely to order diagnostic tests including serological studies and brain imaging to rule out medical and/or neurological causes for symptoms. Because presenting complaints are suggestive of physical illness, it is crucial to rule out the presence of any underlying medical illness that might explain the symptoms. This careful medical attention to the patient's somatic symptoms serves two purposes: it reassures the doctor that the person does not likely have an undetected medical illness, and it reassures the patient that his or her concerns are being taken seriously. As a rule of thumb, once the diagnosis of a somatic symptom disorder is considered, the physician should avoid any diagnostic procedure that is invasive and puts the patient at risk for additional pain or complications. At the same time, physicians should continue to regularly consider undiagnosed physical illness. Patients with somatic symptom disorder challenge the clinician's skill, as the clinician needs to remain vigilant to detect undiagnosed disease and avoid overordering of tests and treatments. Relying on checklists may help clinicians ensure that the standard of care is provided.

Factitious Disorders

Similarly, when a diagnosis of factitious disorder is under consideration, invasive or traumatic procedures or treatments with a likelihood of serious adverse side effects should be avoided. Otherwise, such procedures may lead to iatrogenic complications or additional factitious symptoms and signs. For example, a patient who had an intravenous pyelogram developed an "allergic" reaction to the dye and went into feigned respiratory arrest. At the same time, even though the etiology of the symptoms is factitious, the patient might, in fact, be physically ill and need treatment. For instance, patients who surreptitiously bleed themselves can develop a genuine anemia from the blood loss.

If a factitious disorder is suspected, a careful laboratory review can distinguish fabricated illness from reality. One patient who reportedly was diagnosed with hemophilia was discovered to have no evidence of this on his laboratory tests. When confronted with this finding, he claimed the lab was in error, and the doctor was very apologetic. Repeat testing again confirmed he did not have hemophilia, and upon confronting him further with this news, he fled the hospital.

ETIOLOGY

Predisposing (genetics, neurobiology, cognitive and social functioning), precipitating (illness, infection, trauma, or abuse), and perpetuating (including primary and secondary gain, physiological processes such as inflammation) factors all appear to play a role in the etiology of the somatic symptom and related disorders. Advances in understanding neurobiology and neuroimmunology are contributing to improved understanding of the etiology of these disorders.

Somatic Symptom Disorder

Central to the somatic symptom disorders is the question, why is it that some people are more sensitive to physical symptoms and pain than others? The following cases illustrate two ends of the spectrum (see Figure 10.2). In the first case, a builder required intravenous sedation in the emergency room for pain after stepping on a 7-inch nail. After cutting away his boot, doctors unexpectedly found the nail had passed between his toes. In the second case, a construction worker saw his dentist for a complaint of a toothache. An x-ray revealed that the man had unknowingly shot himself in the head with a nail gun that misfired. While extreme, these cases illustrate different degrees of somatic awareness and symptom amplification. Researchers have observed a limited relationship between symptoms and the severity of disease in a number of conditions, including allergic reactions, arthritis, and cardiovascular disease. If an injury or the extent of disease does not in itself account for the severity of symptoms experienced by an individual, what other factors are involved?

Emerging data from **functional neuroimaging** suggest that people who report high versus low pain sensitivity have corresponding differences in brain activation of the anterior cingulate, somatosensory, and prefrontal cortex. Additionally, cognitive processing centers in the brain influence the assessment of incoming signals from the periphery of the body, determining if they meet a threshold of conscious awareness. Interestingly, imaging studies also show that imagined pain activates the brain in a similar way to actually experiencing the pain directly.

Abnormalities in **serotonin function** have been found in both pain perception and in functional somatic syndromes, such as irritable bowel syndrome and fibromyalgia. Additionally, the norepinephrine, glutamatergic, and dopamine systems appear to play a role in pain mediation.

Perception of pain involves peripheral sensory nerves, which send pain signals to the dorsal horn of the spinal cord and cerebrum via the thalamus. This signaling causes physiological and behavioral responses following a painful event. In turn, descending pathways from the cerebrum and periaqueductal gray matter to the spinal cord inhibit the pain perception. Through a process likely involving N-methyl D-aspartate (NMDA) receptors and central sensitization, trauma can lead to hypersensitivity or a decrease in pain threshold. Disruptions in **pain pathway structure and function** may contribute to the process of symptom amplification.

Inflammation likely plays a key role in symptom amplification. In response to an illness, the body may produce proinflammatory cytokines in both the periphery and the central

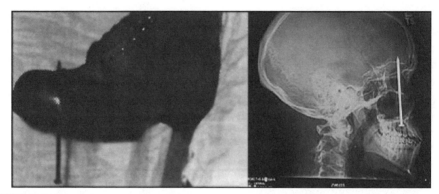

FIGURE 10.2 Variations in symptom perceptions elicited by nails. The picture on the left demonstrates somatic amplification; reprinted by permission from Fisher JP, Hassan DT, O'Conner N. Minerva. Br Med J 1995; 310:70, with permission from BMJ Publishing Group Ltd. The picture on the right exemplifies somatic deamplification; reprinted with permission from Associated Press, Wide World Photos 1/16/05. Figure reproduced from Psychosomatic Medicine 69:850–854 (2007) http://www.psychosomaticmedicine.org with permission by Lippincott Williams & Wilkins.

nervous system that contribute to feeling "sick." Nonspecific cytokine-induced illness symptoms and behaviors include fatigue, anhedonia, aches, and mood changes. While typically these symptoms go away when the illness resolves, subjective illness symptoms and behaviors may persist in individuals with a **chronically activated immune system from prior sensitization or noninfectious trauma (i.e., abuse)**. This is also referred to as a glial scar. Studies have shown an incremental association between inflammatory biological markers and de novo major depression, such as C-reactive protein, which can be measured in patients with somatic symptom disorder and illness anxiety disorder.

Psychodynamic theory suggests that many individuals with somatic symptom disorder have difficulty in directly expressing emotions, such as anger, depression, and anxiety. When faced with a stress or conflict they may express their **emotional pain indirectly** through physical pain or symptoms. Dr. Henry Maudsley, a British psychiatrist, captured this process poetically in his statement, "Grief that finds no vent in tears makes other organs weep."

There is still significant stigma associated with seeking mental health care in many **cultures**. Seeking medical care for physical symptoms may seem less threatening and still allows the individual to receive needed care and attention.

Conversion Disorder

Conversion symptoms are thought to serve the purpose of resolving an emotional **conflict without the conscious awareness** of the patient. An exploration of environmental stressors or changes in life situation often reveals the etiology of the symptoms. Once the symptoms have appeared, the patient may reap secondary gains of sympathy, attention, and support that might otherwise not be forthcoming. These secondary gains may maintain or prolong the conversion symptoms. For instance, one widowed man with nonepileptic seizures who lived in New York appreciated that his son flew repeatedly from California to help manage his refractory condition. Another woman with nonepileptic seizures became so attached to her epilepsy support group that she was unable to make clinical improvements in her symptoms. Conversion symptoms also demonstrate the intricate dynamic connection between the mind and the body. For instance, in the condition of pseudocyesis, emotions likely influence hormonal secretions that then lead to physical symptoms.

Illness Anxiety Disorder

Patients with illness anxiety disorder, like those with somatic symptom disorder, experience somatic amplification. Concerns often have an **obsessive** quality, with a compulsion to check with doctors, family, friends, and Internet sources for reassurance. The clinical similarities between illness anxiety disorder and obsessive-compulsive disorder have led some researchers to conclude that illness anxiety disorder and obsessive-compulsive disorder share a similar etiology, likely including impaired function in the orbitofrontal–cingulate–striatal circuit. Family studies have shown a higher frequency of illness anxiety in patients with obsessive-compulsive disorder and in their first-degree family. Although there appears to be a **genetic predisposition** to illness anxiety disorder, experience with a disease or an ill loved one may precipitate an episode. For instance, those who recover from a serious disease (e.g., heart attack or cancer) may become fearful of relapse and interpret normal somatic sensations (e.g., muscle aches or gas pains) as evidence of illness. The belief that the individual will find a doctor to diagnosis and cure their symptoms may perpetuate the illness.

Body Dysmorphic Disorder

Patients with body dysmorphic disorder likely have **a genetic predisposition** to **obsessional** thinking, given the higher frequency of body dysmorphic disorder in families of patients with obsessive-compulsive disorder. The emotional and biological changes associated with adolescence may serve as precipitating factors. The displacement of underlying anxiety into morbid overconcern about appearance may perpetuate the disorder into adulthood by permitting the person to avoid issues of intimacy or sexuality. Alternatively, the focus on perceived faults in appearance leading the individual to avoid social contacts may protect against a fear of rejection. Rather than consider any psychological shortcomings, such as low self-esteem, the individual can avoid social interactions and blame the avoidance on defects in his or her appearance.

Factitious Disorder

Since patients with factitious disorders tend to flee abruptly from care, these disorders are difficult to study systematically; we rely greatly on pooled case reports for etiology. Factitious disorders likely represent a multidetermined clinical entity. During childhood, many of these patients or their close family members experienced a serious illness. Some patients report holding a grudge against the medical profession, often the result of some real or perceived medical mismanagement. An occupational association may exist, since many patients report having worked as nurses, laboratory technicians, and other health professionals. Patients with factitious disorder also frequently report that they have had an important relationship with a physician, and some report that a physician seduced them.

Patients with factitious disorder frequently have **borderline personality disorder**. Some researchers have suggested that factitious disorder is an extreme form of borderline personality disorder. A history of **abuse** is frequently reported in patients with factitious disorder as well as those with borderline personality disorder. A familial pattern may exist in the relationship between factitious disorder and factitious disorder imposed on another. Victimized children may continue the factitious disorder by simulating illness themselves, in the same way that a subset of people who are victims of abuse may go on to perpetrate abuse later in life. Many of the underlying psychological issues found in patients with factitious disorder are present in borderline personality disorder, including chronic feelings of emptiness and boredom, intolerance of being alone, idealization and devaluation, constant anger, and poor impulse control. In patients with both diagnoses, the self-destructive tendency to "act out" takes the form of self-inflicted wounds and provocation of unnecessary procedures or surgeries, which may seem nearly suicidal.

TREATMENT

Early intervention can reduce patient suffering, diminish the potential for chronicity, decrease the risk of unnecessary treatments and iatrogenic harm, and help preserve the doctor–patient relationship. The earliest interventions for somatic symptom disorders often occur in nonpsychiatric settings, where patients typically come to medical attention. Given that it is not unusual for undiagnosed physical illness to be later identified in patients initially diagnosed with somatic symptom disorders, collaboration and communication between the psychiatrist and referring physician can help provide the best care possible for the patient and minimize medical errors on both sides.

With individually tailored treatment, specific illnesses and their degree of severity can be addressed, to maximize patients' chances of recovery. General principles of treatment planning for patients with somatic symptom disorders include the taking of a careful history for depression and bipolar illness, schizophrenia, neurocognitive syndromes, and personality disorders. A careful medical and parallel psychosocial history must be taken to uncover exacerbating events, ameliorative situations, and the state of the patients' functioning in work and relationships. These lines of exploration can reveal the variables that treatment planning can then address. There is an increasing array of evidence-based treatments to help patients learn to live with bothersome somatic symptoms and better tolerate the physical and psychological distress of somatic symptom disorder. Medication and psychotherapy can each play a role individually and jointly, with the exact mix of therapies depending on the patient's illness profile, preferences, personality style, and personal strengths.

Somatic Symptom Disorder

The psychiatrist, acting concurrently as a consultant with the primary care provider, will usually suggest that the patient maintain ties with only one primary physician and avoid contact with other physicians not familiar with the patient. This limitation should minimize overprescribing of medications and procedures, including unnecessary surgery. All physicians working with these patients should be prepared for long-term involvement; empathy with the patient's suffering is essential.

Successful treatment is particularly problematic in patients who are obtaining secondary gain, such as disability or workers' compensation. While quick settlement of compensation issues is best, this is often impossible given the adversarial nature of some proceedings.

There is evidence that medication and psychotherapy are each moderately effective for reducing somatic symptom disorders and associated pain symptoms. Several classes of antidepressants seem to provide significant pain relief even in patients who do not have a depressive syndrome, including **serotonin and norepinephrine reuptake inhibitors** (SNRIs), and **tricyclic antidepressants** that mostly affect the noradrenergic system (i.e., desipramine) (see Chapter 16, Pharmacotherapy, ECT, and TMS). Certain anticonvulsants that are **alpha-2-delta ligands**, such as pregabalin and gabapentin, are helpful in reducing central pain syndromes. Low doses of glutamatergic agents, such as **ketamine,** are also being investigated for their potential to reduce central sensitization. The prescription of analgesics that are physically addicting is discouraged, in part because they can disrupt sleep architecture and worsen physical symptoms.

Cognitive-behavioral therapy and physical **relaxation interventions** appear moderately helpful in treating the symptoms of somatic symptom disorder. Treatment is generally focused on alleviating, rather than eliminating, the patient's symptoms and minimizing the social and occupational consequences. Inpatient treatment may be necessary for detoxification if narcotic misuse or abuse is present. Outpatient regimens can include group therapy, educational instruction, and physical therapy,

Conversion Disorder

Treatment of the patient with conversion disorder involves a joint undertaking by the referring doctor, usually a neurologist, and the psychiatrist. It is important that a thorough medical workup be completed. In the absence of a demonstrable underlying disorder that accounts for the patient's symptoms, the patient should be confidently reassured that no serious illness has been found. When a relationship is identified between trauma, conflict, or stressors, a variety of treatment modalities can be suggested.

Psychotherapy can be presented to the patient as focusing on "stress management." Doing so often helps the patient to understand and accept the intense conflicts and emotions that may be producing or maintaining the symptoms. Once insight is gained into these psychological factors, the patient's symptoms usually subside. Family therapy may be indicated to address contributory stressors such as abuse, marital or family conflict, or dependence. Some patients may respond better to relaxation techniques employed in a behavioral approach than to more psychodynamic approaches. Experiencing the "mind–body" dissociation of **hypnosis**, or the induction of a trance-like state, may be helpful for some patients. Additionally, training patients in self-hypnosis with suggestions for symptomatic improvement may sometimes be useful in alleviating symptoms.

In cases of fixed postures, weakness, or gait abnormalities, **physical therapy** allows patients to preserve their dignity and self-respect while physically improving from conversion symptoms. Physical therapy also treats the disuse atrophy and contractures that may develop when neurological conversion symptoms have been quite prolonged and persistent.

Pharmacotherapy is indicated to treat comorbid depressive, anxiety, or psychotic conditions. Brief treatment with anxiolytic medications such as **benzodiazipines** can be a useful adjunct that facilitates the psychotherapeutic process. Intravenous amobarbital infusions have been used as well.

Illness Anxiety Disorder

Selective serotonin reuptake inhibitors (SSRIs) and cognitive-behavioral therapy have the most empirical support for treatment of illness anxiety disorder. Pharmacotherapy may also help by reducing comorbid anxiety and depressive symptoms. An adequate pharmacological trial with an SSRI requires daily medication for at least 8 weeks. Pharmacological therapy should start low and go high, as patients with anxiety may be particularly sensitive to medication side effects (so start low), but higher doses may be more effective than lower doses. The latter phenomenon has been observed among patients with obsessive-compulsive disorder as well; this similarity in treatment responsiveness may reflect a similar underlying etiology.

Cognitive-behavioral therapy reduces symptoms and improves general functioning by teaching the patient techniques to modify dysfunctional thoughts and behaviors (see Chapter 17, Psychotherapy). Patients learn to recognize that not every physical symptom indicates serious disease, and that being healthy does not necessarily mean being symptom-free. Patients with illness anxiety disorder are often remarkably aware of their bodies, to the point that symptoms that would not reach the threshold of awareness for most people sound internal alarms of concern for them. Cognitive-behavioral therapy includes teaching techniques for distraction and relaxation. Psychoeducation may be helpful for patients with chronic illness who develop illness anxiety symptoms. They should be educated about the illness and guided in adjusting to limitations and disabilities. For example, the post-myocardial infarction patient who fears that every instance of chest pain indicates a new attack may benefit from learning the difference between angina and infarction. These patients should also be taught how to differentiate activities that are potentially dangerous (e.g., shoveling snow in extremely cold weather) from those that are not (e.g., mildly strenuous sexual relations).

It is generally helpful to focus treatment on the emotional stressors and the dysfunctional cognitions and behaviors that exacerbate and/or perpetuate illness anxiety disorder rather than on the symptoms themselves. It may be useful to schedule regular appointments with patients in a time-contingent rather than symptom-contingent manner, allowing sufficient time during each visit for patients to discuss their problems. Once the diagnosis of illness anxiety disorder is made, it is also important to limit the repetition of tests and avoid unnecessary treatment that can lead to iatrogenic complications.

Body Dysmorphic Disorder

Cognitive-behavioral therapy and SSRIs have the most empirical support for the treatment of body dysmorphic disorder. **Cognitive-behavioral therapy** techniques are used to identify and challenge the patient's cognitive distortions about their appearance and help them to develop more adaptive patterns of coping rather than unnecessary surgeries, excessive mirror checking, picking, and camouflaging behaviors. Supportive and insight-oriented psychotherapies do not appear to be effective for the treatment of this disorder. **SSRIs** may be effective first-line pharmacological treatment. Although antipsychotics are indicated for patients with the somatic type of **delusional disorder**, there is no convincing evidence supporting the use of antipsychotic medications in body dysmorphic disorder.

Factitious Disorder

Effective interventions have not been identified for patients with factitious disorder. It has been difficult to evaluate the effect of a full course of treatment for these patients because treatment tends to be terminated prematurely by the patient's departure. For children or adolescents with factitious disorder, early intervention appears helpful.

One overall goal of treatment is to prevent patients from undergoing unnecessary and potentially dangerous or invasive procedures. Another goal is to sufficiently engage patients so that they receive care in only one facility, where staff members can become familiar with them and follow them over time. This strategy may prevent factitious disorder from progressing into persistent Munchausen's syndrome. One way to achieve this is to acknowledge to patients that their need to fabricate illnesses means that they are indeed very seriously ill with a psychiatric disorder. It is helpful for the entire medical staff to regard these patients as being truly very ill and in need of intensive psychiatric care. Patients may be able to accept their true diagnosis when it is discussed within the context of a supportive relationship. Once patients feel that they are understood and begin to understand their own motivation, they may no longer have the impulse to feign new symptoms.

In suspected cases of factitious disorder imposed on another, it is necessary to involve the appropriate **government agencies** responsible for the welfare of children, because the traumas inflicted on children through an adult's feigning of their illness are tantamount to child abuse. Long-term monitoring of the child and siblings is often necessary and may include removal of children from the care of the offending parent(s). It is also critical to recognize that parents may be inadvertently labeled as having factitious disorder imposed on another when faced with having a "sick child"; this situation may manifest especially when a real medical illness with diverse manifestations is a widespread risk in the community and when that disease does not yet have adequate diagnostic tests to confirm the presence or absence of disease (e.g., Lyme disease). Accusations of factitious disorder imposed on another not uncommonly occur in the context of a divorce in which the medical care of the child becomes a focus of the marital discord. In this situation, careful re-education of the parents about the rationale for the medical doctor's conclusions and what is deemed best for the child is essential to prevent false accusations of factitious disorder imposed on another and unjustified legal intrusion.

SELECTED READINGS

Barsky, A. J. Forgetting, fabricating, and telescoping: the instability of the medical history. *Archives of Internal Medicine* 162:981–984, 2002.

Barsky, A. J., and D. K. Ahern. Cognitive behavior therapy for hypochondriasis. *JAMA: Journal of the American Medical Association* 291:1464–1470, 2004.

Barsky, A. J., and J. F. Borus. Functional somatic syndromes. *Annals of Internal Medicine* 130: 910–921, 1999.

Barsky, A. J., E. J. Orav, and D. W. Bates. Somatization increases medical utilization and costs independent of psychiatric and medical comorbidity. *Archives of General Psychiatry* 62:903–910, 2005.

Coghill, R. C., J. G. McHaffie, and Y. F. Yen. Neural correlates of interindividual differences in the subjective experience of pain. *Proceedings of the National Academy of Science USA* 100: 8538–8542, 2003.

Dimsdale, J. E., and R. Dantzer. A biological substrate for somatoform disorders: importance of pathophysiology. *Psychosomatic Medicine* 69:850–854, 2007.

Fallon, B. A., A. I. Qureshi, G. Laje, and B. Klein. Hypochondriasis and its relationship to obsessive-compulsive disorder. *Psychiatric Clinic of North America* 23:605–616, 2000.

Fliege, H., G. Scholler, M. Rose, H. Willenberg, and B. Klap. Factitious disorders and pathological self-harm in a hospital population: an interdisciplinary challenge. *General Hospital Psychiatry* 24: 164–171, 2002.

Fröhlich, C., F. Jacobi, and H. U. Wittchen. DSM-IV pain disorder in the general population: an exploration of the structure and threshold of medically unexplained pain symptoms. *European Archives of Psychiatry and Clinical Neuroscience* 256:187–196, 2006.

Greeven, A., A. J. L. M. van Balkom, S. Visser, J. W. Merkelbach, Y. R. van Rood, R. van Dyck, A. J. Van der Does, F. G. Zitman, and P. Spinhoven. Cognitive behavior therapy and paroxetine in the treatment of hypochondriasis: a randomized controlled trial. *American Journal of Psychiatry* 164:91–99, 2007.

Harding, K. J., N. Skritskaya, E. Doherty, and B. A. Fallon. Advances in understanding illness anxiety. *Current Psychiatry Reports* 10(4):311–317, 2008.

Kinns, H., D. Housley, and D. Freedman. Munchausen syndrome and factitious disorder: the role of the laboratory in its detection and diagnosis. *Annals of Clinical Biochemistry* 50(Pt 3):194–203, 2013.

Krahn, L. E., J. M. Bostwick, and C. M. Stonnington. Looking toward DSM–V: should factitious disorder become a subtype of somatoform disorder? *Psychosomatics* 49:277–282, 2008.

Krahn L. E., L. Hongzhe, and M. K. O'Conner. Patients who strive to be ill: factitious disorder with physical symptoms. *American Journal of Psychiatry* 160:1163–1168, 2003.

Kroenke, K. Efficacy of treatment for somatoform disorders: a review of randomized controlled trials. *Psychosomatic Medicine* 69:881–888, 2007.

Kroenke, K., M. Sharpe, and R. Sykes. Revising the classification of somatoform disorders: key questions and preliminary recommendations. *Psychosomatics* 48:277–285, 2007.

Kroenke, K., E. E. Krebs, and M. J. Bair. Pharmacotherapy of chronic pain: a synthesis of recommendations from systematic reviews. *General Hospital Psychiatry* 31(3):206–219, 2009.

Libow, J. A. Child and adolescent illness falsification. *Pediatrics* 105:58–64, 2000.

Marks, D. M., M. J. Shah, A. A. Patkar, P. S. Masand, G.-Y. Park, and C.-U. Pae. Serotonin-norepinephrine reuptake inhibitors for pain control: premise and promise. *Current Neuropharmacology* 7(4):331–336, 2009.

Moene, F. C., E. H. Lanberg, K. A. Hoogduin, P. Spinhoven, L. I. Hertzberger, R. P. Kleyweg, and J. Weeda. Organic syndromes diagnosed as conversion disorder: identification and frequency in a study of 85 patients. *Journal of Psychosomatic Research* 49:7–12, 2000.

Pasco, J. A., G. C. Nicholson, L. J. Williams, F. N. Jacka, M. J. Henry, M. A. Kotowicz, H. G. Schneider, B. E. Leonard, and M. Berk. Association of high-sensitivity C-reactive protein with de novo major depression. *British Journal of Psychiatry* 197(5):372–377, 2010.

Phillips, K. A. Body dysmorphic disorder: the distress of imagined ugliness. *American Journal of Psychiatry* 148:1138–1149, 1991.

Phillips, K. A., and E. Hollander. Treating body dysmorphic disorder with medication: evidence, misconceptions, and a suggested approach. *Body Image* 5:13–27, 2008.

Phillips, K. A., W. Menard, C. Fay, and R. Weisberg. Demographic characteristics, phenomenology, comobidity, and family history in 200 individuals with body dysmorphic disorder. *Psychosomatics* 46: 317–325, 2005.

Rogers, R. *Clinical Assessment of Malingering and Deception*, 3rd ed. New York: Guilford Press, 2008.

Schreier, H. Munchausen by proxy defined. *Pediatrics* 110(5): 985–988, 2002.

Schweitzer, P. J., U. Zafar, M. Pavlicova, and B. A. Fallon. Long-term follow-up of hypochondriasis after selective serotonin reuptake inhibitor treatment. *Journal of Clinical Psychopharmacology* 31(3):365–368, 2011.

Sheridan, M. S. The deceit continues: an updated literature review of Munchausen syndrome by proxy. *Child Abuse and Neglect* 27:431–451, 2003.

Stephenson, J. Patient pretenders weave tangled 'web' of deceit. *JAMA: Journal of the American Medical Association* 280:1297, 1998.

Thomson, A. B., and L. A. Page. Psychotherapies for hypochondriasis. *The Cochrane Database of Systematic Reviews* 2008; 1.

Wessely, S., C. Nimnuan, and M. Sharpe. Functional somatic syndromes: One or many? *Lancet* 354: 936–939, 1999.

Psychological Factors Affecting Medical Conditions

SARA SIRIS NASH, LUCY HUTNER, AND EVE CALIGOR

Patients with physical illness face numerous psychological challenges. Underlying psychiatric conditions, including depression and anxiety, may be exacerbated during acute or chronic medical illness, and new psychiatric problems can emerge. Personality traits may become exaggerated and usually effective coping skills may become distorted, impairing the patient's ability to manage medical illness, including hospitalizations, acute illness flairs, and chronic pain, and even interfering with the patient's adherence to treatment regimens. By understanding the psychological challenges faced by patients who are medically ill, physicians can help their patients cope with both the illness itself and treatment. In order to do so, those who practice medicine must pay attention to the human aspects of their patients, specifically their emotions, behaviors, and relationships. Recognizing these complex and varied psychological issues, physicians can integrate their knowledge of human emotion and behavior into their day-to-day medical management of patients. Chronic illness, chronic pain, and adherence to treatment are all conditions in which psychological factors play a particularly important role.

DIAGNOSTIC FEATURES

The DSM-5 diagnosis of psychological factors affecting other medical conditions focuses attention on the interplay of psychological and behavioral factors with medical illness (see DSM-5). This diagnosis is included under the umbrella of somatic symptom and related disorders (see Chapter 10, Somatic Symptom and Related Disorders). Patients with this diagnosis have at least one psychological or behavioral factor that is adversely influencing their medical condition. These factors include psychological distress, interpersonal problems, coping styles, and maladaptive health behaviors. It is important to distinguish psychological and behavioral factors affecting medical illness from an adjustment disorder, in which maladaptive psychological and behavioral symptoms result directly from the presence of a medical illness. Several other conditions are on the differential: mental disorders due to another medical condition, in which the underlying medical illness itself, through set physiological pathways, results in the presence of psychiatric symptoms (see Chapter 5, Neurocognitive Disorders and Mental Disorders Due to Another Medical Condition); somatic symptom disorder, in which the patient is excessively distressed about a physical symptom; and illness anxiety disorder, in which neither an underlying medical condition nor somatic symptoms may be present, but the patient is preoccupied with concern about having a serious illness (see Chapter 10, Somatic Symptom and Related Disorders).

PSYCHOLOGICAL REACTIONS TO PHYSICAL ILLNESS

All patients with medical conditions experience psychological reactions to their illness. The reactions that a patient has vary according to both the nature of the illness and the nature of the patient. Relevant aspects of the illness include its severity and chronicity, as well as the site and nature of the symptoms. Relevant patient characteristics include age, level of maturity, character style, previous experience with illness, and social supports. A psychodynamic approach to patients' behaviors, personality structures, conflicts, and relationships is essential to the care of medically ill individuals. Understanding patients' and physicians' reactions, as well as identifying the meanings of illness for these individuals, can have an important and beneficial impact on treatment.

A person's psychological reactions to being ill and the ability to cope with illness can play an enormous role in determining a patient's quality of life during an illness and also have a powerful effect on medical course and outcome. Some responses to illness are adaptive, allowing patients to tolerate being sick and facilitating their adherence to treatment. Other reactions may be maladaptive and concomitantly can cause great distress and interfere with management.

General Psychological Responses to Physical Illness

Regression, denial, anxiety, depression, and anger are general responses to illness that are common to all human beings and originate in the various meanings that people attribute to physical illness, the fears typically raised by being ill, and the mechanisms commonly used to cope with the illness.

Regression
Clinical Features
Regression is a nearly universal psychological reaction to being ill in which people revert to more **childlike ways of thinking and behaving**. Importantly, illness places the individual in a situation of dependency, which replicates the developmental stressors of early childhood. Because of this, it is common to observe regression to less reality-based thinking and the use of more primitive defenses. It is important to recognize that some degree of regression is adaptive, especially in the more acute phases of an illness. **Adaptive regression** reduces the psychological stress of illness and hospitalization by making it easier for the patient to assume a dependent role and to relate positively to physicians and other care providers. Regressed patients are likely to idealize their physicians, viewing them as powerful, good, all-knowing people who always have their best interests in mind. The **idealization** of caretakers provides powerful protection against anxiety and worry for patients, who must put their physical and emotional well-being into the hands of strangers. Strain and Grossman (1975) identified seven broad categories of psychological stress faced by hospitalized patients that both demonstrate and explain these behaviors. These categories

include (1) the basic threat to narcissistic integrity; (2) fear of strangers; (3) separation anxiety; (4) fear of the loss of love and approval; (5) fear of the loss of control of developmentally achieved functions; (6) fear of, loss of, or injury to body parts; and (7) reactivation of feelings of guilt and shame, and fears of retaliation for previous transgressions.

While a moderate amount of regression can be adaptive, regression can become maladaptive when it takes a more extreme or long-lasting form, as is illustrated in the case example in Box 11.1. Extreme regression in patients can produce overly **demanding** behavior during hospitalization. Such patients may refuse to undergo necessary procedures or comply with treatment, or they may become excessively **passive** and unwilling or even unable to do anything for themselves. They may be classified as "difficult" or "hateful," and their demanding, regressive behavior may alienate physicians, nurses, and even family members, whose withdrawal may further escalate patients' demands for gratification of their dependency needs.

Excessive or unduly prolonged regression can become especially problematic once the acute phase of an illness has passed and it is time for patients to take more responsibility for their care and their lives. They may fail to leave the **sick role** behind, remaining passive and disabled and refusing to comply with further medical treatment. Their regressed role may have become so gratifying or, conversely, so demoralizing that they lose motivation to recover. Even after they have been discharged from the hospital, they may continue to behave in a regressive manner, failing to resume their usual activities or responsibilities

---

BOX 11.1
CASE EXAMPLE OF REGRESSION

A 50-year-old woman was admitted to the hospital with a mild heart attack. She was usually a domineering matriarch who ran her household and her family real estate business by barking out orders and attacking anyone who tried to give her advice. Her internist and her family feared that she would be a truly "impossible" patient. However, to everyone's amazement, she was a model patient in the critical care unit. She followed the physicians' medication and activity orders, cooperated with diagnostic procedures, and interacted pleasantly with the nursing staff when they helped her use the bedpan and wash and dress herself. This patient regressed from her usual domineering attitude to a more childlike, passive demeanor, in which she unquestioningly put her faith in her caretakers, assuming that they knew best, and followed their instructions. However, even after she was transferred out of the critical care unit, she spent her entire hospital stay in bed, refusing to participate in cardiac rehabilitation. She constantly called on nurses and visiting relatives to help her with even the smallest requests. After being released from the hospital, she continued to be demanding and passive, doing nothing for herself and insisting that her family attend to all of her needs. She refused to take walks or otherwise increase her tolerance for exercise, as her physicians had recommended, and would not resume her usual household or business responsibilities. She seemed unable to re-acclimate from her regressed role.

and relying on family members to take care of their needs. Such patients often have difficulty adhering to outpatient follow-up treatment recommendations.

Interview and Management

If regression is interfering with a patient's cooperation with medical recommendations or recovery from illness or both, either during hospitalization or after discharge, intervention is necessary. The first step is for the physician to **explore** the reasons for and meanings of the behaviors with the patient (see Box 11.2, General Interviewing and Management Guidelines in the Medical Setting). This discussion can begin with the physician's commenting on the patient's behavior and inquiring about it: "I notice that you are relying very heavily on the nursing staff. For example, you are still asking for assistance when you go to the bathroom. Are you feeling afraid to do more on your own?" The regressive behavior may remit in some patients after their conscious fears have been alleviated by **education** and **reassurance**.

If discussion and reassurance fail, the physician may find it useful to **set limits** and/ or create a **behavioral contract**. Ongoing individual work with the patient and meetings with the patient's family are usually helpful, because the physician can correct interactions with family members that reinforce the patient's regressive behaviors. If a

---

BOX 11.2

GENERAL INTERVIEWING AND MANAGEMENT GUIDELINES IN THE MEDICAL SETTING

- Do not underestimate the power of the physician–patient relationship. Some of the strongest "medicines" available are taking time to talk with the patient and showing your concern for him or her.
- Ask the patient how he or she is coping with the illness.
- Ask specifically about practical problems resulting from the illness, such as family or marital, financial, and job-related problems.
- Inquire specifically about emotional effects, including anxiety and depression, and the use of alcohol or other substances. Introduce these subjects by saying that these are common feelings and behaviors in patients who are trying to cope with medical illness.
- Speak with the patient's family. They can be a crucial source of information for the physician and a valuable source of support for the patient.
- When recommending treatment, assume out loud that adherence will be a problem. Invite the patient to work out a strategy with you for approaching this challenge.
- When a patient is asking for reassurance that you cannot offer, remember that it may be therapeutic to simply inquire about and listen to the patient's feelings.
- Remain aware of your own feelings about the patient, and use these reactions in service of the patient's care.

maladaptively regressed patient is in the hospital, the physician should work with staff to help them kindly, but firmly, set limits on the patient's behavior.

Denial

Clinical Features

Denial is an unconscious psychological defense mechanism in which the existence or significance of a painful or frightening situation is kept out of the patient's conscious awareness. It is a way of **warding off feelings of anxiety, depression, or despair** until they can be dealt with more comfortably. Some degree of denial is an extremely common reaction to medical illness. A moderate degree of denial need not be a problem and can even be adaptive at times. For example, for the woman who has discovered a lump in her breast and who has scheduled a biopsy in 2 days' time, denial of the possibility of cancer may help her manage better until a definitive diagnosis can be made. Indeed, in the acute phase, denial can mitigate severe anxiety, panic, or despair and can help the patient maintain a calm and hopeful attitude. For the patient with chronic medical illness, mild denial may also help to ward off depression.

However, severe denial can pose serious problems. It can lead to a **delay** in seeking treatment and to **refusal** of necessary interventions or diagnostic tests. If the same woman described above discovered the breast mass but decided against having a biopsy or bringing her finding to medical attention because she determined she could not possibly have cancer, this would be an example of pathological, or maladaptive, denial. In chronically ill patients, maladaptive denial often causes the patient to refuse to take medications or make necessary lifestyle modifications. As with patients experiencing regression, patients in denial can also benefit from education, support, and appropriate reassurance, as illustrated in the case example presented in Box 11.3.

BOX 11.3
CASE EXAMPLE OF DENIAL

A 27-year-old man with AIDS was admitted to the hospital with shortness of breath and cough and was diagnosed with *Pneumocystis carinii* pneumonia (PCP). This was his fourth hospitalization this year for opportunistic infections. He reported that he had not been taking his antiretroviral medications for the last several months because he felt his HIV disease was "just not that bad." A psychiatric consult was requested to help the infectious disease team with management of the patient's denial. During the first several visits, the patient blandly maintained that he did not feel that he would die of AIDS and that antiretroviral HIV medications were not necessary. The medical team decided to keep him in the hospital for an extended period so that he could complete his treatment for PCP and be educated about the potential lethality of his disease. After several visits, the patient revealed to the psychiatrist that he was terrified to die alone, because his extended family was still in his native country. The psychiatrist empathically supported his point of view and validated his concerns. The patient eventually called his sister, arranged for her to come to visit him, and agreed to follow-up care with the AIDS team.

Interview and Management

When denial is mild and does not interfere with the management of the illness, physicians should generally respect patients' needs to defend themselves in this way. The physician should follow the patient's lead, indicating his or her availability to discuss matters with the patient but not pressuring the patient to do so. For the patient whose denial is interfering with treatment, a more active approach is needed. Rather than resorting to direct confrontation, the physician should "chip away" gradually at the denial by introducing **new information** to the patient about his or her illness. After presenting one piece of information, the physician should watch for the patient's reaction to and retention of the material before introducing the next piece of information. In this way, the physician can diagnose feelings of anxiety or depression underlying the denial and help the patient deal with these feelings as soon as they arise, as the case example in Box 11.3 illustrates.

More pressing situations in which the patient's denial is leading to frankly dangerous or life-threatening behavior (e.g., refusal of necessary treatments) require that the physician challenge the patient's defenses by confronting the denial. Patients often react to such a **confrontation** with powerful feelings of anger, anxiety, panic, or depression. Some patients react by threatening to leave the hospital against medical advice or becoming suicidal. Other patients rapidly slip back into even more rigid denial, sometimes of psychotic proportions, which is often accompanied by enormous hostility and even threatening behavior.

These reactions present serious management problems and should be treated as a potential emergency. Physicians and staff members should maintain a calm but firm attitude toward such patients, and family members, if available, should be enlisted to help calm the patient and perhaps even convince the patient to comply with necessary treatments. In the case of psychotic denial, the patient may lack the capacity to give informed consent, in which case a health care proxy should be invoked.

In emergency situations, ensuring the safety of the patient, the staff, and other patients takes the highest priority. If the patient is threatening to leave or to commit suicidal or violent acts, **one-on-one constant supervision** with maximal levels of observation and, if necessary, the involvement of the hospital security staff should be arranged immediately. Low dosages of antipsychotic medications or benzodiazepines may improve the patient's impulse control and help the patient to feel calmer, less threatened, and less hostile.

Anxiety

Clinical Features

Anxiety is essentially an **alarm reaction** that warns an individual of incipient danger. Being ill stimulates many fears, and most medically ill patients suffer from some degree of anxiety during the course of their illness. Cognitive manifestations of anxiety include fear, worry, and ruminative thoughts. Somatic symptoms include palpitations, sweating, dizziness, shortness of breath, hyperventilation, tremulousness, and mild agitation. It goes without saying that one must rule out a physical cause for these symptoms before attributing them to anxiety (see Chapter 6, Anxiety, Obsessive-Compulsive, and Stress Disorders).

A mild degree of anxiety may be adaptive because it keeps patients alert to potential dangers that they may encounter and may therefore enhance adherence to treatment. However, moderate to severe anxiety in medically ill patients can pose a significant problem. In the acute setting, extreme anxiety can interfere with patients' ability to absorb information, follow instructions, or cooperate with necessary diagnostic procedures and therapeutic interventions. In some illnesses, anxiety can even pose a direct physiological risk. In a patient who has had an acute myocardial infarction, for example, extreme anxiety can lead to tachycardia and increased blood pressure, which can increase the work of the heart. In a patient who is having an asthma attack, feelings of panic can result in hyperventilation and intensify respiratory distress. Excess anxiety in chronically ill or convalescing patients can interfere with rehabilitation and recovery and lead to unnecessary chronic invalidism.

Interview and Management

The first step in managing anxiety is for the physician to clarify with patients the **specific content** of their fears. Frequent sources of anxiety include fears of death, disability, or dependence on others. Once the sources of anxiety have been identified, the physician can plan appropriate interventions. Anxious patients are commonly confused about what has happened to them medically, and they may be worrying about unfounded concerns. For example, many patients incorrectly assume that a diagnosis of cancer means that they are terminally ill; that a diagnosis of heart failure means that the heart has permanently "failed;" or that a diagnosis of uncomplicated myocardial infarction means that they will be unable to return to work or resume sexual relations with their partner. In many cases, physicians can reduce a patient's anxiety by simply correcting distortions, giving more **accurate information**, and providing realistic reassurance.

Patients may also have reasonable, well-founded fears about their medical status. These patients benefit from **realistic reassurance** that emphasizes the range of available treatments. It is crucial that physicians let anxious patients know that they will "stick by" them through the ups and downs that lie ahead. The physician's positive attitude, calm demeanor, ongoing concern, and availability are powerful antidotes. For example, a physician might say to a patient who has been recently diagnosed with breast cancer, "I understand that being told you have breast cancer can be very frightening. Let me assure you that we have excellent treatments available. I will go over the options with you in detail and will help you make decisions at each step along the way." Allowing patients to ask questions, as well as simply sitting and "being with" the patient can also have a profoundly powerful effect on anxiety.

If the interventions of exploration, clarification, education, and reassurance are incompletely successful and the patient continues to suffer from moderate to severe anxiety, the judicious use of medications may be indicated. In general, when prescribing medications to patients who are medically ill, the physician must be particularly cognizant of the effects that each medication might have. Drug–drug interactions, inhibition or induction of the cytochrome P450 system, and adverse effects such as orthostatic hypotension, sedation, and cardiac effects all need to be taken into account.

For treatment of anxiety, first-line medications include the **selective serotonin reuptake inhibitors** (SSRIs). The side effects of SSRIs tend to be relatively mild, are often transient, and are generally well tolerated by medically ill patients (see Chapter 16, Pharmacotherapy, ECT, and TMS). **Benzodiazepines** may also be used on a short-term basis (i.e., for several days to several weeks). Lorezapam is often a good choice for medically ill patients because it has no active metabolites, bypasses hepatic oxidation, has a medium length half-life, and generally does not cause the rebound anxiety associated with shorter-acting benzodiazepines such as alprazolam. Particular caution should be taken for elderly patients, for whom benzodiazepines can result in oversedation, confusion, and falls. In addition, benzodiazepine agents can produce paradoxic agitation in patients with preexisting brain disease (such as traumatic brain injury) and the elderly. When benzodiazepines are discontinued, the dosage should be tapered, rather than abruptly stopped, to prevent withdrawal, which can be life threatening. If, after a few weeks, a patient continues to be significantly disabled by anxiety, the physician should more fully clarify the sources of the anxiety, both conscious and unconscious, making a thorough search for physical factors (especially medications) that may be exacerbating the anxiety, and developing a clarified diagnosis. Such an evaluation paves the way for a comprehensive treatment plan.

Depression

Clinical Features

Whereas anxiety is essentially an alarm reaction that warns an individual of incipient danger, depression is an emotional response to what is commonly experienced by the patient as a loss (for which the depressed person often feels in some way responsible). It should not then be surprising that depressive feelings are common psychological reactions to physical illness, as illness itself represents a form of **loss** for most patients. Patients experience many different kinds of losses, ranging from the loss of certain physical abilities, to the loss of bodily integrity, to the loss of organs or limbs. **Feelings of loss of control** are virtually universal among hospitalized patients, who must adhere to hospital rules and routines, wear proscribed hospital attire, and are sometimes unable to independently control the most basic of bodily functions. Most patients find that they cannot do some of the things that had previously been an important part of their identities (e.g., fulfilling family roles, taking care of professional responsibilities, and participating in recreational and social activities). Even in the best of circumstances, all medical patients suffer an important loss—the loss of their sense of being healthy.

When speaking about depressed feelings with medically ill patients, the physician should actively evaluate for a full-blown **major depressive episode.** Though it is easy to err in either direction, depression tends to be underdiagnosed in medically ill patients. This error occurs, in part, because of the commonly held misconception that it is "expected" for people who are physically ill to be depressed. Although there are important biological correlates between certain disease states (such as pancreatic cancer, or certain paraneoplastic syndromes, for example) and depressive symptoms, major depression in medically ill patients should never be considered "normal," and it must be aggressively identified and treated.

Interview and Management

Distinguishing between a *depressive reaction* and a *major depression* in a medically ill patient can be difficult. The difficulty is compounded by the tendency of the neurovegetative symptoms of depression (including anorexia, lack of energy, and insomnia) to overlap with many of the symptoms of both medical illness and the side effects of commonly prescribed medications. The characteristics in Box 11.4 can be helpful in identifying symptoms in the medically ill as those of a major depressive episode.

Undiagnosed major depression in medically ill patients can lead to **nonadherence** with treatment and a poor medical outcome. Patients tend to withdraw into themselves and become passive and uncommunicative. They may feel apathetic about their care and often relinquish decision-making responsibilities to others. They may eat poorly and lose weight, further compromising their medical condition. For some depressed, medically ill patients, certain behaviors (e.g., not taking medications, not communicating with physicians) reflect an unarticulated wish to be dead. Such patients should be considered to have suicidal ideation and should be evaluated and treated accordingly (see Chapter 12, Suicide).

BOX 11.4

CHARACTERISTICS OF MEDICALLY ILL PATIENTS SUFFERING FROM MAJOR DEPRESSION

- Display a lack of interest in their medical management
- Have a personal or family history of affective disorder
- Have pervasive and long-lasting symptoms
- Describe an inability to enjoy anything at all
- Suffer from a profound sense of being "bad" or guilty
- Have thoughts of committing suicide

For medically ill patients who are having depressive symptoms but are not suffering from a major depression, the physician should explain that some depressed feelings are not uncommon in people who are ill and that, for many people, feelings of depression are a way of coming to terms with what is happening to them and are often transient. The physician should keep in mind that patients often feel guilty or angry at themselves, believing that they have brought on the illness. Such concerns should be sought out and addressed. The physician might say, "Most people have a theory about how or why they have become ill. What are your ideas about why this has happened?"

The approach to patients with depressive symptoms requires the physician to establish a differential diagnosis, as depressive symptoms can be the manifestations of a major depressive disorder, demoralization (as seen in adjustment disorders with depressed features), or even a hypoactive delirium (see Chapter 5, Neurocognitive Disorders and Mental Disorders Due to Another Medical Condition). A **complete psychiatric evaluation**, including a detailed personal and family history of mood disorders, is essential. As certain medical illnesses and many commonly used medications can result in mood symptoms, a complete workup for **other medical causes** of depression is also critical.

Interventions should begin with **clarifying** what is depressing the patient. **Correcting distortions** and offering support and appropriate **reassurance** come next. The physician should not be too cheerful, nor tell the patient to "pull yourself up by your bootstraps," because either of these attitudes will quickly alienate the depressed patient. Instead, a sympathetic but professional attitude and an air of quiet optimism are more helpful. The physician might say, for example, "I know it's tough to live with torticollis and that the pain sometimes makes it really hard to get through the day. Fortunately, there is good news. Your disease does not seem to be progressing, and there are many available treatments that we haven't even tried yet. Also, let me assure you that most people find the first months the most difficult. After that, things tend to get easier." If these first-line interventions fail and the patient remains consistently depressed for several weeks or demonstrates suicidal thoughts or behavior, the diagnosis of a major depression should be reconsidered.

Medically ill patients who are suffering from a major depression usually require a combination of **medication** and **psychotherapy**. The SSRIs are the antidepressants of choice for medically ill patients, given their favorable efficacy and limited side effect profile. Other commonly used options include serotonin-norepinephrine reuptake inhibitors (SNRIs). The physician can take advantage of a particular medication's side effects for clinical purposes. For example, a patient whose depressive symptoms include insomnia and anorexia might benefit from the use of the antidepressant **mirtazapine**, whose clinical effect often includes sedation and increased appetite. Patients with low energy and lethargy might benefit from a more activating antidepressant, such as **bupropion** or **sertraline**. **Low-dose stimulants**, such as methylphenidate, also have their place in the treatment of depressed medically ill patients. Although they must be used with caution because of cardiac effects (such as tachycardia), they can elevate mood relatively quickly and may also increase energy and appetite in wasted, cachectic patients.

Anger and Agitation

Clinical Features

Many patients experience anger about being ill, but some patients become enraged and, in an effort to feel less helpless, guilty, or afraid, lash out at the people around them. These patients can become **hostile, suspicious**, and **accusatory** toward family members and medical staff. They may get into power struggles and instigate arguments, even with their physicians. For instance, a patient who developed a painful duodenal ulcer repeatedly lashed out at his wife for nagging him and causing him "stress." Unfortunately, the result of this behavior was to alienate his wife just at the time he most needed her and wanted comfort and reassurance from her. A more extreme example is the patient who was hospitalized following a myocardial infarction and who believed that the complications were caused by medications inappropriately prescribed by his intern. This patient refused all medications and went into a rage whenever the intern attempted to enter his room or examine him.

The first priority in managing an agitated patient is to **determine the cause.** Agitation due to an underlying **medical condition** should be ruled out first (see Chapter 5, Neurocognitive Disorders and Mental Disorders Due to Another Medical Condition). In this case, what appears to be "anger" may actually be a physiological effect of physical illness causing pain, or a neurocognitive disorder such as hyperactive delirium. In general, these patients will manifest other signs and symptoms of delirium, such as inattention, disorientation, and waxing and waning levels of consciousness.

The physician should also evaluate for the presence of an underlying dementia, particularly in elderly patients. **Dementia** can cause disinhibition, agitation, and low frustration tolerance, especially in the unfamiliar hospital setting. Paranoid or delusional patients may also exhibit agitation related to false beliefs about their care.

Last, it is crucial to rule out **substance intoxication or withdrawal** as a cause of symptoms (see Chapter 7, Substance-Related and Addictive Disorders). For example, a 45-year-old man was intimidating medical staff by repeatedly refusing procedures and screaming at care providers when they walked into the room. It was only several hours later, in the face of persistent tachycardia, hypertension, and tremor that the diagnosis of alcohol withdrawal was made. The common medical causes of agitation are listed in Table 11.1.

The physician should then turn his or her attention to primary psychiatric etiologies of an anger reaction. Patients with mood disorders, such as major depression or mania, may commonly present with an element of anger and low frustration tolerance. Patients with psychotic disorders may present with agitation, paranoia, and extreme suspiciousness. Cognitively impaired patients, including patients with dementia or traumatic brain injury, may present with anger or agitation symptoms. Also, patients with severe character pathology, such as borderline personality disorder, narcissistic personality disorder, and histrionic personality disorder, may manifest anger as part of their set of maladaptive coping skills, especially in the regressive environment of the hospital.

TABLE 11.1 Medical Causes of Agitation

Medications

Anticholinergic medications

Antidepressants

Antihistamines

Antiparkinsonian medications (e.g., L-dopa, bromocriptine, amantadine)

Chemotherapeutic agents (e.g., cyclosporine, procarbazine)

Corticosteroids and ACTH

Digitalis

Isoniazid

Muscle relaxants

Nonsteroidal anti-inflammatory agents

Opiates (e.g., meperidine, pentazocine)

Sympathicomimetics

Substance-induced (Intoxication or Withdrawal)

Alcohol

Amphetamine

Anabolic steroids

Cannabis

Cocaine

Hallucinogens

Inhalants

Phencyclidine

Sedative-hypnotics

Endocrine and Metabolic Disorders

Cushing's syndrome

Hepatic encephalopathy

Hypercalcemia

Hypercapnia

Hyperthyroidism

Hypocalcemia

Hypoglycemia

Hypothyroidism

Hypoxemia

Paraneoplastic syndrome

Porphyria

Neurological Disorders

Central nervous system malignant disease (primary and metastatic)

Cortical dementia (early manifestation)

HIV infection (AIDS encephalopathy)

Infection (e.g., viral encephalopathy)

Multiple sclerosis

Porphyria

Stroke

Subarachnoid hemorrhage

(continued)

TABLE 11.1 Continued

Subcortical dementia (e.g., Huntington's disease)

Temporal lobe epilepsy

Trauma (e.g., post-concussion syndrome)

Connective Tissue Disorders

Systemic lupus erythematosus (lupus cerebritis)

Temporal arteritis

Deficiency States and Toxins

Folate deficiency

Niacin deficiency

Heavy metal poisoning (e.g., lead poisoning)

Vitamin B_{12} deficiency

Interview and Management

Safety is of paramount concern, in order to prevent the patient from hurting himself or herself or caretakers. It is best to **minimize conflicts** and help the patient feel in control of what is happening. The physician should try to circumvent power struggles and capitulate to the patient's demands (e.g., for a change in a primary nurse or for additional portions of food) whenever possible. If confrontation is necessary, physicians should **acknowledge the patient's concerns and anger** but not argue about whether the behavior is reasonable. It may be helpful to ask family members to be present when the physician meets with the patient.

Patients who are frankly delusional should be managed like any patient with an acute psychosis (see Chapter 4, Schizophrenia and Other Psychotic Disorders, and Chapter 13, Violence). Acute interventions include **adequate supervision, behavioral interventions,** and **antipsychotic drugs**.

Personality Traits and Medical Illness

An individual patient's response to a physical illness is powerfully affected by his or her **personality traits**. *Personality traits* refer to an individual's characteristic and automatic self-protective mechanisms and are not typically pathological. However, sometimes, due to the regressive pull of medical illness and hospitalizations, personality traits may become so exaggerated that the patient may appear to have a personality disorder. This is in part because many of the personality disorders are exaggerated versions of normal personality traits. The distinction between a personality disorder and a gross and transient exaggeration of normal personality traits is difficult to make in the medical setting. Sometimes the distinction can only be made over time (see Chapter 8, Personality Disorders, for interviewing techniques and more detailed treatment of individual personality disorders).

By assessing a patient's personality style, the physician will gain a greater understanding of how being ill is affecting this particular person and consequently garner useful clues for management. Following this strategy can be enormously beneficial: the relationship between patient and medical staff may be enhanced, hospitalization and treatment may proceed more smoothly, adherence to treatment may be improved, and the patient may experience less distress and learn to cope more effectively with the illness.

A useful schema for assessing patients' personality traits in the medical setting classifies personality styles under seven general categories: dependent, controlled, self-dramatizing, long-suffering, suspicious, superior, and aloof (Kahana and Bibring 1964). A modified version of this schema, along with suggestions for management approaches, is described here.

Dependent Personality Traits
Clinical Features
People with dependent personality traits have a **fear of abandonment** and frequently harbor **unrealistic expectations of boundless care**. In part, because of their unrealistic expectations, they are often disappointed and frustrated by others, particularly caretakers. In the medical setting, these patients can be quite **demanding**; they seem to need special attention and limitless care from the staff. These are the patients who infuriate the nursing staff by "leaning" on the call button; they are often avoided during rounds because they won't let the staff "get out the door."

Interview and Management
For hospitalized patients, routine nursing and medical care provides a fair amount of dependency gratification, and for some dependent patients, this routine care may be enough to satisfy their expectations. The staff can enhance these beneficial effects by communicating their willingness to provide care and by acknowledging the patient's need for reassurance. Even something as simple as the physician's saying, "I understand that it is difficult for you to be in the hospital, away from your family," can provide psychological support.

For the patient who demands excessive amounts of time from physicians and nurses, **gentle limit-setting** can be helpful. Before limits are set, they should be expressed in a way that shows the staff's concern for the patient. For example, the physician might say, "I understand that it is difficult for you to be alone here in the hospital, and I have asked the nurses to check on you every half hour. On your end, I ask that you refrain from using the call button unless there is an emergency. I am concerned that if you continue to ring the nurses as frequently as you have been, they might be slow to respond if there were an emergency." Dependent patients usually do well when interactions with the staff are relatively predictable and **consistent**. Physician visits should take place at a prearranged time, have an expected duration, and be conducted in a structured manner.

Controlled Personality Traits
Clinical Features
Patients with controlled, or compulsive, personality traits tend to be **self-disciplined, orderly, and conscientious**. These patients need to feel that they have as much information as possible about their circumstances and that they are **in control** of what is happening to them, as is illustrated in the case example in Box 11.5. In moderation, controlled traits can result in a "model" patient. However, it can be problematic when these traits become exaggerated. Patients with compulsive personality traits can become **oppositional**, insisting that they know best and should be in charge of their own management. Other patients with these traits become paralyzed by **indecision**. When they are under stress, people with controlled personality traits rely heavily on routine. Any perceived break in the routine (e.g., if a medication is not given at its scheduled time or if the physician is late in getting to the office to see them) may be a cause for extreme anxiety.

Interview and Management
Management strategies for patients with compulsive personality traits should be designed to give these patients as much control over what is happening to them as possible. They should

---

BOX 11.5

CASE EXAMPLE OF A PATIENT WITH CONTROLLED PERSONALITY TRAITS

A 58-year-old tax attorney was admitted to the hospital with nausea, anorexia, and jaundice. Abdominal imaging revealed a pancreatic lesion that was worrisome for a malignancy. When the team came into his room to talk with him about his diagnostic and treatment options, they found him with a laptop on his lap, having researched his disease on the Internet through the hospital's wireless network. He received the news without apparent emotion. He asked many questions about the exact size and nature of the lesion, explaining that the information would help him make a reasoned decision about his care.

---

be provided with thorough **explanations** of all medical procedures. Test results should be delivered promptly, even when reporting that a routine blood test was normal. Patients with compulsive personality traits respond well to active **participation in their own care** and should be invited to help plan the treatment and management of their condition. For example, patients can be taught to change their own dressings, monitor and chart their urine output, or obtain their blood glucose levels and calculate their insulin requirements.

Finally, patients with compulsive personality traits are gratified by the medical staff's taking note of their exacting standards. A comment such as "I can see that you are a highly intelligent and discerning person. Am I right to assume that you will want to be promptly informed about all test results?" can be a more effective anxiolytic than a benzodiazepine for these patients.

Self-Dramatizing Personality Traits

Clinical Features

Self-dramatizing patients tend to be charming, imaginative, seductive, and emotionally engaging. They talk about themselves, their experiences, and their symptoms in an exaggerated and dramatic style that is typically lacking in detail. They have an accentuated need to be considered attractive or admired for some outstanding quality, especially by people in positions of authority, such as physicians. In the medical setting, these patients can be initially gratifying to care for, but they can become demanding over time. Their **need to feel "special"** leads to feeling slighted when they do not receive the attention they desire. When illness itself or the experience of being in the hospital leaves these patients feeling unattractive, self-dramatizing patients may invite **undue familiarity** with the medical staff by presenting themselves in a manner that is charming or seductive. Self-dramatizing patients often respond to the stresses of illness by **denying the seriousness** of their condition and instead using it to obtain **special attention and sympathy**.

Interview and Management

To effectively manage medical patients with self-dramatizing personality traits, the staff must carefully straddle the line between being too reserved and being too familiar in response to the patient's need for attention and admiration. If invitations of familiarity are received with too much reserve, patients may feel painfully rebuffed. On the other hand, the slightest friendly comment can cause the self-dramatizing patient to "fall into" an emotional overinvolvement with a caretaker, which inevitably leads to the patient's disappointment, hurt, and anger. The best approach for a physician is to help the patient feel important and admired only in ways that are appropriate to a physician–patient relationship, for example, by spending time listening to the patient's concerns and explaining test results or by commenting favorably on the devotion shown by family and friends.

Long-Suffering Personality Traits

Clinical Features

Long-suffering patients usually have a lifelong history of perceived suffering, whether caused by illness, failed relationships, or other adversities. They typically have been involved in **self-sacrificing relationships** and often perceive themselves as burdens to others. They are inclined to disregard their own discomfort, live in the service of others, and appear to be modest and humble, although they may display their suffering in an exhibitionistic manner. These people want love and acceptance but feel that they do not deserve it. Thus, their suffering becomes a way to punish themselves and at the same time maintain their self-esteem, by getting the attention and love they crave. When they become ill, people with long-suffering personality traits respond by viewing their condition as a much-deserved punishment and as a legitimate way to gain attention. Beneath the self-flagellation and complaints of these patients are implicit demands for attention and control. It is as if the patient were saying, "See how I suffer. You have to love me and take care of me because I suffer so."

Long-suffering patients may be perplexing at first. They complain and appear to request sympathy, yet they systematically and emphatically **reject all reassurance and encouragement**. The physician may offer advice or point out improvements, but the patient may counter by demonstrating how the advice is useless and the improvements illusory. Then the patient will complain even more pitiably. This type of interaction often leaves the medical staff feeling frustrated, drained, and irritated.

Interview and Management

Successful management of the long-suffering patient is predicated on understanding that the patient wants to be told that his or her suffering is appreciated rather than reassured that it will end. In order to convey this message, the physician should **acknowledge the patient's suffering** with comments such as "It must be tough having to be hooked up to an IV day and night" or "Chest tubes are quite painful." Doing so will gratify the patient and leave him or her feeling that the physician is appreciative and understanding. Encouraging comments to the effect that things are going well are not particularly helpful in this situation. In recommending treatment or diagnostic tests, it is best to frame the recommendation in terms of its potential benefit to others. One might recommend hip replacement surgery to a long-suffering grandmother by saying, "This is a major operation, and there is a demanding recovery period. Nevertheless, I am recommending that you consider hip replacement because it would allow you to resume babysitting for your grandchildren. I understand that your daughter really counts on your help."

Suspicious Personality Traits

Clinical Features

Suspicious patients are mistrustful of others, grossly oversensitive to slights, and feel they see malevolence where none actually exists. Suspicious patients **fear becoming vulnerable** to others, which they assume will result in their being taken advantage of or hurt. A medical illness, with all its implications for dependency on others, represents a crisis for suspicious patients. They might, for example, suspect the staff of being negligent in caring for them; suspect medical personnel of concealing important information from them; or suspect the hospital of exploiting them by hospitalizing them in order to supply medical students with patients "to practice on," to conduct research, or simply to make money. Feeling under attack, they may respond in kind. As their suspicions and anxiety grow, so does the likelihood that such patients will either lash out at those around them with angry accusations or withdraw completely.

Interview and Management

It is most important that these patients receive **detailed information** about the nature of their condition and all plans to treat it, including the potential risks and benefits associated with proposed medical interventions. It is almost inevitable that these patients will feel they have been slighted or mistreated in some way, and they will complain to their physicians about their experiences. Physicians should respond to patients' reports with calm, courteous, but not overly friendly concern. The best course of action is not to try to dispel or dispute patients' suspicious thoughts, which may only reinforce them, but rather to **acknowledge their concerns** by making a statement such as "I see that you have little confidence in our staff or in myself. I can appreciate that this puts you in a very uncomfortable position." The way is then paved for enlisting patients' cooperation by suggesting that, for the time being, they tolerate the unpleasant situation.

Superior Personality Traits

Clinical Features

Patients with superior personality traits are typically self-important, self-centered, and condescending to others. This attitude may be superficially cloaked in a patronizing "humility." In the medical setting, these patients often insist on being taken care of by the most important specialists or the chief of the medical service, as is illustrated in the case example in Box 11.6. They often idealize a few "special" staff members but are rude and depreciative toward others. Superior patients behave as if they are **entitled to special treatment**. They expect their requests and needs to be met automatically and believe that hospital rules or routines do not apply to them.

BOX 11.6

CASE EXAMPLE OF A PATIENT WITH SUPERIOR PERSONALITY TRAITS

A 60-year-old man was admitted with liver failure and was undergoing evaluation for a liver transplant. He began the interview by citing a long list of his accomplishments, including positions such as CEO of several companies and head of several charitable boards. He went on at length describing his "fully actualized life" and his family as "the best I could imagine." He added, "I haven't met a single actual doctor here yet," even though he had been admitted for several days and has been followed regularly by house staff and junior attendings. When the psychiatrist clarified this, the patient explained, "Well, I meant, of course, the head surgeon of the transplant program." The psychiatrist recognized his narcissistic defenses and aimed to project outward confidence and expertise during their meeting.

Interview and Management

The management of patients with superior personality traits involves understanding that their grandiosity protects them from a fragile sense of self-esteem. These patients are most comfortable and supported when they feel that they are being appreciated as people with special attributes and achievements. To this end, it is helpful to behave in a **particularly respectful manner** with these patients and to inquire about their professions or other accomplishments. To most effectively take care of these patients, the medical staff should **emphasize their own expertise** and demonstrate self-confidence. This attitude is usually reassuring to patients with superior personality traits, because they need to believe that they deserve—and are receiving—"the best." If this approach fails, the patient's deprecation should be met without defensiveness. If the patient is complaining about being taken care of by the house staff, it is often worthwhile to invite the participation of a senior consultant or ward attending.

Aloof Personality Traits

Clinical Features

People with aloof personality traits are unemotional, remote, reserved, and reclusive. They appear to be distant and uninvolved with other people and everyday life. In the medical setting, these patients tend to keep to themselves. They typically limit contact with the medical staff to a bare minimum, rarely asking questions and frequently avoiding eye contact. Their attitude toward their illness may be one of apparent detachment. They seem equally uninterested in and unaffected by hospital routines. They may appear to be odd or eccentric (e.g., preoccupied with certain dietary habits or religious concerns).

Interview and Management

In managing these patients, the physician must respect and accept their intense need for privacy and interpersonal distance. These needs are usually intensified during illness and hospitalization. It is not helpful to be overly friendly or warm or to attempt to draw out the patient; such behavior may be experienced by the patient as an intrusive demand and can lead to even further withdrawal. It is best to maintain an **attitude of tempered interest** and consideration, without requesting that the patient reciprocate. A common mistake is to respond too respectfully to the aloof patient's need for privacy (e.g., by skipping the patient's room on rounds, not asking necessary questions about the medical history and symptoms, or omitting parts of the physical examination). It is important to spend enough time with the patient to provide adequate medical care.

PSYCHOSOCIAL FACTORS AFFECTING A MEDICAL CONDITION

Clinical Features

In both the medical and the popular literature, discussions of psychological factors affecting medical illness frequently involve the concept of stress. **Stress** is best defined as the internal emotional reaction, or distress, that a person experiences in response to a given situation or condition, which is the **stressor**. To refer to a given set of conditions as "stressful" implies that the individual's capacity to cope comfortably with and adapt to these conditions has been surpassed.

According to this definition, stress is subjective. What constitutes stress is defined not only by the stressor but also by the person who is being stressed. This approach means that what is stressful for one person may not be particularly stressful for another. Whether an event is experienced as stressful is determined both by the meaning of the stressor to the individual and by his or her ability to cope. These factors, in turn, are affected by the individual's personality, life circumstances, and social supports. For example, a hysterectomy may be extremely stressful for a chronically lonely young woman who was looking forward to having a family, but the operation might not pose as much of an emotional challenge to a postmenopausal woman who is happily married and has teenage children. Sometimes, the factors that determine whether an event is experienced as stressful may not be apparent unless the physician knows the patient and understands his or her psychological makeup. For example, a fiercely independent person who is laid off from a job may find it extremely stressful to be unable to work and to have to collect unemployment compensation, whereas someone who is dependent and passive may find unemployment to be a relief. The attitude of the person's spouse or family toward the layoff will also affect how stressful the experience is for the person.

Increased life stress has been associated with the onset and exacerbation of numerous medical problems, although the exact mechanisms that link stress and disease are extremely complex and incompletely understood. In considering the relationship between stress and illness, it is crucial to keep in mind that physical illness is, itself, stressful and may set in motion a vicious circle: life stressors leave an individual vulnerable to illness; illness generates even greater stress; and greater stress leaves the individual even more physically vulnerable.

Illness often introduces new stressful conditions into patients' lives as well. Social supports appear to buffer the effects of stress: a person with solid social supports is less vulnerable to the emotional and physical sequelae of stressful life events, including medical illness, than the socially isolated individual. Unfortunately, illness can sometimes disrupt the lives even of patients who have solid social supports (e.g., marital tensions are relatively common when one spouse is ill; losing a job because of illness frequently means losing not only income but also a valuable social network). Such disruption leaves the patient more vulnerable to the stresses of physical illness.

In thinking about the mechanisms by which stress affects a person's health, it is important to keep in mind that not all stress-related medical problems are stress-related physiological responses. **Stress-related physiological responses** are the direct result of psychological stress and distress on a person's physiology and physical health. These responses are not behaviors resulting from stress.

The case example in Box 11.7 illustrates a situation in which the initial impression might be a stress-related physiological response, but the most accurate diagnosis is psychological factors affecting other medical conditions. When alcohol, nicotine, or drug use is a contributing problem, the additional diagnosis of a substance-related disorder should be given.

Interview

When interviewing a patient suffering from a medical condition, it is important to take into account the role of stress. The first stress to consider is the illness itself. After taking the history, the physician should explore with the patient **how stressful the illness has been** for the patient and the patient's family. Asking a question such as "How are you coping with all of this?" gently invites the patient to open up a bit. The extent to which the illness is causing secondary problems for the patient (e.g., family tensions, sexual dysfunction, financial or job-related problems) should be clarified. These factors may place

---

BOX 11.7

CASE EXAMPLE OF PSYCHOLOGICAL FACTORS AFFECTING OTHER MEDICAL CONDITIONS

A patient with hypertension and atherosclerotic heart disease had been asymptomatic with medical management. His wife of 30 years left him, and during the next 6 months, he developed angina. Before his physician assumed that the stressful marital separation was physiologically related to the angina, she took a careful history, in which it was revealed that since the patient's wife had left him, he had been smoking more, drinking alcohol, and using drugs to self-medicate his distress. He had gained weight and stopped exercising. He had stopped taking his medications. He had had a recurrence of high blood pressure, but this had not been detected because he postponed his regular checkup. Any combination of these maladaptive behaviors could account for his angina.

---

additional pressures on the patient and the family, making it harder for all of them to cope with the illness.

The next step is to assess the role that psychosocial stressors have played in causing the patient's medical problems. The physician should inquire about **recent life changes or stresses** that are temporally related to the onset or worsening of the condition. Asking specific questions about **financial problems, job-related problems, marriage, and family matters** is helpful. Other recent illnesses in the family or problems with children may also be significant. Most stressful life situations fit into one of these categories, and asking about each one specifically in an open-ended way will help patients to talk about them. Patients may not have regarded these situations as stressful until the physician inquires about them. The physician might ask, "How have things been going for you on the job?" If the patient proceeds to talk about massive layoffs, the physician might comment, "That must be very stressful for you." Most patients will "pick up the ball" and either concur or state that they had not really thought about it. The patient may say, "Now that you mention it, things have been pretty tense lately."

When a patient's medical condition has deteriorated during a period of psychosocial stress, it is important to evaluate the mechanisms by which the stressors have affected the medical condition. The nature of the stressors should be clarified in detail, as well as the ways in which the patient has or has not been able to cope with them. The physician should ask about **symptoms of anxiety and depression** and should tactfully inquire about **maladaptive health behaviors** that may be reactions to stress. It can be helpful to say something such as "You've been under an awful lot of stress over the past few months. Many people in this type of situation resort to trying to comfort themselves with alcohol. Have you found yourself drinking more recently?" or "Typically, people take their medications less reliably during stressful periods. Have you found anything like this happening to you?" Questions framed in this way make it clear that such maladaptive behavior is common and that the physician is accustomed to hearing about it. These questions also communicate an attitude of tolerance on the part of the physician. This approach will make it easier for the patient to be honest about behaviors that the patient is ashamed of or about fears that the physician will disapprove of the patient.

It is important to collect **parallel history** by asking the same questions of the patient's family. People close to the patient may be able to provide information that the patient is unaware of or reluctant to reveal. One has to make the mistake of forgetting to speak with family members only once to remember to do so forever after. Consider again the patient with angina, discussed in Box 11.7, whose wife had left him. It would be common for the physician to assume that such a patient had "broken through" his previous medication regimen. The solution, based on this assumption, would be to increase the dosages of old medications or to add new medications, only to have the patient develop side effects and perhaps even toxicity. At this point, the physician might receive a phone call from the patient's daughter, to say that she suspects that the patient stopped taking his medication when his wife left the house. Box 11.8 describes a case illustration of the importance of a careful, thorough evaluation of the role of stress in a medical condition.

It is extremely common for patients who become ill to describe having recently been under a lot of stress. But it is also important to understand that stress may *not* have played a significant role, even if the patient currently feels stressed or believes that the medical problems are stress related. It is a common belief in the United States that too much stress is "bad." People tend to take it for granted that stress can cause ill health and exacerbate preexisting medical problems. Many patients and their families overestimate the role of stress in illness. Physicians should be alert to this possibility, because patients and their families may suffer unnecessary feelings of guilt or self-blame for their illnesses and may have painful feelings of personal failure or responsibility. The role of stress in the course of an illness varies depending on the disease, the patient's biological vulnerability to disease, and the patient's psychological and physiological vulnerability to stressful events.

BOX 11.8

CASE EXAMPLE OF THE EVALUATION OF THE ROLE OF STRESS IN A MEDICAL CONDITION

A patient in her late 40s with long-standing multiple sclerosis suffered an acute exacerbation of her disease 9 months after the death of her husband. Any of a number of factors may have affected this patient, all of them factors that need to be considered in the differential diagnosis. The patient might be suffering from a stress-related physiological response to having lost her husband, which would affect her immune system and result in increased autoimmune activity and an exacerbation of her symptoms. She might be reacting to the loss of her husband by not taking her maintenance medication as often as she should or by taking a "devil may care" attitude about her health. Her husband may have been responsible for making sure she took her medication as prescribed. The patient's increased fatigue, weakness, and mental slowing might be, in part, symptoms of depression. In order to determine which of these possibilities was the basic problem, the physician asked careful questions in a concerned, tolerant, and open fashion. The results of this inquiry, along with appropriate physical findings and laboratory tests, helped the physician formulate an appropriate treatment plan.

Management

An accurate assessment of the role of stress will determine which medical and psychosocial interventions should be made. Careful assessment can spare the patient unnecessary diagnostic procedures and trials of medications, as well as unnecessary self-blame. If none of these factors seem to be a major issue (e.g., if the patient has many social supports, is financially secure, and appears to be coping well but is nonetheless blaming herself for "letting stress get the better of me"), a different approach is needed. The treatment for the unnecessary guilt and self-blame is a combination of **education** and **reassurance**. A physician is in a powerful position in this regard, and just a few helpful words of explanation and encouragement can make an enormous difference to patients. One might say to the patient described in Box 11.8, "Believe it or not, people tend to overestimate the role of stress in this kind of situation. You are coping very well with the loss of your husband, and it may be that stress is not even playing a significant role in this exacerbation. It may have happened anyway, regardless of what was going on in your life. This may just be an unfortunate coincidence. It leaves you with an awful lot on your plate right now, but, as I said, I am impressed with how well you are handling everything." Patients in this situation usually feel supported and are relieved to hear that the physician does not blame them for having become ill and does not expect them to blame themselves.

PSYCHOSOCIAL ASPECTS OF CHRONIC ILLNESS

Clinical Features

Learning to live with a chronic physical illness presents a psychological challenge for patients and their families. Most people rise to this challenge and are able to adapt after a period of time, although there are always some ups and downs in the process. Sound medical management, including an ongoing relationship with a physician who provides information, guidance, and psychological support, facilitates the adaptation. Patients who are unable to make the adjustment to chronic illness may suffer many serious consequences. If a patient is having unusual difficulty in making the adjustment to a chronic illness, the physician should make it a primary focus of management to help the patient cope and adapt successfully.

Patients who are unable to adapt are at high risk for chronic problems with adherence, which may take the form of underuse or overuse of medications. These patients may delay seeking treatment during exacerbations, which may result in unnecessary hospitalizations and periods of acute illness. They may be too quick to panic when their symptoms change, which may lead to overuse of medical services, especially the emergency room. Such patients may resort to "doctor shopping," which can interfere with the development of an ongoing relationship with one medical practitioner.

All of these factors make it likely that patients who are having difficulty adapting to chronic illness will be subjected to unnecessary diagnostic procedures, which can bring potential complications. Because of problems with motivation, patients who are having difficulty adapting to chronic illness are usually poor candidates for physical and vocational rehabilitation programs; they are more likely than other patients to suffer from impaired self-esteem, depression, and anxiety. Greater than usual tensions at home and disruption of family life are common. The multiple medical and psychosocial complications faced by such patients are illustrated by the first part of the case described in Box 11.9.

BOX 11.9

CASE EXAMPLE OF PSYCHOSOCIAL ASPECTS OF CHRONIC ILLNESS

PART 1. DEPRESSION, ANXIETY, AND DOWNWARD SPIRAL

A 48-year-old disabled fireman, who lived with his wife and 17-year-old daughter, had been in good health until he injured his back 4 years earlier by falling backward in a broken lounge chair. This injury led to chronic low back pain that was not relieved by repeated spinal fusions. Conservative medical management had been recommended, including nonsteroidal anti-inflammatory medication, physical therapy, and exercise. Because he was still faring poorly 4 years after the initial injury, he was referred for psychiatric consultation. When the psychiatrist first saw him, the patient's mood was extremely depressed. He said that he was in constant pain, which preoccupied him day and night. He complained of insomnia and was unable to concentrate. He was extremely anxious and spent most of his waking hours ruminating about his financial concerns. His appetite was poor, but because he was inactive and ate mostly snack foods, the patient had gained 30 pounds since his injury. He spent most of his time in the ground-floor den, which he had made into his bedroom, lying on the couch and watching television. He had not complied with recommendations for physical therapy and exercise, and he rarely left the house. The patient had left his job as a fireman and was receiving temporary disability compensation. He felt inferior to his wife, who was now bringing in more money than he was. He revealed that he had always thought of his wife, who was a senior vice president at a computer company, as more intelligent than him. He had thought of himself as "handy" because he took care of the house and maintained the cars. Now that he was earning less money and was unable to take care of the house or the cars, he felt deprived of his customary role in the household. This change left him feeling useless and unnecessary.

The patient's predominant reactions to developing chronic pain were to become depressed and anxious. He was unable to cope effectively with his physical symptoms and with the psychosocial changes that followed. Most disturbing to him were his concerns about his financial future and the changes in his role in the family. He was left feeling helpless, useless, inferior, and unable to cope and adapt. He was spiraling downward.

PART 2. MANAGEMENT

The patient was referred to a psychiatrist, who recommended the addition of short-term psychotherapy on a weekly basis for several months, along with an antidepressant and an anxiolytic, to the patient's regimen of nonsteroidal anti-inflammatory agents. In psychotherapy, the patient discussed his feelings of inferiority and related them to the recent changes in his role in the family. He and the psychiatrist also discussed,

(continued)

in concrete terms, what he might do to establish a new set of roles for himself. The patient decided to begin taking care of the bills and household paperwork and to cook the family's dinner. The psychiatrist encouraged him to pursue more intensive physical therapy and regular workouts and pointed out that losing weight and being fit and more active would help him to feel better about himself.

The psychiatrist also met with the patient and his wife several times and helped them to clear up misunderstandings that existed between them. The patient's wife was able to tell her husband that he was only imagining that she was recoiling from physical contact with him and that, in fact, she longed for physical affection. She assured him that she was comfortable with being the major breadwinner for the time being and was getting satisfaction from being able to do this for her family. The psychiatrist made suggestions to help the couple learn to communicate more openly with each other. She also recommended that they engage in more affectionate physical contact, without pressuring them to resume specifically sexual activities. At the same time, the psychiatrist discussed the logistics of how to have sexual relations without putting stress on the patient's back. This concern weighed heavily on the patient and, as it turned out, even more so on his wife. It had been part of the reason why they had stopped having sex.

Over the course of the next few months, the patient's depression gradually remitted. His previous good spirits returned, and he slowly began to regain his self-esteem. He was able to sleep and concentrate and discovered that by losing weight and exercising regularly he could increase his range of activities. He resumed his habit of maintaining the family cars and moved out of his den and back into the second-floor bedroom to sleep with his wife. He was on the road to adapting to his chronic illness.

In the course of adapting to chronic illness, patients must make many changes. The exact nature of these changes varies according to the illness, its severity and course, and the patient's psychology and personality, phase of life, previous experience with illness, and social responsibilities and supports. Some of the changes are external changes in daily routines and activities, and others are internal changes in the patient's view of himself or herself in relation to the world. External changes can be as minor as having to remember to take an antihypertensive agent daily or as major as having to give up a profession or the ability to ambulate independently. Internal changes may range from having to accept an increased awareness of a physical vulnerability to losing aspects of the self that have been important sources of self-esteem or a sense of identity. Patients must find new ways to define who they are and to experience themselves as valuable.

In addition, larger social patterns and technological advances in treating illness may also significantly impact the psychological impact of a particular illness. For example, in the early days of the epidemic, infection with the human immunodeficiency virus (HIV) and the development of acquired immunodeficiency syndrome (AIDS) tended to invoke powerful psychological reactions in patients, their families, their health care providers, and the greater population. Many factors contributed to these emotional reactions. HIV infection was seen as a "death sentence," as it tended to end in devastating physical deterioration. The illness tended to affect young people in their prime. HIV infection is contagious, and one of the primary routes of transmission is through sexual contact. The relative ineffectiveness of early measures for the prevention and treatment of HIV also played a role. In addition, because the populations at highest risk include men who have sex with men, people who use intravenous drugs, and people who work in the sex industry, some people's reactions were biased against these groups.

It is important to note, however, that several factors promoted significant change over the past years. Treatment advances prolonged the lifespan of many patients with AIDS and decreased morbidity. Community outreach programs emphasized prevention, substance dependence treatment, and early HIV testing and counseling. Advocacy groups promoted the rights of those living with HIV and helped to address stigma. In turn, what first appeared as a devastating illness with a certain outcome of early death started to shift to an adjustment of living with a challenging chronic illness. In particular, survivor guilt and renewal of vocational and social identity started to become preeminent psychological concerns.

When first given the diagnosis of a chronic illness, many people have a hard time fully appreciating what they have been told. There is usually a period of shock or denial, when the patient may feel that "the whole thing just doesn't seem real." Patients usually assume that the problem will resolve or that a cure can be found. When this fails to happen, many patients visit specialists and seek out traditional or nontraditional treatments in the hope of finding a cure. Over time, as these efforts fail to resolve the problem, many patients feel worried, anxious, and fearful and develop seemingly hypochondriacal preoccupations about their medical problems. Patients may also feel angry, guilty, demoralized, and depressed. Most patients will go through many if not all of these emotions at some point in the course of adjusting to a chronic illness.

In order to adapt successfully to chronic illness, patients must shift their focus away from trying to eradicate the illness and toward trying to live with it. Rather than looking for a cure, the emphasis is now placed on **adapting** to the illness and on minimizing disabilities and psychosocial complications. The initial process is often experienced as "giving up hope" and can be painful. Over time, most patients come to see things from a more positive, active perspective, viewing themselves as involved in a challenging struggle to live with the illness. The patient who continues to feel hopeless and "down" over an extended period of time is the exception and may be suffering from a major depression. Patients' personality traits may also effect how they experience their illnesses. Regardless, it is not "normal" for someone with medical problems to develop a major depression. The effective treatment of affective illness in chronically medically ill patients can have a positive impact on their overall illness course, as the second part of the case in Box 11.9 illustrates.

Interview

When interviewing a patient who is suffering from a chronic illness, it is important to find out how the illness has affected the patient's life. Specific questions should be asked about the impact the illness may have had on the patient's **job, finances, family roles and responsibilities, sex life, recreational activities, and social life**. The physician may begin by asking, "Have you been able to continue to work?" If the patient answers affirmatively, the physician should ask for more detailed information, such as "How hard

---

BOX 11.10

PRIMARY AND SECONDARY GAIN FROM BEING ILL

Primary gain and *secondary gain* are terms that were introduced by Sigmund Freud and that remain highly relevant to medical practice today. Primary gain is a situation in which unconscious psychological factors play a role in causing an illness or a symptom. The physical symptoms are psychologically determined and are seen as a response to an unconscious conflict. For example, patients with conversion symptoms may express unconscious desires, fears, and conflicts in physical symptoms (see Chapter 10, Somatic Symptom and Related Disorders).

A young man who is right-handed develops a functional paralysis of his right arm after having an argument with his father. Though the young man loves his father and feels he should be respectful toward him, he is also very angry. Deep down, he has fantasies of striking his father and severely injuring him, perhaps even killing him. These thoughts are unacceptable or "conflictual" to the young man because they are in conflict with both his love for his father and his own internal code of good behavior. Because of their unacceptable or conflictual nature, the fantasies remain unconscious, repressed, and out of his awareness. Instead, the young man develops a functional paralysis of his arm, as if to ensure his unconscious mind that he is incapable of hitting his father, while at the same time he punishes himself for his unacceptable unconscious impulses by weakening himself. All of this goes on outside of the young man's awareness. When he presents to the emergency room, he truly will not know why his arm has become paralyzed.

Secondary gain refers to the benefits a patient is able to glean from an illness or a symptom. These benefits or gains are considered "secondary" because they develop after the illness or symptom presents and because they are not part of the etiology of the condition. Secondary gain can powerfully affect the course of a medical condition by interfering, more or less directly, with the patient's motivation to make a rapid or full recovery.

Examples of secondary gain from illness include the "taken-for-granted" stay-at-home mother who gets extra attention and affection from her husband and children when she develops viral pneumonia; the "stretched-too-thin" business executive who obtains a sanctioned reprieve from her professional and family responsibilities during medical hospitalization for acute appendicitis; and the "at-the-end-of-my-rope" paralegal who is working at two jobs and who receives workers' compensation benefits after a freak accident in his workplace leaves him with a concussion.

It can be helpful to think of the secondary gain of medical illness in terms of patients' efforts to cope by getting what they can out of the situation they find themselves in. This approach implies that secondary gain is not the cause of illness, avoiding the customary confusion that to talk about secondary gain is to say that the

(continued)

medical condition is "psychogenic." This approach also avoids the accusatory tone frequently used when it is recognized that factors of secondary gain are playing a powerful role in the course of a patient's medical condition.

While, by definition, secondary gain is never the cause of physical illness, in many circumstances it can interfere with adaptation to illness. As a result, while patients are largely unaware of the role that secondary gain may be playing in their illness, it is the job of the treating physician to identify these factors. In this extremely common clinical situation, it is the physician's goal to be aware of and try to minimize internal resistance on the patient's part that conflicts with his or her motivation to make the fullest possible recovery. The need for this type of intervention should be assessed in all patients suffering from physical illness.

has it been for you to continue working?" "Have you had to make any changes on the job because of your illness, or have there been any problems?" "Has this made things tight for you financially?" The physician should inquire about how the patient and the family are coping with the changes that illness brings. Specific questions should be asked about problems with demoralization, depression, anxiety, and substance abuse. The physician might introduce these topics by saying to the patient, "Often, when people are trying to adapt to a chronic illness, they go through painful periods of feeling demoralized or even depressed. Other people become very anxious. What has your experience been?" After exploring this topic with the patient, the physician can go on to say, "It's also very common for people who are trying to cope with chronic illness to turn to alcohol or sedatives for relief. Have you found any of these things happening to you?"

Asking specific questions will bring to light problems that many patients will not volunteer without an invitation. Through this process one can identify areas in which helpful interventions can be made. The disabled fireman described in Box 11.9, Part 1, confided, in response to a question from the physician, that he and his wife had not had sexual relations in several years. In fact, he feared that his wife was repulsed by any physical contact with him. Physical therapy, vocational counseling, treatment for depression and anxiety, or marital and individual counseling can help the patient who is having trouble adapting. Asking patients about their lives and their difficulties is, in and of itself, a therapeutic intervention. For most patients, the opportunity to talk with a trusted physician about their problems and concerns and to receive support and guidance is powerful and highly valued "medicine."

Patients usually have a theory, often unfounded, about why they developed their illness; frequently they believe they are responsible for it. Patients may believe that they have become ill because they subjected themselves to too much stress, did not eat right, or did something bad for which they are being punished. Some patients blame their spouse, if there are marital problems, or their job, if it is stressful. It can be helpful to discuss these beliefs in order to **correct distortions** and alleviate unnecessary fear, guilt, and blame. Failure to do so can cause enormous distress and even depression, as well as unnecessary marital or vocational disruption.

It is useful for the physician to ask patients if they know other people who have the same illness. Patients often base their expectations for themselves on what they have seen happen to others. These expectations tend to be particularly powerful when a patient develops the same illness that has affected a parent or sibling. Similarly, patients who become ill at an age at which a deceased parent or sibling became ill or died generally assume that they, too, have been dealt a death sentence. If they are encouraged to talk about such matters, most patients will experience enormous relief.

Patients with high-risk behaviors (e.g., smoking cigarettes or eating a high-cholesterol diet) often feel particularly self-critical when they become ill. A common error on the part of physicians is to shy away from discussing patients' concerns, fearing incorrectly that talking about them will only make the situation more painful for the patient. This approach reflects the unfounded belief frequently held by physicians that they have little to offer patients who are struggling with realistic regret. If a patient has a chronic progressive illness, such as Parkinson's disease, and is worried about further deterioration, physicians may sidestep the patient's desires to discuss the fears. Here again, physicians may feel that they have nothing to offer and that talking about a painful inevitability will only make matters worse. This is not necessarily true. Many patients feel much better after they have **shared their realistic concerns** with an empathetic, supportive physician. One might say something as simple as "Parkinson's can be a tough disease to live with. Sometimes people go through periods of feeling down or worrying about the future. How has it been for you?"

Physicians play a critical role in helping their patients make a successful adaptation to chronic illness. In order to do so, physicians must deal with their own feelings about chronic illness. Many people become physicians in order to "help" and "cure" other people. They often share patients' expectations that physicians should be able to "fix" things. Such expectations on the part of physicians can lead to feelings of frustration and dissatisfaction when they are dealing with patients with a chronic illness. These feelings, in turn, can cause physicians to unduly blame themselves or patients or even to inadvertently push the patient out of treatment.

Management

There are many things physicians can do to help patients adapt to chronic illness. First, patients need to be **educated** about their illness and, whenever possible, given **responsibility** for day-to-day management decisions. For example, patients who have diabetes can check their urine or serum glucose and adjust their insulin dosages accordingly. Patients with asthma can titrate the precise frequency of inhalers. Patients should be helped to anticipate the predictable fluctuations in their symptoms and taught how to distinguish these fluctuations from an exacerbation that requires medical intervention.

In addition to education and guidance, patients suffering from chronic illness need **emotional support**. A positive relationship with a physician who is sympathetic and available makes a big difference. The physician should get to know the patient's family members, because they can often provide information or raise concerns that the patient will not, and because they are likely to need the guidance and support of the physician as much as the patient does. It is easy to underestimate the powerful and positive effect of physician–patient and physician–family relationships on helping patients cope with and adapt to chronic illness.

The case of the fireman with low back pain described in Box 11.9 illustrates the management of a patient who is having difficulty adapting to chronic illness.

PSYCHOLOGICAL ASPECTS OF CHRONIC PAIN

One significant type of chronic-illness burden is chronic pain. Indeed, chronic pain and its sequelae can be tremendously challenging—for patients and their families, as well as for their physicians. The group of patients with chronic pain is a highly heterogeneous one; it includes individuals of all ages who suffer from many different physical and psychiatric problems and who have varying degrees of psychosocial supports and stressors. Examples include an elderly widower who is socially isolated and dependent on alcohol and who suffers from rheumatoid arthritis; a 40-year-old fireman, married and the father of four, who strained his back and now suffers from chronic low back pain; an unemployed young woman with chronic pelvic pain of undetermined etiology; and a 50-year-old married businesswoman suffering from a painful diabetic neuropathy. These people have many more differences than similarities. What they do share is the challenge of adapting to life with chronic pain.

Most experts consider a pain syndrome to be chronic if it has lasted for 6 months or longer. Chronic pain syndromes are subclassified as malignant or benign, according to whether or not they are due to a malignant disease. The psychological issues involved and the management strategies employed are often different for benign and malignant chronic pain syndromes. Patients with an excessive response to their pain symptoms are diagnosed with somatic symptom disorder, with a specification indicating that the disorder is "with predominant pain." Severity criteria differentiate between mild, moderate, and severe forms of the illness, and it is considered persistent if severe symptoms and significant impairment have lasted more than 6 months. In addition, DSM-5 identifies the presence of genitopelvic pain/penetration disorder. Some pain disorders may also fall under the category of a mental disorder due to another medical condition.

Clinical Features

Malignant chronic pain is pain due to cancer or its treatment. The two main causes are direct tumor invasion with compression of tissue (usually bone or nerve tissue) and treatments for cancer, including chemotherapy, irradiation, and surgery, which frequently lead to painful destruction of nerve fibers in peripheral pain pathways. For many cancer patients, pain serves as a constant reminder of a life-threatening illness. It is also one of the primary risk factors for depression and a wish for hastened death in terminally ill patients. Approaches to the treatment of chronic malignant pain emphasize physical and psychological comfort and, as much as possible, **relief of pain**. Narcotics are used liberally and are limited only by side effects. However, in recent years, there has been renewed attention to the subtleties of treating patients with prior substance dependence. Cancer patients are encouraged to speak up actively. New pain may indicate progression of the disease, which requires evaluation, and new or increased pain is always an indication for the titration of narcotic regimens.

Benign chronic pain can be caused by many medical conditions, including (but not limited to) degenerative spinal disease, trigeminal and postherpetic neuralgias, diabetic neuropathy, arthritis, chronic headache, myofascial syndrome, fibromyalgia, or reflex sympathetic dystrophy. Patients are usually preoccupied with their pain, feel that it has become the focus of their lives, and are in great distress. As a result of their pain, patients have suffered significant psychosocial disruption, including depression, anxiety, substance abuse, marital problems, and difficulties at work.

The basic management approach for chronic benign pain is different from that for malignant pain. For chronic benign pain, the emphasis is on increased activity through physical therapy or graded exercise and on return to function. The use of narcotics is discouraged if possible. The fireman with low back pain described in Box 11.9 exemplifies many aspects of what can happen to patients with chronic pain before they get the help they need. At the time that he presented to the psychiatric consultant, the patient was totally preoccupied with his pain, had given up all his usual activities, was not working, and was virtually housebound. He was anxious and depressed, alienated from his wife and daughter, felt terrible about himself, and felt hopeless and fearful about his future.

While this patient fared better than most, his experience illustrates how patients with chronic pain typically find themselves locked into a vicious cycle of steady psychosocial deterioration and intensification of pain. Caught in this trap, patients tend to become increasingly depressed and preoccupied with their pain, as the rest of their lives become progressively disrupted. Patients may lose their jobs, be at odds with loved ones, and give up all hobbies and interests. Pain can become the focus of the patient's world. Life can be reduced to a series of visits to medical specialists, looking for a "cure." Or patients may become virtually housebound, doing little except focusing on pain and medications.

The etiology of chronic pain is complex and, for many patients, involves an interaction between medical and psychosocial factors. Once a patient has developed a chronic pain syndrome, psychosocial factors play a major role in the course of the syndrome, in a variety of ways. Different people have different pain thresholds, and a person's pain threshold will vary over time, depending on the person's mood, level of anxiety or fatigue, use of drugs and alcohol, prior experience with pain, and other factors. Patients who cope well are likely to experience less pain. Patients who are unable to cope and adapt are at risk for many secondary psychosocial problems that can intensify pain, interfere with treatment adherence, and make it even more difficult to cope. Depression and **substance abuse** often become problems. The most common substances of abuse are prescription narcotics, but abuse of alcohol and benzodiazepines is also quite common in patients with chronic pain. Full-blown **major depression** is common. In fact, the presence of depressive symptoms at some point in the course of chronic pain is nearly universal. **Secondary social problems**, such as family tensions and breakups, loss of social supports, vocational difficulties, and financial problems, commonly result from chronic pain. This type of psychosocial disruption often makes it more difficult for patients to comply with medical management and adapt to chronic pain.

Another way that psychological factors can play a role in chronic pain is by providing **secondary gain** (see Box 11.10). Patients might enjoy getting solicitous attention from family, friends, and physicians; might be relieved to have fewer demands made on them at work; or might discover that they are eligible for medical disability and, for example, can afford to stay home with young children. Factors of secondary gain will interfere with a patient's motivation to make a full adjustment to the pain syndrome, because the gratifications or gains provided by being sick or disabled can outweigh, in the patient's mind, the gratification of making a more successful adaptation.

Interview

All patients with chronic pain require a thorough medical and psychiatric evaluation. It is important for the physician to take a detailed history of the quality of the pain and the functional and psychosocial impairment that it causes. Patients should also be asked about past and present symptoms of depression and about use or abuse of substances, including narcotics, benzodiazepines, and alcohol. This inquiry is best prefaced by explaining that these are routine complications of chronic pain. The physician might say, "Many people suffering from chronic pain turn to narcotics, tranquilizers, or alcohol to help them get by. What has your experience been?"

CASE EXAMPLE OF CHRONIC PAIN MANAGEMENT

The psychiatrist prescribed duloxetine for the patient presented in Box 11.9 to treat depression and to provide analgesia, as well as low dosages of the benzodiazepine diazepam on a short-term basis to reduce the patient's anxiety, provide antispasmotic properties, and help him sleep at night.

The patient's self-esteem began to return as his depression resolved and as he began to be more active and take on more responsibility. As he and his wife began to communicate more directly, she was better able to provide emotional support and help him adjust to his chronic pain. When he started to feel better, his motivation to comply with physical therapy and exercise increased greatly, and he undertook an ambitious exercise program. Exercise and antidepressants for analgesia made his pain more bearable and contributed to his overall adjustment to his condition. By taking a biopsychosocial approach and addressing the patient's difficulties from as many angles as possible, the psychiatrist was able to help him successfully cope with and ultimately adapt to his physical condition and the psychosocial changes it brought.

It became clear in the course of the patient's treatment that secondary gain had contributed to his difficulty in adapting to his chronic back pain. In the end, the patient did not return to the fire department, even though he was offered a desk job. He opted instead for long-term disability. When it became apparent that he would not be returning to his job, the patient, in fact, felt quite relieved. Over time, he acknowledged that in recent years he had become progressively disenchanted with the fire department and unhappy in his job. He had very much wanted to move to another, less expensive, less hectic region of the country but had felt obliged to remain with the fire department until he reached retirement. Perhaps most important to the patient, his daughter was about to begin college, and he did not want her to move far away to attend school.

Leaving the fire department and being on disability meant that the patient could afford to sell his house and relocate his family to a small southern town that afforded the less harried, less expensive lifestyle he had been yearning for. The move also enabled his daughter to attend the college of her choice and still live at home. The patient was able to take advantage of the opportunity afforded by his back injury and pain and to get out of a situation in which he felt trapped—namely, a job that he wanted to leave and that deprived him of the freedom to relocate with his daughter. That the patient obtained such benefits from his illness in no way implies that factors of secondary gain were the cause of his chronic pain or that he was malingering. Rather, the patient had a physical problem that, in the end, gave him certain advantages; or, to put it another way, he simply made the best of a bad situation. On the other hand, the difficulties the patient faced in adapting to his pain

(continued)

were increased by the role the pain played in offering the patient a way out of an oppressive situation.

If the patient had been told that he was eligible for long-term disability only for as long as he remained severely disabled, it probably would have been much more difficult for him to make the kind of physical and psychological progress that he did make. If this had been the case, the physician would have done well to intervene, with the goal of minimizing the patient's internal resistance to making the fullest possible recovery. His dissatisfaction with his job and with the prospect of separating from his daughter would have needed to be addressed, which would have entailed exploring the aspects of these situations that were hard for him. Such a line of inquiry would probably have led to a new and deeper understanding of his feelings about his job and his daughter's leaving home. Such an understanding may in itself make a situation more acceptable to a patient; insight into a problem can be enough to reduce the gratification a patient obtains from being ill and can facilitate physical improvement and adaptation. In many cases, however, understanding is only the first step in the intervention. It is often also necessary to actively help patients to find practical solutions to their problems that do not rely on ongoing, severe physical and psychological disability.

Two years after he first met with the psychiatrist, the patient sent her a New Year's card to thank her and to say that he and his family were doing well. He wrote that he had come to see his back pain as a chronic disability that he could live with. He was no longer depressed or anxious but continued to take duloxetine for analgesia. He expressed satisfaction in having been able to adjust to his pain physically and psychologically, and he reported that he was enjoying his new life.

Unfortunately, treatment does not always proceed so smoothly. It is worth noting that the patient in this case had a number of important factors working in his favor. He had always functioned well in the past. He had a good work history and a good history of close, long-lasting relationships with others. Though he had psychological conflicts around separation and masculinity, he had a healthy, well-integrated personality. He had a number of excellent social supports, including a loving wife and daughter who were willing to support him emotionally and financially for as long as he needed. He had been employed at the same job for 25 years and had excellent medical and disability benefits. Even at his lowest point, he did not develop problematic substance use.

Patients with chronic pain often do not appear to be in pain and do not have the signs of autonomic arousal characteristic of patients with acute pain. These factors can lead the physician (and others) to believe mistakenly that the pain is not "real" and to assume that the patient is malingering or suffering from a primary psychiatric disorder. Many patients with chronic pain are sensitive about this and enter the physician–patient relationship defensively. When interviewing patients with chronic pain, physicians should emphasize that they understand that the patient's pain is genuine. The physician may say, "I know that many people with chronic pain have the experience of being told that their pain isn't real or that it's 'all in their heads.' I want to assure you that I know your pain is very real, as is your suffering."

Management

Patients and physicians must have **realistic expectations** about the treatment of chronic pain. Otherwise, both are likely to become frustrated and disappointed. Physicians should tell their patients that they understand the magnitude of the problem and the difficulties of treatment. It is helpful to mix **encouragement** with **tempered expectations**. Patients can be helped to anticipate a positive outcome but should also know that the work will proceed slowly and the gains will be hard-won. After consulting with the fireman described in Box 11.9 for the first time, the psychiatrist said, "I am confident that I can help you get back on your feet. But you have to expect that things will improve slowly and at the price of a fair amount of hard work and perseverance on your part. If you are able to accept this, you will be successful."

Patients should be educated about the role of psychological factors in the exacerbation of pain and the need to include these factors in the treatment plan. They should be helped to understand that secondary depression and substance abuse are common complications that must be treated. It is extremely important to emphasize that attending to psychological factors does not mean that the patient is weak or that the pain is not real. Over time, it will be necessary to help the patient make the transition from looking for a cure to managing with and adapting to a chronic problem.

Most patients with chronic pain require lengthy treatment. As a result, most physicians try to avoid prescribing narcotics for these patients, although in some cases it is inevitable. Antidepressants such as **duloxetine**, an SNRI, or **tricyclic antidepressants** (TCAs) are frequently prescribed, along with nonsteroidal anti-inflammatory agents. Anticonvulsants, such as **gabapentin** or **carbamazepine**, appear to be particularly effective for neuropathic pain, such as postherpetic or trigeminal neuralgia. In addition, nonpharmacological treatments such as hypnosis, meditation, or acupuncture may be helpful.

The use of antidepressants as analgesics is often a cause for confusion for patients and physicians. It may be unclear whether pain or depression is being treated. It has been clearly demonstrated that TCAs have analgesic effects that are independent of their antidepressant properties and that they can be effective in a wide variety of pain syndromes. TCAs tend to be particularly effective in the management of neuropathic pain, headache, facial pain, and arthritis. Antidepressants such as duloxetine have a separate indication for fibromyalgia and diabetic neuropathy. The efficacy of the SSRIs in the treatment of chronic pain remains equivocal. SSRIs are generally not used as first-line medications for analgesia in the treatment of chronic pain. For at least some patients, antidepressant medications are effective as analgesics at approximately half of the standard antidepressant dosage, but other patients may require the full antidepressant dosage. In non-depressed patients, it is important to emphasize that the medication is being used as an analgesic, not as an antidepressant. Otherwise, the patient may feel misunderstood and even insulted, thinking that the physician secretly believes that the patient is depressed or that the pain is "all in the patient's head." The treatment of the disabled fireman referred to previously in Box 11.9 is described in Box 11.11, illustrating the potential usefulness of antidepressant medication in chronic pain management.

When patients first develop a pain syndrome, they often hope that the pain will go away (i.e., that it will either resolve on its own or that a cure will be found). Over time, as the pain does not improve, many patients become depressed and anxious. Preoccupation with the pain is common, and many patients appear to be hypochondriacal. During this phase, patients often visit many physicians. While the process described thus far could apply to a patient diagnosed with any chronic illness, patients with chronic pain tend to have a particular experience as they go from physician to physician. Each new physician makes new promises and offers new hopes for relief, but ultimately, all of these "fall through." This process happens over and over again, leading the patient to feel increasingly frustrated, depressed, despondent, and angry.

The physician often has the same experience as the patient. There are initial feelings of optimism and hope of being able to succeed where previous physicians have failed, but these give way to feelings of increasing frustration and disappointment as all efforts fail to provide the patient with significant relief. It is not uncommon at this point for physicians to lose interest in the patient and to withdraw from the patient's care. The patient may experience this withdrawal as a painful rejection. Physicians may also be tempted to respond to the situation by blaming the patient, becoming suspicious that the patient's pain is not "real" or that the patient "doesn't want to get well." Recognition of such feelings by the physician can prevent inappropriately acting on them, deepen the physician's understanding of the patient's emotional experience, and ultimately improve the physician's care of the patient.

PSYCHOSOCIAL ASPECTS OF ADHERENCE

Clinical Features

One of the most powerful influences that psychological factors have on the course of a patient's medical illness is the effect they have on whether or not a patient follows medical advice. Adherence to medical advice or treatment becomes an issue when medications are prescribed, tests are indicated, or ongoing follow-up is needed. Adherence is also an important factor when a patient must modify high-risk behaviors, such as smoking cigarettes or being grossly overweight, that pose a serious threat to health.

Physicians often incorrectly assume that adherence to medical advice is the rule. About 50% of patients with chronic illness and up to 90% of patients with acute illness do not take their medications as prescribed. Adherence to taking medications tends to be particularly low when the patient does not have symptoms of a disease (as is often the case with antihypertensive or prophylactic medications). Perhaps most important in terms of overall health costs, adherence to a physician's recommendations for modifying risk factors tends to be exceedingly low.

While certain patients are at higher risk for not adhering to medical treatment than others, no one is immune (not even physicians and medical students). Among the groups of patients who are at especially **high risk for poor adherence** to medication are those patients who do not know why a particular medication is being prescribed or how they are supposed to take it. Patients who do not know in advance what side effects can be expected are also less likely to be adherent. Others at risk are patients who cannot afford medications, those who have cultural or religious biases against taking medications, and those whose families are opposed to the use of medications. Pill burden, the number of pills required each day, as well as the total number of daily doses in a day can also have profound effects on patients' adherence. Organizing a schedule around a patient's daily activities can help reduce problems. Patients with psychiatric disorders due to another medical condition; patients with primary psychiatric disorders, including psychotic, depressive, and anxiety disorders; as well as patients with neurocognitive disorders may also be especially vulnerable to nonadherence. Patients with maladaptive emotional and psychological reactions to illness, such as extreme denial, regression, and anger, can also be at risk.

Interview and Management

While individual circumstances and patient characteristics require specific interventions, some general treatment strategies can improve the adherence of many patients. The first strategy is the physician's placement of adherence high on the list of clinical problems to be addressed. Patients should be informed that poor adherence is extremely common and that they must work with the physician to combat this almost inevitable intrusion into the treatment.

When first prescribing a medication for a patient, the physician might say, "I am going to give you a medication that will help control your blood pressure. Controlling your blood pressure will lower your long-term risk of having a stroke or developing heart disease. This kind of medication needs to be taken daily. Believe it or not, even though it may not sound hard, many people find it difficult to take a pill every day on a long-term basis, especially when the problem being treated does not cause any symptoms." Such an introduction will make it easier for the patient to answer honestly when the physician inquires about adherence. The physician might go on to say, "Tell me your thoughts about starting medication, and then let's talk about how we can make it as easy as possible for you to take it reliably." Patients should be educated about the risks and side effects that can occur from irregular use of medications. When prescribing an SSRI, for example, a physician might want to remind the patient that these medications require daily use, and that "as needed" usage for anxiety or depression can actually result in a rebound or worsening of symptoms.

During follow-up visits, the physician should praise favorable results and **explore adherence problems** with the patient without reprimanding the patient or making moral judgments. The physician might say, "I can see from the number of pills still in the bottle that you've been finding it difficult to take your medication regularly every day. As I mentioned when you started the medicine, this is a very common problem. Let's talk about this to see if we can figure out together why you are having difficulty."

The medication and the recommendations given to the patient about taking it also affect adherence. The regimen should be made as **simple** as possible. Possible **side effects** should also be anticipated and discussed with the patient. The physician should provide the medication's brand name and its generic name, along with the indications, expected benefits, and length of time it will take before any benefits are felt. Writing out dosage schedules clearly and going over them with the patient is extremely important. For those who are taking numerous medications, the physician should suggest that the patient make a chart and use a pill box. Before the patient leaves the office with a new prescription, the physician should check again to make sure that the patient understands how to take the medication and that the patient's questions about it have all been answered. It is helpful to review information about medications when a family member is present. The support and participation of care partners who understand the benefits of the patient's medications can play a significant role in improving adherence.

Patients are more likely to adhere if the physician–patient relationship is positive. In fact, the **therapeutic alliance** may be the most powerful and reliable factor affecting adherence. Regularly scheduled appointments for monitoring adherence and progress are helpful, and patients should be encouraged to call with questions or concerns about their illness or its treatment. Physicians should foster a **collaborative atmosphere** between themselves and their patients. Patients who are actively involved in making decisions about their treatment are more likely to adhere to it. If there is a choice of treatments, the options should be reviewed with the patient, and the one that is most desirable (e.g., on the basis of side effects or cost) to the patient should be chosen. If medications need to be evaluated over time or dosages need to be titrated, the patient should be involved in the process. For example, the patient who is starting a new medication for prophylaxis of migraine headaches should be asked to keep a log of symptoms (e.g., frequency, severity, and duration of headaches) and side effects and to review the log with the physician at the next visit. This information then becomes part of the process in which the physician and the patient decide together about whether the patient is taking the right medication and the most effective dosage.

REFERENCES CITED

Kahana, R. J. and G. L. Bibring. Personality types in medical management. In Zinberg, N., ed. *Psychiatry and Medical Practice in a General Hospital*. New York: International Universities Press, 1964.

Strain, J. J., and S. Grossman, eds. *Psychological Care of the Medically Ill: A Primer in Liaison Psychiatry*. New York: Appleton-Century-Crofts, 1975.

SELECTED READINGS

Breitbart, W., and J. C. Holland (eds.). *Psychiatric Aspects of Symptom Management in Cancer Patients*. Washington, DC: American Psychiatric Press, 1993.

Breitbart, W., B. Rosenfeld, H. Pessin, M. Kaim, J. Funesti-Esch, M. Galietta, C. J. Nelson, and R. Brescia. Depression, hopelessness, and desire for hastened death in terminally ill patients with cancer. *JAMA: Journal of the American Medical Association* 284:2907–2911, 2000.

Cohen, M. A., and D. Chao. A biopsychosocial approach to psychiatric consultation in persons with HIV and AIDS. In Cohen, M. A., and J. M. Gorman, eds. *Comprehensive Textbook of AIDS Psychiatry*. New York: Oxford University Press, 2008.

Cohen-Cole, S. A., and C. Haupe. Diagnostic assessment of depression in the medically ill. In Stoudemire, A. S., and B. S. Fogel, eds. *Principles of Medical Psychiatry*. Orlando, FL: Grune and Stratton, 1987.

Epstein, L. A., and P. R. Muskin. Consultation-liaison psychiatry. In Sharfstein S. S., F. B. Dickerson, and J. M. Oldham, eds. *The American Psychiatric Publishing Textbook of Hospital Psychiatry*. Baltimore, MD: American Psychiatric Publishing, 2009.

Fogel, B. S., and C. Martin. Personality disorders in the medical setting. In Stoudemire, A. S., and B. S. Fogel, eds. *Principles of Medical Psychiatry*. Orlando, FL: Grune and Stratton, 1987.

Groves, M. A., and P. R. Muskin. Psychological responses to illness. In Levenson, J. L., ed. *The American Psychiatric Press Textbook of Psychosomatic Medicine*. Washington, DC: American Psychiatric Publishing, 2005.

Irwin, M. R., and H. Strausbaugh. Stress and immune changes in humans: a biopsychosocial model. In Gorman, J. M., and R. M. Kertzner, eds. *Psychoimmunology Update*. Washington, DC: American Psychiatric Press, 1991.

Molnar, G., and G. A. Fava. Intercurrent medical illness in the schizophrenic patient. In Stoudemire, A. S., and B. S. Fogel, eds. *Principles of Medical Psychiatry*. Orlando, FL: Grune and Stratton, 1987.

Nash, S. S., L. K. Kent, and P. R. Muskin. Psychodynamics in medically ill patients. *Harvard Review of Psychiatry* 17:389–397, 2009.

Schlozman, S. C., J. E. Groves, and A. D. Weisman. Coping with illness and psychotherapy of the medically ill. In Stern, T. A., G. L. Fricchione, N. H. Cassem, M. S. Jellinek, and J. F. Rosenbaum, eds. *Massachusetts General Hospital Handbook of General Hospital Psychiatry*. Philadelphia: Mosby/ Elsevier, 2004.

Stoudemire, A. S., M. B. Moran, and B. S. Fogel. Psychopharmacology in the medically ill patient. In Schatzberg, A. P., and C. B. Nereroff, eds. *The American Psychiatric Press Textbook of Psychopharmacology*. Washington, DC: American Psychiatric Press, 1995.

Stoudemire, A. S., and T. L. Thompson. Medication noncompliance: systematic approaches to evaluation and intervention. *General Hospital Psychiatry* 5:233–239, 1983.

/// 12 /// Suicide

BRIAN ROTHBERG AND ROBERT E. FEINSTEIN

Suicide is a major public health problem, both in the United States and abroad, and suicide prevention is a priority for the field of psychiatry. In the United States in 2010, suicide was the **tenth leading cause of death** in the general population and the **third leading cause** of death among the 15- to 24-year age group (Centers for Disease Control and Prevention, 2012; see Box 12.1). Rates in the United States have recently been **increasing**: over the past decade, suicide rates among middle-aged Americans rose by nearly 30%. Recent suicide deaths in active-duty U.S. soldiers have outnumbered combat deaths in Afghanistan.

Underlying psychiatric diagnoses clearly play a major role in the etiology of suicide. It has been repeatedly observed that many individuals who complete suicide see a physician in the month immediately preceding the event. This pattern makes it particularly important for physicians to be aware of how to conduct an effective assessment of suicide risk.

CLINICAL FEATURES

Suicide is defined as an intentional self-inflicted death. A **suicide attempt** is defined as a potentially self-injurious act committed with at least some wish to die, whether or not any injury occurs. Individuals with **suicidal ideation** have thoughts about killing themselves. Suicidal ideation may vary in seriousness as reflected in the details of the suicidal plan and the degree of suicidal intent. **Suicidal intent** is the intensity of the wish to die. Suicidal thoughts can be present without intent, in which case the thoughts are referred to as **passive** suicidal ideation. The **lethality** of suicidal behavior is the objective danger to life associated with a particular action. Lethality is distinct from and may not always coincide with an individual's expectation of what is medically dangerous. **Deliberate nonsuicidal self-harm** is the willful self-inflicting of painful, destructive, or injurious acts without the intent to die. Many patients who engage in nonsuicidal self-harm state that they feel a sense of "relief;" for example, a patient who was angry at a friend felt much better after cutting herself with a razor.

Patients with suicidal thoughts or behavior commonly feel frustrated, helpless, or hopeless. They tend to become extremely pessimistic when their repeated attempts to solve problems appear to have failed. They may verbalize feeling like a burden on others. Suicidal individuals often have a style of thinking that can be described as tunnel vision, leading them to believe that suicide is the only solution to their problems. They are

---

BOX 12.1

EPIDEMIOLOGY OF SUICIDE IN THE UNITED STATES

- Since the 1990s, suicide rates have ranged between 10.7 and 12.4 suicides per 100,000 persons.
- There are approximately 25 suicide attempts for each completed suicide in the general population.
- In 2010, the Centers for Disease Control and Prevention reported that 38,364 persons commit suicide annually (11 suicides per 100,000 persons).
- Men complete suicide at a rate four times that of women (79% of all suicides are males).
- Women attempt suicide approximately three times more often than men.
- The rate of suicide for women typically peaks in middle adulthood (ages 45–49) and typically declines slightly after age 60.
- Older white men (65 years of age and above) are at the highest risk with a rate of approximately 31 suicides per 100,000 persons each year.
- Between 1991 and 2009, suicide death rates from firearms among males 45 to 64 years of age were greater than all other suicide mechanisms combined.
- Older persons attempt suicide less often than younger persons, but are more often successful (approximately four suicide attempts for one completed suicide).
- Suicide is estimated to cost $34.6 billion a year in combined medical care and work loss.

Adapted from Centers for Disease Control and Prevention, National Center for Injury Prevention and Control. Suicide prevention, 2012. http://www.cdc.gov/ViolencePrevention/pdf/ Suicide_DataSheet-a.pdf

---

frequently angry, self-punishing, and harshly self-critical. They may describe themselves as stupid or worthless and say they deserve to die.

THE INTERVIEW

Screening

All psychiatric assessments should include screening for recent suicidal ideation and past suicide behavior (see Box 12.2). It is useful to keep in mind the characteristics of individuals who commit suicide in identifying high-risk patients who should be evaluated with particular care (see Box 12.3).

Safety

Once a patient is identified as currently suicidal, their safety becomes the first priority, keeping in mind that a balance needs to be struck between keeping the patient

BOX 12.2
COLUMBIA-SUICIDE SEVERITY RATING SCALE, SCREEN VERSION

1) WISH TO BE DEAD
Person endorses thoughts about a wish to be dead or not alive anymore, or a wish to fall asleep and not wake up.

Have you wished you were dead or wished you could go to sleep and not wake up?

2) SUICIDAL THOUGHTS
General nonspecific thoughts of wanting to end one's life or commit suicide.

Have you had any thoughts about killing yourself?

If YES to Question 2, ask Questions 3, 4, 5, and 6. If NO to Question 2, go directly to Question 6.

3) SUICIDAL THOUGHTS WITH METHOD (WITHOUT SPECIFIC PLAN OR INTENT TO ACT)
Person endorses thoughts of suicide and has thought of at least one method during the assessment period. This is different than a specific plan with time, place, or method details worked out. For example, "I thought about taking an overdose but I never made a specific plan as to when, where, or how I would actually do it…and I would never go through with it."

Have you been thinking about how you might kill yourself?

4) SUICIDAL INTENT (WITHOUT SPECIFIC PLAN)
Active suicidal thoughts of killing oneself with some intent to act on such thoughts.

Have you had these thoughts and had some intention of acting on them?

5) SUICIDAL INTENT WITH SPECIFIC PLAN
Thoughts of killing oneself with details of plan at least partially worked out and with some intent to carry it out.

Have you started to work out or worked out the details of how to kill yourself? Do you intend to carry out this plan?

6) SUICIDE BEHAVIOR
Have you ever done anything, started to do anything, or prepared to do anything to end your life? For example, collected pills, took pills, obtained a gun, gave away valuables, wrote a will or suicide note, took out pills but didn't swallow any, held a gun but changed your mind or it was grabbed from your hand, went to the roof but didn't jump.

From Posner, K., D. Brent., C. Lucas, M. Gould, B. Stanley, G. Brown, P. Fisher, J. Zelazny, A. Burke, M. Oquendo, & J.J. Mann. Copyright 2008 The Research Foundation for Mental Hygiene, Inc.

BOX 12.3

CHARACTERISTICS OF INDIVIDUALS WHO COMMIT SUICIDE

- Past history of suicide attempt

MOST COMMON MEANS
- Males: firearms
- Females: poisoning

RACIAL STATISTICS
- Caucasian males have the highest suicide rate, followed by Native Americans, and then African-American males.

RELIGIOUS
- Protestants and atheists have the highest rates.
- Catholics and Orthodox Jews have the lowest rates.

MARITAL STATUS
- Those who are divorced, separated, or widowed have the highest rates.
- Those who are married rank among the lowest.

CONTACT WITH PHYSICIAN
- Those recently discharged from inpatient psychiatric hospitalizations (highest risk is in the first month past discharge)

MEDICAL COMORBIDITIES
- The most common nonpsychiatric diagnoses are cancer, chronic obstructive pulmonary disease, and chronic pain.
- Patients undergoing renal dialysis have a suicide rate 400 times that of the general population.

PSYCHOSOCIAL FACTORS
- History of physical and sexual abuse
- Family history of suicide
- Financial difficulties

PSYCHIATRIC DIAGNOSES
- Depressive disorders
- Alcohol and other substance use disorders
- Psychotic disorders
- Cluster B personality disorders
- Panic disorder

---

safe and respecting their dignity and personhood. If patients reveal thoughts of self-harm, death, and hopelessness in an outpatient setting, the physician must inquire about plans to end their lives. If an imminent threat is present, help from law enforcement may need to be enlisted to ensure the safe transition to a higher level of care. On an inpatient unit, the surroundings and level of supervision of suicidal patients will need to be regulated to ensure that they do not have the opportunity to harm themselves.

Obtaining the History

As with all patients, the history-taking portion of the interview with a suicidal patient begins with an effort to establish a therapeutic **alliance**. In the case of acutely suicidal patients in an emergency room setting, providing physical comforts such a warm blanket if they are cold, or food and fluids if they are hungry, can be helpful in establishing an alliance. The physician should explain that the main purpose of the interview is to find out what drove the patient to desperation. A careful history should be taken to explore the events that may have incited the emergence of suicidal thoughts or behavior.

In presenting their history, suicidal patients may minimize or deny their intentions and may provide a narrative that leads the physician to greatly underestimate the gravity of the clinical situation. The physician must be careful not to collude with the patient's denial about the seriousness of the symptoms or behaviors (see Box 12.4). For example, a patient being evaluated for a questionable suicide attempt may have ingested 10 benzodiazepine sleeping pills and later claim, "I wasn't suicidal. I was just trying to go to sleep." While the overdose was not pharmacologically dangerous, it may be psychologically revealing of serious suicidal intention. Clinically, this suicide attempt is an important warning sign that should be taken as seriously as an ingestion of 50 lethal pills. The denial of suicidal intention needs to be questioned and the meanings of the patient's suicidal crisis explored. The physician should encourage the patient to describe all of his or her feelings before, during, and after the attempt (see Box 12.5).

Collateral information obtained from family members, treating providers, and other people with whom the patient has had recent contact may be crucial in evaluating a suicidal patient, by broadening the scope of the physician's understanding of the patient's attitudes, beliefs, and behaviors (see Box 12.6). Understanding both the subjective and objective timeline of the course of events will provide an opportunity to compare the patient's psychological understanding of the events with evidence from friends, family, police, or emergency medical technicians (EMT). If the patient is still unable to gain access to his or her feelings and make sense of the events, the physician should consider changing from an individual approach to a crisis-family model, in which family members are invited to tell their versions of the events in the presence of the patient. This approach may be effective in breaching the blockade of the patient's denial and allowing the open expression of feelings.

Risk Assessment

Although physicians are not able to predict which individuals will eventually complete suicide, there are factors known to place people at a particularly high risk. The Columbia Suicide Severity Rating Scale (C-SSRS; Posner et al. 2011) provides a **reliable and validated objective assessment of suicide risk** (see Box 12.2). The scale measures the **severity and intensity of suicidal ideation**, as well as suicidal behavior and the **lethality of actual suicide attempts**. The scale has been shown to have **predictive validity**, but it cannot provide a definitive risk estimate. It is essential to use it in combination with clinical assessments and judgments.

Suicidal Ideation

Suicidal ideation varies in its degree of risk. The intensity of ideation, including frequency and duration of thoughts, should be assessed. More frequent and more long-standing

---

BOX 12.4

SAMPLE QUESTIONS AND ADDITIONAL INTERVIEWING TIPS FOR SUICIDAL PATIENTS

- Use the terms *suicide* or *suicide attempt* to help the patient realize that you want to hear about the painful details.
- Ask about the frequency, intensity, duration, and specificity of thoughts.
- Always ask about method.
  - "How are you thinking about killing yourself?"
  - "Do you have access to (method)?"
  - "What to you think will actually happen if you use (method) to kill yourself?"
- "Have you thought about when or where you would kill yourself?"
- Always ask about multiple methods, although patients most often will not consider multiple methods.
- "What are your reasons for wanting to die?"
- Ask about protective factors.
  - "Even though you've had a very difficult time, something has kept you going."
  - "What are your reasons for living?"
- How did the patient end up accessing care?
- Did the patient initiate getting help?
- Was it by random chance that the patient was found after the attempt?
  - "How did you get to the hospital?"
  - "Did you call someone?"
- Did the patient take active steps to prevent discovery or rescue?
  - "Did you take steps to try to prevent your discovery or rescue when you made the suicide attempt?"
  - "Did you time the attempt or otherwise make it difficult for someone to find you?"
- "How do you feel about surviving?"
- "Did you learn anything helpful about yourself or others from the behavior?"
- What was the patient's perception of lethality of his or her behavior?
  - "Did you think that what you did would kill you?"

---

suicidal ideation predicts higher risk. Uncontrollability of thoughts, the absence of deterrents (such as religious beliefs, responsibility for dependent family members), and the reasons for the suicidal ideation are relevant to the risk assessment as well. **Deliberate planning** of a destructive act for which the patient has the means suggests a high risk. Patients who view suicide as a **solution** to a specific problem are at high risk. For example, a man wanted to kill himself to get away from a job that was particularly stressful after he was unable to find other work for some time. Patients who have not made a plan and are ambivalent about hurting themselves have a lesser risk. Patients with ambivalent

---

BOX 12.5

SAMPLE QUESTIONS FOR ASSESSING AN OVERDOSE

- "Can you describe what happened and how you were feeling the day before you took the pills?"
- "When did you take the pills?"
- "Who was there?"
- "How did you take the pills?"
- "One at a time or all together?"
- "What were you thinking and feeling at the time?"
- "After you took the pills, what happened?"
- "Who did you tell?"
- "How did they find you?"
- "How did you get here for medical treatment?"
- "How did you feel when you didn't die?"
- "What do you wish had happened?"

BOX 12.6

CASE EXAMPLE ILLUSTRATING THE UTILITY OF COLLATERAL INFORMATION WHEN CONDUCTING A RISK ASSESSMENT

A 65-year-old man was brought to the emergency room by police officers. They had picked him up on a nearby elevated highway. The patient told the physician in the emergency room that he had been walking "to calm my nerves" after an argument that evening with his daughter about his need for psychiatric care. He denied that he was depressed or suicidal. His self-care was poor, and he appeared anxious but was able to respond appropriately during the interview. The physician was curious: if the patient had been out on the highway, only for a late evening walk, why did the police officers bother to question him and take him to the emergency room for further evaluation?

The officers who had brought in the patient were located and interviewed. They said that the patient had been halfway over the elevated highway railing when they first saw him. He tried to jump over the railing as the police approached. They saved him, and when he became angry and assaultive they had to handcuff him to bring him into the emergency room.

When the patient was confronted with these facts he acknowledged that he had been depressed, feared he was becoming demented, and worried that he would become an unfair burden on his daughter. He preferred to die rather than "lose [his] mind" and become a burden. He required psychiatric hospitalization. Evaluation revealed that he did not have dementia. Instead it was determined that he was simply depressed, and he was successfully treated for a major depressive episode.

or fleeting thoughts or fantasies are at low risk, particularly if they have no intention of action. For example, a person who makes a superficial cut on her wrist and then calls a family member appears ambivalent about committing suicide.

Suicidal Behavior

A history of past suicide attempts is a risk factor for future suicide. Risk is increased by more **serious,** more **frequent,** or more **recent** attempts. The physician should inquire about past suicide attempts and self-destructive behaviors, including specific questioning about suicide attempts that were **interrupted** by an outside circumstance or person or **aborted** by the patient. Examples of the latter would include putting a gun to one's head but not firing it, driving to a bridge but not jumping, or creating a noose but not using it. The physician should also explore details about the **precipitants, timing, intent,** and **consequences** as well as the medical **lethality** of the attempt. The patient's consumption of **alcohol and drugs** before the attempt should also be ascertained, since intoxication can facilitate impulsive suicide attempts but can also be a component of a more serious suicidal plan. The physician should question the patient about the outcome of each attempt and the patient's reaction to surviving the suicide attempt. If the patient has had many attempts, explore in detail the "worst" suicidal episode, as well as the first and last attempts. Finally, in patients who have not made a suicide attempt, inquiry should be made about **preparatory acts or behaviors**. The behavior might be in preparation for a particular suicide method (e.g., purchasing a gun or pills) or for death (e.g., giving away belongings, writing a suicide note).

Psychiatric Symptoms and Diagnoses

Psychotic patients who are suicidal in response to delusions or to **command auditory hallucinations** are at particularly high risk. It is important to ask about **previous psychiatric diagnoses** and treatments, including illness **onset and course,** psychiatric **hospitalizations,** as well as **treatment for substance use disorders** (see Differential Diagnosis, later in this chapter). Specific symptoms such as **impulsivity, hopelessness, fearfulness, or apprehension,** whether or not focused on specific concerns, increase risk. Contact with caregivers can provide relevant information and help in the planning for treatment. With patients who are currently in treatment, the strength and stability of the therapeutic relationships should be assessed, as a positive therapeutic alliance may be protective.

Psychosocial History

Patients who are suicidal are persons **"in crisis."** A crisis is defined as a situation in which a person faces an obstacle to important life goals that seems insurmountable through the use of customary methods of problem solving or coping behavior. During the ensuing period of disorganization or crisis, a variety of abortive attempts are made to solve the problem. Eventually, some kind of adaptation is achieved, which may or may not be effective. The crisis model assumes that the patient was previously in a state of equilibrium and analyzes how equilibrium can be restored. This process may involve simply replacing or reinforcing internal or external supports that may help the patient return to the previous equilibrium or status quo. The physician will need to help the patient through the crisis until the risk for suicide has subsided or is resolved.

Establishing a **baseline** of behavior—that is "who this person is" when not in crisis—will further the working alliance, as well as help reorient the patient to his or her healthier self (see Box 12.7). Under normal circumstances, a person has a stable internal

---

BOX 12.7
AREAS TO COVER IN OBTAINING A PSYCHOSOCIAL HISTORY

PSYCHOSOCIAL SITUATION

- Acute psychosocial crises
- Chronic psychosocial stressors
- Employment status
- Living situation
- Family constellation
- Cultural or religious beliefs

INDIVIDUAL STRENGTHS AND VULNERABILITIES

- Ability to cope with stress
- Ability to tolerate psychological pain
- Ability to satisfy individual needs

---

psychological equilibrium and receives emotional and other kinds of support from a network of relatives, friends, and other persons. This enables the individual to participate in and enjoy the normal activities of daily living as well as to cope with the daily stressors of everyday life. Suicidal symptoms can develop when internal or external stressful events disturb this equilibrium. The suicidal patient is often not aware of these stressors or may deny that they exist. It may be important to ask the patient to describe, in minute detail, their feelings about themselves, interactions, and events that occurred immediately before, during, and after the suicidal thoughts or behavior, in order to ascertain the stressful events.

Possible stressors include financial difficulties or changes in socioeconomic status, legal difficulties, actual or perceived interpersonal conflicts or losses, housing problems, job loss, educational failure, family discord, domestic violence, and past or current sexual or physical abuse or neglect. Stressors can be psychological events such as feelings of hopelessness, anxiety, fearfulness, recent or impending humiliation, or feelings of shame or apprehension. Stressors may be acute or chronic. Usually, the individual with suicidal impulses is experiencing several chronic and acute psychosocial stressors. The physician should explore the patient's employment history, current living situation, including whether there are children in the home, the makeup of the family, the quality of those relationships, and cultural or religious beliefs about death and suicide.

Family History
The following information should be obtained about family members: suicide or suicide attempts, mental illness, and substance abuse. When suicides have occurred in first-degree relatives, it is often helpful to learn more about the circumstances, including the patient's involvement. The patient's childhood and current family environment may also be relevant, since many aspects of family dysfunction may be linked to self-destructive behaviors. Such factors include a history of family conflict or separation, parental legal trouble, and family substance use.

Physician Reactions

Suicidal patients are among the most challenging patients for physicians to treat and can evoke anxiety in even the most experienced clinicians. Suicidal patients can activate a clinician's own latent emotions about death and suicide, leading to a number of defensive responses on the part of the clinician, ranging from **avoidance**, to **minimization** of the significance of suicidal symptoms, to **overestimation** of the patient's capabilities (creating unrealistic and overwhelming expectations). Conversely, the physician may become enveloped by the patient's sense of helplessness and despair and feel **discouraged** about the patient's capacity to improve. Physicians sometimes **worry excessively** that a suicidal patient might die and fear that their medical career will be ruined if the patient commits suicide. Physicians sometimes feel **angry** with manipulative suicidal patients. Some physicians imagine that they can keep suicidal patients alive through heroic measures. Such **rescue fantasies** can lead to misguided treatment decisions. When patients make suicide attempts or succeed in committing suicide, physicians may feel **guilty** and responsible.

DIFFERENTIAL DIAGNOSIS

Over 90% of individuals who die by suicide have at least one psychiatric disorder. **Mood disorders** are particularly associated with an increased risk of suicide during a **depressive episode**. Patients with depression are more likely to commit suicide if they have **panic attacks, insomnia**, or **alcohol or drug abuse**. Those who are recovering from depression who gain energy may be at increased risk as well. It is estimated that approximately 15% of patients who require hospitalization for a major depressive episode are at lifetime risk for committing suicide.

Patients with **schizophrenia** are estimated to have a lifetime risk of about 4%. Suicide may occur more frequently during the early years of this illness, and the time immediately after hospital discharge is a period of heightened risk. Although psychotic symptoms are often present at the time of an attempt or completed suicide, suicide may occur during periods when psychotic symptoms are improving. Sometimes suicide occurs in patients with schizophrenia when additional depressive symptoms are present. Suicide risk may paradoxically be increased in those who have insight into the implications of having a psychotic illness, particularly if this insight is coupled with a feeling of hopelessness.

Alcohol and other substance use disorders are associated with an increased risk for suicide—approximately six times that of the general population. Recent or impending interpersonal losses and comorbid psychiatric disorders have been linked to suicide in alcoholic individuals. Suicide is also more likely to occur among alcoholics who suffer from depressive episodes than in persons with major depression or alcoholism alone.

Compared to the general population, individuals with **personality disorders** have an estimated risk for suicide that is about seven times greater. Specific increases in suicide risk have been associated with borderline and antisocial personality disorders. Personality disorders have been identified in approximately 30% of those who commit suicide. **Medical comorbidities** must be assessed and factored into the suicide assessment. Acute or chronic medical illnesses may be one of the core factors creating a sense of a foreshortened future and a burden on family and friends. In particular, chronic diseases such as diabetes mellitus and renal failure requiring long-term dialysis are associated with an increased risk of suicide.

ETIOLOGY

Neurobiological Factors

Although psychiatric disorders infer an increased risk of suicidal behavior, many patients with psychiatric disorders, including major depression, never attempt suicide. Research has increasingly focused on identifying additional predisposing factors. A 4- to 10-fold increase in suicidal behavior has been observed in first-degree relatives of suicidal individuals. This familial transmission appears to occur independent of the familial risk for psychiatric disorders. **Impulsivity** seems to be an inherited trait that makes individuals more vulnerable to suicide. Ongoing research is trying to identify genetic markers for such vulnerability.

Several lines of evidence suggest that **serotoninergic dysfunction** is associated with increased **suicide risk**. For example, lower levels of the serotonin metabolite 5-hydroxyindoleacetic acid (5-HIAA) have been found in the cerebrospinal fluid of individuals who have made more lethal suicide attempts, and postmortem brains of individuals who completed suicide have abnormal serotonergic function localized to the ventromedial prefrontal cortex.

Psychosocial Factors

Family Influences

Suicidal behavior may serve as a means of communication between family members. Threats of suicide are sometimes used to gain power and control over other family members. Suicidal symptoms may be a sign of serious underlying family problems. For example, a woman repeatedly attempted suicide by talking pills. These attempts began when she was 7 years old and continued until she was 25 years old. Therapy revealed that the attempts occurred after episodes of sexual abuse by her father.

Societal Influences

Cultural influences vary widely and can greatly affect attitudes toward suicide and violence. Citizens of Japan traditionally have viewed suicide as an **honorable solution** to a disgraceful situation, whereas many other cultures consider suicide a dishonorable act. Media reports of people who commit suicide can precipitate "**copycat**" suicides. Suicide contagion can spread through a school system, through a community, or, in the case of a celebrity suicide, nationally. To prevent this phenomenon, it has become customary for schools or media to downplay suicide reports.

TREATMENT

Motivation for Treatment

The physician must determine whether the patient is willing to follow through with treatment and whether he or she is capable of it. Some high-risk suicidal patients are incapable of engaging in therapy because the severity of their symptoms impairs their ability to think. Patients with dementia or psychosis who cannot plan ahead or take action may not be able to engage in treatment. Other patients may lack the motivation to follow through. The physician should elicit patients' thoughts and feelings and observe their actions to assess their motivation for change.

Therapeutic Settings

Outpatient Treatment

Outpatient treatment of a suicidal patient should be attempted only when the physician is certain that the patient wants help and has a fully available support system. The potential for a reemergence of suicidal thoughts must be discussed with patients and their support system. A detailed plan for how to manage suicidal acts should be developed. Plans should include ways to recognize precipitants, stress, and other early warning signs that suicidal ideation might reemerge. Patients need to have detailed plans of what to do if symptoms occur. They should be instructed to use 24-hour help hotlines; to enlist the help of family, friends, or current treating providers; or to find the nearest emergency room if they and their support system cannot manage their symptoms. A psychiatric hospitalization should be readily available if outpatient treatment fails.

For many patients **crisis intervention** in combination with monitoring from the patient's psychosocial support system is the safest approach. The physician helps to mobilize the individual's social network and promote adaptive coping mechanisms to reestablish equilibrium. The overall goal is to foster feelings of hope in the patient by beginning the problem-solving process. Supportive measures to provide stabilization include encouragement and praise for use of behaviors that have previously worked. Psychotherapy can facilitate the acquisition of new understanding, new cognitive or interpersonal skills, or the modification of relationships. These changes can contribute to reaching a new and potentially better equilibrium.

Hospital Treatment

All **psychotic** patients should be strongly considered for hospitalization after a suicide attempt. Hospitalization should also be considered for patients whose suicide attempt was **violent, near lethal**, or **premeditated**; if precautions were taken to **avoid rescue** or discovery; if the patient **regrets surviving;** and if the patient still has a **persistent plan** and/or **intent**. Hospitalization should also be strongly considered for all **male patients older than age 45** years who have made a suicide attempt, especially if they are suffering from the new onset of psychiatric illness and if they have limited family or social support, including lack of a stable living situation. Hospitalization is also generally indicated for patients after a suicide attempt if they display severe agitation, refuse help, or have a change in mental status requiring further workup in a structured setting. A multimodal approach can be used during hospitalization to address the psychiatric and psychosocial issues that led to the suicidal behavior (see Box 12.8).

Hospitalization may be necessary even in the absence of a suicide attempt if a patient describes a specific plan with high lethality and suicidal intent. Hospitalization should be considered if suicidal ideation is present in a patient who is **psychotic** or who has a history of **past attempts**, particularly if near lethal. Hospitalization may be the safest option in patients with other contributing **medical conditions** (e.g., an acute neurological disorder, cancer, infection), patients who have not responded to outpatient treatment, and patients who are no longer able to cooperate with outpatient treatment. Hospitalization may be helpful for patients with **limited family or social support**, including the lack of a stable living situation; patients with ongoing problems in their relationship with their therapist or physician; or those with **lack of access** to timely outpatient follow-up. Hospitalization also may be necessary if a patient with suicidal ideation feels that he or she will inevitably act on those impulses.

BOX 12.8

CASE EXAMPLE ILLUSTRATING HOSPITAL TREATMENT FOLLOWING A SUICIDE ATTEMPT

A 55-year-old married storeowner, who had been undergoing outpatient treatment for depression and alcoholism, was admitted after taking a serious overdose of his antidepressant as well as alcohol. A number of immediate stressors were identified, including his wife's diagnosis of breast cancer, his oldest daughter's marriage (who managed the store) and her plans to move away, the patient's recent worry that he might have prostate cancer, and feelings of hopelessness about his persistent depression. Consultation with the patient's outpatient psychiatrist helped the team focus on the need for family assessment (which had never occurred before), medical evaluation, and medication adjustment.

The patient tended to put on a cheerful front and function "normally" at the store and with friends and family. He hid from everyone his increasing despair and his recent workup for prostate cancer, not wanting to further burden his family. These feelings overwhelmed him and led to the suicide attempt.

The therapeutic goal was to discuss the events preceding his overdose and their meaning, as well as his fears about his wife's life-threatening illness, his daughter's move, and his possible cancer. Individual and group insight-oriented psychotherapy were essential for this patient, as was family therapy conducted jointly by his inpatient psychiatrist and a social worker. The nursing staff played an important role by encouraging the patient to socialize during his free time rather than sit and read in his room. For this patient, the inpatient milieu served as a safe place to confront his fears and his maladaptive defenses and coping style, including his alcoholism, while also providing much support. In addition, his prostate condition could be assessed.

Within 10 days the patient was ready for discharge. He felt supported in dealing with his new diagnosis of prostate cancer as the discharge plan included a referral to the cancer center as well as individual psychotherapy and pharmacotherapy, as well as family therapy.

Pharmacotherapy

Antidepressants

Suicidal symptoms are commonly associated with depressive disorders. The **selective serotonin reuptake inhibitors** (SSRIs) are often used as first-line treatments. While there is some concern that SSRIs might be associated with increased risks of aggressive or impulsive acts, including suicide, the risk of not treating a depressed suicidal patient with medication outweighs the possible risk from the medication. The U.S. Food and Drug Administration (FDA) has issued a **black-box warning** stating that individuals less than 25 years of age who take these medications may experience increased suicidal ideation and/or behavior particularly in the first months of taking an antidepressant. As treatment begins, baseline levels of anxiety, agitation, and sleep disturbance should be determined.

Physicians should carefully monitor patients for increasing suicidal symptoms. Patients should be seen frequently, particularly at the beginning of treatment. The FDA recommends weekly visits for the first month, bi-weekly for the second month, and at least one visit in the third month for those who are 24 years of age and younger. Analysis of data regarding those over 24 years of age has shown that the net effect of antidepressant use in patients ages 25 to 64 appears to be moderately protective against suicidal ideation and more strongly protective for adults age 65 and older.

Other Medications

Lithium may reduce the risk of suicide attempts in patients with mood disorders. Some patients will not want to take it because of its side effects and requirement of blood level monitoring. Its potential lethality in overdose should also be taken into consideration when prescribing lithium. Although **mood-stabilizing anticonvulsants** can be helpful for manic excitement or irritability, impulsivity associated with personality disorders, and impulse control disorders, there is no established evidence that these medications directly reduce suicidality. Of the second-generation antipsychotics, **clozapine** has been the most studied; evidence shows a reduction in suicidal behavior in schizophrenic patients.

Benzodiazepines

Benzodiazepines have no demonstrated short- or long-term antisuicide efficacy. Acute suicide risk that is associated with severe anxiety, panic attacks, agitation, and severe insomnia, however, can be reduced with short-term benzodiazepine treatment. Patients should be monitored for worsening depression or worsening aggressive and dangerous behaviors. Monitoring of benzodiazepines is particularly important when they are used for an extended period, especially in patients with borderline personality disorder and head injury, as benzodiazepines can disinhibit patients and increase aggressive behaviors.

Electroconvulsive Therapy (ECT)

Evidence exists that ECT reduces suicidal ideation. ECT may be particularly helpful in suicidal depressed patients who are not eating and thus are in imminent danger, who have not responded to medications, or who are pregnant.

Psychotherapy

Psychotherapy can play a vital role in the management of suicidal behavior. Techniques common to all psychotherapies, such as forming an **empathetic therapeutic alliance** and **instilling hope**, can help alleviate suicidal symptoms. Suicidal patients may benefit from individual treatment, group treatment, or a combination of both. **Psychodynamic psychotherapy** techniques can identify suicidal patients' predominant psychological defenses and modify their pathological functioning. Dialectical behavioral therapy uses cognitive-behavioral therapy (CBT) and other techniques to treat suicidality in patients with borderline personality disorder (see Chapter 17, Psychotherapy).

Family therapy can be extremely effective in treating suicidal symptoms that arise within the context of a transaction between family members. It is often necessary to treat the entire family because other members may have the capacity to break the pathological interaction. Family therapy for suicidal patients usually combines psychoeducational, strategic, and structural approaches (see Chapter 17, Psychotherapy).

Chronic Suicidality

Some patients develop a lifelong daily pattern of suicidality. The treatment of such patients is geared toward the underlying severe personality disorder or refractory psychosis or mood disorder. If the patient is amenable to treatment, it is usually long term and multi-modal, although sometimes with brief, intermittent, and problem-focused interventions. Psychodynamic psychotherapy, CBT, family therapy, and pharmacotherapy may be used in inpatient or outpatient settings. Treatment may last for several years in an outpatient or institutional setting, including long-term psychiatric facilities or a group home.

LEGAL ISSUES

Confidentiality

In caring for suicidal patients, physicians sometimes struggle with conflicting responsibil-ities to respect patient autonomy and protect patients from self-harm, which can require the disclosure of protected health information. The concept of "imminent" danger is a key to physician decision-making in these cases. The Health Information Protection and Portability Act (HIPPA) allows for breaches of doctor–patient confidentiality, in limited circumstances. The Department of Health and Human Services has issued guidelines for physicians around breaches of confidentiality (Rodriguez 2013): "The HIPPA Privacy Rule protects the privacy of patients' health information but is balanced to ensure that appropriate uses and disclosures of information still may be made when necessary to treat a patient, to protect the nation's public health, and for critical purposes such as when a provider seeks to warn or report that persons may be at risk of harm because of a patient." Physicians must use their best clinical judgment to decide if a suicidal patient has passed the threshold of posing an imminent risk to themselves and to notify the appropriate individuals. Physicians may need to review the statutes of their state to clarify the mean-ing of "imminent risk" as defined by state-specific legislation.

Involuntary Commitment

In most states, any physician can involuntarily detain a patient in an emergency room. When medically necessary to save the life of another person or the patient, patients can initially be held against their will for 72 hours. This is not a punitive measure, but rather an effort to provide essential emergency psychiatric care and treatment. Many patients who are involuntarily committed will protest at first, but in time, usually they will come to appreciate receiving appropriate psychiatric care. Committed patients are entitled to legal representation, and they retain all of their civil rights with regard to participating in treatment decisions, including taking or not taking medication. Some states also allow involuntary hospitalization when patients are "gravely disabled." The criteria for **gravely disabled** applies to patients who are not able to care for themselves (e.g., patients with ill-nesses such as schizophrenia or bipolar disorder). Gravely disabled patients are unable to perform the basic functions of life, such as feeding themselves, finding shelter or a place to live, or getting medical treatment.

REFERENCES CITED

Centers for Disease Control and Prevention, National Center for Injury Prevention and Control. Suicide prevention. http://www.cdc.gov/ViolencePrevention/pdf/Suicide_DataSheet-a.pdf

Posner, K., G. K. Brown, B. Stanley, et al. The Columbia Suicide Severity Rating Scale: initial validity and internal consistency findings from three multisite studies with adolescents and adults. *American Journal of Psychiatry* 1168:1266–1277, 2011.

Rodriguez, L. (2013, January 15). Message to our nation's health care providers. U. S. Department of Health and Human Services. http://www.hhs.gov/ocr/office/lettertonationhcp.pdf

SELECTED READINGS

American Psychiatric Association. Practice guideline for the assessment and treatment of patients with suicidal behaviors. *American Journal of Psychiatry* 160:1–60, 2003.

Cavanagh, J. T., A. J. Carson, M. Sharpe, and S. M. Lawrie. Psychological autopsy studies of suicide: a systematic review. *Psychological Medicine* 33:395–405, 2003.

Feinstein, R., and R. Plutchik. Violence and suicide risk assessment in the psychiatric emergency room. *Comprehensive Psychiatry* 31:337–343, 1990.

Joiner, T. E., Jr. The trajectory of suicidal behavior over time. *Suicide and Life Threatening Behavior* 32:33–41, 2002.

Joiner, T. E., Jr., Y. Conwell, K. K. Fitzpatrick, T. K. Witte, N. B. Schmidt, M. T. Berlim, M. P. Fleck, and M. D. Rudd. Four studies on how past and current suicidality relate even when "everything but the kitchen sink" is covaried. *Journal of Abnormal Psychology* 114:291–303, 2005.

Mann, J. J., and D. Currier. Understanding and preventing suicide. In Stein, D. J., D. J. Kupfer, and A. F. Schatzberg, eds. *The American Psychiatric Publishing Textbook of Mood Disorders*. Arlington, VA: American Psychiatric Publishing, 2006.

Mann, J. J., and D. M. Stoff. A synthesis of current findings regarding neurobiological correlates and treatment of suicidal behavior. *Annals of the New York Academy of Science* 836:352–363, 1997.

Maris, R., A. Berman, and M. Silverman. *Comprehensive Textbook of Suicidology*. New York: Guilford Press, 2000.

Paris, J. Predicting and preventing suicide: do we know enough to do either? *Harvard Review of Psychiatry* 14(5):233–240, 2006.

Posner K., M. A. Oquendo, M. Gould, B. Stanley, and M. Davies. Columbia Classification Algorithm of Suicide Assessment (C-CASA): classification of suicidal events in the FDA's pediatric suicidal risk analysis of antidepressants. *American Journal of Psychiatry* 164:1035–1043, 2007.

Rudd, M. *The Assessment and Management of Suicidality*. Sarasota, FL: Professional Resource Press, 2006.

Rudd, M. D., T. Joiner, and M. H. Rajab. *Treating Suicidal Behavior: An Effective, Time-Limited Approach*. New York, Guilford Press, 2001.

Shea, S. C. The chronological assessment of suicide events: a practical interviewing strategy for the elicitation of suicidal ideation. *Journal of Clinical Psychiatry* 59(Suppl 20):58–72, 1998.

Shneidman, E. S. *Autopsy of a Suicidal Mind*. New York: Oxford University Press, 2004.

Stone, M., T. Laughren, M. L. Jones, M. Levenson, et al. Risk of suicidality in clinical trials of antidepressants in adults: analysis of proprietary data submitted to US Food and Drug Administration. *British Medical Journal* 339:b2880, 2009.

/// 13 /// Violence

ROBERT E. FEINSTEIN AND BRIAN ROTHBERG

Violence is a major public health problem. It lies within the province of psychiatry when the perpetrator has a psychiatric illness. Violent ideation and aggressive behavior can be manifestations of psychiatric illness. Violent acts committed by individuals suffering from mental illness must be distinguished, however, from the commission of violent crimes and institutionalized violence, such as terrorism or war. Psychiatric patients are more likely to be victims of violence and crimes than perpetrators. In fact, psychiatric patients are 2.5 times more likely to be attacked, raped, or mugged than individuals in the general population. Among individuals with schizophrenia and other psychoses, however, there is a small but significantly higher risk of homicide: 0.3%, compared with 0.02% in the general population. This association between psychosis and violence is strongest in people with comorbid substance use disorders, and most of the excess risk of violence associated with schizophrenia and other psychoses appears to be mediated by substance use (Fazel et al. 2009).

CLINICAL FEATURES

Violence can be defined as an individual's use of verbal threat, intimidation, or physical force with the intent to cause property damage, personal harm, or death to another person. Violent behavior can be categorized according to its level of organization: it can be classified as disorganized and impulsive, or organized and premeditated.

Agitated, disorganized, affective, impulsive violent behavior tends to be manifested as irritability, panic, or anger. Often this is expressed as confusion, insomnia, verbal outbursts, temper tantrums, or unfocused physical violence. Agitation, emotional outbursts, or anger may result in significant psychological harm to others, serious destruction of property, or physical violence. Patients can act passively or "bottle up" their feelings, only to explode later. They often have little or no insight into their aggressive behavior. This kind of violence is associated with delirium, other neurocognitive disorders, such as those due to Alzheimer's disease and traumatic brain injury; impulse control disorders, including intermittent explosive disorder; substance-related disorders; psychotic and mood disorders; and some personality disorders.

Individuals who engage in **organized, predatory, premeditated violence** are usually not mentally ill, although some of these individuals may have severe personality disorders, particularly antisocial personality disorder. Such people may derive predatory sadistic pleasure from scaring other people or putting them in a humiliated or weakened position. They do not typically benefit from psychiatric treatment.

THE INTERVIEW

Safety

Patients with acute aggressive or violent impulses are typically experiencing a turbulent emotional crisis, which leaves them fragile, volatile, and determined to take action. These circumstances present a clinical challenge. The physician will not be able to conduct a useful psychiatric interview if he or she feels threatened. Thus, potentially violent patients need immediate attention and evaluation to determine their risk of imminent violence and their need for medication, seclusion, or physical restraint in order to **establish a safe environment**. The evaluation begins by observing the patient's appearance and behavior (e.g., self-care and hygiene, level of consciousness, physical signs of agitation, intoxication, withdrawal, other medical illness, or intellectual disability) from a distance for at least 30 seconds. Such evaluations must be conducted in a safe location, such as the holding area in an emergency room or the quiet room in an inpatient psychiatric service. In outpatient settings, high-risk patients should be interviewed in an open public space with other staff nearby and readily available. Patients commonly present with friends and family. If it appears that they will help calm the situation, they should be allowed to stay; if not, they may be asked to leave.

The next step in establishing a safe environment will depend on the patient's current **behavioral phase of agitation.** As the intensity of violent symptoms increases, persons may progress through four different phases of behavior, ranging from least to most dangerous. When clinicians are attuned to the early phases of violent behavior their interventions can diffuse the progression of the patient's behavior to more dangerous phases.

Calm Phase

Patients who are in the calm phase appear relaxed, alert, and fully conscious. They exhibit a level of good self-care and engage in normal social interactions. The physician can proceed with the interview of a patient in this phase without any additional precautions.

Psychomotor Agitation Phase

Patients in the psychomotor agitation phase may present with **constant questioning and chatting** as well as **increased physical activity**, such as pacing or foot tapping. Psychic agitation often accompanies the physical hyperactivity and is experienced by patients as anxiety, diffuse uneasiness, **increased tension**, or confusion. These internal states can be observed in patients' anxious, angry, or sad facial expressions. Patients in this phase often exhibit **approach–avoidance behavior**. They may walk up to another person and glare in a hypervigilant or paranoid manner and then walk away.

The physician should display an empathic, nonjudgmental, and **nonconfrontational attitude** when approaching a patient who is in the psychomotor agitation phase. Good eye contact and a relaxed body position with arms and legs uncrossed and visible will convey a nonthreatening stance to the patient. The patient may be calmed by initial nonthreatening questions, such as "What is your understanding of why you are in the hospital?" or "Who thought you needed to come to the emergency room?" Some patients may be able to provide very good but limited information (e.g., the person may have slept on the streets for the last several days during a delusional episode and may be cold and

> **BOX 13.1**
>
> ## CASE EXAMPLE OF MANAGEMENT IN THE PSYCHOMOTOR AGITATION PHASE
>
> A 45-year-old man with a diagnosis of posttraumatic stress disorder came to the outpatient center worried about whether his service dog would be allowed to stay with him. Within a few minutes he became restless, fidgeting in his chair, tapping his foot, then pacing while looking highly anxious. A staff member said, "You seem worried. . . . How can I help?" The patient explained his fears of being separated from his dog. The staff member reassured him that he could arrange for his dog to be a certified service dog, which would allow the dog to accompany him to every visit. He was also told that a psychiatrist would be out to see him in 15 minutes. The patient was relieved and waited calmly for his appointment.

hungry). Other patients may be able to provide the name of a specific medication that has been helpful in the past under similar circumstances. The interview may also allow the patient to ventilate some of the feelings underlying the agitation, which may in turn allow him or her to access usual coping mechanisms to regain control of behavior (see case example in Box 13.1).

Verbal Aggressive Phase

The threatening behavior of patients in the verbal aggressive phase should serve as a clear warning that a **violent attack could be imminent**. Such patients tend to be defensive and may start **yelling or cursing**. They may question authority and become increasingly **insistent and demanding**. For example, a male inpatient started cursing and glaring menacingly as he approached the nursing station, stating that he did not have to follow the rules and yelling that he wanted to speak to the doctor in charge. He continued his yelling as he followed the staff around the unit.

Patients who seem to be on the verge of losing control should be approached in a **calm but firm** manner. The physician needs to be self-protective while also protecting the patient. The door of the interview room should be kept open so that the patient does not feel trapped and can leave the room rather than become assaultive. The physician should stay about **1.5–3 feet away** from an agitated patient (at least one leg length), out of reach of explosive kicks or punches. A **standing position at a 45-degree angle** with one foot forward shows respect for the patient, avoids "squaring off," and allows the physician to leave the situation safely if need be. Trained personnel should be nearby to help restrain the patient if violence erupts.

Once patients have progressed to the verbal aggressive stage, supportive verbal interventions are usually not effective. Escalation of violent behavior can sometimes be prevented by the use of **verbal directives,** which are short, firm, nonthreatening commands, such as "Please stop cursing. I cannot help you when you are yelling at me." or "Please sit down and tell me what is bothering you." Communication should be clear and firm from the start. The physician's questions should be directed at exploring the reasons for the patient's rage and loss of control, as well as **empowering** the patient to identify and use his or her usual coping mechanisms to stay in behavioral control. Patients may need to be reoriented if they are confused. It is important to try to **minimize misinterpretation** by the patient. The physician should be active and indicate that something will be done to relieve the acute agitation. A delay or half-hearted attempt to control the patient's agitation may result in violence, since the patient may realize that the clinician is unable to exert control.

Should the patient continue to escalate verbally, the interview should be **terminated**. The patient may be offered a **"time-out"** in a "quiet room." Quiet rooms have few furnishings and no hazardous objects. They offer open access and are closely monitored by staff. Patients may also be offered nonsedating, calming drugs at any time before, during, or after the interview (see Medication Treatment, later in this chapter, and case example in Box 13.2). The primary goal of medication is to calm patients sufficiently to participate in their treatment. If possible, medication choices should be discussed with patients. Offering limited options (i.e., two choices) can empower but not overwhelm them. Intramuscular medications can be administered to patients who are acutely out of control and refuse to take oral medications. Ultimately, any intervention preventing violence should be considered successful, including abruptly terminating an interview when the risk of violence is increasing.

Physical Aggressive Phase

Patients in the physical aggressive phase are **intimidating**. They may begin to "air box," attempt to **assault** others physically, throw things, grab at people, or **destroy property**. Unless **verbal commands** have an immediate effect, a **"show of force"** to offer medication is the next step (see Box 13.3). If the patient refuses medication, the show of force may need to proceed to the administration of **involuntary medication**. **Physical seclusion or restraints** are sometimes necessary to re-establish a safe environment. Only a team of **well-trained staff** should undertake secluding or restraining a patient. The overall principle governing seclusion and restraint is to use the least restrictive alternative available to treat the episode. Once the patient is in restraints, medication will generally be chosen and administered.

Placing patients in seclusion or restraints are procedures that both staff and patients usually find unpleasant. Once patients have regained control, they may feel **guilty** about losing control or worry that the staff will punish them. They can be reassured that the staff will continue to help them maintain control and can be approached if they become concerned about losing control. Some patients may be resentful of the seclusion or restraints. It is helpful to remind them that seclusion and restraints were used so they would not hurt

---

BOX 13.2

CASE EXAMPLE OF MANAGEMENT IN THE VERBAL AGGRESSIVE PHASE

A 35-year-old woman diagnosed with schizophrenia stopped taking her medication and became increasingly psychotic. Her family brought her to the emergency room. She repeatedly left her assigned room and approached the nurse's station, asking when she was going to be released and staring at staff. Her behavior escalated to screaming, "Let me out of here. . . . I need to be seen now!" The nurse approached the patient standing at a 45-degree angle. She said loudly and firmly, "Sit down! . . . Calm down!" She offered the patient medication. The patient sat down and agreed to take the medication; a physical assault was averted.

BOX 13.3

CASE EXAMPLE OF MANAGEMENT IN THE PHYSICAL AGGRESSIVE PHASE

A young man recently hospitalized on an inpatient unit complained that people were spying on him, following him, and threatening him. He began kicking the furniture, throwing things at other patients, and running up and down the hall, shouting, "Get away from me....I didn't do anything." As a show of force, several male and female staff members surrounded the patient. With others standing beside her, one staff member announced, "I have others staff members here with me to help you regain control of yourself and make sure nobody gets hurt. We would like you to drink some medication but can give you an injection if that is what you would prefer." The man calmed down and took the medication orally. He also agreed voluntarily to go into the quiet room for his own protection, thus avoiding the need for restraints.

---

themselves or others. The post-violence phase presents the opportunity to reduce guilt over the previous episode and review alternative coping styles to prevent future episodes.

Obtaining the History

The psychiatric interview can formally begin once the patient no longer feels the need to take an aggressive action and is able to participate in a thoughtful discussion. The first priority will be to establish a **working alliance**. The physician can explain in a non-judgmental fashion that the main purpose of the interview is to find out what drove the patient to anger, aggression, or violence. For example, "What has been happening that led you to react in an angry or violent way?" (see Boxes 13.4 and 13.5 for additional suggestions). During the initial stages of the interview, the physician should express the desire to become an ally who will help the patient understand the precipitants of the violent crisis, resolve his or her anger, and develop a treatment plan. The patient may sense the physician's genuine intention to help him or her find ways to stay in behavioral control. It is important to be an empathic listener, to validate the patient's experience, and to clarify that one of the main goals of the interview is to develop an understanding of the patient's current situation. If the patient is able to talk, discussion should focus on understanding the precipitants of the agitation. The interview can progress to exploring possible strategies to help the patient regain behavioral control. Calm questioning by an unruffled, confident physician helps agitated patients remain engaged and in control.

Patients who are angry or violent are often defensive and may **deny their violent intentions** or **minimize the seriousness of threats.** Although some aggressive events are less life threatening than others, the physician must be careful not to collude with the patient's denial about the seriousness of the situations and the need for treatment. For example, a patient committing intimate partner violence may make excuses, saying, "She provoked me." Not all potentially violent situations are imminently dangerous. Intervening early during angry verbal stages increases the chance of preventing future violence. A detailed assessment of psychological, social, and cultural circumstances surrounding each violent episode will allow the development of well-planned treatment interventions.

BOX 13.4
INTERVIEWING GUIDELINES

- Interview angry or violent patients in a safe environment.
- Staff, security, or police should be nearby to intervene, if needed.
- Begin the interview by focusing on the recent crisis (e.g., "Why do you think that you are feeling angry or violent now?")
- Identify factors that may have immediately precipitated the aggressive or violent symptoms.
- Explore the meaning of the present violent symptoms and how they have evolved over the past 6 weeks.
- Develop the timeline of recent events contributing to violence.
- Explore the relationship between past violence and present symptoms.
- Address the patient's efforts to minimize difficulties and obscure his or her intentions.
- Obtain collateral information from family, friends, the treating providers, past medical records, and police.
- Self-monitor for reactions that might affect your judgments.
- Direct the focus of the interview toward risk assessment, treatment, and prevention.

Recent History

Initial history-taking should focus on acute risks before going on to explore long-standing difficulties. It can be helpful to develop a timeline of the patient's **most recent** threats or aggression, going back, in reverse chronological order, through the 6 weeks immediately preceding the violent episode. The physician should explore the events that incited the emergence of aggressive behaviors, as well as the meanings of these events to the patient. Approaching aggressive patients from the perspective that they are persons "in crisis" (see Chapter 12, Suicide) provides a focus on violent symptoms as resulting from a stressful or impulsive event that disturbs the person's previous equilibrium. The patient is often not consciously aware of stressors or may deny that they exist. Asking the patient to describe, in minute detail, the interactions and events that occurred immediately preceding, during, and after the violent situation usually results in identifying the stressors. Determining the precipitants to their aggressive behavior helps many patients to be focused, calmer, and willing to discuss their problems.

External life events, such as legal or financial difficulties, or problematic substance use are the most common precipitants of an aggressive episode. Stressors can also be psychological events, such as a disturbing dream, a surge of emotion or impulsive anger, or a response to worsening hallucinations or intensifying delusions. Interpersonal stressors or conflicts, such as an argument about substance use or marital strife leading to the contemplation of divorce, may also play a role.

It is important to understand the dynamic personal meaning that may be underlying the violence. The same events can affect individuals differently, depending on the context, the individual's phase of development, and how a person interprets or adds meaning

> ## BOX 13.5
> ### SAMPLE INTERVIEW QUESTIONS
>
> - "What was your most recent act of aggression or violence?"
> - "Do you have guns, other weapons, or access to other means for hurting others?"
> - "Are substances involved when you become violent?"
> - "At what age did your violent acts begin?"
> - "How frequently did those acts occur?"
> - "Have there been common stressful events preceding the acts?"
> - "Has there been a recurring pattern of escalation preceding violence?"
> - "Have any of your violent actions resulted in arrests, legal actions, or incarceration?"
> - "Do you have a history of recklessness or other impulsivity?"
> - "What medical or psychiatric diagnoses do you have (that are associated with violence)"?
> - "Is there a family history of violence, child or elder abuse, or gang involvement?"
> - "How do you usually deal with stress?"
> - "Do you drink or use drugs when stressed?"
> - "Do you blame others for your problems?"
> - "Do you stop taking your medications when you're feeling stressed?"
> - "Do you tend to expect that the worst will happen?"
> - "How do you tolerate psychological pain?"
> - "What has helped you tolerate stressful situations in the past?"
> - "What do you do to cope?"
> - "Do you seek contact with family, friends, professionals, or programs to ask for help?"

to them. For example, violence precipitated by excessive drinking as compared with violence that occurs when an affair is discovered has very different meanings to those who are involved and will require different interventions.

Important collateral information should be obtained from family members, treating providers, and other people with whom the patient has had recent contact, including the police. When assessing for imminent violence risk, an exemption in the Health Insurance Portability and Accountability Act (HIPPA 1996) permits contact with collateral informants without the patient's consent. Information should be collected from as many collateral sources as possible.

Past History
The focal past history of violence obtained from the patient and collateral sources centers on looking for the **repetitive dysfunctional patterns** that are currently being relived in

the current crisis situation. Clinicians should inquire about past stressors or traumas; prior incidents and hospitalizations related to violent events; a prior history of psychosis, bipolar disorder, and substance abuse; and other seminal events from past psychosocial, family, occupational, and medical histories. The physician should also explore the **past circumstances** of all aggressive behavior, including the **target**, the **patient's state**, and the **environment** during the violent episode. The **precipitating factors, intensity, frequency, nature, and context** of the violent acts deserve special inquiry.

Psychosocial History

When a patient has a strong, healthy family and supportive network, the members of the network can be mobilized to reduce the risk of violence. They can provide a buffer against stressors, help resolve problems, and offer concrete resources or support. Unfortunately, some networks are the cause of the problem (as in domestic violence situations). A toxic support system, such as a family inciting violence or enabling substance abuse, may make the patient's problems worse. Networks that are hostile, angry, or toxic to the patient may need to be excluded from care.

The support network's interest, competence, and availability should be assessed during the interview. To get a detailed view of a **support network**, it is useful to develop an ecological map, which is a trigenerational genogram detailing the current household, relevant marriages, divorces, illnesses, and deaths. The ecological map also includes other potential community supports, such as health care providers, religious organizations, friends, and community programs, such as Alcoholics Anonymous.

Physician Reactions

Even physicians who are very experienced working with violent patients can feel intimidated, bullied, threatened, and **afraid**. These feelings may evoke angry responses in the physician, or unconscious wishes to retaliate against the patient. Inappropriate physician behaviors can result, including verbal confrontations and unnecessary orders for sedation, intramuscular medications, seclusion, or restraints. The best protection against these behaviors is the physician's self-awareness, consultations with others, and careful consideration of the optimal responses for the patient's benefit.

Some violent patients discuss their symptoms so rationally and with such perceptiveness that the physician may feel moved to be overly protective, for example trying to help the patient avoid arrest or prosecution. Once patients are able to express remorse for violent acts, physicians should avoid a stance of being either overly sympathetic to the patient's suffering, at one extreme, or wishing to punish the patient at the other.

Inexperienced clinicians, particularly those still in training, can sometimes be distracted by their concerns about supervisors' and colleagues' expectations. This concern can result in their inattention to cues of potential danger. Particularly when interacting with new patients, the physician should be prepared to evaluate potential risk for violence even if that is not the patient's presenting complaint.

RISK ASSESSMENT

The assessment of dangerousness is generally understood to be the best effort at determining the probability of a violent episode within a few hours to a few days. Determining imminent risk involves appraisal of several risk variables, each of which can be viewed on a continuum from highest to lowest risk. The greater the preponderance of higher-risk variables, the more likely the risk of imminent dangerousness (see the VASA, a standardized violence risk assessment tool; Feinstein and Plutchik 1990). The aggregation of many variables in one patient, each individually conferring moderate risk, will tend to place the patient in a high-risk category.

Current Behavior

Observation of current behaviors is particularly useful for predicting who may become violent in a matter of minutes to hours.

Current Ideation

Patients who express a specific plan to kill or hurt a specific person within a specific time frame are the highest risk. Patients suffering with command auditory hallucinations or delusions involving killing or hurting someone (e.g., a patient who is commanded by God to kill) are also relatively high risk. A **nonspecific** plan (e.g., "My partner is going to get it!") or target (e.g., "I want to kill all liberals") represents a more moderate risk. Ambivalent wishes to hurt others or damage property, or unfocused rage and belligerence carry lesser risk.

Recent Behavior

There is a similar continuum of recent behaviors that correlates with violence risk. Imminent dangerousness of the highest probability is associated with patients who have made an intentional serious assault on another person; patients who have exhibited recent violent behavior, had homicidal ideation or psychosis with violent content, *and* had access to weapons (i.e., guns and knives); and patients with homicidal ideation or recent violent behavior comorbid with a severe substance use disorder, psychosis, bipolar disorder, impulse control disorders, or a severe personality disorder. Patients who commit physical assaults without weapons (e.g., beatings causing an emergency room visit) carry slightly lesser risk. Violent acts without serious physical consequences (e.g., slapping, punching, or pushing) need to be taken seriously, but their perpetrators are less imminently dangerous. Individuals who damage only property and not persons carry lesser risk.

Past History of Aggression

A past history of violence is the best predictor of future violent behavior, but it does not predict the timing of any future events. A detailed history of the lifetime patterns of violence, anger, and impulsiveness is essential for understanding the patient's potential for future violence. Individuals who have committed violent acts in the past and have been arrested for assaultive behavior represent the highest risk. People who carry weapons or have access to weapons are of relatively high risk. A criminal record of any kind, chronic problems with authority, a history of impulsive or unpredictable behavior, or a childhood history of frequent changes in living situation confers moderate risk of future violence.

Support Systems

Assessing both the quality and the abilities of the patient's support network is another important variable in assessing imminent risk for violence in vulnerable patients. Networks comprised of competent helpers who are strongly committed and readily available to the patient can diminish the imminent risk. On the opposite end of the spectrum are families who show little interest in helping their ill family members, either because they are toxic networks or because they are simply exhausted by many failed attempts to help. Support networks of moderate help are those that may be interested but may not be competent, such as young children who are asked to care for their ill parents, or family caretakers who are overwhelmed by their own problems. Sometimes, families are interested and competent but not available, as they have to work or have other responsibilities.

Substance Use

Problematic substance use is often the largest amplifier of violence. The risk of violence increases when any form of substance use is involved. In general, patients with violent impulses who are either intoxicated or are in withdrawal have the most extreme risk for imminent violence. Some drugs of chronic abuse, such as alcohol and methamphetamine, consistently increase the risk of violence, whereas other drugs, such as marijuana, have more varied effects. Individuals who chronically abuse or compulsively binge on drugs or alcohol are at greater long-term risk of imminent dangerousness than those who occasionally use recreational substances in a more controlled fashion.

Ability to Cooperate with Treatment

The clinician's perception of the patient's ability to cooperate with treatment is an important factor in the risk assessment. Patients who can take an active role in arranging, planning, and participating in their treatment present the lowest risk of imminent violence. Patients who passively accept treatment recommendations without active involvement in planning as well as patients who have demonstrated a limited capacity to participate in previous treatments represent higher risk. Patients who are not able to participate, refuse to cooperate, or have been previously uncooperative are of highest risk and will most likely require admission to an inpatient psychiatric facility.

Neurological and Other Medical Conditions

There is ample evidence of the association between certain neurological and medical disorders and an increased risk of violence. Neurological disorders associated with risk of violence include disorders involving damage to the frontal lobe and other deep brain structures. A partial list includes seizure disorders, brain tumors, and neurocognitive disorders due to traumatic brain injury, stroke, delirium, and Alzheimer's disease.

ETIOLOGY

Neurobiological Factors

The neurobiological mechanisms mediating aggression are not well understood. Impulsivity seems to be an inherited trait that makes individuals more vulnerable to violence and, as in suicide risk, the serotonin neurotransmitter system appears to be involved.

Low levels of the serotonin metabolite 5-hydroxyindoleacetic acid have been found in the cerebrospinal fluid of those with aggressive behavior. Other major neurotransmitters linked to aggression include gamma-aminobutyric acid (GABA), glutamate, dopamine, and noradrenaline.

Social Factors

Societal factors known to increase rates of violence include increased population density, poverty, ethnic heterogeneity, residential instability, unemployment, and weak community ties. Rates of violence have consistently decreased during times of economic prosperity and war, and increased during times of economic recession or collapse.

Cultural Factors

Cultural influences may affect the incidence of violence. American culture as reflected in the media, including the Internet, video games, television, film, and popular music, has become increasingly violent in content. This proliferation of media violence has been accused of encouraging the likelihood of violence, although there is little strong data to support this view. The pervasiveness of guns in America has also led to high homicide rates compared to those in countries that are more restrictive of gun access.

Treatment

Crisis Formulation
Each of the factors identified as contributing to the violent episode should be described in detail (see discussion of a crisis in Psychosocial History, Chapter 12, Suicide). The clinician should prioritize the treatment of each factor according to (in this order) (1) what needs immediate attention (e.g., intoxication, command auditory homicidal hallucinations), (2) those issues that can be treated over a longer period (e.g., poor coping skills, family disruptions, impulsivity), and (3) other factors that are most difficult or unlikely to be significantly modifiable (e.g., personality disorders or neurocognitive disorders secondary to traumatic brain injury). Once the priorities for treatment are decided, the specific treatment approach for each factor should be developed.

Therapeutic Settings
Violent patients should be treated in the least restrictive setting that is necessary to keep them safe from harming others. Regardless of setting, the treatment should provide psychoeducation, address substance use disorders, and include communication with and use of the patient's support system. In addition, care should be coordinated with the patient's other health care providers. At times, it may be necessary to involve the police for the safety of others.

Hospital Treatment
Hospitalization should be considered in the following situations: (a) the patient has homicidal ideation directed at a specific person; (b) the patient is psychotic and the hallucinations or delusions have homicidal or violent content; (c) the patient has had a recent violent episode or displays severe impulsivity and agitation and is refusing help; (d) the patient has had a recent violent episode and displays severe impulsivity and agitation; (e) the patient has a change in mental status that includes homicidal ideation or violent

behaviors requiring further workup in a structured setting; (f) the patient with a psychiatric illness describes premeditated violence with a specific plan, directed at a specific person; (g) the patient describes premeditated violence and is known to have access to multiple means to commit violence; (h) the patient continues to have a risk of violence despite outpatient treatment.

The first goal of inpatient treatment is safety. The next goal is identification and treatment of the multifactorial causes of violence. Typically, this includes treating familial conflicts and systemic problems; mobilizing the healthy part of the support network to prevent future violence; addressing substance abuse, as well as psychiatric and other medical illnesses; teaching coping skills designed to prevent violence; and developing a safety discharge plan (see Box 13.6) that includes outpatient referrals.

Outpatient Treatment

A structured intensive outpatient or partial hospitalization program, or frequent outpatient visits, are viable alternatives to an inpatient stay when safety can be maintained by a strong support network that is interested, competent, and available for supervision of the patient's treatment. Patients are especially at risk for recurrence of violence in the 30 days after the initial outpatient or emergency room evaluation for violence, or in the 30 days after discharge from an inpatient setting. To prevent recurrence of a violent crisis, outpatient treatment should include the negotiation of a detailed outpatient safety plan prior to the patient's release from the emergency room or inpatient unit. It is essential to set a time for a follow-up conversation with the patient in the first week after the initial

---

BOX 13.6
VIOLENCE PREVENTION SAFETY PLAN TO BE REVIEWED 1 WEEK AFTER DISCHARGE

- Make sure the patient's immediate environment is safe, without weapons or other means to hurt others.
- Review all current or new stressors since discharge.
- Review early warning signs of increasing risk of violence (e.g., substance use, isolation).
- Review coping strategies to diffuse dangerous impulses (e.g., relaxation techniques, exercise, distraction).
- Using the ecological map, review the support network of who can be called to help, such as friends and family (and their relevant contact information).
- Review information on how to access and use a 24-hour crisis hotline.
- Use prescribed medications to help to control symptoms.
- Review plans for outpatient psychiatric programs, including psychotherapy, to facilitate the acquisition of new understanding, new cognitive or interpersonal skills, or the modification of relationships.
- Review the names and contact information for specific mental health professionals and programs (e.g., Alcoholic Anonymous) to be contacted for treatment.

contact or discharge from the hospital. A safety plan is not "contracting for safety," which has not been shown to offer any benefits. Instead, safety plans include details of what to do if symptoms recur (see Box 13.6).

Pharmacotherapy

Psychopharmacological strategies for treatment of violence differ according to whether the medication is for the treatment of acute violence or for the prevention of episodes in patients with chronic aggression. The treatment of acute aggression or agitation involves the judicious use of sedative-anxiolytics or low doses of second-generation antipsychotics. The treatment of chronic aggression is guided by underlying diagnoses and specific target symptoms.

Antidepressants

The SSRIs have been used to treat **aggressive, impulsive, and violent** symptoms, particularly in individuals with head injuries. Low doses are recommended initially, and patients should be watched for exacerbation of their symptoms as doses are raised to therapeutic levels.

Mood-Stabilizing Agents

Lithium carbonate has been shown to reduce impulsive aggression to extremely low levels during the course of treatment for some aggressive or violent patients. There is no established evidence that **mood-stabilizing anticonvulsants** directly reduce the risk of violence. However, these medications are effective as a treatment of mood disorders associated with violence. Mood stabilizers can target irritability or anger, the impulsivity associated with personality disorders and impulse control disorders, and violent behavior associated with traumatic brain injury, seizures, dementia, or an intermittent explosive disorder.

Antipsychotics

Second-generation antipsychotics are replacing mood-stabilizing medications as the preferred treatment of aggression. Those available parenterally can be useful in an acute setting (see Chapter 16, Pharmacotherapy, ECT, and TMS). First-generation antipsychotics are equally effective but may be less well tolerated because of side effects. Antipsychotics are contraindicated in the treatment of agitation and violence due to sedative-hypnotic withdrawal because they lower the seizure threshold.

Beta-Adrenergic Receptor Antagonists

The role of the central noradrenergic system in facilitation of aggression suggests that agents with adrenergic blocking property should exhibit anti-aggressive activity. Both propranolol and nadolol, which are beta-adrenergic receptor antagonists, reduce aggressive behavior in patients with traumatic brain injury or chronic neurocognitive disorders and in some violent psychotic psychiatric inpatients. Use of these medications often requires high doses and must be carefully monitored for the side effects of hypotension and bradycardia.

Benzodiazepines

Benzodiazepines have no demonstrated short- or long-term antiviolence efficacy. However, benzodiazepines are the treatment of choice in agitation and violence **due to sedative-hypnotic withdrawal**. They may also be effective adjunctive agents for highly anxious psychotic patients or in the treatment of panic attacks, agitation, and severe insomnia. **Lorazepam** is particularly useful, as it is available for **intramuscular** administration. Patients treated with benzodiazepines should be carefully monitored for worsening depression, especially when prescriptions last for a period of days. Close monitoring of patients with borderline personality disorder, trauma, or head injuries is required, as benzodiazepines can disinhibit these patients and, paradoxically, increase aggression.

Psychotherapy

Psychotherapy can play a vital role in the treatment of violent behavior, although there are no violence prevention–specific psychotherapies. Crisis intervention, cognitive,-behavioral or psychodynamic treatments, anger management, and family therapy are all useful psychotherapies. They can focus on treatment of the primary psychiatric disorders or medical conditions and on some symptoms (e.g., impulsivity or irritability) associated with the violence (see Chapter 17, Psychotherapy).

Legal Issues

There are several difficult legal and clinical considerations when treating violent patients. While laws regarding these issues vary by state, the basic concepts underlying them are similar.

Involuntary Commitment

All states have laws guiding involuntary hospitalization or outpatient certification. Such action is taken when patients with psychiatric disorders present an imminent danger to themselves or to others (see Chapter 12, Suicide).

Confidentiality, Duty to Warn, and Duty to Protect

In most states, the law recognizes that protecting the lives of other people takes precedence over confidentiality. Physicians are usually exempt from confidentiality requirements when they become aware that the patient is likely to commit violence or homicide. In situations in which other people are potentially at risk, the clinician is allowed to discuss the patient with all necessary collateral informants (e.g., family members, friends, health care providers, police). This disclosure does not require the patient's consent. As with many situations involving violent patients, this decision requires clinical judgment and a risk–benefit assessment that weighs the effects of infringing on patient confidentiality versus fostering the safety of others.

In some cases, patients may not want to reveal violent impulses, intentions, or behavioral plans until the clinician reassures them that the information will be kept completely confidential. The following statement is an appropriate response to such questions: "Our communications are usually confidential, unless there is a danger to others or to yourself. Under those circumstances, I cannot keep your intentions a secret." This response is reassuring to most patients, and it frees the clinician to take necessary steps to prevent the loss of life, including disclosure of the patient's intentions to anyone who might need to know.

While state laws requiring notification of potential victims of their risk from a homicidal patient vary widely, the two **Tarasoff** decisions have become national standards for clinical practice (Tarasoff v. Regents of University of California, 17 Cal.3d 425, 131 Cal. Rptr. 14, 551 P2d 334 [1974, 1976]). Both cases refer to the situation in which a man who had confided his intention to kill to a University of California therapist murdered Tatania Tarasoff. In the first Tarasoff case, the court found the university and the therapist guilty of a failure to warn Ms. Tarasoff or her family that her life was in imminent danger, declaring, "The protective privilege ends where the public peril begins." This case became the precedent for the therapist's **"duty to warn" all potential victims of life-threatening danger from a homicidal patient**. A second Tarasoff ruling, in 1976, gave therapists a broader alternative to the **"duty to warn,"** referred to as the **"duty to protect."** The clinician can take an alterative pathway and protect others from violence by providing *"reasonable care"* to potential victims under the second Tarasoff ruling: *"When a therapist determines, or should determine, that his patient presents a serious danger of violence to another, he incurs an obligation to use reasonable care to protect the intended victim from danger." Reasonable care* means that the physician must try to prevent violence by taking actions such as hospitalizing the violent patient or prescribing outpatient partial hospital treatment, crisis intervention, or other appropriate outpatient care.

Following the second Tarasoff ruling, "duty to protect" statutes were passed in all but 13 states, although many state laws reflect ambivalence. Some states require that a violent threat be clearly foreseeable, and that the duty is extended only to "reasonably foreseeable victims" and not to the general public. Other states have laws known as "Tarasoff-limiting statutes," prescribing specific criteria that typically include a requirement for a credible threat to have been made against an identifiable victim.

REFERENCES CITED

Fazel, S., G. Gulati, L. Linsell, J. R. Geddes, and M. Grann. Schizophrenia and violence: systematic review and meta-analysis. *PLoS Medicine* 6(8), August 2009.

Feinstein, R., and R. Plutchik. Violence and suicide risk assessment in the psychiatric emergency room. *Comprehensive Psychiatry* 31:337–343, 1990.

SELECTED READINGS

Citrome, L. Interventions for the treatment of acute agitation. *CNS Spectrum* 12:8–12, 2007.

Feinstein, R. E., and A. Snavely. Crisis intervention, trauma, and intimate partner violence. In Rakel, R., and D. Rakel, eds. *Textbook of Family Medicine*, 8th ed., pp. 1022–1036. Philadelphia: Saunders, 2011.

Friedman, R. A. Violence and mental illness—how strong is the link? *New England Journal of Medicine* 355:2064–2066, 2006.

Hiday, V. A. Putting community risk in perspective: a look at correlations, causes and controls. *International Journal of Law and Psychiatry* 29:316–331, 2006.

Kung, H., D. Hoyert, J. Xu, and S. Murphy. Deaths: final data for 2005. *National Vital Statistics Reports* 56, January 2008.

Otto, R. K., and K. S. Douglas. *Handbook of Violence Risk Assessment. International Perspectives on Forensic Mental Health*. New York: Routledge, 2010.

Simon, R. I., and K. Tardiff. *Textbook of Violence Assessment and Management*, 1st ed. Washington, DC: American Psychiatric Publishing, 2008.

Umukoro, S., A. C. Aladeokin, and A. T. Eduviere. Aggressive behavior: a comprehensive review of its neurochemical mechanisms and management. *Aggression and Violent Behavior* 18:195–203, 2013.

14

Child, Adolescent, and Adult
Development

JONATHAN A. SLATER, KATHARINE A.
STRATIGOS, AND JANIS L. CUTLER

A nearly infinite number of tasks accompany the complex devel-
opment of human beings over a lifetime. Of primary importance are the tasks pertaining
to emotional, social, and cognitive function, gender identity, and sexuality at each stage
of life.

These tasks naturally change as the individual passes through infancy, the toddler
years, the preschool years, the latency years, adolescence, adulthood, and old age. The
somewhat arbitrary and oversimplified divisions of the life cycle into childhood, adolescence, and adulthood are best understood as general stages that overlap with one
another, not as phases that have discrete beginnings and endings. In order to understand
the developmental vulnerabilities inherent in each stage that may affect a person or give
rise to psychiatric disorders, it is first necessary to understand the normal developmental
progression of each stage.

NORMAL AND ABNORMAL LIFE DEVELOPMENT

Approach to the Study of Development

It is useful to understand patterns of normal mental functioning that occur throughout
the life cycle in order to recognize psychiatric illnesses, predict the effects of these illnesses, and suggest treatment strategies. Table 14.1 provides an overview of the five particular areas that will be addressed: neurodevelopmental, psychosexual, psychosocial,
cognitive, and attachment.

Patterns of Development

Psychological development occurs at different rates during the various stages of life. From
infancy through young adulthood, mental functioning is characterized by enormous
change and progression, and major shifts in functioning can occur virtually overnight.
Rapid progression in one area can be associated with stress and often causes regression

TABLE 14.1 Overview of Major Developmental Theories

Theorist	Area of Focus	Why Important?	Clinical Example
Gessell	Biological development and milestones	To monitor for appropriate biological development, screen for developmental disabilities	A 1-year-old child typically can stand, cruise, clap hands, use pincer grip, and say one recognizable word.
Freud	Psychosexual development	To understand unconscious conflicts and the impact that early experiences can have on later emotional development	A toddler refuses to wear a coat in the winter, representative of other struggles over autonomous urges and control seen during the "anal" phase.
Erikson	Psychosocial development	To understand an individual's development within the social context over the lifespan	A 10-year-old boy develops low self-esteem as a result of failing classes because of a learning disability ("industry versus inferiority").
Piaget	Cognitive development	To understand cognitive development and the child's abilities and subjective understanding of the world	A 4-year-old girl thought she developed a stomachache because she was "bad" (lack of appreciation of cause and effect, characteristic of preoperational stage)
Ainsworth, Bowlby	Attachment	To understand the early development of attachment and the implications for later relationships	A 1-year-old child who is separated from the mother will protest her departure and cry, then run to her affectionately upon her return (secure attachment).

in another area. For example, a previously even-tempered 3-year-old might abruptly, and seemingly without effort, give up her diapers but then almost immediately become much more clinging and dependent, a phenomenon that can be quite confusing to unsuspecting parents.

Although abrupt discontinuities are characteristic of the development of children and adolescents, there are also continuous aspects of behavior such as individual temperament. **Temperament**, which is generally considered to be inherited, is observable from birth in the way a person tends to behave. Temperamental traits include activity level, distractibility, persistence, regularity, mood, sensory threshold, intensity of emotional expression, adaptability to change in routine, and the tendency to approach or avoid novel situations (Chess and Thomas 1995). For example, an infant who becomes hyperaroused in response to novel stimuli may manifest this tendency in somewhat different ways at various developmental stages and even as pathology at a later stage of life. An infant who has behavioral inhibition may have intense stranger anxiety as a 1-year-old, separation anxiety as a 6-year-old, and vulnerability to panic attacks as an adult. Other traits that are fairly continuous over developmental periods are intelligence, motor coordination, musical talent, and a predisposition to certain physical symptoms.

Adults tend to have more stable and persistent emotional lives than do children and adolescents. Shifts and adjustments do occur, albeit gradually in adults, and their development can be seen in slowly evolving patterns.

Effects of Stress and Trauma on Development

Everyone encounters periods throughout the life cycle of particular emotional vulnerability to certain stressful and traumatic events. When such events occur during vulnerable stages of childhood, they may profoundly affect the developmental course of that person's life. **Physical illness** and the **loss of a parent** are particularly severe stresses for most children and adolescents. For example, children who are hospitalized many times before age 4 seem to have a higher incidence of emotional problems later in life. Repeated hospitalizations later in the course of development do not seem to have the same lasting effects.

Regression, which is the reappearance of behaviors and coping mechanisms that were used at a younger age, is a common response to stress for children as well as adults. Regression can occur in one or more areas of functioning. For example, a 5-year-old boy who had remained dry at night for over a year began wetting his bed when his parents separated, but otherwise moved ahead in his daily life at school and with friends. Periods of developmental vulnerability may be associated with the first appearance of psychiatric disorders, which may be identified during childhood or later in life.

INFANCY: BIRTH TO 12 MONTHS OF AGE

Developmental Progression

Affect Regulation

The infant has several specific needs that must be met by the caretaker. First, the infant requires physical sustenance in the form of nourishment, cleanliness, and warmth. The infant's emotional needs are at least as important. A crucial role of the caretaker is to modulate the intensity of the child's feelings. The caregiver's empathic responsiveness guides the child toward the appropriate emotional response and appropriate amplitude of response. The infant smiles, and the parent smiles back. A mother calms her infant's harsh cries with soft soliloquy and gentle stroking. In such ways, infants turn to their caregivers for the soothing that they are innately receptive to, facilitating their developing capacity for self-regulation.

The infant also follows the caretaker's cues to learn to identify emotions and associate them with specific types of experiences in an appropriate way. Emotional signals are used extensively in the infant–caregiver relationship. Consistent nurturing by an empathic caregiver allows the infant to develop trust in an environment in which emotional and physical needs are met. Adequate responsiveness by the caregiver is necessary for the child to develop what **Erik Erikson** has referred to as **basic trust** (i.e., the feeling of the self and others being essentially "all right"), which is a precursor to the development of a sense of identity and mastery (see Table 14.2). This reciprocal relationship also lays the groundwork for the development of empathy.

By the second half of the first year, infants seem to realize that they can share their inner emotional experiences with others. This revelation, which involves coordination and, at times, synchronization, of affective and mental states, is referred to as intersubjectivity. Now the infant can share a focus of attention, called **joint attention**, and the infant's eyes will follow a pointing finger and look back at the adult for a facial cue to validate that he or she is looking at the correct location. As infants realize that they can share a subjective state with their caregivers, they begin to "read" the emotional signals of others in order to modify their behavior, a phenomenon known as **social referencing**. The infant will acquire information about unfamiliar or ambiguous situations by observing

TABLE 14.2 Erikson's Stages of Psychosocial Development

Stage	Age	Phase of Life	Task of the Life Phase	Key Question or Concept
1	Birth–18 months	Infancy	Basic trust versus mistrust	Is my world trustworthy and dependable?
2	18 months–3 years	Toddler	Autonomy versus shame and doubt	With increased independence, will I be able to do things by myself and develop self-control?
3	3–6 years	Preschool	Initiative versus guilt	Can I engage and succeed in challenging tasks without becoming overly frustrated and then guilty?
4	6–12 years	School-age	Industry versus inferiority	Do I have the ability to do the work that I need to succeed (e.g., schoolwork)?
5	12–18 years	Adolescence	Identity versus role confusion	Who am I and what is my role?
6	19–40 years	Adulthood	Intimacy versus isolation	Will I find lasting, meaningful relationships or will I be alone?
7	40–65 years	Adulthood	Generativity versus stagnation	How will I contribute to the next generation?
8	65 years+	Adulthood	Ego integrity versus despair	Have I lived a good life? Am I fulfilled and do I accept my life as I have lived it?

the caregiver's face for signs of happiness, interest, fear, or anger. For example, the infant may look toward the parents for approval before crawling over an unfamiliar surface or smiling at an approaching stranger.

Attachment

The nature of the newborn infant's first task is social: to ensure the devoted attention of a loving caretaker. Infants enter the world with the genetically determined ability to gain such attention, first by crying and later by using facial expressions, especially eye contact, to actively engage and hold the interest of others. Infants selectively attend to the human face and voice over other competing stimuli. Adults seem to respond instinctually to the infant's efforts, adjusting their voices and facial expressions to imitate those of the infant. At approximately 2 months of age, as the infant becomes more alert and curious about her or his surroundings, parents perceive the infant as behaving "more like a baby." The infant's increased eye contact and vocalizations and, most importantly, the **social smile**, feel like a well-deserved reward to the parents for the sleepless nights and endless diapers. Infants keep their caretakers involved—in fact, captivated—by their developmental progression. Video recording of infants and their caretakers has recently elucidated the remarkable subtlety and harmony of the early social interaction between parents and infant, and how both parent and infant respond dynamically and continually to cues from the other (Koulomzin et al. 2002).

An impaired infant (e.g., an autistic infant who avoids eye contact) may not elicit the same degree of bonding from the caretaker. In the past, this lack of parental responsiveness was mistakenly seen as the cause of autism, but it is now recognized that **autism**

BOX 14.1

THE STRANGE SITUATION

A 12-month-old boy, accompanied by his mother, enters the room and begins to explore the toys. When the stranger walks in, the boy leans backward against his mother. When the mother quietly leaves the room, the boy immediately runs to the door calling for her. He is increasingly upset and not comforted by the stranger. By the time his mother returns, he is crying, but stops almost immediately when he sees her. He quickly resumes exploring the room and showing her different toys. Of note, securely attached infants show little distress at home when their mothers leave the room to move around the house. Secure attachment is related to the mother's sensitivity to her infant's communications, the mother's prompt and effective responses to her infant's distress, sensitive physical contact (holding and rocking), and synchronous face-to-face interactions.

---

spectrum disorders are neurological conditions that have secondary effects on the parent–child relationship.

Ainsworth initially described 3 forms of **attachment** between infants and their mothers: **secure, avoidant, and resistant** (Ainsworth et al. 1978). Infants with a **secure attachment style** who are separated from their mother will cry and call for her. They will be consoled and soothed upon her return and resume their play activities. A vivid description of a securely attached child observed using the "Strange Situation" paradigm is provided in Box 14.1 (Main 2000). In this experimental model the infant is observed when separated from his or her mother, placed briefly with a stranger, and then reunited with the mother.

Object Permanence

Jean Piaget, a psychologist who described **cognitive** development, observed that infants see themselves in an "egocentric" way, as if all events were determined by their own thoughts and actions (see Table 14.3). He also described the **sensorimotor** period of the first 2 years, when children are **preoccupied with exploring objects with their hands and mouth**. An object will only have meaning when it is with the child, and will be **forgotten when it is out of sight**. Before the development of memory, symbolic thinking, and language, objects essentially do not exist for the child unless the child can see them. The attainment of **object permanence** at approximately **8 months** of age is a major cognitive achievement. When infants who are between the age of 5 and 7 months are presented with an object that is then removed or hidden, they will either cry or turn their attention to other things. Their world is one in which objects are constantly "appearing" and "disappearing," as if they never existed or no longer exist. Objects have no past and no future. Just a month later, however, a remarkable thing happens—infants begin to search for an object in the spot where they saw it disappear. Out of sight is no longer out of mind.

Stranger Anxiety

The emotional reaction referred to as stranger anxiety is closely tied to these cognitive developments. Before the age of 7–9 months, infants may react indiscriminately or

TABLE 14.3 Piaget's Stages of Cognitive Development

Age	Stage	Description
Birth–2 years	Sensorimotor	Intellectual development arises from infants' actions on objects (e.g., things fall if they are hit off the table). Use of reflex patterns and chance discoveries (trial and error), followed by repetition of an act to cause a desired outcome (e.g., infant puts thumb near mouth and, with sucking reflex, learns to suck thumb, then repeats this discovered behavior)
2–7 years	Preoperational stage	Intelligence is symbolic (i.e., language), but thought processes are intuitive rather than logical. Concepts: "egocentrism," i.e., the inability to see things from another's perspective.
7–11 years	Concrete operations	Intelligence is symbolic (language) and logical, but concrete. Concepts: conservation of mass, creating categories, and reversibility; "de-centering," i.e., the ability to use multiple perspectives to solve a problem
12+ years	Formal operations	Abstract thinking Concepts: make and test hypotheses, think about possibilities, introspective

"neutrally" to strangers, although they may recognize and perhaps smile more at familiar faces. Stranger anxiety is caused by the ability to recognize someone who is unfamiliar, and thus infants now may react with **distress when their caregivers leave or a stranger approaches**. At this point, babysitting becomes more difficult. Caregivers feel that they are quite special in the infant's life, and that substitutions are not acceptable. The evolution of stranger anxiety develops, not coincidently, just as attachment to major caregivers solidifies (see Table 14.4 for a summary of infant development and Box 14.2 for an infant case example).

Developmental Vulnerabilities

Since the crucial task of the first year of life is the development and solidification of the attachment between infant and caretaker, this relationship is the most vulnerable area with regard to possible disruption by physical illness, developmental disability, or parental psychopathology.

Physical Illness and Caretaking Relationships

The infant's physical growth is the earliest concrete sign for parents that they are adequately caring for their newborn infant. Parents eagerly await the physician's findings about changes in length and weight and how their infant compares with others on standard growth charts during early "well baby" visits. Common disruptions in growth, such as colds and other minor illnesses, can contribute to parental demoralization if physicians are not sensitive to these concerns. Box 14.3 illustrates parental response in a case of serious physical illness during infancy.

TABLE 14.4 Infant (Birth to 12 Months) Development

Neurodevelopmental (e.g., Gesell)	Cognitive (e.g., Piaget)	Psychosexual (e.g., Freud)	Psychosocial (e.g., Erikson)	Attachment (e.g. Bowlby)
1–2 months Visual attentiveness to others Increased vocalizations (squeals) Supports head and chest	**1–4 months** Repetitions of simple acts for their own sake Objects are "out of sight, out of mind"	Oral stage (passive): Puts everything in his or her mouth Any sudden change of position, falling, loud noise causes anxiety	Trust versus mistrust	
2–4 months Depth perception Smiles Primitive reflexes decrease Babbling (imitates speech sounds) Reaches for object				
4–6 months Smiles to mother's face/voice Hand–eye coordination Increased vocalizations Sits with support, then alone Prehensile grasp (uses whole hand)	**4–6 months** Repetition to produce desired effects	Oral stage (active): Aggressive, biting		
7–12 months Cruising (walk with support) Grasp with thumb and finger First word	**7–12 months** Searches for vanished objects (object permanence) Repetition of past actions Simple problem-solving			**7–9+ months** Stranger anxiety **12 months+** Four attachment styles based on "the strange situation" (infant's reaction to being with a stranger then reunion with mother): ○ Secure ○ Avoidant (avoid parent upon reunion) ○ Resistant/ambivalent (anxious, not easily soothed) ○ Disorganized (inexplicable, odd, disoriented behavior in parent's presence)

Modeled on Theories of Development chart by Clarice Kestenbaum, MD, Department of Psychiatry, Columbia University College of Physicians and Surgeons and New York State Psychiatric Institute.

BOX 14.2
INFANT CASE EXAMPLE

Just several hours following her birth, Hannah gazes toward her mother's face and recognizes her voice. Several days later she can identify the scent of her mother's breast milk. By 2 months of age she begins to realize that her mother will feed her or change her diaper if she cries. She is able to lift her head up while on her stomach and look around, tracking objects that move through her visual field. By 3 months of age Hannah sleeps through the night and smiles at her parents. At 4 months she readily reaches for, grasps, and places in her mouth objects that interest her, and she solicits attention by vocalizing. Her sense of basic trust is solidifying. At 6 months Hannah recognizes her name, takes her first bites of solid food, and drinks from a "sippy" cup. She "babbles," using more consonants. She realizes that she is an autonomous being, separate from her parents. Appreciating how her bodily actions influence objects around her, she enjoys hitting the mobile over her crib and watching it move. At 7 months of age Hannah sustains a standing position holding onto her crib when she is helped up. She enjoys looking at herself in the mirror and is extremely social with people who are familiar to her. She easily transfers objects from one hand to the other and rolls over both back to front and front to back. She incorporates repetitive vowel and consonant strings into her vocalizations and says "ba-ba." If an object she likes is momentarily covered, she understands that it is hidden and will look for it. At 8 months of age, to her parents delight, Hannah identifies her mother as "ma-ma" and father as "da-da." She complies when told "no." At 9 months she is adept at crawling and pushes herself up to a sitting position on her own. Her language incorporates more vowels and the normal rhythm of speech. Her emotions are more differentiated and her happy and determined temperament more apparent. At 11 months of age she "cruises" while holding on to the side of the couch and at her first birthday party she is walking independently, enjoying "peek-a-boo," picking up Cheerios with a "pincer" grasp, and pointing to individual animals in a new book.

Psychopathology
Developmental Disorders

The developmental disorders observed in infants include **motor disorders**, in which activities requiring motor coordination, such as crawling or walking, are delayed; **communication disorders**, in which speech or expressive or receptive language is delayed; and **autism spectrum disorders** (see Chapter 15, Child and Adolescent Psychiatry). Most of these disorders are associated with severe deficits in language and social functioning. Autistic children may seem "different" to their parents from an early age (e.g., the infant may make poor eye contact, be less social and verbal, and/or not point to objects of interest). Parents may say that they find it difficult to bond with the infant, and that the infant seems qualitatively different from their other children when they were the same age.

BOX 14.3

PARENTAL RESPONSE TO PHYSICAL ILLNESS DURING INFANCY

When infants become seriously ill, parents may have greater difficulty in reestablishing their sense of confidence in themselves and the infant. During a chronic illness, relationship patterns can become dramatically distorted. When parents do not believe in the vitality of their infant, they may treat the infant in a drastically altered manner. If the parents feel guilty, they may fail to set appropriate limits, such as not letting the infant fuss for a few minutes when going to sleep. If the parents feel angry about their own helplessness, they may divert the anger toward the infant who engages in the normal bedtime fussing. When parents are able to nurse the infant through a medical crisis, whether minor or major, their confidence in the infant's ability to weather stress is renewed and the relationship is set back on course.

An infant who received a lung transplant at 16 months of age had spent only 2 months at home before he was admitted to the hospital, where he spent the next 14 months. Following the transplantation, which was performed at a tertiary care medical center to which he had been transferred, the medical staff became concerned about the lack of time that his parents spent with him. It almost seemed as if they had "dropped him off" to have a transplant. The infant was alone in his hospital room for long stretches of time, unlike many of the other children, whose parents literally hovered by their bedsides and never left. The staff wondered whether this behavior constituted neglect. After the infant was discharged to go home, it became apparent that the parents had been completely misjudged. They became model parents, "never skipping a beat," according to their pediatrician. In reviewing this infant's life history, one can see that these parents had never had the opportunity to bond with him, because he had been admitted to the hospital in an extremely compromised state so soon after birth. His mother had been completely overwhelmed and had not been given the chance to "feel like a mother." Also, she felt that she did not have a role in his care because, out of necessity, a multitude of nurses had cared for her infant. A follow-up meeting with this family when the child was 3 years old found a beaming father, who was proud of and loving toward his son, describing his toddler as "just like any other 3-year-old," except for some speech and language problems.

Parental Psychopathology

Disruption of the parent–infant bond due to parental impairment (e.g., depression in the mother) or loss can lead to a depressive response in the infant, which may be manifested by feeding and eating disorders or by attachment difficulties in infancy or early childhood. Avoidant/restrictive food intake disorder is a feeding disorder that often occurs during infancy or early childhood for which there is no identifiable physiological explanation. Infants with this disorder usually begin to gain weight when they are admitted to the hospital. Infants with reactive attachment disorder have a significant deficit in

---

BOX 14.4

CASE EXAMPLE OF DISORGANIZED ATTACHMENT

A 14-month-old boy and his mother (currently depressed with a history of sexual abuse and trauma) are observed during separations and reunions in the "Strange Situation." Upon separation from his mother, the child screams at the door. Upon her return, he walks away from her and raises his hand to his mouth in a fearful manner. He then walks toward his mother with a dazed smile on his face and hits her. He tries to climb into her lap and then freezes and falls silent.

---

social relatedness and attachment behavior caused by pathological care, such as neglect or abuse. These infants tend to bond indiscriminately to strangers in the hospital and to lack normal stranger anxiety.

Disorganized attachment (Main 2000) is fairly common in abused children and the children of severely traumatized mothers and may culminate in chronic issues in attachment. Some clinical manifestations may include contradictory behaviors (e.g., the infant moving toward the mother and away from her); the infant freezing and showing slowed movements, disorientation, and confusion; and the infant's apprehension toward the parent (see case example in Box 14.4). Infants with chronic attachment issues may develop problems in forming future relationships and a propensity toward depression.

THE TODDLER: 1 TO 3 YEARS OF AGE

Developmental Progression

Toddlerhood begins around 12 months of age, when the infant begins to walk, or "toddle." This occasion marks a motoric discontinuity of remarkable proportions. Children are often elated by their ability to be mobile in this novel way and revel in their exploration of the world from this new vantage point.

Emergence of Autonomy

Whereas the task of the infant is to become attached to the caregiver, the task of the toddler is to become a **socially detached, separate, autonomous being**. This **separation-individuation** process has been described in great detail by **Margaret Mahler** and generally begins with what she referred to as the **practicing** subphase, in which the child practices recently acquired skills with compulsive repetition. Even the most dedicated parent finds it trying to help the child climb up the slide 50 times or to clean up a mess after the toddler insists on eating independently.

During the "terrible twos," a term commonly used to describe this phase, the toddler can be experienced quite negatively by caregivers. It is helpful for caregivers to keep in mind that this **contrary behavior** is a necessary part of the child's establishment of her or his own autonomy. Just as the nature of the tasks that the child must master has changed from infancy, the caregivers' tasks have also shifted considerably. The caregiver must allow the toddler to explore the world and become independent but also protect the child from the perils of the real world.

Ambivalence

Both parents and children struggle with many conflicting emotions during the toddler years. Parents who are delighted to glimpse the growing, independent child may feel sadness at losing their adoring, compliant baby. Similarly, the toddler **alternates between clinging to and pushing away caregivers**. The child feels sadness at losing the caretakers and wants to "refuel" with them but also wants to be on her or his own. The child may so desperately want to be independent that the caregiver's help may be rejected even when it is needed. Mahler labeled this struggle the **rapprochement crisis.**

Tantrums may be precipitated in a toddler if the child becomes frustrated when attempting to comply with the plethora of adult demands and requests. These demands address every aspect of the child's daily life, including meals, dressing, toilet routines, and bedtime, and they come at a time when toddlers are beginning to see themselves as autonomous beings. Because pleasing their parents is important to toddlers, who thrive on parental love and approval, they may be afraid that an angry parent will abandon them or withdraw love.

Sigmund Freud held the perspective that children's main developmental tasks include gradually gaining control over their sexual and aggressive impulses. He referred to toddlerhood as the **anal stage,** since this area of the body is symbolic of the child's growing mastery over his or her body and actions. Power struggles between caregiver and child may occur around toilet training. Caregivers who are overly controlling or critical of a child in the "terrible twos" may set the stage for future problems.

Erikson's description of these children as struggling with a wish for **autonomy** and yet a tendency toward **shame and doubt** reflects the same issues that were identified by Freud and Mahler. Overly critical caregivers tend to make children feel shameful and insecure rather than confident and autonomous. Children need to feel that they will not lose caring by having a mind of their own. They should be encouraged and praised. Children who are shamed in their quest to begin exploring their autonomy may develop self-esteem problems.

Decentering and the Acquisition of Symbolic Thought

During toddlerhood, a "decentering" process occurs cognitively, whereby children learn to see themselves as one of many objects in a world where there are laws of cause and effect. **Symbolic function**, the understanding that one thing can represent another, is a second cognitive milestone that occurs during this time. **Symbolic play** is one aspect of this developmental progression; for example, a little girl may pretend to sleep, cuddling with her teddy bear and closing her eyes. **Language** is another important aspect of this symbolic capacity. One result of the interrelationship between the emotional and cognitive lines of development is that temper tantrums may lessen as verbal expressiveness increases. This effect has implications for language-impaired children, who may have more behavioral problems even as adults.

Internal Representations

As cognitive skills evolve, the child's ability to hold onto stable images of others also evolves. The development of **internal representations** (i.e., stable images of other people that exist within the child's memory) is an important part of this process. The child's *inability* to carry mental images of caregivers seems to contribute to the **separation anxiety** to which toddlers are particularly prone. Thus, a child cannot be comforted by the image of the mother when separated from her if the child cannot evoke a mental representation of the mother and understand that she has not just "disappeared."

Children of this age tend to experience other people and themselves as completely good or completely bad. They are **unable to reconcile contradictory feelings** toward the same person. The "good" loving mommy and the "bad" angry one seem to be two different people. This instability makes angry feelings particularly frightening for them.

At age 24–36 months, the child's ability to integrate conflicting feelings about the same person improves dramatically. This developmental milestone is called **object constancy,** and the child can carry a more stable image of the parent in mind, even when separated. The child establishes **stable internalized object relations**, which are the child's composite emotional memories of interactions with the prototypical person (e.g., the parent). Toddlers now more confidently allow significant others to come and go, since they are able to hold onto stable images of others in their minds. The mother with whom a child is affectionate at one moment and angry the next is recognized as one and the same person. Because the child is now able to tolerate this ambivalence, the child can trust further that the mother will return if she leaves her or his presence. It is not a coincidence that the age at which children may enter nursery school is also when they have usually acquired object constancy.

More prolonged separations, as when parents go away for a long vacation, can be especially difficult for children age 2–3 years, especially if they are left with adults with whom they are unfamiliar. By age 3–3 1/2 years, most children are able to master such separations easily, although they are always vulnerable to regression and increased sensitivity during a stressful separation, such as a medical hospitalization. While they are mastering the anxiety of separateness from caregivers, children tend to become attached to a **transitional object**, such as a stuffed animal or a special blanket, to serve as an intermediary that symbolically represents the parent(s). The ability to be comforted by a transitional object is one of the first steps in the use of symbols, and it further exemplifies the interplay between emotion and cognition (see Table 14.5 for a summary of toddler development and Box 14.5 for a case example of a toddler).

Establishment of Gender Identity

Freud first noted **infantile sexuality**. Self-stimulation of the genitals begins early and continues throughout the toddler years. **Gender identity**, the sense that one is a girl or a boy, is established by 2–3 years of age. Interestingly, this is the age at which the child is able to recognize herself or himself in a mirror. It is not uncommon for little boys and girls to notice the difference in their external genitalia. Parents might explain to girls that they have special organs (e.g., the vagina is on the inside and cannot be seen) that will one day allow them to have a baby.

Developmental Vulnerabilities

As during infancy, the main area of vulnerability in the toddler's emotional development is the caretaker–child relationship and attachment. Whereas separations between infant and caretaker exert their most profound impact by disrupting the growing preverbal attachment, separations between toddlers and caretakers have a much more direct effect on the child. For instance, sudden, prolonged separations of 2- and 3-year-olds from their parents may result in behaviors that resemble mourning (e.g., if the child must be medically hospitalized and separated from parents).

Transient Symptoms

Bedtime fears are frequent in toddlers and may be exacerbated by nightmares. **Fears of monsters, robbers, or of being alone** are especially common. Until toddlers have mastered

TABLE 14.5 Toddler (1–3 Years) Development

Neurodevelopmental (e.g., Gessell)	Cognitive (e.g., Piaget)	Psychosexual (e.g., Freud)	Psychosocial (e.g., Erikson)	Attachment (e.g. Bowlby)
13–18 months	**11–18 months**	Anal stage:		Typical toddler alone
Mouthing stops	Trial and error	Issues of		in unfamiliar setting
First spoken language	exploration	emerging control		(e.g., in hospital)
Gestures to	Develops spatial	and autonomy		Stages:
communicate needs	relations	symbolically enacted		1. Protest (hopeful
Walks and runs		in ambivalence over		calling and crying)
independently		toilet training		2. Despair (listless,
16–24 months	**18–24 months**	Mahler: separation	Autonomy versus	crying)
Horizontal	Internal	and individuation	shame and doubt	3. Detachment
pencil stroke	representations of	Oppositional stage:		(settle into new
Ongoing toilet training	the external world	◦ "Terrible twos"		place, may avoid
Throws ball overhead	Object constancy	◦ Everything is "no"		parent upon
24–36 months	Beginning of	◦ "Battle of the		reunion)
Understands ~800	conceptual thought	potty"		
words (by 3 years)	(e.g., words			
Draws a circle	symbolize real			
Rides a tricycle	things, symbolic play			
	with dolls)			

Modeled on Theories of Development chart by Clarice Kestenbaum, MD, Department of Psychiatry, Columbia University College of Physicians and Surgeons and New York State Psychiatric Institute.

separation anxiety, they may be frequent visitors in their parents' bedroom, motivated by the need to be reassured that their parents are still there in case they are needed. Problems in separating at bedtime are often handled best with a story and a ritual, which are comforting to children in this age group. The parents should honor the toddler's requests for leaving a night light burning and having a particular door open (usually, the bedroom door) or closed (usually, the closet door). Phobias, particularly toward animals, may emerge but tend to pass. Children are more likely to manifest anxiety in behaviors, such as **increased oppositional or clinging behavior**, moodiness, and sleep or appetite disturbances.

The child in this age group also has a more vulnerable sense of bodily security and may be upset by the inevitable skin cuts and scrapes. In most cases, with empathic parental responses, these fears and anxieties gradually diminish over the next year or two as the child progresses emotionally and intellectually. Overall, toddlers' coping mechanisms are unstable, as they are relatively newly acquired. Therefore, their reliance on such "external" means of comfort as people or transitional objects is greater. Box 14.6 describes the response to physical illness in the toddler.

Psychopathology
The psychopathology that is first noticeable in the toddler years includes many of the diagnostic entities mentioned in infancy, including **motor disorders, communication**

BOX 14.5
TODDLER CASE EXAMPLE

By Tina's second birthday she is using two- to three-word phrases and understanding fairly complex sets of commands from her parents ("Put your toys in the trunk"). She is also responding "no" more frequently as she establishes her autonomy and separateness from them. She does not yet have the coping skills to postpone gratification or to use her words to express fully what she feels, and she experiences the ambivalence of both wanting and rejecting help at the same time. Her use of the pronoun "me" to say what she wants reflects her growing self-conception. By age 2½ Tina throws a ball with reasonable accuracy, holds a cup of juice, feeds herself, turns the pages of a book, and helps to dress herself. She retains the mental image of objects and is able to conjecture and plan. She plays with dolls in such a way that they symbolize people and imitate adult behavior. Her play represents a microcosm of a world in which she is in control, helping her develop a sense of mastery and cope with anxiety over the unknown. She can be the princess or the dragon-slayer, and exert the control she lacks in real life. Her healthy attachment to her parents allows her to feel secure that they will be there when she needs them, which she has learned from their expectable parental responsiveness. As she ventures off to explore the world, she returns frequently to "refuel." The bedtime story has become a reassuring ritual that helps her to separate from her parents into the nighttime world, which can be scary at times. Her imagination can be both a source of fear and security, and her favorite stuffed animal serves as a "transitional object" to hug during the night.

BOX 14.6

RESPONSE TO PHYSICAL ILLNESS IN THE TODDLER

Accepting the "sick role" involves the ability, in a sense, to regress and accept nurturing care, even for an adult. For a toddler, that need is tempered by the pride taken in newly acquired skills, such as feeding, going to the bathroom, dressing and undressing, and having ever-increasing bodily control. Therefore, illness and hospitalization in particular present threats to the child's strivings toward autonomy and control. A practical application of a developmental understanding is that toddlers should bring transitional objects with them when being admitted to the hospital. A sheet from the child's crib at home may be comforting because it surrounds the child with a familiar sight, smell, and texture. The young child's life is dominated by concrete sensations. Children sometimes revert to using a pacifier during a hospitalization. This temporary regression provides an additional transitional object. Sucking on the pacifier soothes the child during an overly stressful experience.

disorders, autism spectrum disorders, and reactive attachment disorder. An intellectual disability (intellectual developmental disorder) may also be first suspected in young children. Many of these disorders may become more evident as toddlers have greater contact with other children and differences become more noticeable, especially in social settings. **Hyperactivity, impulsivity, and heightened distractibility** (compared with same-age peers) may also become apparent during the toddler years. Some children with these traits may later be diagnosed with attention-deficit hyperactivity disorder.

THE PRESCHOOL CHILD: 3 TO 6 YEARS OF AGE

Developmental Progression

The Autonomous Self and the Emergence of Morality

As a result of positive social interactions with caregivers, the child begins to understand the word *we*. By age 3 years this internalization is applied to new relationships. The child has the sense that caregivers are "with" him or her even when they are absent, so that there is an **enhanced sense of mastery and control**. The emotional core that the child brings from the toddler years will serve as a template for future relationships.

This stage corresponds roughly to **Erikson's age of initiative versus guilt** or **Freud's Oedipal stage** (see Table 14.6). In this phase, language blossoms, and so the child has new means of expressing thoughts and feelings. Also, evolving at the same time is the understanding that people may have relationships with each other outside of the child's relationship with them. The classic example is that the mother and father have their own relationship with each other from which the child feels excluded (**triadic relationships**). The child is able to use initiative in actively exploring the world and has less of the defiant quality seen in the earlier toddler phase. The potential danger in this phase, according to Erikson, is that excessive guilt might result if the child is overwhelmed by aggressive feelings (e.g., anger associated with extreme sibling rivalry). During this period

TABLE 14.6 Preschool (3–6 Years) Development

Neurodevelopmental (e.g., Gessell)	Cognitive (e.g., Piaget)	Psychosexual (e.g., Freud)	Psychosocial (e.g., Erikson)	Attachment (e.g. Bowlby)
3–4 years	**2–4 years**	Oedipal stage:	Initiative versus	Child with
Examines	Preoperational	Competitive	guilt	disorganized
picture books	thought:	relationships		attachment:
Hops on one foot	∘ Intuitive rather			∘ Role reversing
Rules of grammar	than logical			behavior with
Draws a square	∘ Egocentric			parent, e.g.,
4–5 years				demanding or
Understands 2000				parent-like
words by 5 years				∘ Fearful of
Draws a triangle				separations

Modeled on Theories of Development chart by Clarice Kestenbaum, MD, Department of Psychiatry, Columbia University College of Physicians and Surgeons and New York State Psychiatric Institute.

children renounce their earlier grandiose self-confidence that they could be "master of the universe" and temper ambitions with reality. Children bury their infantile wishes in the unconscious, permitting the emergence of the superego, or **conscience**, an internal agency that guides them morally and produces guilty feelings when they have done something "wrong." This newly formed superego can be rather harsh, as seen in children's tendency to believe that illness is a punishment for misdeeds. For example, a 5-year-old who was told that his heart was failing and that he would need to get a new one (i.e., have a transplantation) was heard to comment that he wished he had not been so naughty. He asked his parents, "If I promise to be good, would my heart get better?"

In the evolution of thought between ages 3 and 6 years, children become more fully aware of the feelings and rights of others. Parental and social values are grasped, and a sense of morality develops. Internal moral standards start to take shape, accompanied by a sense of self-discipline. Children begin to recall aloud or to themselves parental prohibitions (e.g., "don't touch electrical outlets"). This process is facilitated by parents' ability to approach discipline in a fairly consistent and firm but not overly punitive manner.

Imaginative Play

As a number of social and cognitive developmental lines converge, children can now **play cooperatively**, inhibiting impulses to be aggressive or selfish. The preschooler's make-believe play is crucial for the later development of adult modes of thinking and relating emotionally to others, thus representing a continuous line of development. Play is thought by some to be a prototype for imagination in adults. If a child does not have the ability to play, the child's social and academic functioning will probably be impaired from an early age. Play may be viewed as a microcosm of the world, in which the child has enhanced control over events and outcomes and may practice different responses and skills. It can also be a means by which children anticipate future events and replay past events in order to diminish anxiety and enhance mastery. Imaginary playmates are common and should not be a cause for concern. To the contrary, significant early childhood psychopathology can be associated with the inability to play imaginatively.

Parental tasks include encouraging play by providing a conducive atmosphere and facilitating social involvement with other children. The child will learn about sharing and reciprocity, skills that will be needed during the school years. The preschool years are a time for parents to help secure a base for their children, who will soon be leaving the nest to enter school. Encouragement, love, and guidance help to consolidate an early sense of self that is competent and confident. These years are often among those most fondly remembered by parents. They observe their preschoolers becoming "little people" who can carry on animated conversations as language development flourishes and truly share activities with adults, such as going to the movies and playing board games.

The Evolution of Magical Thinking

By age 3 years, the child has reached the stage that Piaget described as a **preoperational level** of cognition, during which the child becomes **aware of time as a continuum** with a past, present, and future. Even though the child may refer to all past events as occurring "yesterday," this perspective is a major shift from the child's earlier sense of existing only in the present. The world, however, is still a confusing place for the preschooler, who has not yet grasped more complicated issues of relative size and space, or cause and effect. For instance, one 3-year-old who had to have repeated cardiac biopsies became fearful that too much of her heart would be removed, causing it to fall into her stomach.

> ### BOX 14.7
> ## PRESCHOOLER CASE EXAMPLE
>
> Paul is a miniature person at age 3 years, toilet trained, dressing himself independently, and speaking in full sentences, although he often makes mistakes with pronouns. He can be logical, but is still easily distracted and prone to magical thinking; for example, he worries that he became sick because he misbehaved. Attending nursery school is a major step for him. He is making friends, learning to share, and following rules. Shy as a toddler, he remains shy in nursery school but is increasingly receptive to playing with other children with the help of his sensitive and nurturing teacher. He loves to dress up like an astronaut and role-play with his peers. He also likes to wear biking clothes like his father and go out on a ride sitting on a "trailer bike" that is attached to the back of his father's bicycle. He is strong enough to sit upright and hold onto the bars. Part of this behavior reflects his growing identification with his father. Much of his conception of what it means to be a "boy" he has derived from both explicit and implicit messages and expectations from his parents and the world around him. Paul sleeps in his own bed by himself, though he occasionally wets the bed or has a bad dream that brings him into his parents' bedroom. Paul is reading by the time he is ready for first grade. He can carry on a conversation about just about anything, and has a personality of his own.

The preschooler's world is still infused with a great deal of magic, which may, at times, blur the line between fantasy and reality, as the following bedtime incident involving a 5-year-old boy demonstrates. One night when a breeze from the window gently rattled the bedroom blinds, the boy jumped out of bed and ran out of the room. In the hallway, he laughed nervously, admitting that he had suddenly become worried that a monster was behind the blinds, even though he "knew" that there was "no such thing as monsters." He was reluctantly coaxed back into his room when his parents offered to accompany him over to the blinds to take a look. He was noticeably relieved to see that nothing was there (see Table 14.6 for a summary of preschool development and Box 14.7 for a preschooler case example).

Evolution of Sexuality

Preschool children may exhibit aggressive and sexualized behavior toward parents or other children in their play, where strivings for mastery and competition are often seen. Children become interested in storytelling and fairy tales, which often reflect their own fantasies, such as wanting to be a mommy or daddy. This fantasy may include a certain degree of "showing off," especially in a coy manner.

Sexual behavior is not uncommon in preschoolers and may include a wide continuum of behaviors, including touching their own genitalia or those of others, interest in looking at naked people, inquiring about sexual organs and acts, watching people on the toilet, expressing interest in pregnancy and birth, showing other children their genitalia, an interest in their own feces, and "playing doctor." These behaviors may indicate problems if they seem to preoccupy the child relative to other activities or if there is any history of childhood sexual abuse. Many of these behaviors may continue into the young school-age years.

Developmental Vulnerabilities

Psychopathology in preschoolers includes the **communication disorders**. Entry into school often allows such language problems to be identified, because the child is in an environment of adults and children who are not familiar with her or his idiosyncratic means of expression. **Selective mutism**, in which the child will not speak in specific social situations but does not have a communication disorder, can also become evident. Children with **attention-deficit hyperactivity disorder** may begin to clearly differentiate themselves from other children who are better able to tolerate the transition into more structured class settings. **Anxiety disorders** may also manifest themselves at this age. **Specific phobias** are often seen in this age group and may be directed at animals, naturally occurring phenomena such as storms, or specific situations such as riding in an elevator. **Posttraumatic stress disorder** may result from an acute event in which there is a sudden, brief exposure to a trauma (e.g., a schoolyard shooting) or from a chronic situation (e.g., chronic physical or sexual abuse of a child). **Adjustment disorders,** which are by definition transient, may result from a specific event, such as an illness, parental divorce, move, or birth of a new sibling, and may be manifested in mood or behavioral changes. The **elimination disorders** occur in this age group (e.g., enuresis). **Gender dysphoria** (see DSM-5) may have its onset during this time period. Box 14.8 describes the response to physical illness in the preschooler.

THE SCHOOL-AGE CHILD: 6 TO 11 YEARS OF AGE

Developmental Progression

The school-age years, or middle childhood, begin at age 6 years and end with puberty. As their social world expands beyond the family to include friends and teachers, children at this age find it easy to be physically apart from their parents. The tasks of this period include developing a **sustained sense of mastery and competence, morality, and stable self-esteem** (see Table 14.7).

Acquiring Competence

Erikson underscored the importance of social processes for children of elementary school age when he described this period as one in which children must either achieve **industry** or suffer from **inferiority**. During this period, children leave the world of their parents and are taught the fundamental skills that are prerequisite to becoming productive members of society, such as being literate and having a functional understanding of society.

As they watch their children proceed through this stage, parents should be protective but not intrusive in order to facilitate their children's continued socialization and development of morality, academic skills, and autonomy. A major determinant in the development of a sense of competence is the manner in which important people react to the child's growing abilities and successes. Responses that affirm and validate these developing skills facilitate self-esteem. Through encouragement and acknowledgment of their attempts at mastery, whether in schoolwork, athletics, or music, children come to recognize their talents as real and part of themselves. As a result of this process, the exhibitionism of preschool children is transformed into a sense of **pride and mastery**.

TABLE 14.7 School-Age (6–11 Years) Development

Neurodevelopmental (e.g., Gessell)	Cognitive (e.g., Piaget)	Psychosexual (e.g., Freud)	Psychosocial (e.g., Erikson)
Mastery of games, sports	Concrete operations:	Latency stage:	Industry versus inferiority
Increasing independence	◦ Rules of logic, categories, serial ordering	◦ Strengthened conscience	
Academic skills		◦ Same-sex peers	
Increasing independence	◦ Reversibility	◦ New adult role models (e.g., teacher, coach)	
Capacity for judgment	◦ Conservation of mass	◦ Empathy, altruism	

Modeled on Theories of Development chart by Clarice Kestenbaum, MD, Department of Psychiatry, Columbia University College of Physicians and Surgeons and New York State Psychiatric Institute.

BOX 14.8
RESPONSE TO PHYSICAL ILLNESS IN THE PRESCHOOLER

The regression that sometimes accompanies illness can be anxiety provoking for the preschooler, who, like the toddler, is still striving to become independent. The unconscious fantasies typical of preschoolers, such as the fear of bodily mutilation as punishment, may exaggerate fears associated with surgery, because young children typically attribute external events to their own internal thoughts and feelings. With respect to surgery, unconscious fears and wishes often modulate a child's conscious worries. The normal developmental concerns of a 3- to 5-year-old include the fear of bodily mutilation, as well as the struggle with angry feelings when a parent will not allow the child to do as he or she pleases. For these reasons, a surgical procedure may be seen as the actualization of an intense fear, a punishment for being bad, or a retribution for angry feelings toward a parent.

An appreciation of the defense mechanisms used in childhood is crucial to understanding reactions to illness and devising appropriate intervention strategies. A child with cystic fibrosis who ties her stuffed animals down to give them injections and at the same time soothes them demonstrates regression, repression (of unconscious fears and wishes), identification with the aggressor, and transformation of passivity into activity. The child identifies with the more powerful physician, who is in control, but also empathizes with the helpless stuffed elephant, which she soothes. Allowing the child to play out the procedure on a doll beforehand fosters both intellectual and emotional mastery. By acting out this scenario repeatedly, the child helps master the anxieties associated with treatment of her chronic illness and turns a passive experience into a more active one. Interventions designed to bolster this function would be supportive of the child's developing ego, which can easily be overwhelmed by anxiety. Interestingly, interventions aimed at helping to prepare the parents and allay their anxiety usually also decrease anxiety in the child. Likely this is because these interventions fortify the parents and may prevent the "emotional contagion" sometimes seen between parent and child.

Hobbies represent an intermediate step between play and work, requiring realistic planning and preparation.

Evolving Coping Styles and Morality

While preschoolers are prone to becoming overwhelmed by stressful external events and manifesting these feelings by withdrawal and other behavioral disturbances, middle school children have an expanded repertoire of coping responses and defense mechanisms. They are more **emotionally flexible** and better able to take care of themselves. Essentially, this is a time in which ego functions grow and consolidate, allowing children to **tolerate frustration and delays** in the gratification of their wishes and desires.

Temperamental characteristics, such as shyness, level of activity, persistence in approaching tasks, resilience, and quality of mood follow children through this period and beyond. Temperament may have important influences on achievement during this phase of life.

As children approach adolescence, their idealization of parental figures that characterized the preschool years is transformed into an appreciation of the values for which their parents stand. An intermediate stage in this transition is the **idealization of other role models**, such as sports heroes and teachers. Children also look to their peers for positive feedback and a sense of belonging. If they receive support and encouragement, their self-esteem becomes more stable and is less shaken by failures or disappointments. The child's needs for independence and attachment are both satisfied by **group affiliations**, which also serve as the arena in which children first perform or compete with others.

The conscience evolves during this period, developing more mature determinants, including **empathy**, internal guilt, and a concern for what is morally right. As children's social development progresses, their relationships become based on mutual respect. Although younger children follow rules handed down to them by authority figures, children between the ages of 7 and 8 years begin to see rules as agreements made between all interested parties that can be changed if a consensus is reached. At this point, justice becomes an operative force rather than an act of simple obedience. When a child truly identifies with parents or authority figures, rules are followed independently and without the need for external enforcement. Along the way, children's ambivalence about their parents may mediate their following of rules, such that a child may be angry with her or his parents and disobey them, but then later feel guilty and comply. In this way, cognitive, social, emotional, and moral lines of development intertwine.

Reading, Writing, and Arithmetic

During the school-age years, children progress markedly in the cognitive sphere. Piaget identified the stage of **concrete operations** as beginning at approximately age 7–8 years and concluding when children reach preadolescence, at approximately age 11–12 years. Examples of concrete operations include **joining** (e.g., mother and father together equal parents); **ordering** (i.e., the ability to arrange numbers in a sequence or objects in order of increasing size); **conservation** (i.e., the understanding that the properties of an object are not changed if its location or position is changed); and **classification** (i.e., the ability to arrange objects according to color or shape). Children also understand the concept of **reversibility** of operations, that operations have opposites (e.g., subtraction is the reverse of addition). Children are able to understand the **concept of numbers** instead of only being able to recite them. The concepts of spatial **measurement** (e.g., the length of a line), time, and speed also fall into the category of concrete operations.

Piaget demonstrated the concept of conservation with the following experiment: children of various ages watch a fixed amount of liquid being poured from a beaker into either a taller, thinner container or a shorter, wider container, causing the height of the water level to change. When asked whether the amount of water had changed, children of 4–5 years of age said that there was more water in the beaker with the higher water level (preoperational thinking). Children who had attained concrete operational thinking knew that the amount of water had not changed (see Table 14.3).

Gender Differentiation

A crucial aspect of this period is the further development of gender identity. Children tend to turn to the same-sex parent and to identify and share in more culturally defined, gender-specific activities. The precise form of this identification depends on the specific sociocultural context. Children also usually prefer same-sex peers at this age, although their interest in opposite-sex children never disappears. Boys and girls seem to differentiate into opposing camps. Members of both genders tend to join gender-specific groups and clubs. Gender-specific behaviors and tendencies are observed, and it remains unclear to what extent these differences can be attributed to inborn divergences or to cultural influences. In general, boys are drawn to "rough and tumble" play, especially play involving competitiveness and prowess, while girls seem to mature more quickly and use more diplomatic, verbal means of persuasion in their play. Boys tend to cluster in larger groups that are organized around a common interest or goal, while girls focus more on the interpersonal aspects of relationships, such as sharing confidences, interacting within smaller groups, and operating by consensus rather than dominance. At the same time, not all boys and girls fit comfortably into these general patterns. Children with atypical preferences may feel different from other children and be seen as different by their peers, which may lead to ostracism. Some children may eventually emerge with a stronger sense of self despite their differences, while others will suffer from diminished self-esteem.

Sexual Curiosity and Modesty

Children are initially socialized about sexuality through experiences with their parents. Children learn how to feel about their bodies from the direct and indirect lessons that their parents teach them in subtle but influential ways. They also learn about sexuality and physicality within a relationship by observing the way in which their parents interact with each other.

Freud initially dubbed this developmental phase **latency**, because he believed that the sexual curiosity present in earlier childhood became dormant, not to be reactivated until adolescence. Recent observations suggest that this is not completely true. Instead of being dormant, the sexual interests and preoccupations of latency-age children are more likely simply concealed from adults.

When children enter school, they begin to learn social etiquette. Teachers and classmates reinforce standards for what is appropriate with regard to toileting and showing one's body. By fourth or fifth grade, most children are **extremely self-conscious** about having their underwear show, let alone being seen naked, especially by the opposite sex. As adolescence approaches, children may be uncomfortable during physical examinations, and physicians should be sensitive to this. Children often begin to exhibit increased modesty about their bodies in the presence of their parents and may prefer to bathe in private. Box 14.9 provides a case example of a latency-age child.

BOX 14.9
CASE EXAMPLE OF A LATENCY-AGE CHILD

Laura enters first grade as an eager but apprehensive 6-year-old. She will leave fifth grade as an accomplished reader of literature and a competitive sports team member. During each of the intervening years she will lose an average of four baby teeth, grow an average of 2 ½ inches, and gain about 7 pounds. Laura gravitates toward friendships with girls, though she enjoys competing athletically with boys. Her cognition develops dramatically through these years as she applies a growing appreciation for cause and effect and the rules of nature not just to academics but also to life in general. Laura retains large amounts of information (she is able to recall 6–7 digits) and can group objects and categorize information. She uses concepts such as conservation of mass to override conclusions based solely on appearance, such that when two identical balls of clay are molded into different shapes, Laura understands that their weight remains the same.

Laura's moral development is marked by refinements in her ability to experience empathy, which is seen in her wish to help others. She increasingly takes on independent jobs around the house. As a result of positive feedback from parents and peers, as well as her acquisition of skills in the classroom, in the social arena, at home, and in extracurricular pursuits, Laura has a sense of pride and confidence in herself. Her ability to inhibit selfish impulses (at times) and to use greater self-control and respect for others heralds a successful adolescence and the development of mature relationships with peers. Her exposure to the community-based interests of her parents has shaped Laura's interests in this area. As a result of growing math skills and a sense of responsibility, she begins to handle money in the form of a weekly allowance. By the time she is in fifth grade she has a sense of modesty and privacy, which is seen during her annual visit with the pediatrician. She has moved away from seeing her parents as her only role models and now has a collection of singers, athletes, and dancers whom she idealizes.

As a "tween" caught between childhood and adolescence, Laura takes sexual education class in school. Her parents have broached this topic as well and are making clear their limits on which movies and television shows she can watch. Laura has become keenly aware of the "popular" and "not so popular" groups in school, and the shifting loyalties of friendships are a source of frustration and upset for the first time. Her parents find themselves in a new role as they try to find the right balance between intervening on Laura's behalf and letting her work through challenges on her own. They remain actively involved in her schoolwork and have contact with her teacher. The preadolescent girl that emerges from elementary school shares many of the temperamental qualities of the preschooler that entered first grade, yet much has changed physically, socially, and cognitively.

Developmental Vulnerabilities

Potential dangers during this phase of life are related to the child's ability to successfully navigate pressures to perform academically and socially. School can be a trying place for children of this age, especially if they feel incapable of meeting the expectations of parents and teachers or of competing with peers. For some children, accomplishments may become the only priority. If parents or coaches place too much emphasis on winning competitions rather than on having fun and building skills, children may suffer significant self-esteem problems, feeling they do not measure up. This corresponds with Erikson's stage of industry verses inferiority. Box 14.10 describes the response to physical illness in the school-age age child.

Psychopathology

Children who have **specific learning disorders** or **attention-deficit hyperactivity disorder** often first manifest problems when they enter school. When appropriate interventions are not made promptly, children may deviate from the normal course of development, failing to acquire the skills and self-confidence necessary for entry into the occupational world and suffering from diminished self-esteem. **Communication disorders** and specific learning disorders can interfere with mastery of academic tasks for the school-aged child. **Obsessive-compulsive disorder** is especially likely to be first diagnosed in this age group. **Anxiety disorders**, for example, **posttraumatic stress disorder**, may be seen in children at this age. Disorders affecting mood (bipolar and related disorders, and depressive disorders including disruptive mood dysregulation disorder) can have their onset in the school-aged child. **Adjustment disorders**, which can be associated with mood and behavioral changes as well as anxiety, can also occur (e.g., start at a

---

BOX 14.10

RESPONSE TO PHYSICAL ILLNESS IN THE LATENCY-AGE CHILD

Physicians caring for latency-age children with serious medical illnesses can use their knowledge of developmental progressions to help the children adjust. Because these children are in the process of becoming increasingly competent and autonomous, they will appreciate receiving booklets and DVDs that explain the illness, anticipated procedures, and treatments. Their interest in peer groups can be turned to advantage by encouraging contact with other children who have similar illnesses. Physicians and parents should not make the mistake, however, of assuming that latency-age children have the same understanding of illness that they have. Both regression and variable progress along cognitive or emotional lines can result in misunderstandings and worries. For example, a bright, mature 8-year-old boy surprised his parents with a remnant of magical thinking when he developed the flu during his first ice-skating expedition. He was convinced that the skating had made him sick, "like getting car sick," because he felt fine before he started skating, became progressively nauseated and weak while skating, and became febrile and vomited at home that evening.

new school). **Tic disorders** occur in this age range. Simple tics are particularly common in school-age boys and are usually transient.

ADOLESCENCE

Adolescence is a time of great change. It begins with **puberty**, the period of sexual maturation in which the primary sex organs develop and become capable of reproduction and secondary sex characteristics appear (such as facial hair in boys and breast enlargement in girls). Girls usually mature 2 years earlier than boys. There are "late developers" in both sexes, which can have profound consequences for self-esteem, as adolescents place great importance on body image, comparisons with peers, and sexual attractiveness.

Developmental Progression

Achieving Independence Through Groups
As they develop socially, children in early adolescence tend to identify with groups in order to deal with the anxieties associated with the **lack of a coherent sense of individual identity**. The teenager may also form early love relationships in an attempt to clarify her or his self-image by having it reflected by a partner.

Adolescents often exhibit a **lack of tolerance for difference**, which can be seen in their cliques and prejudices. This intolerance may be a way to protect teenagers from the anxiety of not knowing who they are. Adults may remember the "in" crowds and the "outsiders" and how, as teenagers, they desperately tried to figure out what was "cool" and what was not. Being part of a fairly homogenous group (e.g., with regard to ideals and behavior, as well as enemies) may soothe the unsettling feeling of not being sure of who one is or what one will become. Adolescents feel pressure to remain faithful to the group; tests of loyalty are not uncommon and may be intense.

Young adolescents usually rely on external praise to feel good about themselves, making them particularly **vulnerable to criticism**. Parents are characteristically de-idealized in early adolescence, as adolescents begin to see them more objectively. This distancing may be associated with feelings of irritation and frustration with parents (i.e., as if the adolescent has been "let down" by the parents). Adolescents may idealize other adults or the parents of friends, allowing them to retain a sense of support as they separate and individuate from their own parents. As achieving autonomy becomes an all-important goal for adolescents, they may be propelled into oppositional behavior. This defiance tends to be mitigated by a continued need for parental support. These conflicting feelings often result in **alterations between rebelliousness and neediness**, which can become painfully evident in the face of stresses, such as illness.

In the middle years of adolescence, the adolescent typically ventures out of the peer group to form a relationship with single others, as they further refine their identity. The tasks of this phase include separating from the family, establishing intimate relationships, beginning to take responsibility for one's life, and learning to weather the feelings of anxiety or loneliness that may accompany these transitions. It is generally not until late adolescence (age 18–22 years) that the peer group's influence recedes in relation to the importance of the significant other. Until then, the task of separating from parents is often worked out more in friendships than with lovers, as the peer setting is more acceptable for obtaining support and sharing experiences.

Consolidation of Identity and Growing Emotional Maturity

Erikson referred to this stage as one of **identity versus role confusion**. He believed that the adolescent searches for present-day meaning in skills mastered earlier. The early adolescent may be relatively unfocused and confused about roles and expectations in less structured settings. Early in puberty, young adolescents tend to experience more anxious or depressed feelings than they had previously and may find it difficult to enjoy themselves. Because their sense of identity is evolving and unclear, young adolescents may have difficulty in trusting themselves or others or in viewing themselves highly. They tend to look to peers for self–definition, which partially explains the intensity of fluctuating relationships with friends.

Parents continue to play an important role in the adolescent's life. Empathic and protective responses that provide support but allow for independent growth can facilitate adjustment during this phase of life. The major psychological tasks of adolescence involve what has been referred to as the **second phase of separation-individuation**, one goal of which is to achieve psychological autonomy from the parents. As in the toddler's phase of separation-individuation, parents must be able to tolerate the increasing disengagement of the adolescent. The adolescent's de-idealization of the parents and the accompanying growing autonomy and emergence of sexual identity may cause a **mourning reaction in parents,** who may long for the latency years. Parents' abilities to work through their own adjustment are important to the adolescent's successful passage through these years. Pathological separation difficulties in the parents may predispose the adolescent to the same problems. Healthy parents are able to relish their adolescent's achievement without having their own self-esteem compromised and without trying to quash the process of separation.

The age of 16–17 years is regarded as the **midpoint of adolescence,** when the earlier feelings of omnipotence become tempered by adulthood, which looms ahead. By this time, adolescents have grown accustomed to the bodily changes that heralded puberty and tend to be less anxious about their bodies and more focused on the future. This adjustment usually takes about 2 years from the onset of puberty.

Adolescents in this age group tend to feel less anxious or depressed and are perhaps more trusting of others than during pubescence. They tend to identify with a more diverse group of mentors and idealized adults and appear more content and upbeat. Middle adolescents also often have feelings of arrogance, defiance, and superiority alternating with feelings of deflation, compliance, and inferiority. Their self-image is more coherent but still has a certain degree of instability, especially when their independence is challenged. Arguing with adults may bolster their sense of autonomy while incorporating values in a manner that appears less dependent on authority figures. For similar reasons, middle adolescents typically have difficulty being appreciative of adults. As the adolescent's **identity is consolidated**, behavior and motivation becomes more consistent and future career plans and value systems may be embraced. As adolescents make the journey into young adulthood, they must abandon grandiose dreams and fantasies and begin to develop more realistic conceptions of possible future roles and accomplishments. The process of developing a more realistic self-assessment has been described as a second "decentering" process.

The establishment of intimate relationships is another crucial milestone. Erikson thought that the establishment of a stable identity was a prerequisite to the development of intimate relationships. Also, if adolescents have not fully resolved issues involving separation from their parents, the establishment of intimate relationships with others may be affected.

Acquisition of Abstract Thought

Piaget's stage of **formal operational, or abstract thinking** becomes apparent between 12 and 16 years of age. This achievement probably reflects central nervous system maturation during this time. Now the adolescent can hypothesize about things that have not yet happened or evaluate hypotheses with which she or he disagrees. Adolescence is a time of philosophizing and of taking **pleasure in ideas**. Parental values remain important during this phase of life, but considerable thought and revision is given to parental value systems as adolescents evolve their sense of identity and ethics.

The development of **creativity** manifests itself predominantly during adolescence, although prerequisites to the ability to initiate the creative process occur earlier during childhood. Some of the impetus for creativity may derive from the autonomy and identity development that occur during adolescence. Table 14.8 provides a summary of adolescent development.

Gender-Related Issues

The onset of menarche is a time of intense feelings for adolescent girls, who may be surprised or even hide its occurrence. If a girl is uninformed she may be confused or frightened about what has happened. The first ejaculation in boys may be similarly experienced. These first demonstrable signs of sexual reproductive function can stir up conflicting feelings, including embarrassment, anxiety, or guilt, since this function was "prohibited" during latency. Distorted perceptions about these experiences and bodily functions are extremely common at this age and complicate matters for the early adolescent.

Early adolescent boys are generally concerned about the size of their penises and will overtly or subtly make comparisons. They are fond of "dirty jokes" but have limited interest in actual sexual contact. Most adolescent males place a premium value on muscular strength and athletic prowess. Smaller or nonathletic boys may fear that they appear "feminine."

TABLE 14.8 Adolescent Development

Neurodevelopmental (e.g., Gessell)	Cognitive (e.g., Piaget)	Psychosexual (e.g., Freud)	Psychosocial (e.g., Erikson)	Attachment
Female, 10–11 years Onset of puberty, growth spurt, breast growth	Formal operations: ∘ Ability to plan ∘ Make and test hypotheses	Second phase of individuation: ∘ Separation from parents	Identity versus role confusion: Evolve in social, sexual, and vocational roles	Former disorganized attachment: May have difficulty forming trusting, positive relationships with others
Female, 11–13 years Menstruation, pubic and axillary hair growth	∘ Abstract thought ∘ Consider various possibilities in the future	∘ Identity formation ∘ Same-sex peer group		
Male, 12–16 years Onset of puberty	∘ Introspection	∘ Sexual exploration		
Male, 13–17 years Enlargement of penis, voice change, period of maximal physical growth		**Late adolescence** Intimacy with romantic partner		

Modeled on Theories of Development chart by Clarice Kestenbaum, MD, Department of Psychiatry, Columbia University College of Physicians and Surgeons and New York State Psychiatric Institute.

Young adolescent girls often share sexual secrets with one or two close friends, and their friendships tend to be more intense. While the social role for young adolescent girls has changed significantly, adolescent girls in Western cultures may experience a conflict between making the needs of others a priority and focusing on their own needs and wishes. This conflict can carry over into adulthood as young women struggle with the conflicting roles of a professional life and a family life.

Sexuality

Young adolescents generally do not actively pursue sexual partners. Masturbation is common among young adolescents. Peers are usually the main source of information about sex. There seems to be a lower incidence of teenage pregnancy when parents discuss sexuality with their teenagers. Approximately 10% of young men and 25% of young women have homosexual experiences or interest, and homoerotic activity and interest may be more interwoven with heterosexual activity for women (Pedersen and Kristiansen 2008). Whether with heterosexual or homosexual partners, first sexual experiences for boys tend to raise anxieties about performance and competition with peers, fears of intimacy, and guilt. Adolescent girls tend to have more concerns about whether relationships will continue.

Risk-Taking

Adolescents tend to engage in risk-taking behaviors (see Box 14.11 for a case example of an adolescent). For example, the Center for Disease Control and Prevention's Youth Risk Behavior Surveillance System in 2011 found that that 24.1% of teens had ridden in a vehicle driven by someone who had consumed alcohol; 18.1% reported current cigarette use; 38.7% reported current alcohol use; 39.9% reported lifetime marijuana use (ever used marijuana);

BOX 14.11

ADOLESCENT CASE EXAMPLE

Andrew is a 14-year-old freshman in high school. He is beginning to enter puberty, though he has not hit his growth spurt yet. In school Andrew is able to make and test hypotheses, consider multiple perspectives and various possible solutions to problems, and think about abstract concepts (e.g., the philosophies of historical figures). Andrew has a group of boys with whom he socializes on the weekends. The boys idealize their tight group. While they still look to their parents for guidance, they turn more and more to each other to provide models for how to act and what to do and say. They have some interest in girls, and a couple of Andrew's friends have had short-lived relationships with girls. Andrew and his friends sometimes dare each other to do "crazy things." One night the boys trespassed into an abandoned lot and climbed to the top of a tall water tower. On the way down, they had a contest to see who could jump from the highest rung. Andrew's friend jumped from halfway up and fell on his leg screaming. He had broken his leg. Later that evening in the hospital waiting room the boys had difficulty explaining to their parents what had happened, as they were themselves perplexed.

47.4% reported having had sexual intercourse; and among the 33.7% of currently sexually active students, 39.8% reported not using a condom during their last intercourse.

The adolescent's brain changes significantly from childhood into adulthood. High-risk behavior and impulsive decision-making in teenagers may have neurophysiological correlates. In particular, the teenage brain is remodeled over the course of adolescence (Powell 2006). Gray matter tends to thicken in childhood, and then a process of thinning occurs in a wave traveling from the occipital region of the brain to the frontal region, finishing by early adulthood (Giedd 2008). This process is completed earlier in females, which suggests that aspects of **executive function** that originate in the prefrontal cortex may mature more quickly in females. The thinning of gray matter itself is postulated to occur by a process of **synaptic pruning**, which removes unnecessary connections. White matter is increasing at the same time that gray matter is decreasing, which may also play an important role in cognitive maturity. Adolescents also appear to have higher relative activity in the limbic region (e.g., nucleus accumbens) as compared with the prefrontal cortex (Casey 2008), which is correlated with the increase in risky behaviors seen in this age group. In addition, emotional reactivity is exaggerated in adolescents compared to children and adults. The progressive maturation of frontolimbic, frontotemporal, and frontostriatal networks in the transition from childhood to adulthood may be responsible for the increased ability to inhibit impulses (Rubia et al. 2006).

Developmental Vulnerabilities

Psychopathology
Recent studies have disputed earlier notions that adolescence is necessarily a tumultuous, unstable period. In fact, approximately 80% of adolescents function normally. An adolescent whose rebelliousness includes severe disturbances in conduct, mood, or drug abuse should not be dismissed as merely going through a stage. The adolescent in turmoil needs help.

In males, the main developmental vulnerability is that the cultural emphasis on "machismo" may lead to rebellious, self-destructive behavior that threatens connections; in females, the priority of maintaining connections may lead to the denial or suppression of autonomous needs. Box 14.12 describes the response to physical illness in the adolescent.

ADULTHOOD

Developmental Progression

Adult life begins when adolescence ends, which is usually in the early 20s. Adult life is characterized somewhat more by stability than by change. However, various patterns of evolution occur throughout adulthood in each of the developmental lines discussed for children and adolescents (i.e., social, emotional, and cognitive function, gender-related issues, and sexuality). As in children, these changes may lead to psychological growth and maturity, but may also result in conflict, regression, and psychiatric symptoms.

Gratification in Work and Love
The main social developmental tasks for adults take place in the realms of work and intimate relationships. The degree to which adults achieve fulfillment in these two areas varies widely.

BOX 14.12

RESPONSE TO PHYSICAL ILLNESS IN THE ADOLESCENT

Physical illness affects adolescents when it results in delayed physical or sexual maturation. This delay may be due to medications (e.g., chronic steroid use), genetic anomalies, or chronic illness (e.g., cystic fibrosis). The adjustment to chronic illness seems to be enhanced if the adolescent is able to accept that in some ways he or she will be "different." This is obviously particularly difficult in this age group. The mother of a 13-year-old female heart transplant patient put this conflict succinctly: "It's a 50–50 thing. Yes, you're normal. But yes, you had a heart transplant. If you don't accept the fact you had a transplant and take your medicine, you can't be normal." Psychological adjustment seems to be facilitated when adolescents take an active role in their recovery and maintenance, whether this involves physical therapy, medication, or other treatments. With proper education and support, most 12-year-olds are capable of taking their own medication. Taking a more active role reinforces the adolescent's strivings for autonomy and helps to counter the regression accompanying the stress of illness.

This conflict between regression (e.g., the wish to be cared for) and autonomy may be acted out (e.g., when adolescents refuse to take medication as a way of exercising their autonomy but then have an exacerbation of their illness and must rely on others even more). Regression can also cause the adolescent to retreat to earlier modes of magical thinking. In general, however, adolescents are able to view illness with a more sophisticated perspective in which they see themselves and their behavior (e.g., adherence to prescribed medication) as playing a role in their recovery. In addition, adolescents are able to understand that different symptoms can be associated with the same illness, and the illness can be seen with a longitudinal view that includes different stages, including an onset, middle course, and ending. When the adolescent reaches the stage of formal operations, she or he has acquired an understanding of the inner processes and anatomy of the body, and causality is understood with respect to biological processes.

It is important to remember that physical illness can be used as a way of avoiding many of the conflicts of the adolescent's world, such as fear of the transition into adulthood, social and sexual anxieties, or family difficulties. Staying ill may provide adolescents with secondary gain by allowing them to avoid scenarios that cause anxiety or fear.

In adolescents, self-image is so dependent on body image that the physical manifestations of chronic illness can have devastating effects on self-esteem. For example, a 16-year-old girl had a relapse of a soft tissue sarcoma of the right leg but refused amputation because of the disfigurement. That she would probably die

(continued)

without the treatment meant nothing to her because she felt that she looked so abnormal that her life was "hopeless" anyway.

The connection between body image and self-esteem may also be affected as chronically ill adolescents measure their ideal image of themselves ("ego-ideal") against where they realistically stand or will stand with regard to interpersonal, educational, and occupational goals. The extent to which adolescents perceive that they will not live up to expectations may negatively impact self-esteem. Low self-esteem, in turn, may cause physical symptoms to become worse.

The separation from friends during a hospitalization can be quite stressful for the adolescent, who craves these attachments. The separation from parents may also precipitate loneliness. The adolescent with a chronic illness has the reality of the illness superimposed on the typical adolescent sensitivity to feeling different or rejected. As a result, self-esteem problems can be exacerbated, as well as body image and the ability to feel "normal."

A shift from play to work accompanies the developmental course from childhood into adulthood. Advanced schooling serves as an intermediate step, particularly college and postgraduate studies, including professional training. The transition to the "real" world of work is a major one. Adults who are able to negotiate this step well have completed adolescence with a secure sense of themselves as competent people and with the capacity to relate to others in a stable manner. Joining the work force requires making a commitment to a chosen career path. This step can cause anxiety for people who have concerns about separation and independence and for those who have difficulty in giving up the grandiose adolescent fantasy that anything is possible.

Achieving a **successful work life** is one of the ultimate tests of an individual's ability to join society as a productive member. Work can be a source of much gratification in the financial, intellectual, and social realms, among others, and can contribute to personal growth. Like latency-age children whose view of themselves as competent grows each time another task is mastered, adults can grow significantly in self-confidence with successful work experiences.

Failure in work may have devastating consequences. Work can be a source of much frustration and disappointment. Even individuals who were successful students can be vulnerable to injured self-esteem resulting from failures in work, as the case example in Box 14.13 illustrates. For many adults, failure can occur at any transitional stage in a career. A promotion or job change that requires different strengths or abilities may suddenly bring to the forefront previously unrecognized areas of weakness or conflict. For instance, a bright, conscientious high school teacher, who inspired her students with her enthusiasm and intellectual curiosity, was rewarded with a promotion to an administrative position. In this position, she was plagued by disorganization and interpersonal conflicts that she was unable to resolve. This difficulty is an example of the "Peter principle," which is the tendency for society to keep promoting workers until they get to a level at which they cannot function fully. It can be the source of failure and loss of self-esteem for many adults, particularly in middle age. Some adults have conflicting responses to

---

BOX 14.13

CASE EXAMPLE OF FAILURE AT WORK

A male attorney who had completed each aspect of his training with the highest honors at the best schools found that what had been strengths in his academic pursuits (i.e., attention to detail, willingness to put in long hours, and perfectionism) became liabilities at work. His inability to set priorities and cut corners left him exhausted, overwhelmed, and unable to keep up with the workload. Interpersonal difficulties surfaced as well. He felt both intimidated by and contemptuous of authority figures, and these conflictual feelings left him unable to deal appropriately with his superiors. Instead, he veered between being overtly ingratiating and covertly aggressive. While silently complying with a partner's refusal of his request to take off a week after the birth of his first child, he expressed his resentment when he cavalierly encouraged law students spending the summer at the firm to give up law and go to medical school. As he became increasingly aware of his difficulties, his confidence in himself as a lawyer plummeted; this caused his work performance to deteriorate even further.

---

success, which may be partially related to unresolved guilt about competitive issues and which may result in self-sabotage to avoid success.

The establishment of **mature, committed, intimate love relationships** is the other key social developmental task in the transition from adolescence to adulthood. Commitment to a monogamous relationship requires that adults relinquish their fantasies of the "perfect" mate. Identity consolidation is essential, as well, including coming to terms with sexual orientation and values. Finally, the adult must have a capacity to tolerate closeness and dependence while preserving a sense of autonomy.

A major milestone for many adults is **parenthood**. Becoming a parent together with a loving partner can be a source of enormous fulfillment. Parenthood is also an opportunity for significant psychological growth and mastery. Adults have the satisfaction of providing their offspring with a childhood that is in some way an improvement over their own, not to mention the joy of seeing the world again through the wondrous eyes of a growing child.

Parenthood significantly changes the adult child's relationship with his or her own parents. New parents can enjoy sharing the experience with their own parents of raising offspring, gaining a better appreciation for the challenges and demands that their parents met in raising them. If new parents feel insecure in their parental roles or in their separateness from their own parents, intergenerational conflict or overinvolvement may result.

Unplanned pregnancies and unwanted children can be the source of tremendous grief and stress. For all of the joy they can bring, children are, by their very nature, demanding of parents' time and energy. These demands, and the conflicts they may exacerbate or reawaken, can be stressful even for the most emotionally mature, socially supported, and financially secure couples. For single parents or parents struggling with abusive or otherwise impaired partners, social isolation, or poverty, those demands may be overwhelming. Physicians should be aware that parenthood can be a time of particular stress and that parents under stress are at high risk for psychiatric disorders, as well as committing child abuse.

As was discussed above, each phase of child development requires different parental responses. The parents of infants face the task of taking care of a completely helpless, dependent human being; this responsibility can often arouse intense fears and anxieties. The parents of toddlers and adolescents witness their children's struggles with sexual and aggressive impulses, as well as conflicting yearnings for dependence and autonomy. Just as a promotion or job change might highlight a previously unrecognized area of weakness in adults, the developmental transitions of children may precipitate crises in parents who lack the flexibility and coping skills to adjust their parenting style to their child's needs.

For adults who do not have children, there may be other issues. For instance, women who delay childbearing while they develop their careers may find the failure to conceive to be particularly painful and accompanied by guilt and self-blame. The onset of menopause for these women can precipitate strong feelings of grief and loss. A healthy adjustment frequently involves redirecting the urge for what Erikson described as the "generativity" of middle age into activities other than parenthood that can serve a similar function and allow one to guide and mentor the next generation.

Emotional Maturity

Much of adult emotional development can be regarded as an evolution of ego strengths. A crucial aspect of ego functioning is the unconscious deployment of defense mechanisms to maintain emotional stability (see Chapter 17, Psychotherapy). Once most persons reach adulthood, they have the ability to use mature defenses (e.g., sublimation, humor, and altruism). These defenses may be observed in emotionally mature behaviors, such as patience, flexibility, and responsibility, lack of impulsivity, capacity for empathy, and acceptance of ambivalence in themselves and others.

Cognitive Awareness

In the realm of cognitive function, young adults have fully reached Piaget's stage of formal operational thinking, which permits **self-reflection**. Impairments in intellectual function or delays in cognitive development will interfere with this process.

Aging involves a decline in certain cognitive capacities, especially memory and problem-solving abilities. At the same time, there seems to be an increased ability to conceptualize, put ideas into a context, and accept situations that may seem paradoxical. Some observers have, therefore, described a further stage of intellectual development beyond Piaget's stage of formal operations that is essentially characterized as being more practical.

As adult development progresses, major shifts in the **perception of time** occur. Children live in the present, without much ability to reflect on the past or anticipate the future. Adults can do both, and begin to understand that their life trajectory does not involve unlimited time. Death becomes a more real phenomenon as adults experience the loss of friends and family and note their own physical deterioration.

Sexual Function and Dysfunction

Satisfactory sexual functioning is central to, and closely associated with, emotional and social well-being. Conflicts in this realm may involve sexual orientation, the integration of sex with companionship, and sexual inhibitions at any stage of the sexual arousal cycle, from desire to arousal to orgasm.

Sexual dysfunctions tend to have multiple causes. **External relationship difficulties** (e.g., disagreements over money) or **internal emotional conflicts** (e.g., excessive guilt or anxiety with regard to sexuality) may be causes, as may be a history of **sexual trauma** or physiological abnormalities. The latter may be caused by **medications** or medical disorders, most commonly **diabetes** and **cardiovascular disease**. Psychiatric disorders, particularly depression, can be associated with a change in sexual functioning.

Physicians can play an important role in assessing their adult patients' sexual functioning. In screening for dysfunction, the physician should be aware that the diagnosis of physical causes could be a great relief for patients who are afraid to raise their concerns. In addition, **education and information can be very helpful** for many patients who do not have physical reasons for their difficulties. Because many adults have conflicts and worries with regard to sexuality, the physician's nonjudgmental attitude and acceptance of a wide range of sexual practices may be helpful in contributing to the patient's personal acceptance and improved functioning.

Premature ejaculation (see DSM-5) and **female orgasmic disorder** (delay or absence) (see DSM-5) are two common sexual disorders that tend not to have an identifiable physical etiology. **Behavior therapy** has been extremely effective for these disorders. Physicians should refer patients who are suffering from these problems and other sexual dysfunctions that do not respond to medical and educational interventions to therapists who are trained in appropriate techniques.

Developmental Vulnerabilities

The transition from late adolescence to adulthood may be an ambivalent one due to uncertainty about a career and difficulties developing intimate relationships. Adolescents may mourn the many losses that are necessary as they make the transition into adulthood and may feel an emptiness in their lives that was once filled by their relationship with their parents. This provides a counterpoint to the eager anticipation of the freedoms that adults enjoy. Cultural and economic factors, such as a poor job market, can also affect this process and exacerbate the young adult's ambivalence.

Problems in this age group result from conflicts about work, love, school, or family. Many of these conflicts cause short-term anxiety or depression, but more serious problems with work inhibition or depression also occur as perhaps biological vulnerability interfaces with environmental factors. Many of these symptoms may be acute or short-lived and may cause the late-adolescent concern that is out of proportion to the actual severity of the problem. Chronic problems may develop in the late adolescent as earlier unresolved issues become extrapolated into a new developmental phase. A person who had separation problems as a toddler and who experienced difficulty in developing a sense of independence in early and middle adolescence may later find it difficult to leave home and attend school or to develop intimate relationships with others. If adequate coping skills were not learned earlier, problems may develop as adolescents leave the home.

As life proceeds, significant stresses may be imposed by financial responsibilities, such as mortgages, shifts in the work place and marketplace, problems in interpersonal and marital relationships, and uncertainty about whether the chosen life path has been the correct one. These concerns can precipitate a "midlife crisis," which may be more accurately labeled a period of reflection, or reassessment, during which adults may wonder whether their lifestyle, job, and relationships are the ones that were most desired. These questions were first confronted in late adolescence and now appear again.

Psychopathology

Many psychiatric disorders appear initially during the period of young adulthood through the 30s, including the **mood** and **anxiety disorders**. **Schizophrenia** typically begins in late adolescence but can also occur in the 20s. The manifestations of **personality disorders** and **eating disorders** are generally present by early adulthood, although patients may not present for treatment until years after the problem begins. Responses to physical illnesses during adulthood are discussed at length in Chapter 11, Psychological Factors Affecting Medical Conditions.

OLD AGE

Developmental Progression

As adults approach old age, the stability that they have achieved over the preceding 40–50 years must, in some respects, give way to great change. At the same time, the range of individual approaches to a life phase is more varied during old age than at any other time. The age at which people become "old" may be as early as their late 50s or early 60s or as late as their 70s or 80s. Some people seem "old before their time," and others remain active, vigorous, and "youthful" into their 80s. These variations result from individual differences in people's capacity for adapting to and interpreting the psychosocial, cognitive, sexual, and physical changes that accompany old age. Box 14.14 describes the response to physical illness in the elderly.

Changing Relationships

One of the main changes for the elderly results from alterations in their social realm. The constellation of important people in the elderly individual's life changes, for several reasons. First, since most people have retired from work by the time they are in their 70s, their circle of colleagues with whom they had had daily contact at work is virtually eliminated. While relationships with some of those people may be maintained, the former character of those interactions, which focused on joint goal-oriented, productive work, will never be the same. **Retirement** generally leaves the elderly more involved with

---

BOX 14.14

RESPONSE TO PHYSICAL ILLNESS IN THE ELDERLY

As with children and adults, the elderly may have a whole range of responses to physical illness, which depend in large part on their psychological makeup, previous experiences with illness, and current developmental state. One of the challenges for physicians in caring for the elderly is understanding the needs and wishes of individual patients. It is crucial to avoid making assumptions about their fears or wishes with regard to death. Physicians should be wary of distortions resulting from the patient's resemblance to the physician's parents or grandparents. This caution is particularly important if a patient refuses further treatment. The physician should recommend a thorough psychiatric evaluation for such a patient rather than simply assume that the refusal makes sense for anyone in their 70s or 80s.

and reliant on family and friends. For those who are financially secure, retirement allows them to spend their time as they wish, in leisure and pleasurable pursuits, charitable work or other activities aimed at benefiting society at large, or increased time with family and friends. This release from the constraints of a daily work routine can be liberating for some elderly persons, but it can also precipitate feelings of loss, guilt, anxiety, and purposelessness. Elderly people without adequate savings or retirement income are beset by an additional set of worries with regard to supporting themselves.

The passage of time is inevitably accompanied by the **deaths of family members and friends**. In earlier stages of adulthood, most people must grieve and work through the loss of their grandparents and, later, their parents. For the elderly, death becomes more commonplace and closer to home, because many of those lost will be of similar age or even younger. These losses serve as reminders of one's own mortality, as well as sources of grief and survivor guilt. Death and illness inexorably whittle away at the social network that has been put into place over a lifetime. Even elderly persons who are resilient, flexible, and optimistically willing to reach out and develop new friends cannot easily replace intimate relationships that have spanned decades. Some losses, especially of a spouse or a child, are particularly difficult for the elderly to accept.

The social configuration of the elderly is also affected by their **changing roles** in relation to others. An elderly person is no longer a boss or supervisor, a family wage earner, a head of a household of dependent children, or even, in some cases, a financially or physically independent, self-sufficient adult. Elderly men and women with children relinquish many of these roles to their middle-aged offspring, who are in their "prime." Those who are childless may worry about who will take care of them if and when they become unable to take care of themselves. The shifting roles can reawaken conflicting feelings about dependence and autonomy. Children may even come to represent powerful parental figures in the perceptions of the elderly. The capacity of middle-aged children to tolerate these changing roles can affect the adjustment of the elderly person. The case example in Box 14.15 illustrates these developmental issues faced by the elderly.

Positive aspects of old age include the satisfaction of seeing one's children—and other members of the younger generation for whom one served as a support or mentor—functioning as healthy, happy, and competent adults. Adults who found parenthood to be fraught with conflict and stress are sometimes better able to find gratification in being a grandparent and great-grandparent.

Gradual Decline

Physical and cognitive capacities continue to decline during old age. Elderly persons realize that life is finite and that more years have been lived than are left to live. This fact is often brought into stark relief when close friends and relatives die. The inevitable real losses, such as the deaths of loved ones, accompany these other symbolic role losses in stature and prominence.

In old age, reminiscence tends to become a more central feature of one's reflection on life. One may recall hopes that were never fulfilled, perhaps in a nostalgic way, and reflect on one's life course with a critical eye.

Sexuality in the Elderly

There is much variation in the degree to which the elderly remain sexually active. For some, sexuality remains an important part of life and of loving relationships. For others,

---

BOX 14.15

CASE EXAMPLE OF RESPONSE TO AGING

A 74-year-old retired physician and mother of two nursed her husband through several years of declining health. He died several months before what would have been their 50th wedding anniversary. She had enjoyed a full, gratifying career, a strong, intimate marriage, and a close circle of friends. By the time she became a widow, however, many of her friends had died or were too ill to be active. Turning for companionship to her two daughters, who were both physicians with families, she became hurt and rejected when she found that their busy lives left them with little time to spend with her. In psychotherapy, she explored her fears that she had been a "bad mother" for "abandoning" her children to continue to practice medicine at a time when few women with young children worked outside of the home and that she was now being "punished" by their lack of interest in her. Her therapist helped her reframe her children's preoccupation with their own challenging careers and growing families as evidence that she had done a good job in raising successful, independent women, who had chosen to follow her career path. Through therapy, this woman realized that she had been a pioneer in many ways; this perspective allowed her to contemplate her life course with the sense of inner peace and satisfaction that Erikson referred to as integrity.

---

sexual desire fades, perhaps because a partner is lost or because there is a decreased capacity for sexual gratification due to physical infirmity. For women, the decline in estrogen associated with menopause can cause a number of physical changes, such as an absence of vaginal lubrication during arousal, which may interfere with sexual functioning. Men as well as women must come to terms with the changing physical appearance of their own bodies and of their partners' bodies.

As with younger adults, information and education can sometimes be quite helpful. In particular, elderly men can be informed that they might very well retain the capacity to achieve orgasm without an erection, and elderly women experiencing vaginal dryness and discomfort can be encouraged to use lubrication during sexual intercourse. The class of phosphodiesterase type 5 inhibitors (e.g., sildenafil citrate, tadalafil) is usually well tolerated and effective for men with erectile disorder (see DSM-5). Finally, it is crucial that physicians not assume that their elderly patients are sexually inactive. Such an assumption may not only be based on social prejudices but also on the age difference between the younger physician and the older patient.

Developmental Vulnerabilities

Erikson theorized that elderly persons who are unable to achieve a sense of integrity are at risk for feeling "disgust" and despair. Individuals who are relatively isolated and lacking in outside interests may be more vulnerable to a poor outcome, as illustrated by the case example in Box 14.16.

BOX 14.16

CASE EXAMPLE OF POOR ADJUSTMENT TO AGING

A 72-year-old divorced man had worked for over 40 years as a window washer. His retirement, which was precipitated by increasing difficulties with his balance, represented a loss of the stable source of self-esteem in his life. He was an isolated, somewhat mistrustful man who had maintained a caring but emotionally distant relationship with his daughter, having separated from her mother when she was only 3 years old. He had been a conscientious, steady worker who took great pride in a job well done. After retirement, he filled his days by listening to country and western music on the radio and watching sporting events on television. These pursuits left him feeling unproductive and despairing as to the lack of meaning or purpose in his life, and he complained, "There's no point any more."

Psychopathology

The most prevalent psychiatric disorders in elderly persons are the neurocognitive disorders, particularly the dementias. It is a misperception that the elderly are more susceptible to mood and anxiety disorders than are middle-aged adults. Most psychiatric disorders appear by age 40–50 years. However, perhaps because of an increase in chronic medical illnesses and a lack of social supports, which are two risk factors for suicide, the incidence of suicide increases among the elderly.

As has been pointed out, the elderly are not immune from conflicts and psychic pain. Psychotherapy and carefully monitored pharmacotherapy, when indicated, can be extremely helpful. Old age is not a contraindication to adequate psychiatric treatment.

REFERENCES CITED

Ainsworth, M. D. S., M. C. Blehar, E. Waters, and S. Wall. *Patterns of Attachment: A Psychological Study of the Strange Situation.* Hillsdale, NJ: Lawrence Erlbaum Associates, 1978.

Casey, B. J. *The adolescent brain: vulnerability to anxiety and depression.* Grand Rounds presentation at Cornell Weil Medical College, September 2008.

Centers for Disease Control and Prevention (CDC). The Youth Risk Behavior Surveillance System, 2011. http://www.cdc.gov/HealthyYouth/yrbs/index.htm

Chess, S., and A. Thomas. *Temperament in Clinical Practice.* New York: Guilford Press, 1995.

Giedd, J. N. The teen brain: insights from neuroimaging. *Journal of Adolescent Health* 42:335–343, 2008.

Koulomzin M., B. Beebe, S. Anderson, J. Jaffe, S. Feldstein, and C. Crown. Infant gaze, head, face and self-touch at 4 months differentiate secure vs. avoidant attachment at 1 year: a microanalytic approach. *Attachment and Human Development* 4:3–24, 2002.

Main, M. The organized categories of infant, child, and adult attachment: flexible vs. inflexible attention under attachment-related stress. *Journal of the American Psychoanalytic Association* 48:1055–1096, 2000.

Pedersen, W., and H. W. Kristiansen. Homosexual experience, desire and identity among young adults. *Journal of Homosexuality* 54:68–102, 2008.

Powell, K. Neurodevelopment: how does the teenage brain work? *Nature* 442:865–867, 2006.

Rubia, K., A. B. Smith, J. Woolley, C. Nosarti, I. Heyman, E. Taylor, and M. Brammer. Progressive increase of frontostriatal brain activation from childhood to adulthood during event-related tasks of cognitive control. *Human Brain Mapping* 27:973–993, 2006.

SELECTED READINGS

American Academy of Child and Adolescent Psychiatry. *Your Child.* New York: Harper Collins, 1998.

Bailey, J. M., and R. C. Pillard. A genetic study of male sexual orientation. *Archives of General Psychiatry* 48:1089–1096, 1991.

Blos, P. *On Adolescence.* New York: Free Press, 1962.

Erikson, E. H. *Childhood and Society.* New York: W. W. Norton, 1950.

Freud, A. The concept of developmental lines. *Psychoanalytic Study of the Child* 18:245–265, 1963.

Freud S. Three essays on the theory of sexuality. In *The Standard Edition of the Psychological Works of Sigmund Freud,* J. Strachey, ed. and trans. London: Hogarth Press, 1905.

Gilligan, C., H. Hartman, and E. Kris. The genetic approach. *Psychoanalytic Study of the Child* 1:11–30, 1945.

Hesse, E., and M. Mai. Disorganized infant, child, and adult attachment: collapse in behavioral and attentional strategies. *Journal of the American Psychoanalytic Association* 48:1097–1127, 2000.

Mahler, M. S. On the first three subphases of the separation-individuation process. *International Journal of Psychoanalysis* 53:333–338, 1972.

Martin, M., F. R. Volkmar, and M. Lewis, eds. *Lewis's Child and Adolescent Psychiatry: A Comprehensive Textbook,* 4th ed. Baltimore: Williams & Wilkins, 2007.

Nemiroff, R. A., and C. A. Colarusso, eds. *New Dimensions in Adult Development.* New York: Basic Books, 1990.

Oldham, J. M., and R. S. Liebert, eds. *The Middle Years: New Perspectives.* New Haven, CT: Yale University Press, 1989.

Savin-Williams, R. C., and G. L. Ream. Prevalence and stability of sexual orientation components during adolescence and young adulthood. *Archives of Sexual Behavior* 36:385–394, 2007.

Smith, A. M., C. E. Rissel, J. Richters, A. E. Grulich, and R. O. de Visser. Sex in Australia: sexual identity, sexual attraction and sexual experience among a representative sample of adults. *Australian New Zealand Journal of Public Health* 27:138–145, 2003.

Topál, J., G. Gergely, A. Miklósi, A. Erdohegyi, and G. Csibra. Infants' perseverative search errors are induced by pragmatic misinterpretation. *Science* 321:1831–1834, 2008.

Tyson, P., and R. Tyson. *Psychoanalytic Theories of Development: An Integration.* New Haven, CT: Yale University Press, 1993.

Vaillant, G. E. *The Wisdom of the Ego.* Cambridge, MA: Harvard Press, 1993.

Winnicott, D. W. Transitional objects and transitional phenomena: a study of the first me possession. *International Journal of Psychoanalysis* 34:89–97, 1953.

15

Child and Adolescent Psychiatry

DANIEL T. CHRZANOWSKI, ELISABETH B.
GUTHRIE, MATTHEW B. PERKINS,
AND MOIRA A. RYNN

PSYCHIATRIC ASSESSMENT OF CHILDREN AND ADOLESCENTS

In the psychiatric assessment of children and adolescents, the physician has three goals. The first is to determine whether **psychopathology** is present. Realization of this goal requires familiarity with not just psychiatric disorders but also child and adolescent development (see Chapter 14, Child, Adolescent, and Adult Development). What degree of hyperactivity or impulsivity is abnormal in a 5-year-old? Or in a 15-year-old? How does a middle school–age child describe his or her identity? What about a high school student? Does a child's detailed description of an imaginary friend reflect impaired reality testing? What of similar thought content in an adolescent?

Second, the physician generates and substantiates a **differential diagnosis** and **case formulation**. As with adults, the physician assessing children and adolescents will consider a range of diagnostic possibilities, including particularly disorders that are more prevalent earlier in life (e.g., separation anxiety disorder), disorders that persist into adulthood but first present earlier in life (e.g., learning disorders, attention-deficit hyperactivity disorder), and disorders whose presentation may differ earlier in life (e.g., obsessive-compulsive disorder, generalized anxiety disorder). In the case formulation, the physician should keep in mind the full array of biological, psychological, and social considerations relevant to patients of all ages, with particular attention to the stability and security of psychosocial systems, as well as the patient's developmental strengths and vulnerabilities.

Third, the physician develops an initial **treatment plan**, elements of which may very well comprise further assessment (e.g., medical evaluation, laboratory testing, collateral history, psychological assessment). Throughout the psychiatric assessment process, the physician should aim to build rapport with the patient and family and, in a larger sense, create a positive interface between the mental health care system and the people who need its services.

The psychiatric assessment of children and adolescents typically includes interviews, rating scales, medical evaluation, and, when indicated, psychological assessment.

THE INTERVIEW

As with the psychiatric assessment of adults, the foundation of an assessment of any child or adolescent is the clinical interview (see Chapter 1, Psychiatric Assessment and Treatment Planning, and Chapter 2, The Psychiatric Interview). In fundamental ways, interviews conducted for the purpose of assessing a child or adolescent psychiatrically are similar to those conducted in the assessment of an adult. The physician clarifies the problems to be assessed, explores what events led to the clinical presentation, elicits relevant past history, and conducts a mental status examination (see Table 15.1). There are, however, important differences between interviews conducted to assess an adult and interviews conducted to assess a child or adolescent.

Whereas the assessment of an adult patient *may* include interviews with other informants, the assessment of a child or adolescent patient *always* includes **multiple informants**. Children and adolescents are legally, financially, and developmentally more dependent on the systems in which they live than are adults. The guardian of a minor patient must give informed consent for evaluation and treatment. Informed consent entails, at a minimum, discussion of relevant privacy practices, as well as therapeutic options, together with their potential benefits and risks. In the case of an adolescent patient (typically, 12 years of age or

TABLE 15.1 Components of the Comprehensive Psychiatric Assessment

Identifying information
  Age
  Gender
  With whom the patient lives
  Locus of legal custody and medical decision-making
  Type of educational program
  Grade in school
Sources of information (both individuals and documents)
Chief complaints (a multitude of perspectives is the rule)
History of the present illness or situation (with particular emphasis on *why now?*)
Past psychiatric history (diagnoses—including substance use—and treatments)
Medications and allergies
Medical history
Developmental history (beginning with the environment in utero)
Educational history (including results of any past psychological testing)
Family psychiatric history
Psychosocial history
  Family composition
  Cultural context
  Languages spoken
  Religious affiliations
  Any history of moving, migration, trauma, abuse, neglect, legal difficulties
Mental status examination
Case formulation
Differential diagnosis
Initial treatment plan

older), the physician should obtain the adolescent's assent for evaluation and treatment, in addition to the legal guardian's consent. Along with the legal and financial realities, developmental considerations necessitate the involvement of parents and other important adult figures. The ability of children and adolescents to present a complete history is variable and depends on their cognitive, emotional, and social development. Therefore, parents as well as other important caregivers in the family (unless a difference is being emphasized, parents, caregivers, and legal guardians will be referred to as "parents"), teachers, counselors, and other significant adults are critical informants in any psychiatric assessment. The utility of this approach is illustrated in Box 15.1.

Conducting clinical interviews with multiple informants requires the physician to schedule **multiple evaluation sessions** (see Figure 15.1). It is not unusual for the psychiatric assessment of a child or adolescent to require three or more separate sessions, usually in the following order: one interview with the parent, a second with the child or adolescent patient, and a third with the parent, with or without the minor patient. The actual sequence and composition of sessions will vary, in large part with the developmental age of the identified patient.

Children

Interview with the Parents

In the evaluation of children (preadolescents, generally younger than 12 years of age), the first session is usually conducted with the parents, alone, to gather relevant history.

BOX 15.1

CASE EXAMPLE OF THE UTILITY OF COLLATERAL INFORMATION IN THE EVALUATION OF CHILDREN

The mother of a 9-year-old boy presented for evaluation of her son's school avoidance and irritability. She described her son as having grown increasingly irritable, particularly in the evening, at homework time, and in the morning, before school. His irritability had been resulting in oppositional behavior including tantrums and, ultimately, refusal to go to school some mornings. She wondered if her son was having trouble concentrating, and worried that he sometimes seemed hopeless. He had not had any significant disturbance in sleep, appetite, or energy. Asked what he thought was going on, the boy would only say, "school is boring," and that he sometimes got "stomachaches." With parental consent, the physician contacted the school for additional information. The child's teacher described similar outbursts, frequent requests to visit the school nurse, and deterioration in academic performance, all with onset in the fourth grade. She expressed concern that the child did not seem to understand what he read. As interviews with his mother and teacher provided critical information about the boy's relatively concrete and externalized complaints, the physician was able to begin to focus the differential diagnosis to include a learning disorder and to consider additional evaluations (see Box 15.6).

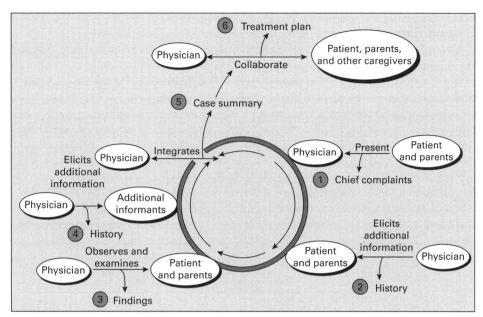

FIGURE 15.1 Steps in assessment and treatment planning. (1) The child or adolescent patient and parents present the chief complaint or, as is often the case, *chief complaints* to the physician. The presenting problems, therapeutic setting and developmental age of the patient determine the order of interviews. (2) As the interviews proceed, the physician elicits additional information from the patient and parents in order to obtain the history of the present illness, the past psychiatric history, medical history, developmental history, educational history, family psychiatric history and psychosocial history. The physician often incorporates appropriate rating scales. (3) Findings from the physical examination, mental status examination (including how the patient relates to both the physician and the parents), laboratory tests, academic reports, and past psychological assessments are collected. (4) The physician elicits additional history from relevant informants (e.g., teachers, counselors, previous mental health providers, and speech pathologists). Again, the physician often incorporates appropriate rating scales. (5) The physician then integrates all of the information and generates a descriptive and diagnostic impression. (6) Together, the patient, parents, and other relevant caregivers develop a theoretically sound, evidence-based, and feasible treatment plan.

(Only one parent may be involved, but for simplicity the plural, "parents," will be used.) This history includes not only the parents' perspective on the **presenting difficulties** (range and duration of symptoms; relevant stressors and systems changes; type, place, and degree of impairment) but also the child's **past psychiatric history, medical history, developmental history, family psychiatric history, and psychosocial history**—elements of which may not be appropriate to discuss with the child present. Having this information in advance allows the physician to contextualize and focus the interview with the child, whose insight and other cognitive capacities may be relatively and appropriately limited.

In addition, the physician should ask about the child's **strengths and likeable qualities**. This conveys the physician's interest in the whole child, not just psychopathology. It affords the physician a window into the parents' view of their child. Do they appreciate their child's strengths? Are there things they like about their child? Answers will shed light on the nature of the parent–child relationship, will facilitate the physician's interview with the child and, down the road, may assist in treatment planning.

Given the centrality of important adults and systems in a child's life, the physician should systematically assess the **context** in which the child's difficulties occur, including changes in the family (health, harmony, composition, finances, housing), at school (location, grade level, teachers, class size and structure, academic performance), and with friends (number and quality of relationships, conflict, activities). Additionally, the potential functions of any problematic behavior (e.g., school refusal, aggression, self-injury) should be assessed. Employing the framework of a **functional behavioral assessment**, the physician should consider the following functions: escaping from demand, earning attention, gaining access to tangible goods, and, particularly in the developmentally delayed population, self-stimulation.

Throughout the interview with the parents, the physician should attempt to put them at ease, acknowledge how difficult it can be for parents to bring their child to a psychiatrist, and take care to **avoid blaming the parents** (or even implying blame) for their child's difficulties. Many parents will already be wondering what they have done "wrong." In obtaining the family psychiatric, psychosocial, and developmental history it is useful to start with a relatively open-ended question, such as "Who in the family does your child remind you of? In what ways?" This approach reemphasizes an interest in not only the child's difficulties but also his or her strengths.

Interview with the Child

The child should be interviewed in a second session, with or without the parents, depending on the child's presenting difficulties and developmental age. For example, an 11-year-old boy with depressive symptoms might very appropriately be interviewed without any parental presence, as children generally report their symptoms of depression and anxiety very reliably, whereas a 7-year-old girl with separation anxiety might not tolerate being apart from her mother and alone with the physician during the initial interview. A 4-year-old boy with disruptive behavior might easily separate from his parents, but such "externalizing disorders" (discussed later in the chapter) are usually more reliably described by parents. Furthermore, in the case of both the disruptive 4-year-old and the separation-anxious 7-year-old, the physician may want the opportunity to observe how the parent and child interact and thereby learn how the presenting difficulties may affect or be affected by the dyadic relationship (see case example in Box 15.2).

During the interview, the physician should **clarify the child's understanding** of the purpose of the assessment. Parents are often at a loss as to how to explain a psychiatric evaluation to their children and may have provided little explanation. It is not unusual for children to think of a visit to the psychiatrist as punishment and, potentially, as a harbinger of bad things to come (including the extreme but not uncommon example of removal from the family home by children's protective services). Correcting any distortions will foster the therapeutic alliance. In addition, if the child does not offer a "chief complaint," it can be helpful to offer a modified version of what the physician has already heard (e.g., "I understand that sometimes it's hard for you to get along with the other kids").

The physician should ask early on about the child's **favorite activities or games, interests, and friends**. Doing so is helpful in establishing not only rapport but also the diagnosis (e.g., presence, age-appropriateness, and enjoyment of interests; facility or difficulty with socializing) and later in treatment planning (e.g., in selecting activities, rewards, and settings to advance therapeutic goals). When interviewing the child, the

---

BOX 15.2
CASE EXAMPLE OF THE UTILITY OF OBSERVING INTERACTIONS BETWEEN THE CHILD AND PARENTS

The mother of a 4-year-old boy, Conrad, presented with the complaint that he was biting other children in preschool and at the neighborhood playground. His biting had not resulted in any broken skin, but he had been sent home from preschool several times. His mother was clearly very distressed about his behavior, which she thought might reflect an unhealthy inability to share toys. During the initial interview with the mother alone, she denied symptoms of separation anxiety, other significant aggressive or disruptive behavior, or developmental delays. She described her son as bright and imaginative, and she professed a solid understanding of behavioral principles. Asked specifically about parental responses to the boy's biting, she reported that she and her husband had "tried everything," including rewards (toy cars) for not biting and contingencies (time-outs) for biting. She expressed exasperation over this seemingly intractable behavior. During the second interview, attended by the boy and both of his parents, Conrad grabbed a toy dinosaur, ran to the physician, and, with the toy, "bit" the physician's knee—an action that earned him considerable laughter from both parents. His father then asked Conrad about what had happened with his friend Noah in the elevator of their apartment building. Gleefully, to the obvious if self-conscious amusement of his parents, the child announced to the physician, "I bit Noah...I bit Noah!" The opportunity to observe these interactions between the boy and his parents was invaluable in understanding one function of the presenting problem—namely, earning attention from his parents—and in providing a very relevant foundation for discussion of inadvertent behavioral reinforcement.

---

physician should also obtain the **history** from the child's point of view and, simultaneously, conduct the **mental status examination** (described below).

Activities such as **drawing, playing, and story-telling** will often facilitate the child interview. At a minimum, such activities will reveal important parts of the mental status examination (e.g., the assessment of motor function, attention, impulse control, intelligence, and judgment) and allow the child to engage more readily with the physician, by virtue of their familiarity and because talking is often easier if children are simultaneously doing something. More substantively, these activities can serve as developmentally appropriate media through which the physician can learn about the presenting difficulties through the mind of the child, as the case example in Box 15.3 illustrates.

Play is facilitated by having toys in the office, including a dollhouse, dolls, puppets, and board games. Helpful techniques include following the child's lead, stepping in and out of the play (i.e., the physician steps out of the play scenario and asks the child's advice about how his or her assigned character should respond, thereby gaining fuller insight into the child's perspective in any given situation), and "marking" (i.e., explicitly pronouncing) emotions. Unstructured drawings, such as Winnicott's squiggles (Winnicott

> ### BOX 15.3
> ## CASE EXAMPLE OF DRAWING AND STORYTELLING DURING THE EVALUATION OF A CHILD
>
> A 6-year-old girl, Ellen, was brought for psychiatric evaluation of "melt-downs" that had been occurring episodically for several months. Her parents, who presented together for the first interview, described her as having had an easy temperament since infancy. She had adjusted well to the birth of her younger brother 4 years ago, to the school she had attended for over 2 years, and to a new house and neighborhood 1 year earlier. They denied any recent stressors in the family or at school, and noted that the behavioral episodes, characterized by a mix of intense sobbing and trembling, usually while lying on the floor, occurred only at home. Ellen had continued to excel at school and, for this reason, together with a self-acknowledged tendency to minimize problems, her parents had been reluctant to seek professional help or "label" her as having a "problem." During the physician's interview with the child, she immediately gravitated toward drawing. She drew her pet cat, Tommy, who, she explained, had moved to her grandmother's house on account of her mother's allergies. With encouragement from the physician, the child elaborated on Tommy's story. Tommy had adapted well to the move and continued to enjoy his same group of friends, who attended his birthday party. At his birthday party, Tommy couldn't find his mother, so he set out looking for her. He found her lying on the floor, and worried that she was sick or even dead. Then Tommy's mother "woke up" and told him that she was fine, that she had been "napping." In a subsequent appointment with the parents, the physician learned that the mother had suffered several episodes of syncope over the preceding year, and that the first of these episodes had been witnessed by the child when she was home alone with her mother. The cardiac and neurological workups had been negative, and the syncope had not recurred in several months, so the parents had not thought to mention the incident to the physician.

1977), have their place, as do structured approaches including draw-a-person and kinetic family drawings. Projective questions (e.g., "If you had three wishes, what would they be?" or "Let's pretend we just heard a loud noise outside. If we were to look through the window, what would we see?") can illuminate the mind of the child and serve as a bridge to more direct discussion between physician and child.

Interview with the Parents and Child
In the third and final evaluation session, the physician discusses impressions and recommendations with the parents and child. Typically, this final session includes time alone with the parents during which the physician can address their concerns without inappropriately exposing the child to issues such as suboptimal parenting strategies and marital discord, as well as any parental concerns about the effectiveness or safety of treatment recommendations.

Adolescents

As in the evaluation of children, the evaluation of an adolescent typically takes three or more interviews. The adolescent should usually be interviewed **alone**. Furthermore, the physician may recommend that the adolescent be allowed to **choose the sequence** of interviews. In so doing, the physician not only respects and promotes the adolescent's typical developmental strivings for separation and autonomy but also potentially learns something about the patient's stage of development, the parent–adolescent relationship, and the quality and severity of symptoms at hand. For example, a 15-year-old girl who cannot leave her mother's side to speak with the physician alone may be struggling with severe anxiety.

In general, the interviews proceed with goals similar to those described in the evaluation of children. There are, however, a few considerations particularly relevant to adolescents. First, adolescents often have a different perspective on why a psychiatric assessment has been sought—a perspective that must be acknowledged explicitly. At a minimum, this difference may require the physician to reconcile **competing chief complaints**. It can, however, pose a challenge to engaging the adolescent in the interview. For example, parents may present with the complaint, "Our son has grown angry and defiant," while the adolescent boy complains, "My parents are the only problem in my life. They won't get off my back. They made me come here." Throughout the assessment, the physician should strive to understand these complaints and the reasons they differ. Of course, this pursuit assumes that the adolescent can be engaged in the assessment at all. It is sometimes helpful to reframe the "problem" as "So, you and your parents have a difference of opinion" and to express genuine curiosity about the difference. Relocating the "problem" from the parents' complaint and the adolescent's reaction to a neutral reflective space is "face-saving" and conducive to collaborative evaluation.

A second consideration that takes on particular importance with adolescents is **confidentiality**. It can be a challenge for the physician to respect the adolescent's confidentiality. A psychiatric assessment leads to and includes discussion of diagnostic impressions and, potentially, treatment recommendations with not only the adolescent patient but also the parents. No treatment can be undertaken without the consent of a legal guardian. This task may require the physician to disclose the signs and symptoms that substantiate diagnostic impressions and indicate treatment. This limitation of confidentiality must be discussed with the adolescent. In addition, the physician should make clear at the outset that confidentiality will be breached if a safety concern arises. In such a circumstance, the physician should attempt to include the adolescent in its disclosure and discussion.

Mental Status Examination

As in the assessment of the adult patient, most data for the mental status examination are collected simply by observation during the interview of the child or adolescent. Select information, however, must be specifically elicited. See Box 15.4 for a description of the elements of the mental status examination of children and adolescents.

Rating Scales

Many efficient and quantifiable measures, also called rating scales, are available to assess children and adolescents for psychopathology in a number of areas, including attention,

BOX 15.4
MENTAL STATUS EXAMINATION

Appearance should include dress, hygiene, height and weight, as well as any dysmorphic features and physical signs of trauma.

Attitude can be described in terms of quality (e.g., cooperative, provocative, guarded) and appropriateness. The latter must be interpreted in the larger context of the psychiatric assessment. For example, the uncooperativeness of a 13-year-old who was "tricked" into seeing the psychiatrist may be at least partly appropriate.

Relatedness refers to amount of eye contact, level of engagement, capacity for reciprocity, and respect of physical boundaries. These parameters should be observed with respect not only to the physician–patient interaction but also interactions between the patient and parents, siblings, and other children or adults.

Motor function warrants observation of handedness, pencil grasp, penmanship, overall level of activity, abnormal movements (e.g., tics, tremors, dystonias), gait, and age-dependent abilities (e.g., hopping on one foot by age 4, drawing a triangle by age 5).

Speech and language are assessed for prosody (musicality, volume, rate, and intonation), fluency, articulation, and developmental appropriateness.

Mood is the patient's subjective description of the current, predominant emotional state. Assessing the mood of young children or children with lower intellectual functioning or a language disorder may require the use of pictorial examples (e.g., as portrayed in "mood charts" or simple drawings of various faces by the examining physician).

Affect is characterized by its quality, amplitude, range, stability, and appropriateness. Any discrepancy with mood should be noted.

Thought process is assessed in terms of organization, goal-directedness, and logic. The significance of findings must be assessed with a developmental perspective. For example, the thought process a 5-year-old child is not expected to be logical.

Thought content is assessed for themes (e.g., worry, fear, low self-esteem, hopelessness, grandiosity, hypersexuality) and basis in reality (e.g., overvalued or delusional material). Depending on the developmental age of the patient, themes may mainly emerge through play and drawing rather than in verbalized self-reflection.

Perceptual disturbances are described in terms of modality (auditory, visual, olfactory, touch), context (place, time), content (i.e., what is seen, heard, or smelled), and intensity (e.g., illusions versus hallucinations).

Suicidal ideation and homicidal ideation are assessed in the same thorough fashion as with adult patients. Additionally, if ideation is present, it is helpful to ascertain where the patient learned about suicide or homicide, as well as the patient's understanding of death (see discussion of the evaluation of suicidal ideation in major depressive disorder).

(continued)

Orientation, attention, and intelligence are assessed with respect to the patient's developmental age. For example, a young child may not know the actual time but may be oriented to seeing the physician after school and before dinner. Span of attention, like motor activity, varies with age, and in younger children is better assessed through play than with more standard techniques (e.g., digit span, spelling in reverse) appropriate for adolescents and adults. Intellectual functioning can be gauged by drawing (e.g., circle by 3 years, "+" or square by 4 years, triangle by 5 years, amount of detail in figure drawings), fund of (developmentally appropriate) knowledge (e.g., knowing first and last names by age 3 years), language, and the type of play the child engages in: parallel play (i.e., simultaneous but separate) is generally present at 2 years of age, while cooperative play (i.e., interactive and integrated) typically develops between 3 and 5 years of age.

Insight and judgment are also assessed through a developmental lens. A school-aged child who is "happy" during the interview may normatively lack the cognitive capacity to recognize that he or she harbors another feeling (e.g., sadness) simultaneously. Or, a child may understand the impact of a particular action (e.g., a time-out for misbehaving) but lack the capacity to reflect on motivations and appreciate that such analysis can lead to greater self-understanding. Such limitations do not indicate "poor" or "impaired" insight but, rather, developmentally appropriate insight.

motor activity, anxiety, mood, and social relatedness. It is sometimes useful to incorporate rating scales into the psychiatric assessment and treatment of children and adolescents. Rating scales are not diagnostic tools. In psychiatric assessment, their utility lies in corroborating diagnostic impressions that are based primarily on the history and mental status examination. Additionally, rating scales establish a quantifiable baseline in both range and severity of symptoms against which therapeutic outcomes can subsequently be compared (see further description of rating scales in Box 15.5 and a case illustration of the clinical utility of rating scales in Box 15.6).

Medical Evaluation

The psychiatric assessment of a child or adolescent should include a medical evaluation, for several reasons. First, it may be necessary to rule out medical causes of presenting difficulties. For example, a drug screen should be routinely incorporated into the assessment of an adolescent with new-onset psychosis. Second, certain psychiatric disorders can be complicated by physiological disturbances that require medical evaluation and sometimes urgent intervention. One such example is a purge-type eating disorder and hypokalemia. Third, medical conditions that increase the risk of adverse effects associated with certain treatment modalities should be identified. A pertinent example is cardiac evaluation of a child with a family history of structural heart disease or sudden unexplained death for whom a trial of stimulant medication is under consideration. Finally, baseline values of physiological parameters should be determined that may be affected

---

BOX 15.5
RATING SCALES

Rating scales can be categorized as either "broadband" or "narrow-band." Broadband rating scales, also known as screening tests, identify issues in an individual that merit further evaluation. The best broadband rating scales are inexpensive, brief, easily assessed, and indicative of a next step if there is a positive result. The positive predictive value of any significant result is directly correlated with the prevalence of the condition in question. Examples of broadband rating scales include the Pediatric Symptom Checklist and the Child Behavior Checklist. Considered the gold standard among broadband rating scales, the Child Behavior Checklist is very commonly used in the assessment of children and adolescents. It is available in various forms, depending on the rater (e.g., parent, teacher, patient) and developmental age of the patient, and it quantifies a range of symptomatology (e.g., anxiety, depression, attention, oppositional behavior, aggression).

Narrow-band rating scales measure symptoms that are relatively specific to a diagnostic entity (e.g., attention-deficit hyperactivity disorder) or category (e.g., anxiety disorders). Results help to confirm the diagnosis and ensure that specific features of the disorder or criteria for the diagnosis are not overlooked. Commonly encountered narrow-band rating scales include the Vanderbilt ADHD Diagnostic Parent/Teacher Rating Scale, the Conners' Rating Scale for ADHD, the Multidimensional Anxiety Scale for Children, the Self-Report for Childhood Anxiety Related Emotional Disorders, the Beck Depression Inventory for Youth, the Center for Epidemiological Studies Depression Scale Modified for Children, and the Reynolds Child/Adolescent Depression Scales. A range of clinically useful rating scales can be found at http://www.schoolpsychiatry.org, a website developed by Massachusetts General Hospital's School Psychiatry Program and MADI Resource Center. For each instrument, the site lists the target age group, who administers and completes the instrument, the estimated time required for completion, and whether or not it is freely available.

---

by psychotropic medications either already in use by the patient or under consideration by the evaluating physician.

Baseline Laboratory Testing

Typically, baseline laboratory tests include complete blood count (CBC) with differential; serum electrolytes, blood urea nitrogen (BUN), and creatinine; urinalysis; liver function tests (LFTs); thyroid-stimulating hormone (TSH) level; and, depending on the patient's age and presentation, lead level, drug screen, and pregnancy test.

Anemia is associated with a wide range of mental status changes, including depression, anxiety, and psychosis. Leukocytosis can reflect infectious or neoplastic processes that can present psychiatrically, whereas leukopenia is an adverse effect of some psychotropic

---

BOX 15.6

CASE EXAMPLE OF THE UTILITY OF RATING SCALES IN THE EVALUATION OF A CHILD

A 9-year-old boy was brought to clinical attention for escalating aggression. He was threatening his mother, fighting with his siblings, and spending less time with his friends. His grades had deteriorated over the preceding 2 years, but he had not been oppositional or aggressive at school. After taking the history and examining the child, the physician asked the teacher and the mother to complete the Child Behavior Checklist. The teacher's and the mother's assessments on the broadband rating scale noted significant difficulties with attention, concentration, and hyperactivity. The mother's report had a significant elevation in the aggression subscale. Considering the history and the distractibility, hyperactivity, and irritability observed in the office, the physician then asked the mother and teacher to complete the Vanderbilt ADHD Rating Scale. Their ratings on this narrow-band scale revealed clinically significant symptoms of inattention and hyperactive/impulsive symptoms, both at home and at school.

The physician's diagnostic impression was ADHD. Treatment with a stimulant was initiated. A month later the mother and teacher again completed the Vanderbilt ADHD Rating Scale, which demonstrated some improvement in hyperactive and inattentive symptoms, but persistent and clinically significant difficulty. The dose of stimulant was increased. A month later the boy was enjoying a more positive attitude about school and earning better grades. His mother noted improved behavior at home. Congruent with the interim history, repeat Vanderbilt ADHD Rating Scale scores were "subclinical."

---

medications (e.g., clozapine). Hyponatremia, which can result from psychogenic polydipsia, the syndrome of inappropriate secretion of antidiuretic hormone (SIADH), or use of carbamazepine, can produce many signs of depression (e.g., depressed mood, irritability, anorexia, and fatigue) and confusion. Hypokalemia, associated with purging and laxative abuse, can present as weakness and produce life-threatening disturbances in cardiac conduction. Impaired renal and liver function, both of which have broad differentials, including iatrogenic, can present with a range of disturbances in mental status. Thyroid disorders can produce symptoms of anxiety, depression, and psychosis and have been associated with attention-deficit hyperactivity disorder and intellectual disability. Serum lead concentration as low as 10 μg/dL puts children at risk for hyperactivity and deficits in executive function. Regular use of, intoxication with, or withdrawal from drugs of abuse can produce an array of behavioral and emotional disturbances. Finally, pregnancy should always be considered in any postmenarcheal girl and definitely ruled out before the nonemergent administration of any medication.

Special Laboratory Testing
Certain presentations and therapeutic considerations indicate additional medical or neurological evaluation. Examples include genetic testing to clarify known causes of

neurodevelopmental disorders (e.g., fragile X, Prader-Willi, Turner, and Klinefelter syndromes), neuroimaging to rule out gross intracranial causes of new-onset psychosis, electroencephalogram (EEG) to assess developmental delay or recent change in mental status, audiogram to assess hearing in the case of speech or language delay, and electrocardiogram (ECG) to characterize individual risk of cardiac adverse effects posed by certain psychotropic medications (e.g., stimulants and antipsychotics).

Psychological Assessment

Psychological assessment is often incorporated into a comprehensive psychiatric evaluation of children and adolescents. Conducted by a qualified clinical psychologist, a psychological assessment can enhance the accuracy and reliability of diagnosis and enrich treatment planning, particularly for children and adolescents with unclear diagnoses, multiple and complex problems, suspected developmental delay, poor school performance, school refusal, or history of poor response to treatment.

A psychological assessment has multiple components, including interviews, behavioral observations, and batteries of psychological tests. Psychological tests can measure achievement (i.e., strengths and weaknesses in various aspects of learning), characterize behavioral problems, determine adaptive behavior skills (e.g., in self-care or social functioning), measure intelligence (i.e., intelligence quotient, or IQ, which is typically subdivided into verbal IQ and performance IQ), characterize personality (e.g., conflicts, drives, and defenses), and examine neuropsychological functions (e.g., perception, attention, and executive functioning). Achievement testing can clarify whether a child with depressed mood, low self-esteem, or behavioral problems is struggling to learn or process information. Intelligence testing can assess whether a significant discrepancy between verbal IQ and performance (or nonverbal) IQ is exacerbating anxiety and social difficulties. A combination of personality and neuropsychological testing can enhance the assessment of reality testing across developmental ages.

PSYCHIATRIC DISORDERS OF CHILDREN AND ADOLESCENTS

The common disorders of children and adolescents are described in four sections that follow the empirically supported organization of DSM-5: **neurodevelopmental disorders** (e.g., intellectual disability, autistic spectrum disorder, and learning disorders); **internalizing disorders** (e.g., mood and anxiety disorders); **externalizing disorders** (e.g., oppositional defiant disorder and conduct disorder); and the additional diagnoses of **schizophrenia** and **personality disorders**. Features of the internalizing group of disorders include prominent anxiety, depression, and somatic symptoms, whereas features of the externalizing group include mostly impulsive and disruptive behaviors. Although attention-deficit hyperactivity disorder (ADHD) was ultimately not categorized as an externalizing disorder in DSM-5, it is presented here within that category. Recognizing its hyperactive and impulsive features, it is often studied and described as a "disruptive behavior disorder" along with oppositional defiant disorder (ODD) and conduct disorder (CD). In addition, "internalizing disorders" in children and adolescents can sometimes present with "externalizing" behaviors (e.g., irritability and temper outbursts in mood disorders, defiant avoidance in anxiety disorders), and neurodevelopmental disorders can present with features of both the internalizing and externalizing groups (e.g., anxiety and depression associated with a learning disorder, behavioral dysregulation with intellectual disability or autism spectrum disorder).

NEURODEVELOPMENTAL DISORDERS

INTELLECTUAL DISABILITY

Diagnostic and Clinical Features

The diagnosis of intellectual disability is reserved for individuals with **significantly sub-average intelligence and impairments** in adaptive functioning that present before age 18 years (see DSM-5). Using IQ scores, intellectual disability is subtyped as mild (IQ 50–55 to approximately 70), moderate (IQ 35–40 to approximately 50–55), severe (IQ 20–25 to 35–40), profound (IQ below 20 or 25), or unspecified (when IQ is unavailable). Despite this categorization, a significantly low IQ is necessary but not sufficient for a diagnosis of intellectual disability; impaired adaptive functioning is also requisite. Approximately 85% of all intellectual disability is mild, 10% is moderate, 3–4% is severe, and 1–2% is profound.

The American Association on Intellectual Disability defines intellectual disability as a state of functioning that begins in childhood, is characterized by limitations in both intelligence and adaptive skills, and reflects the "fit" between the capabilities of the individual and the structure and expectations of the environment. This definition emphasizes the contextual nature of adaptive functioning.

In the first few years of life, a child's failure to meet neurodevelopmental milestones is often referred to as developmental delay. Developmental delay reflects a developmental age (DA) that lags behind chronological age (CA), or a quotient, DA/CA, that equals less than one. In the assessment of developmental delay, five domains of function are considered: gross motor, fine motor, communication, problem solving, and personal-social. The term *developmental delay* should be limited to the first years of life. By the time a child is school-aged, any developmental delay should either have resolved or been clarified diagnostically (e.g., as a specific learning disorder, autism spectrum disorder, communication disorder, or intellectual disability).

Global developmental delay is a term reserved for individuals under the age of 5 years who cannot be reliably assessed. Testing at an older chronological age is indicated to determine the level of intellectual disability more accurately.

Etiology

Half of all cases of mild intellectual disability have identifiable causes, including **genetic syndromes, fetal stressors** (e.g., inadequate placental perfusion, infection, teratogenic exposure) and **perinatal complications**. Approximately 75% of cases of severe intellectual disability have an identifiable cause. **Chromosomal and other genetic disorders** account for approximately 40% of severe cases (fragile X syndrome and Down syndrome are the most common). The mapping of the human genome and discovery of copy number variants have increased our capacity to identify submicroscopic chromosomal changes that result in intellectual disability, so the percentage of cases secondary to genetic alterations is increasing.

Other causes include fetal alcohol syndrome, abnormalities of brain development, inborn errors of metabolism, congenital infections, extremely low birth weight, prematurity, and, less commonly, postnatal trauma or infection. Reflecting a combination of improved child health and the emergence of new disease, the prevalence of severe intellectual disability has changed little since the 1940s. On the one hand, morbidity for low-birth-weight infants has improved, the incidence of Down syndrome has decreased, and phenylketonuria has all but been eradicated. On the other hand, more extremely low-birth-weight infants (with high rates of disability) survive, and HIV and exposure to drugs of abuse are more prevalent.

Treatment and Prognosis

Treatment of intellectual disability is multimodal and targets all aspects of functioning. Associated impairments in hearing, vision, speech, and language must be assessed and therapeutically addressed. Appropriate educational programming should be developed to maximize academic and social potential. All children and adolescents with intellectual disability should have an individualized educational plan (IEP). Opportunities to facilitate social interaction with chronological and mental age–equivalent peers should be promoted. Community, state, and federal programs are often helpful in providing structured recreational activities.

Families require education, support, and often counseling to address the special needs of a child with intellectual disability. Family support is particularly important as children mature and concerns emerge regarding independent functioning, burgeoning sexuality, and possible separation from parents.

Comorbid psychiatric diagnoses are three to four times more common among individuals with intellectual disability than in the general public. Comorbid psychiatric disorders warrant symptom-targeted interventions. **Behavior therapy**, coordinated between home and school, is the treatment of choice. Critically, behavioral interventions must be geared to the mental, not chronological, age of the child or adolescent. Psychopharmacological treatment should be reserved for psychiatric symptoms that are refractory to behavioral intervention. Any change in behavior, such as new-onset aggression, must be fully evaluated to rule out medical precipitants.

The course of intellectual disability is contingent upon the degree of cognitive and functional impairment. In mild intellectual disability, adaptive functioning is highly variable and does not correlate with IQ, but in severe intellectual disability, adaptive functioning and IQ tend to be closely correlated. Across subtypes of intellectual disability temperament varies, but significant impairments in communication may generate frustration and aggressive behavior.

Individuals with mild intellectual disability can usually learn to read but can less commonly read to learn. Consequently, mild intellectual disability is often undiagnosed in early elementary school (when the academic focus is learning to read) and is most commonly diagnosed between the ages of 10 and 14 (by which time children generally must be reading to learn). Adolescents with mild intellectual disability tend to be concrete in their thinking and, as subtle humor and innuendo become more socially normative, often become isolated from their chronological peers. They require guidance and supervision to develop appropriate vocational skills and facilitate social adaptation. Adults with mild intellectual disability generally can be gainfully employed and live independently, but they may need guidance to negotiate social, economic, and other life events.

Individuals with moderate intellectual disability demonstrate developmental delay in early childhood. They do not learn to read beyond a second-grade level but are relatively effective communicators and can maintain conversations about daily activities and other concrete topics. With appropriate vocational training, individuals with moderate intellectual disability can maintain unskilled or semiskilled jobs and take care of themselves, but generally they require a supervised living arrangement.

Individuals with severe intellectual disability commonly have significant delays in language and other forms of communication. Children who do learn to talk have a restricted repertoire of words, and signing may play an important role in communication. Academically, skills rarely exceed the preschool level. Most individuals with severe intellectual disability can attend to their own hygiene, toileting, and self-care but, in need of close supervision, commonly live with family or in a community-based group setting.

Individuals with profound intellectual disability demonstrate significant impairments in infancy that will persist throughout life. Dependence on others for hygiene, feeding, and other aspects of self-care is the rule. With intensive intervention some improvement in self-care may occur, but these individuals require highly structured living environments with constant supervision.

COMMUNICATION DISORDERS

Successful verbal communication rests upon numerous fundamental capacities, including hearing, articulation of speech, phonological processing, grammar, semantics and pragmatics. In order to use language fluently, these components must function together simultaneously and seamlessly. Dysfunction results in a communication disorder. Communication disorders include language disorder (which may have receptive, expressive, or mixed features), speech sound disorder, childhood-onset fluency disorder, and social (pragmatic) communication disorder.

As with specific learning disorders, the diagnosis of a communication disorder requires demonstrable impairment on standardized measures of communication, compared with norms for intellectual capacity. In most cases, intellectual capacity must be measured using nonverbal instruments. Communication disorders generally impair both academic and social functioning.

Language Disorder

The main impairments in language disorder are in the acquisition and use of spoken or signed language to communicate (see DSM-5). Language development requires the normal progression of receptive and expressive skills. **Delayed language acquisition** and **slow rate of language growth** are hallmark features of language disorder. Language disorder is not diagnosed if the difficulty is secondary to autism spectrum disorder, a speech or hearing impairment, or environmental deprivation. Impaired articulation and phonological errors are common, particularly in children under the age of 3 years, and do not necessarily suggest a diagnosis. Associated disorders of speech sound, reading, and writing are frequent; comorbidity with other specific developmental delays is less common. Compared with their peers, children with expressive language disorder have a relatively restricted vocabulary, make more grammatical errors, and struggle to verbalize (or sign) what they desire to express in a timely fashion. These children are often ashamed to express themselves in the classroom or with peers, and social teasing and alienation are common, particularly in the elementary and middle school years.

Speech Sound Disorder

Speech sound disorder is characterized by a child's failure to recognize and subsequently utilize speech sounds (see DSM-5). Difficulties may reside in the accurate production of speech sounds, the omission of speech sounds, and in the cognitive and semantic aspects of language processing that are necessary for building vocabulary and linguistic maturation. Some expressive phonological problems, such as lisping, are common in early development. Speech sound disorder should not be diagnosed if poor articulation is secondary to a medical condition, such as chronic ear infections, hypotonic or incomplete palate, and neurological problems.

Childhood-Onset Fluency Disorder

Childhood-onset fluency disorder (stuttering) is a dysfluency that creates significant psychological distress for an affected child (see DSM-5). Children who stutter have increased physical tension when speaking and have multiple monosyllabic or whole-word repeats that disrupt the timing and rhythm of their utterances. Shame and social avoidance often result and indicate referral for treatment.

Social (Pragmatic) Communication Disorder

This disorder refers to a persistent difficulty in the social use of verbal and nonverbal communication, without the behavioral stereotypies and restrictive interests of autism spectrum disorder (see DSM-5). Youngsters with a diagnosis of social communication disorder have difficulty with social greetings, conversational dialogues that involve turn taking and rephrasing, and other nonscripted interactions. These difficulties result in functional limitations of their communication and socialization for age.

Etiology and Treatment

Every child with a speech delay should receive an audiogram to rule out a **hearing impairment**. A speech and language assessment is likewise indicated to help understand the origins of delay. If the disorder is primarily one of speech, then interventions focus on breathing and oropharyngeal manipulation to promote and improve voice production and word articulation. Communication disorders require multisensory, individualized interventions that help foster understanding and facilitate learning both at school and at home. An affected child's participation in dialogue may be facilitated by providing multiple options for answers. For example, asking, "Do you like the ninja movie or the knight movie better?" is more likely to engage a child with a communication disorder than asking, "Which movie was your favorite?" For severe communication disorders, the use of "augmentative and alternative communication" may be necessary. Although several neurological mechanisms have been implicated, the etiology of childhood-onset fluency disorder, or stuttering, remains unclear. Children with normal language development may experience limited periods of dysfluency, especially when there is a lag between their ability to retrieve and articulate what it is they know they want to say. Cognitive-behavioral interventions are used to address the related social anxiety and distress.

Social (pragmatic) communication disorder shares many features with level I (i.e., mild) autism spectrum disorder without intellectual impairment. Etiology for this disorder is unknown. Interventions include social skills groups, individual therapy that focuses on the rehearsal of social scripts, and milieu interventions that facilitate awareness and implementation of the same.

AUTISM SPECTRUM DISORDER

Diagnostic and Clinical Features

Autism spectrum disorder is characterized by persistent **deficits in social communication and social interaction** (see DSM-5). These deficits include a lack of social-emotional reciprocity, joint attention, facial expression, vocalizations, and motivation to share experience, as usually demonstrated even in toddlers by declarative pointing and shared eye movements. Older children may have interest in social relationships but an inability to negotiate back-and-forth conversation, appreciate nonverbal aspects of communication, make or sustain relationships, or adapt behavior to a variety of contexts. Individuals with this disorder may appear **oblivious to others** and have no interest in or concept of others' needs or experience—deficits that significantly impair social functioning.

Impairments in communication are both verbal and nonverbal. Verbal impairments include delay or failure to acquire spoken language. If language is acquired, it tends to be aberrant in form and function. With the exception of simple requests or directives (e.g., "milk" or "out"), affected children rarely use language spontaneously. Acquired language is generally rote repetition of words and phrases, often used with odd grammatical structure, out of context, and with abnormalities of pitch, intonation, rhythm, rate, and inflection. Idiosyncratic language may be comprehensible to only those closest to the affected child. The capacity to enter into and sustain dialogue to describe, share, and elaborate on experience is lacking. Abnormalities in the social use of language are common and include the inability to appreciate humor, irony, and implied meaning.

A **restricted repertoire of behaviors and interests** is another cardinal feature of autism spectrum disorder. Behaviors may be **repetitious and stereotyped** (e.g., clapping, hand flapping, rocking, swaying, counting, lining toys up in a specific order and direction). A preference for sameness and inflexibility to change can be striking. For example, a child may eat foods of only one color or consistency, or be unable to adapt to any changes in daily routines. Preoccupation with parts of a whole, particularly parts that move (e.g., knobs on a door, wheels on a toy car, or the spinner of a board game), is common. Attachment to a "transitional object" such as a "security blanket" or favorite stuffed animal is usually absent in affected toddlers. When a child with autism spectrum disorder does cling to a particular item, the object may seem odd or unexpected (e.g., a toaster, a rubber band, or a blank video cassette). Some children display inattention, hyperactivity, and impulsivity.

Lastly, individuals with autism spectrum disorder often demonstrate unusual sensation with either extreme insensitivity or excessive sensitivity to temperature, taste, texture, touch, sounds, and smells.

The majority of individuals with autism spectrum disorder have **abnormal cognitive functioning**. Standardized IQ testing may fall in the borderline to moderate range for intellectual disability. When coupled with impairments in adaptive functioning, the comorbid diagnosis of intellectual disability is made. In addition to lower IQ, individuals with autism spectrum disorder demonstrate uneven neurocognitive functioning, with verbal—and particularly social comprehension—skills significantly lower than nonverbal skills. Epileptiform discharges are also a common finding among individuals with autism spectrum disorder, although their significance is unclear.

In mild (level 1) autism spectrum disorder, which was often previously referred to as "high functioning autism" or Asperger's disorder, **language acquisition is timely** and **cognitive impairment is rare**. If intellectual disability coexists with mild (level 1) autism spectrum disorder, it is usually mild. Children with mild (level 1) autism spectrum disorder have intact phonological processing and are able to master vocabulary. Some are even precocious in the ability to master the mechanics of reading. Delays and relative difficulties with visuomotor and visuospatial coordination may impair drawing, writing, and playing sports.

The social deficits of children with mild (level 1) autism spectrum disorder are less apparent during the preschool years. Deficits in social comprehension become increasingly more impairing with maturity. Children may miss the meaning of their peers' jokes; introduce eccentric, incongruent, or redundant topics into conversation; or fail to appreciate nonverbal cues. As schoolwork becomes more abstract and nuanced in middle school, affected individuals tend not to understand fully what they read. Physical awkwardness often limits athletic success, thereby compounding social isolation and rejection. Affected individuals tend to develop relationships with people who are appreciably younger or older.

Individuals with moderate (level 2) or severe (level 3) autism spectrum disorder demonstrate significant delays in verbal and nonverbal communication. All levels of autism spectrum disorder are accompanied by restricted interests and repetitive behaviors.

The course of autism spectrum disorder is **chronic and continuous**. Some children will show gains in certain areas during the school-age years, but others will deteriorate. Language development and ability are the best predictors of outcome. Intensive early intervention with behavior, speech, and language therapies has been shown to result in significant improvements by age 5 years.

Differential Diagnosis

Many individuals with autism spectrum disorder also have intellectual disability. Careful assessment of adaptive functioning, which by definition is impaired in intellectual disability, can be helpful in narrowing the differential. **Communication disorders** can present with features of intellectual disability and complicate the assessment of intellectual potential (i.e., IQ) by depressing scores on standardized tests. Children with **receptive and expressive language disorders** are distinguished from children with autism spectrum disorder by their normal social interactions and capacity to communicate nonverbally. Children with **selective mutism** communicate in selected environments and not in others, whereas a child with autism spectrum disorder has impairment across environments. Autism spectrum disorder can be distinguished from childhood-onset **schizophrenia** by the later onset that is typical of schizophrenia (after age 7) and the generally normal period of development preceding the onset of psychotic symptoms. For unclear reasons, there is an association between autism spectrum disorder and schizophrenia, so their comorbidity must be considered. Developmental regression must be distinguished from sequelae of an infection, metabolic disorder, or space-occupying lesion affecting the central nervous system on the basis of a thorough medical and neurological evaluation.

Etiology

Although autism spectrum disorder likely results from pre- and postnatal interactions with the environment, there is no single etiology or unifying theory. Autism spectrum disorder is found in children with a myriad of genetic syndromes and congenital abnormalities, and research suggests that multiple genes, interacting with each other as well as the environment, contribute to the development of autism spectrum disorder. Recent research regarding vaccinations has found no correlation between MMR or ethylmercury (thimerosal) and autism spectrum disorder. Increased brain volume and head size within the first 3 years of life has been reported, but the significance of this finding remains elusive.

Treatment and Prognosis

Psychopharmacological treatments for autism spectrum disorder should target specific psychiatric symptoms rather than the developmental deviance. For example, risperidone may decrease self-injury, aggression, and agitation in children and adolescents with autism spectrum disorder.

Recent research suggests that early detection, diagnosis, and **psychosocial intervention** can improve outcomes for children with autistic spectrum disorder. A review of early interventions suggests that several focused daily therapies including, among others, parent training, speech-language therapy, applied behavioral analysis, occupational therapy and social skills group therapy are effective in improving communication and lessening symptomatology.

While developmental deviance generally persists into adulthood, the resultant impairment may vary dramatically. Individuals with autism spectrum disorder and moderate to severe intellectual disability (i.e., IQ < 55) have impairments in adaptive and social functioning that preclude independent living. Individuals with mild (i.e., level 1) autism spectrum disorder may not only live independently but also function with relatively less impairment over time. Without the need to participate in physical education, recess, and cafeteria lunches at school or to meet expectations of social conformity in adolescence, individuals once considered "weird" by peers for their obscure interests or odd speech may come to enjoy areas of expertise shared by a small number of like-minded adults and, thereby, a degree of social connection.

SPECIFIC LEARNING DISORDERS

Diagnostic and Clinical Features

Specific learning disorders encompass a heterogeneous group of intrinsic disabilities. As such, "learning disorder" and "learning disability" are commonly used interchangeably. Between 5% and 10% of school-aged children are estimated to struggle with a learning disability. This wide range reflects the heterogeneity of these disorders and controversy surrounding accurate diagnosis. The most widely accepted definition of a specific learning disorder is **academic achievement two standard deviations below** that predicted by IQ. This definition is, however, plagued by problems with both specificity and sensitivity. Offering a qualitatively superior description, the National Joint Committee of Learning Disabilities describes learning disabilities as a heterogeneous group of disorders manifested by significant difficulties in the use of listening, speaking, reading, writing, reasoning, or mathematical abilities.

Specific learning disorders stem from **neurological dysfunction** in perceptual processing or in the manipulation, integration, or synthesis of information. They may be comorbid with sensory impairments (e.g., blindness or deafness) or cognitive impairments (e.g., intellectual disability), but learning disorders are not caused by such impairments. Children with learning disabilities may be of average or even above-average intelligence. Disorders of attention (e.g., attention-deficit hyperactivity disorder) can impair academic achievement and compound co-occurring learning disorders in a generalized fashion, but these are not defined as learning disabilities. As such, attention-deficit hyperactivity disorder is a *disability for learning*, but it is **not** a learning disability. In accordance with the Individuals with Disabilities Educational Act, all children diagnosed with learning disabilities are entitled to an individualized educational plan (i.e., "special education").

The DSM-5 defines a specific learning disorder as difficulties in learning and using academic skills that persist for at least 6 months despite the provision of interventions that target those difficulties. Learning disabilities are best described by their specific impairments, but it is often the case that individuals with a specific learning disorder with impairment in reading meet diagnostic criteria for other specific learning disorders because so much learning is dependent on understanding written language.

Often referred to as reading disability or **dyslexia**, specific learning disorder with **impairment in reading** is characterized by reading accuracy, speed, or comprehension significantly below expectation for educational level or chronological age, as measured in a standardized assessment, despite at least 6 months of targeted intervention (see DSM-5). Impairment in reading is the most common type of specific learning disorder, and the vast majority of affected individuals have problems with phonological awareness (i.e., the ability to recognize and discriminate the smallest individual sounds, or phonemes, that correspond to letters and comprise words). Individuals with problems with phonetic awareness are unable to decode or recognize phonemes rapidly, accurately, and fluently without excessive effort. Children may also have difficulty retaining phonemes in their working memory.

Specific learning disorder with **impairment in written expression** is diagnosed when a child's ability to express himself or herself in writing falls substantially below expectations for the child's intellectual functioning, chronological age, and educational level, despite at least 6 months of targeted intervention (see DSM-5). The production of written words, sentences, paragraphs, and text that convey meaning requires a number of abilities. The individual must know what he or she wants to say, access the requisite communicative words, build those words by correctly pairing phonemes with the appropriate symbols, or graphemes, and produce on paper the desired graphemes in the correct order, spatial orientation, and alignment. Given this array of requisite skills, a variety of specific impairments can result in a specific learning disorder with impairment in written expression.

A diagnosis of specific learning disorder with **impairment in mathematics** is made when a child's mathematical ability as measured on standardized tests falls significantly below that predicted for chronological age, measured intelligence, and educational background; impairs academic achievement; and persists despite at least 6 months of targeted intervention (see DSM-5). As with writing, many skills contribute to mathematical ability, and dysfunction in any or a combination of these skills may result in a specific learning disability with impairment in mathematics. Problems with comprehending the language of mathematics, recognizing mathematical signs and symbols, appreciating and attending to sequential ordering and operations, and grasping spatial orientation may all result in mathematics disorder. A learning disorder with impairment in mathematics is often comorbid with impairments in reading, written expression, or both.

Etiology and Treatment

Specific learning disorders have a **genetic** component. Recurrence rates in susceptible families range between 35% and 45%. The higher incidence in males may in part reflect a referral bias because males have more comorbid disruptive behavior than females. Several genetic loci have been recognized to confer vulnerability for specific learning disorder with impairment in reading. Loci on chromosome 6 have been linked to difficulties in phonological recognition, and loci on chromosome 15 are associated with impairments in whole-word reading. Although some severe cases of reading disorder may be due to single-gene abnormalities, it is unlikely that this mechanism of inheritance is common. Most cases likely result from a confluence of inherited and environmental neurobiological processes.

Functional brain imaging research reveals inefficient brain mechanisms in individuals with specific learning disability with impairment in reading, and highlights the significance of the left temporoparietal cortex in successful and effective reading. When reading new words or new text, all readers recruit areas of the occipital cortex, in addition to the left temporoparietal cortex. When reading familiar material, however, individuals without reading disorder recruit only the temporoparietal region, whereas individuals with a specific learning disorder with impairment in reading continue to recruit additional cortical domains.

Children with a history of language delay or difficulties are at greater risk for a specific learning disorder with impairment in reading and should be followed closely in the early school years. Children with above-average IQ may adeptly compensate for their deficiencies by interpreting nonverbal and nuanced cues; attention to these children's phonological development in kindergarten and ability to recognize phonemes and graphemes in first grade is critical.

Interventions for specific learning disability with impairment in reading include multisensory approaches to teaching phonological processing in a multisensory context and individualized educational planning to address the unique learning profile of affected children. A variety of other interventions have been promoted over the years, including eye-tracking exercises and the use of colored eyeglass lenses, but these approaches have not been proven to be consistently effective.

Since both reading and writing require phoneme–grapheme correspondence and fluency, almost all youngsters with impairment in reading will meet criteria for a specific learning disorder with impairment in written expression. Children with deficits in working memory may be unable to hold in their mind what it is they want to write. A youngster with impairments in fine motor coordination or visuospatial orientation will struggle with the mechanics of writing and, depending on severity, may qualify for a diagnosis of a specific learning disorder with impairment in written expression.

Children are sometimes not taught writing until they have mastered reading. This educational programming delays recognition of children at risk for impairment in written expression. The introduction of writing in kindergarten and prompt recognition of the youngster who struggles with the written word in early elementary school promote early referral and intervention. Occupational therapy is indicated for children with fine-motor coordination or visuospatial difficulties. If motor problems persist, a laptop computer should be introduced in lieu of handwriting. Youngsters with significant working memory impairments should be assessed and, if appropriate, treated for attention-deficit hyperactivity disorder. Underlying phonological and speech sound difficulties must be addressed on an individualized educational level.

Since formal mathematical operations are introduced later in elementary school, diagnosis of specific learning disorder with impairment in mathematics is rarely made before third grade. Interventions should be geared at the specific learning profile of the affected child, with efforts to remediate deficiencies and promote relative strengths in learning.

MOTOR DISORDERS

Diagnostic and Clinical Features

Developmental Coordination Disorder

Developmental coordination disorder is a motor skills disorder that is characterized by significant deficiencies in motor coordination for age and intellectual ability (see DSM-5). The deficiencies are not accounted for by a diagnosis of cerebral palsy or muscular dystrophy. A delay in meeting developmental milestones is usually the presenting complaint. Failure of an infant to hold up his or her head, reach, sit, or walk on time, as well as impairments in eye-tracking, pincer-grasp, latching, suckling and feeding, all suggest a developmental coordination disorder.

Stereotypic Movement Disorder

Stereotypic movement disorder refers to purposeless, repetitive, often rhythmic motor behaviors such as hand flapping or body rocking that interfere with developmentally appropriate daily activities (see DSM-5). These behaviors begin in early development and are often associated with other neurodevelopmental disorders, especially severe intellectual disability. They may be self-injurious in nature, such as self-biting, head banging, or face slapping. More normative self-stimulation behaviors may develop into full-blown stereotypic movement disorders in vulnerable individuals who are socially isolated. Repetitive behaviors are common among individuals with a diagnosis of autism spectrum disorder, for whom the additional diagnosis of stereotypic movement disorder should be made only when the behaviors are self-injurious or sufficiently severe as to warrant specific target interventions. Differential diagnosis for stereotypic movements includes tic disorders, obsessive-compulsive disorder, and movement disorders that are primarily neurological in origin (i.e., clonic and choreaform movements).

Etiology and Treatment

Developmental Coordination Disorder

A full medical and neurological assessment is indicated to rule out etiologies that indicate specific interventions. Because fine-motor skills contribute to the visuospatial abilities necessary for academic achievement, children with developmental coordination disorder frequently have comorbid learning disorders of written expression and mathematics.

Interventions for developmental coordination disorder may address either the presumed underlying deficits or the results of the impairment. Occupational therapy is the most common treatment for the former; an individualized educational plan, with accommodations such as a laptop, for the latter.

Stereotypic Movement Disorder

Interventions for stereotypic movement disorder may include behavioral or psychopharmacological interventions or both, depending on the child and nature of the movement.

TIC DISORDERS

Diagnostic and Clinical Features

Tics are **abrupt, purposeless, recurrent, nonrhythmic motor movements or vocalizations**. They can mimic voluntary movement or speech and can sometimes be suppressed, but they are generally thought to be involuntary. Examples of **simple** tics include grimaces, jerks, coughs, eye blinking, and throat clearing. Examples of more **complex** tics include hitting, touching, obscene gestures (copropraxia), and obscenities (coprolalia). Typically (and especially in children at least 10 years of age), a premonitory sensation or urge (variably described as a "pressure," "itch," or "tingle") precedes and is relieved by the tic. The onset of tic disorders is often prepubertal, and all tic disorders have their onset **before 18 years** of age. They must **not be attributable to the physiological effects of any substance** (e.g., stimulant medication or cocaine) **or another medical condition** (e.g., Huntington's disease or postviral encephalitis).

Children with tic disorders commonly have comorbid psychiatric disorders, including obsessive-compulsive disorder, attention-deficit hyperactivity disorder, major depressive disorder, or autism spectrum disorder, as well as symptoms of impulsivity and aggression. Tic disorders are classified according to the type of tics (i.e., motor and/or vocal) and their duration.

Tourette's disorder is characterized by *both* **multiple motor** *and* **one or more vocal tics** at some time during the course of illness, but not necessarily concurrently (see DSM-5). Tics may wax and wane in frequency but, since the onset of the first tic, have persisted for **more than 1 year**. Although not required for the diagnosis, motor tics often precede vocal tics by 1 or 2 years.

Persistent (chronic) motor or vocal tic disorder is characterized by single or multiple **motor or vocal tics**, *but not both*, that may wax and wane in frequency but have persisted for **more than 1 year** since the onset of the first tic (see DSM-5). The diagnosis of persistent tic disorder requires specification, "with motor tics only" or "with vocal tics only."

Provisional tic disorder is characterized by single or multiple **motor and/or vocal** tics that have been present **less than 1 year** since the onset of the first tic (see DSM-5). Because the course of illness must be less than 1 year, criteria have not been met for either persistent tic disorder or Tourette's disorder.

Differential Diagnosis

Acute and tardive akathisia and dyskinesias are associated with changes in antipsychotic medications. Chorea is associated with Wilson's disease, Huntington's disease, or, in the case of Sydenham's chorea, a recent streptococcal infection. **Stimulant medications** can cause tics. Complex motor tics can sometimes be difficult to differentiate from compulsions; the presence of obsessions can be helpful in the differentiation of a tic disorder from obsessive-compulsive disorder. Stereotyped movements associated with autism spectrum disorders tend not to wax and wane or cause distress but rather to be chronic and soothing.

Etiology

In twin studies, higher concordance rates in monozygotic than in dizygotic pairs indicate a strong **genetic** component in the etiology of tic disorders. The presence of discordant monozygotic pairs suggests the existence of nongenetic factors as well (e.g., lower birth weight). Family studies have shown high rates of heritability for tics, as well as for obsessive-compulsive disorder. That heritability is probably polygenic. The **basal ganglia** have been implicated in the pathogenesis of tics on the basis of their neurophysiological function in integrating sensorimotor information and motor control, their richness in dopamine, and neuroimaging data. The relevance of autoimmune mechanisms triggered by group A beta-hemolytic streptococci (pediatric autoimmune neuropsychiatric disorders associated with streptococcal infection, or PANDAS) remains controversial.

Treatment and Prognosis

Tic disorders have a wide range of severity, impairment, and temporal course. Tics in childhood are most often transient and associated with little impairment. Persistent tics have a broad range of severity and impairment, but when they persist into adolescence, they tend to become less severe and impairing. Tics characteristically decrease or disappear during calm, focused activity and worsen with stress, including illness, fatigue, anxiety, and excitement. Frequently, tics are most severe between 10 and 12 years of age, but diminish or disappear by early adulthood. Unfortunately, as tics diminish, other psychopathology, most commonly **obsessive-compulsive disorder**, may emerge. It has been estimated that among children affected by Tourette's disorder, by early adulthood one-third will be tic-free, one-third will have milder tics, and one-third will continue to have relatively severe and impairing tics.

Psychoeducation and reassurance are the foundation for all treatment of tic disorders. **Habit reversal training**, a modified form of cognitive-behavioral therapy, has been shown to be efficacious. It is founded on a behavioral model in which environmental factors affect tics, and tics affect factors in the environment. Antecedents and consequences are identified and modified to reduce the frequency of tics. Specific therapeutic techniques include awareness training (of both tics and their premonitory urges), competing response training (i.e., the substitution of more socially acceptable behavioral responses to premonitory urges than tics), relaxation exercises, and positive reinforcement.

Although no known medication suppresses tics completely, options include dopamine antagonists and adrenergic agonists. **Haloperidol** and **pimozide** are FDA approved for the treatment of Tourette's disorder, but they can produce significant adverse effects, including sedation, cognitive dulling, and extrapyramidal symptoms. Recent evidence supports the efficacy of risperidone in the treatment of tics, but weight gain and sedation can be limiting. Ziprasidone is another option, but it may prolong the QTc index. In their capacity to reduce tics, clonidine and guanfacine may be as effective as the dopamine antagonists and are especially useful when attention-deficit hyperactivity disorder is comorbid.

INTERNALIZING DISORDERS

BIPOLAR DISORDER

Diagnostic and Clinical Features

The clinical features that define bipolar disorder in children and adolescents are similar to those seen in adults. When present in a child or adolescent, these features can be striking. Some examples of manic behavior include **defying a teacher** and attempting to take over the classroom, engaging in **risky or life-threatening behaviors**, masturbating in a public place, and engaging in unsafe sex with multiple partners. Manic children and adolescents tend to be **overly confident, unable to sit still, and bothered by thoughts that are hard to organize or "moving too fast."** Cardinal signs and symptoms of mania (e.g., euphoria, grandiosity, decreased need for sleep) may be less common in children and adolescents. **Mood instability**, reactivity and **irritability**; aggressive and oppositional behavior; and severe temper tantrums may be more common, if less specific, features of pediatric bipolar disorder.

Chronic mixed affective states may be more typical than discrete episodes of depression and mania. Adolescent-onset bipolar disorder in particular is associated with mixed affective episodes, psychotic features, and a chronic course. Some clinicians and researchers use a broader definition (e.g., including "severe mood dysregulation") that includes individuals who do not meet DSM criteria for the diagnosis of bipolar disorder. Until better diagnostic tools are developed and/or biological markers are identified, the diagnosis of pediatric bipolar disorder will remain a clinical challenge.

Family history can be helpful in making the diagnosis. Bipolar disorder in a first-degree relative confers a four- to sixfold increased risk. **Prepubertal onset** of depression is also suggestive of increased risk for the ultimate development of bipolar disorder. Other features that increase the risk of bipolar disorder include depression with psychotic features or psychomotor retardation and history of antidepressant-induced mania or hypomania.

Treatment and Prognosis

Treatment should be comprehensive and multimodal, involving a team of providers who work with the patient and family. Family-focused, interpersonal, and social-rhythm therapies are designed to decrease stressful interactions with peers, manage high expressed emotion within the family, and help the child or adolescent regulate sleep–wake patterns. The combination of individual and family therapy improves adherence to treatment of both bipolar and comorbid disorders and thus functional outcomes.

The psychopharmacological treatment of bipolar disorder in children and adolescents is very similar to the treatment of bipolar disorder in adults. First-line agents include traditional mood stabilizers such as **lithium** and **valproate**, as well as **atypical antipsychotic** medications. Occasionally, the combination of a traditional mood stabilizer and an atypical antipsychotic improves treatment outcome. The addition of antidepressant medications may be necessary when depressive symptoms do not respond to mood stabilizers alone (see Pharmacotherapy, later in the chapter).

DISRUPTIVE MOOD DYSREGULATION DISORDER (DMDD)

Diagnostic and Clinical Features

Introduced in DSM-5, DMDD emerged as a diagnostic entity partly from the study of and controversy surrounding pediatric bipolar disorder. DMDD is diagnosed in children with **chronic, severe persistent irritability** and **frequent temper outbursts** (see DSM-5). The diagnosis cannot coexist with bipolar disorder, oppositional defiant disorder, or intermittent explosive disorder, and outbursts cannot occur exclusively during a major depressive episode or be better explained by another psychiatric (e.g., neurodevelopmental or anxiety) disorder.

The temper outbursts of DMDD occur on average three or more times per week for at least 1 year, manifest in verbal rages and/or physical aggression toward people or property, and are grossly out of proportion in intensity or duration to the provocation or situation. In between temper outbursts, children with DMDD are observed by others to have a persistently negative (i.e., irritable or angry) mood. The onset of illness must be before age 10 years, and the diagnosis cannot be made before age 6 or after age 18 years. Symptoms must be present in at least two settings (e.g., at home, in school, with peers).

The validity and specificity of DMDD are not yet clearly understood, but follow-up studies have demonstrated a high risk of subsequent depressive and anxiety disorders (hence, DMDD's inclusion among Internalizing Disorders).

Differential Diagnosis

The differential diagnosis of DMDD is broad and includes especially bipolar disorder, oppositional defiant disorder (ODD), and intermittent explosive disorder (IED). In pediatric bipolar disorder, the chief affective disturbance can be irritability, but that irritability is often **episodic**. In contrast, the irritability of DMDD is persistent. Also helpful in differentiating DMDD from bipolar disorder are hallmark features of the latter, such as **elated or expansive mood** and **grandiosity**. Oppositional defiant disorder and DMDD are both characterized by behavior outbursts, but only DMDD has a persistent disturbance of mood between outbursts. As such, most children whose difficulties meet diagnostic criteria for DMDD also meet criteria for the diagnosis of ODD (but DMDD precludes the diagnosis of ODD). Children with IED have severe temper outbursts like those in DMDD, but neither disrupted mood nor a 12-month duration is required for the diagnosis of IED. As with ODD, the diagnosis of IED is not made if criteria for the diagnosis of DMDD are met.

The differential diagnosis of bipolar disorder is also broad, and comorbidity is extremely common. The differential includes DMDD, oppositional defiant disorder, conduct disorder, prescription or nonprescription substance-induced mood disorder, mood disorder due to another medical condition, psychotic disorders (in the event of psychotic features) and, perhaps most common and challenging to differentiate, attention-deficit hyperactivity disorder.

Attention-deficit hyperactivity disorder is defined by inattention, distractibility, hyperactivity, and excessive talkativeness, and it is associated with irritability, temper outbursts, mood lability, and bossiness. These features all overlap with mania. Adding to the difficulty of differentiation of these two conditions, bipolar disorder in children and adolescents may not be clearly episodic. The following relatively specific signs of mania, when present, are most helpful in distinguishing between these two disorders: euphoria, flight of ideas or racing thoughts, decreased need for sleep, and hypersexuality (see Figure 15.2). In addition, symptoms and impairment of attention-deficit hyperactivity symptoms must be present before 12 years of age.

Treatment and Prognosis

Because DMDD is a new diagnostic entity, specific evidence-based treatments do not yet exist. That said, there is much to be drawn from the treatment of other pediatric mood disorders, including severe mood dysregulation and behavior outbursts. It is important to treat comorbidity. While the disruptive behaviors of DMDD may not be better explained by another mental disorder, they can certainly be exacerbated by a number of them (e.g., attention-deficit hyperactivity disorder, specific learning disorder, autism spectrum disorder, separation anxiety disorder, dysthymic disorder). For the treatment of disruptive behaviors and mood dysregulation, mood stabilizers, antipsychotics, psychostimulants, and, to a lesser extent, atomoxatine and alpha-agonists (e.g., guanfacine, clonidine) all can be helpful. Parent management training is indicated for behavior modification. To track progress and refine interventions in both psychosocial and psychopharmacological treatments, the clinician should track the frequency, duration, and intensity of

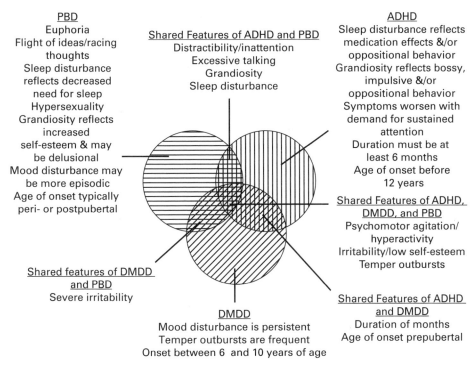

FIGURE 15.2 Pediatric bipolar disorder (PBD), disruptive mood dysregulation disorder (DMDD), and attention deficit hyperactivity disorder (ADHD).

outbursts, together with relevant contextual factors (e.g., antecedents and consequences of outbursts).

Although DMDD is in many ways similar to severe mood dysregulation (or, the broader phenotype of pediatric bipolar disorder), rates of conversion to bipolar disorder are very low. Children with DMDD are at greater risk of developing major depressive disorder and anxiety disorders.

MAJOR DEPRESSIVE DISORDER

Diagnostic and Clinical Features

The clinical presentation of major depressive disorder in children and adolescents often differs from that in adults (see DSM-5). Children often manifest sadness in **irritability, low frustration tolerance, and temper tantrums**. In keeping with a preference for action over words, they are more likely to argue and fight with family and peers than to verbalize sadness or low self-esteem. A child may not understand or relate to the idea of depression and, therefore, may not respond when directly asked if he or she is "depressed." A depressed child will, however, describe changes in relationships with family and friends (e.g., getting into fights more often, less interest in being around people). The child may describe an **inability to focus** on schoolwork and dropping grades. A child with depression may **refuse to participate** in extracurricular activities that he or she once enjoyed. A depressed child may be unable to say anything positive about himself or herself, and may be unusually focused on negative life events, such as the death of a family member.

There may be weight loss or gain, and there are often sleep disturbances, such as difficulty falling asleep or staying asleep. Multiple **somatic complaints** (e.g., fatigue, headaches, and stomachaches) are common. Parents may report a tendency to isolate (e.g., dropping out of school activities, not returning friends' calls, complaining of being bored, and "zoning out" in front of the television) and indifference about appearance (e.g., refusing to bath). **Dysthymic disorder** also occurs in children and adolescents. The requisite duration of symptoms is only 1 year in children and adolescents, and the mood may be irritable, rather than depressed (see DSM-5).

Although **suicide** is infrequent in children under age 12, it is a most serious consequence of major depressive disorder, and all children and adolescents should be assessed for the potential of suicidal ideation and behaviors. The physician should first ascertain the patient's understanding of death—that is, what it means and what happens to people who die. Children as young as age 5 often have a clear concept of death. A child may, however, think that when a person dies, that person is gone for a period of time but can still return. A child with this understanding might think that doing something to harm himself or herself would not lead to a permanent result. Once the level of understanding of death is determined, the physician can tailor appropriate, simple, and direct follow-up questions: "Do you ever wish you were dead?" "Do you think your family would be better off without you?" "Do you think about joining people you know who have died?" "Do you have thoughts of hurting yourself?" "Do you have thoughts of ending your life?" "What have you done to harm yourself?" "How often?" "Did you ever start to hurt yourself and then stop?" "Why did you stop?"

Risk factors for suicide in children and adolescents include impulsivity, aggressive behavior, substance abuse, family history of suicidal behavior, and access to firearms. Access to lethal means such as firearms, medications, and household poisons must be clarified, and parents of a depressed child or adolescent should be instructed to remove them from the home.

In the evaluation of a depressed child or adolescent, the physician must also explore past or present exposure to negative life events, such as bullying, physical or sexual abuse, domestic violence, and parental conflict. Concern for the safety of a child or adolescent may require the physician to contact proper authorities (e.g., children's protective services).

Between 20% and 40% of prepubertal children who present with a major depressive episode later develop bipolar disorder. This possibility is particularly likely if there is a family history of bipolar disorder, psychosis, or medication-induced mania.

Differential Diagnosis

The differential diagnosis of major depressive disorder includes anxiety disorders, disruptive mood dysregulation disorder, oppositional defiant disorder, attention-deficit hyperactivity disorder, adjustment disorder, sleep disorders, and substance use disorders. Medical disorders that should be considered include **hypothyroidism**, **anemia**, and **viral illnesses**.

Treatment and Prognosis

Depression of mild severity is often treated with psychoeducation and supportive psychotherapy—both involving parents of the depressed child or adolescent. Moderate to severe depression should be treated with cognitive-behavioral therapy (CBT), interpersonal therapy, and/or antidepressant medication (see Psychotherapy and Pharmacotherapy sections, later in this chapter). There are various pros and cons to each of these therapeutic modalities, and a treatment plan is best developed collaboratively with the child or adolescent and parents.

One recent study found that the combination of **CBT** and **fluoxetine** produced a more rapid improvement in depressive symptoms than either CBT or fluoxetine alone (March et al. 2004). As such, if depression in a child or adolescent does not respond to a single therapeutic modality (i.e., psychotherapy or antidepressant medication), their combination should be recommended. Once a child has responded to treatment, that treatment should be continued for 6 to 12 months.

ANXIETY, OBSESSIVE-COMPULSIVE, AND STRESS DISORDERS

Diagnostic and Clinical Features

All of the anxiety, obsessive-compulsive, and stress disorders that occur in adults also affect children and adolescents, although their presentation can be different. Anxiety disorders are among the most common diagnoses reported among children and adolescents. Overall, 8.9% of the pediatric population has at least one anxiety disorder. In general, girls are more likely to report an anxiety disorder than boys (see Table 15.2 for epidemiological information for specific anxiety disorders).

Somatic complaints (e.g., headache, stomach ache) are very common among children and adolescents with anxiety disorders, particularly in children under 10 years of age. Visits to the pediatrician may antecede psychiatric assessment. Additionally, anxiety in children may manifest as **crying, tantrums, freezing, or clinging**. Worries and anxiogenic situations tend to be relatively developmentally specific. Children, for example, commonly worry about the dark, separation from parents, bodily integrity, and school. Adolescents more commonly worry about appearance and social or academic performance. Children with anxiety disorders struggle with social skills and suffer from low self-esteem. Avoidance of social, academic, and, more generally, independent settings can adversely impact development. Anxiety disorders in children may cause a great deal of stress in the family. For example, a parent may be late every day for work because of a child's refusal to leave home and attend school.

Diagnostic criteria for the anxiety, obsessive-compulsive, and stress disorders are largely similar across age groups (see Chapter 6, Anxiety, Obsessive-Compulsive, and Stress Disorders). Age-specific differences are highlighted here.

Separation Anxiety Disorder
Children suffering from separation anxiety disorder often present initially to the pediatrician with **somatic symptoms**, such as headaches and gastric distress (see DSM-5). The symptoms become prominent with the anticipation of being separated from the primary caregiver, often the mother. The child typically expresses significant **distress about any separation** from the parent (e.g., leaving for camp, going to school, attending a sleep-over, or even falling asleep alone in a bedroom) and will make every attempt to prevent it with crying, tantrums, and clinging to the parent. The child will express fears about serious harm befalling the parent, such as death or a serious physical injury. The child will also worry about something bad happening to himself or herself and being permanently separated from the caregiver. Parents often find these fears very distressing and may accommodate and thereby inadvertently reinforce the child's behavior by limiting activities and

TABLE 15.2 Epidemiological Characteristics of Disorders of Children and Adolescents

	Prevalence	Onset	Gender
Separation anxiety disorder	2.4%–4.1%	Early onset <6 years	
Generalized anxiety disorder	2.9%–4.6%	School age	
Obsessive-compulsive disorder	0.5%–2.0%	Middle childhood	
Specific phobia		Early childhood	
Social phobia		Adolescence	
Panic disorder		Adolescence	
Posttraumatic stress disorder		Any age	
Major depressive disorder	2% of children 4%–8% of adolescents		Male:female 1:1 in children; 1:2 in adolescents
Bipolar disorder	<1% in children; 0–1% in adolescents		
Disruptive mood dysregulation disorder	2%–5%	6–10 years	Male > female
Attention-deficit hyperactivity disorder	7.8%	<12 years	Male:female 2:1
Oppositional defiant disorder	2%–16%	6 years	Male:female 2:1
Conduct disorder	1%–16%	Childhood onset <10 years	Male:female 3:1–5:1
Specific learning disorder with impairment in reading	4% of school-age children		Male:female 1.5:1–4:1
Specific learning disorder with impairment in mathematics	1% school-age children		
Developmental coordination disorder	6% of children age 5–11 years		
Expressive language disorder	10%–15% of children <3 years; 3%–7% of children >5 years		Males > females
Speech sound disorder	3% of preschool children		Males > females
Childhood-onset fluency disorder	1% of prepubertal children; 0.8% of adolescents		Male:female 3:1
Intellectual disability, mild	0.8%–1.2% of general population; more common among socioeconomically disadvantaged groups	2–7 years, with peak onset at 5 years	Male:female 2:1
Intellectual disability, severe	0.3%–0.5% across all socioeconomic groups	<18 years	Male:female 5:1
Autism spectrum disorder	0.7% (increased substantially over the past 25 years)[1]	<3 years	Male:female 4:1; females generally have more severe cognitive impairment

(continued)

TABLE 15.2 Continued

	Prevalence	Onset	Gender
Childhood-onset schizophrenia	Rare	>7 years and <13 years	Male:female 1:1–4:1
Tic disorders	Transient tics are common; chronic tics may occur in 1%–3% of children; Tourette's disorder 0.05%–0.5%	<18 years, usually before puberty	Transient tics are more common in boys
Pica		1–2 years[2]	
Rumination disorder	Rare	3–12 months; rarely later in childhood[3]	Males > females
Enuresis	5%–10 % of 5-year-olds; 3%–5% of 10-year-olds; 1% of adolescents		Male:female 1:1 between 4 and 6 years; 2:1 >10 years[4]
Encopresis	1% of 5-year-olds		Males > females

[1] Reasons for this remarkable **increase in prevalence** over a relatively short period of time include increased awareness on the part of parents, teachers, and other professionals, resulting in greater identification; diagnostic shift (e.g., children who may previously have been diagnosed with intellectual disability or schizophrenia are now recognized as having autism spectrum disorder); improved access to school-based screening and interventions; and broadening of the diagnostic criteria.

[2] Pica is more common among individuals with **intellectual disability** and is most common among those with severe cognitive impairment. Children of lower socioeconomic status, greater familial disorganization, and little adult supervision appear to be at greatest risk.

[3] An older age of onset is associated with developmental delay.

[4] Diurnal enuresis is more common in females, but rare after 9 years of age.

avoiding separations. Some children with moderate to severe separation anxiety will follow the parent throughout the house and refuse to attend school or to sleep alone.

Generalized Anxiety Disorder

Children with generalized anxiety disorder have many **worries**, such as what will happen if they become sick, if their parents cannot afford their home, or if they fail a test at school (see DSM-5). Usually, worry about one issue leads to worry about others, and the child will often seek reassurance from the parent. Parents often report experiencing great frustration with the child's constant questioning about concerns and **need for reassurance**. They may describe their child as "my 8-year-old going on 108." Parents may attempt to accommodate the worries by avoiding certain topics, limiting the child's exposure to media, and restricting the child's activities.

Obsessive-Compulsive Disorder

Children experience both obsessions and compulsions (see DSM-5). The most common obsessions in childhood are **concerns with contamination and germs** and **fears of something bad happening** to self or others. The most common compulsions are hand washing, cleaning, touching, repeating, and counting. Children often have no insight into the difficulties that their symptoms are causing, and they may suffer from the disorder for several years before it is known to anyone. Such diagnostic delay may be due to denial on the parents' part, as well as the child's ability to conceal the symptoms.

Social Phobia (Social Anxiety Disorder)

The symptoms of social phobia that occur in childhood are similar to those seen in adults, but, as with obsessive-compulsive disorder, children are more likely to have limited insight into the difficulties that the illness is causing (see DSM-5). Children with social phobia usually experience **fear of speaking in front of a group**, such as answering a question in class, eating in front of peers, attending social events, performing in front of people, reading aloud, or writing in front of a group. The school setting is generally very challenging for these children, and school refusal is a most serious complication.

Panic Disorder

Panic disorder rarely occurs prior to puberty. The symptoms of panic disorder in adolescents are the same as those found in adults (see DSM-5). Some adolescents may, however, have difficulty articulating what they are experiencing, and the related impairment may manifest mainly in **maladaptive behaviors** such as refusing to attend school or other defiant behavior.

Specific Phobia

Insight is not required to make the diagnosis of a specific phobia in childhood, but the symptoms must be present for at least 6 months.

Posttraumatic Stress Disorder

Diagnostic criteria are developmentally sensitive in a number of ways (see DSM-5). In children, intrusion symptoms may take the form of repetitive play (rather than memories) that express themes or aspects of traumatic events, frightening dreams with content that is not clearly related to traumatic events, and trauma-specific reenactment in play (rather than dissociative reactions). Additionally, in children 6 years and younger, criteria appropriately emphasize the impact of trauma sustained by primary caregivers and allow for the presence of either persistent avoidance or negative cognitions, not both, as required in older children, adolescents, and adults.

Differential Diagnosis

Comorbidity among anxiety disorders in children and adolescents is extremely common. For example, separation anxiety disorder, generalized anxiety disorder, and social phobia constitute a common triad. Both **attention-deficit hyperactivity disorder** and **depressive disorders** are comorbid in about 30% of children with an anxiety disorder. Depression can be characterized by significant worries, and anxiety and its related impairment can negatively impact self-esteem. An **adjustment disorder** can present with anxiety. The disorder begins within 3 months of an identifiable stressor (e.g., physical illness, parental divorce, birth of a sibling, or loss of a pet), it resolves within 6 months of the resolution of the stressor (and its consequences), and the stress-related disturbance does not meet diagnostic criteria for another mental disorder. In children with separation anxiety disorder, the possibility of **parental anxiety** should be assessed, because anxiety about separation can be bidirectional.

Children with **autistic spectrum disorder** sometimes complain of anxiety about socializing, and parents of these children often describe cognitive rigidity and preference for sameness as "obsessional." For children with markedly impaired sleep, a **primary sleep disorder** should be considered.

Treatment and Prognosis

Early detection and treatment of anxiety disorders may profoundly affect both the course of the disorders and the development of affected children and adolescents. Mild anxiety may resolve with psychoeducation for the parents. Persistent, severe, or impairing symptoms require more intensive treatment. Anxiety disorders in childhood are associated with anxiety, mood, and substance use disorders later in life. In addition, many adults with anxiety disorders report having had anxiety (e.g., separation anxiety disorder) as children. Additionally, anxiety disorders in childhood, especially those comorbid with depression, have been prospectively shown to decrease the likelihood of living independently, working regularly, and attending school in early adulthood.

Both CBT and selective serotonin reuptake inhibitors (SSRIs) are effective treatments for anxiety disorders in children and adolescents. With the exception of clomipramine for obsessive-compulsive disorder, studies of tricyclic antidepressants (TCAs) and benzodiazepines have not shown efficacy. The FDA has approved clomipramine, fluoxetine, fluvoxamine, and sertraline for the treatment of pediatric obsessive-compulsive disorder.

Numerous clinical trials have shown that **CBT** significantly reduces symptoms of anxiety in as many as 80% of clinically referred children. When children are younger or female, or when parents themselves have anxiety, family-based treatments may be particularly effective. CBT alone or in combination with **sertraline** has been found to be particularly efficacious in treating pediatric obsessive-compulsive disorder. A child with obsessive-compulsive disorder might first be treated with CBT alone; if response is inadequate in 4 to 6 weeks, then the combination of CBT and medication should be recommended (Pediatric OCD Treatment Study Team 2004). The combination of CBT and sertraline has also been found to be effective treatment for children and adolescents with generalized anxiety disorder, separation anxiety disorder, and social phobia (Walkup et al. 2008). These findings support the use of CBT and sertraline, either alone or in combination, in the treatment of pediatric anxiety disorders.

SOMATIC SYMPTOM AND RELATED DISORDERS

The most common somatic symptom disorders diagnosed in children and adolescents are **somatic symptom disorder** and **conversion disorder** (also known as **functional neurological symptom disorder**). Diagnostic criteria for somatic symptom disorders are the same in children, adolescents, and adults (see Chapter 10, Somatic Symptom and Related Disorders). The prevalence of somatic symptom disorders in children and adolescents appears to be lower than the prevalence in adults, perhaps in part because children's health care–seeking behavior is mitigated by parents. Irrespective of the prevalence of specific disorders, somatization is a common symptom in childhood when bodily sensations may be substituted for more abstract complaints of worry, sadness, or depression. Disproportionate, preoccupying worry about the seriousness of symptoms may emerge as a source of impairment, especially in adolescence. Similar to adults, female children are significantly more likely to develop a somatic symptom disorder than males.

Diagnostic and Clinical Features

Somatic Symptom Disorder with Predominant Pain

Recurrent abdominal pain and headache are the most common pediatric physical complaints, and in several studies were reported weekly by 10% to 30% of children and adolescents. When complaints of pain are severe, require repeated consultation with the pediatrician, do not diminish with medical reassurance, and result in significant school absence (i.e., weeks), a diagnosis of somatic symptom disorder with predominant pain may be warranted.

Conversion Disorder (Functional Neurological Symptom Disorder)

Conversion disorder that presents under age 10 years is usually limited to gait disturbances or seizures. Psychogenic, non-epileptiform seizures, also known as "pseudoseizures," are complex and may mimic epileptic seizures closely. Further complicating their differentiation, pseudoseizures occur in many individuals with epilepsy.

Illness Anxiety Disorder

Children rarely suffer from illness anxiety disorder, formerly known as hypochondriasis, in which there is anxious preoccupation with having or acquiring a serious illness. When they do, parental anxiety may be a significant contributor, and discerning parental from child symptomatology can prove challenging. Children who meet criteria for a diagnosis of illness anxiety disorder should be closely evaluated for additional signs and symptoms of anxiety.

Differential Diagnosis

The diagnosis of any somatic symptom disorder requires the exclusion of medical conditions that fully explain the presenting difficulties. If a related medical condition exists, it cannot fully explain the degree of distress and impairment. This requirement is particularly important in pediatrics, because children are less articulate and adept than adults at describing symptoms. **A thorough and exhaustive medical and neurological workup is absolutely obligatory**.

The differential diagnosis for somatic symptom disorder with predominant pain and conversion disorder in children includes anxiety and mood disorders, particularly **depressive disorders**. Psychotic disorders with somatic delusions are another consideration. Sexual dysfunction or dyspareunia should be considered when assessing sexually active adolescents.

Children take their cues from their caregivers. **Generalized anxiety disorder**, especially when parental anxiety is extreme, can resemble childhood illness anxiety disorder. Illness anxiety disorder may also mimic **obsessive-compulsive disorder**, with recurrent thoughts of illness and demands for repeated reassurances from medical professionals. In obsessive-compulsive disorder, preoccupations are, however, not limited to illness and disease.

Children occasionally purposefully use physical complaints to avoid school and receive secondary gain from the sick role, which may indicate a diagnosis of **factitious disorder or malingering**.

Etiology

Children vary in their linguistic skills and their insight into internal states of worry, fear, and sadness. When a child or teenager cannot recognize, label, or articulate an internal affective state, psychological distress is often experienced physically. For example, anticipatory anxiety about a separation may be experienced as a "stomachache," or worry over performance on an examination, as a "headache."

A phenomenon known as somatosensory amplification may predispose children to somatoform disorders. Children with somatosensory amplification have heightened awareness of their bodily sensations and may misinterpret bodily cues as ominous or suggestive of illness.

Intergenerational factors may also contribute. Children whose parents have a somatoform disorder have been shown to have more bodily preoccupations and disease phobia than children whose parents do not have a somatoform disorder. Prior somatic complaints and psychosocial stressors (in the family, at school, with peers) have both been shown to predict future somatoform disorders.

Treatment and Prognosis

Treatment should be multidisciplinary, incorporating both physical rehabilitation and psychological and social interventions to address contributing factors. Individual psychotherapy may incorporate cognitive-behavioral techniques, relaxation exercises, guided imagery, and insight-oriented work. Psychoeducation, family therapy, and school consultation may also improve outcomes.

Children and adolescents with chronic medical illnesses may experience physical symptoms in excess of medical expectations and thus may qualify for a diagnosis of psychological factors affecting other medical conditions. Particularly in the case of a chronic pediatric medical condition, effective multidisciplinary treatment facilitates the patient's ability to participate in school and extracurricular activities despite somatic symptoms or pain, acknowledges psychological contributors, supports adherence to psychiatric treatment, and avoids ineffective analgesic treatments.

Somatic symptom disorder with predominant pain and conversion disorder are generally time-limited. Nonetheless, prompt consultation with a child psychiatrist is recommended to assess possible contributing psychological factors.

FEEDING AND EATING DISORDERS OF CHILDHOOD

Anorexia nervosa and bulimia nervosa typically emerge in adolescence (see Chapter 9, Feeding and Eating Disorders). The eating disorders described here present significantly before adolescence.

Diagnostic and Clinical Features

Pica

Pica refers to the **ingestion of non-nutritive substances** on a regular basis for a period of at least 1 month (see DSM-5). The behavior is inappropriate to the developmental level and not part of any culturally sanctioned practice. The substances ingested tend to vary with age. Plaster, wool, ashes, paint, and hair are common among young children. Sand, animal droppings, insects, and leaves are common in older children. Dirt and clay are the most common substances ingested by adolescents and adults.

The age of onset is typically between **1 and 2 years**. Because almost all infants and young toddlers will mouth objects within reach, inadequate parental oversight should be considered responsible for ingestion of non-food items in youngsters less than 2 years of age. Most cases of pica spontaneously remit after a period of a few months. In a minority of cases pica persists into adolescence or adulthood. Complications of pica include lead poisoning, gastrointestinal disturbance, and intestinal obstruction secondary to bezoars. Individuals with pica are also at risk for parasitic infections.

Rumination Disorder

Rumination disorder is characterized by the **effortless regurgitation** of recently swallowed food (see DSM-5). The regurgitated food is often re-chewed and re-swallowed, or spewed out, without associated gastrointestinal symptoms or discomfort. When the disorder occurs in children with developmental delay, it may have a self-stimulating quality. The regurgitation follows a period of normal eating, and structural disease is not present.

Avoidant/Restrictive Food Intake Disorder

Youngsters with this disorder avoid or restrict food intake for a variety of reasons (e.g., extreme sensitivity to sensory characteristics of food, a seeming lack of interest in food or eating) and persistently fail to meet their nutritional or energy needs (see DSM-5). The avoidance or restriction of food results in at least one of the following: failure to achieve expected weight gain (or frank weight loss), significant nutritional deficiency, reliance on enteral feeing or oral supplements, or significant psychosocial dysfunction (e.g., inability to eat with others or consequently to sustain relationships). The restricted food intake is not due to unavailability of food, culturally sanctioned practices, developmentally normal behaviors (e.g., picky eating in toddlerhood), excessive concern with body weight or shape (as in anorexia nervosa), or a concurrent medical condition.

Parents describe feeding problems in approximately 25% of infants under 6 months of age and children aged 2 years, and in 18% of 4-year-olds. Infants may refuse feedings, disengage from feeding prematurely, appear apathetic or withdrawn, have inappropriate or disruptive behaviors during feeding, or develop peculiar feeding habits. Infants and children with a history of prematurity are at greater risk. The onset is usually in the first year of life, and nearly always begins before age 3 years.

Approximately 1% to 5% of all pediatric inpatient admissions are for "failure to thrive," and an estimated half of these cases are the result of feeding problems. In the context of a medical illness or developmental delay, the diagnosis of a feeding disorder is made when the magnitude of the feeding problem far exceeds that anticipated from the medical condition or developmental delay. In such a situation, the diagnosis of a feeding disorder would be supported by a positive change in feeding behavior following psychosocial intervention (e.g., a change in caregiving).

Differential Diagnosis

Pica

Schizophrenia and other psychotic disorders may include delusions that motivate ingestion of non-nutritive items. Kleine Levin, an extremely rare sleep disorder found most often among adolescent boys, is associated with binge eating, occasionally of non-nutritive substances (as well as hypersomnia, irritability, and hypersexuality). Temporal lobe damage can result in Kluver-Bucy syndrome, characterized by abnormal eating behaviors and mouthing of objects, as well as inappropriate affect and inability to recognize familiar people and places.

Rumination Disorder

Gastroesophageal reflux, pyloric stenosis, gastroparesis, and gastritis are gastrointestinal disorders that can present in infancy with recurrent vomiting. They should be ruled out before making a diagnosis of rumination disorder. The normal "spitting up" that most infants experience should be distinguished from rumination disorder by the apparent volitional quality of regurgitation in the latter.

Avoidant/Restrictive Food Intake Disorder

The differential diagnosis for and array of associated conditions with this disorder are broad. Anxiety, obsessive-compulsive, depressive, autistic spectrum, and psychotic disorders must be considered, as well as medical, neurological, structural, and congenital conditions. Avoidant/restrictive food intake disorder can be diagnosed together with any of these conditions if all diagnostic criteria are met and the disturbance requires specific clinical attention. As noted previously, eating disorders characterized by disturbances in perception and experience of body weight and shape (e.g., anorexia nervosa) cannot be diagnosed concurrently.

Etiology, Treatment, and Prognosis

Pica

The etiology of pica is not known. There may be an association between pica and underlying celiac disease. Immediate assessment of and intervention for medical complications of pica are always the first order of business. Educating and advising parents about pica and the need for vigilance in all settings (e.g., home, school, playground) are appropriate. Adolescents with pica should be included in a similar discussion with parents, but more comprehensive additional assessment and intervention may be warranted. Most treatments are **behavioral**, substituting food items for non-food items with positive reinforcement. Spontaneous remission is common among infants, but fatality rates approach 25% among affected children. When the age of onset is later, the disorder tends to have a more protracted course. Repeated misdiagnoses and costly, extensive gastrointestinal evaluations often precede the diagnosis. Weight loss and failure to gain weight in a growing child are frequent complications and can result in clinical "failure to thrive."

Rumination Disorder

The etiology is thought to include gastrointestinal predispositions and psychosocial factors. Understimulation, neglect, parent–child relationship problems, and frustration in caregivers may predispose to and exacerbate the condition. Treatment is tailored to the specific patient and family. For an infant with otherwise normal development, **parent education and nutritional and behavioral interventions** geared at positively reinforcing normal eating behaviors may suffice. If the rumination disorder is the product of larger parent–child relationship problems or parental neglect, couple or family therapy and social interventions to modify parental behavior are indicated. Occasionally, if the rumination disorder appears to be compromising the health of a child with intellectual disability, positive reinforcement combined with mild adverse conditioning may be indicated.

Avoidant/Restrictive Food Intake Disorder

The cause of this disorder is unknown, but temperamental variables in both parents and affected infants or children are likely relevant, in that goodness of "temperamental fit" can affect feeding outcomes. Infants and children with extreme sensitivity to taste, smell, and texture may be at higher risk. Occasionally, food avoidance may represent a conditioned negative response to a prior noxious experience, such as vomiting, choking, or medical procedure. Parents should avoid power struggles over eating and model healthy eating habits for their children at an early age. Successful feeding interactions promote attachment and self-regulation. Unsuccessful interactions leave parents feeling frustrated, inadequate, and worried for the health of their child, and leave children frustrated and hungry.

Early recognition and intervention are important. After a complete medical evaluation, multiple observations should be made of parent–child feeding interactions, as well as feeding interactions between the infant or child and non-caregivers. Provided malnutrition is not acutely life threatening, interventions should be nutritionally informed but primarily **behavioral**. Education and support for caregivers are critical. Meals should be time-limited, and solid foods, if appropriate, should be introduced before liquids. In particular, high-volume, low-calorie liquids such as water, juice, and sweet drinks should be minimized. Environmental distractions during mealtime should be avoided, and positive reinforcement should be provided for the infant or child as well as the caregivers.

In most affected infants and children, feeding improves with intervention, but growth curves often continue to lag, and susceptibility to illness is heightened. Over time, feeding disorders may be complicated by physical, cognitive, and social delays. Approximately one-third of infants with "failure to thrive" develop an intellectual disability.

ELIMINATION DISORDERS

Attaining control of bladder and bowel function is a major developmental milestone for children. Daytime and nocturnal "accidents" are common as children transition from diapers to toileting. When wetting or soiling is developmentally inappropriate and persistent, a diagnosis of an elimination disorder may be warranted.

Diagnostic and Clinical Features

Enuresis
Enuresis is the **repeated voiding of urine** into bedding or clothing by a child with a chronological or developmental age of **at least 5 years** (see DSM-5). The diagnosis requires that the behavior, which is usually involuntary, but can be intentional, occur at least twice a week for at least three consecutive months, or cause significant distress (e.g., embarrassment) or impairment in social or academic functioning. It is not exclusively secondary to a substance (e.g., diuretic) or general medical condition. Enuresis is "primary" in a child who has never achieved bladder control; it is "secondary" in a child who has previously attained bladder control for at least 3 months. There are three subtypes: nocturnal only, diurnal only, and combined nocturnal and diurnal.

The **nocturnal only** type is most common and refers to urination that occurs exclusively during sleep. Voiding usually takes place during the first third of the sleep cycle, sometimes while children dream that they are on the toilet. Because children tend to attain nocturnal dryness later, some physicians do not diagnose nocturnal only enuresis before 6 years of age (but will diagnose diurnal only type as early as 4 years of age). The **diurnal only** type is further divided into "urge incontinence" and "voiding postponement" subtypes. Children with urge incontinence sense the need to void urgently and accidents ensue. Children with voiding postponement are often too preoccupied with other activities to attend to bodily cues. A majority of cases of enuresis are primary and nocturnal. More than half of children who have diurnal enuresis also have nocturnal enuresis.

Encopresis

Encopresis is the repeated (once a month for 3 months) **passage of feces into inappropriate places** in an individual **at least 4 years** of age (see DSM-5). The behavior is not caused by medication, another substance, or a medical condition other than constipation. While encopresis may occur with or without constipation and overflow incontinence, it is involuntary and associated with constipation and overflow in approximately 75% of cases. A minority of children with encopresis do not have constipation, and the encopresis appears to be more volitional in those cases. Encopresis is "primary" in a child who has never achieved bowel control; it is "secondary" in a child who has previously had regular toileting behavior.

Avoidance of toileting, especially in school, at a friend's house, or in public restrooms is common. Children with encopresis often suffer a great deal of ridicule from peers. Some children try to hide soiled clothing or attempt to flush it down the toilet. In a rush to clean up fecal messes a child may inadvertently smear feces; less commonly, fecal smearing is intentional. When a child refuses to use the toilet, parent–child power struggles as well other oppositional and defiant behaviors can ensue.

Differential Diagnosis

Enuresis

A full medical workup is warranted to rule out neurological or genitourinary disorders. **Urinary tract infection**, spinal cord anomalies (e.g., spina bifida, tethered cord), and ectopic ureters can result in both diurnal and nocturnal urinary incontinence. Any condition that results in increased urine output, such as diabetes mellitus, diabetes insipidus, or sickle cell disease, can produce urinary incontinence. Acute stress can result in loss of bladder control that is infrequent and non-recurrent. Children with severe or profound intellectual disability frequently experience urinary incontinence, but it is not deemed developmentally inappropriate.

Encopresis

Gastrointestinal abnormalities, neurological conditions, and metabolic disorders can be causal or perpetuating, particularly in cases of primary encopresis. Children and adolescents with encopresis may have comorbid oppositional defiant disorder or, less commonly, conduct disorder.

Etiology, Treatment, and Prognosis

Enuresis

In the vast majority of cases, the cause of enuresis is not known. There is strong evidence of **genetic predisposition**. Seventy-five percent of all children with enuresis have a first-degree relative with the disorder, and identical twins have a higher concordance rate than fraternal twins. Developmental delays, learning disorders, attention-deficit hyperactivity disorder, and encopresis are associated with enuresis. Difficulties with arousal from sleep may play a role. Enuresis may worsen or recur with stress. Enuresis has a **spontaneous remission** rate of approximately 15% per year. Only 1% of cases persist into adulthood.

Enuresis should be explained to the child in developmentally appropriate terms. In particular, the child should be reassured that enuresis is usually self-limited. If a parent or relative experienced enuresis in childhood, this information should be shared. If a child has both diurnal and nocturnal enuresis, the diurnal component should be addressed first. Children who have "voiding postponement" should be assessed for attention-deficit hyperactivity disorder and treated accordingly.

Behavior therapy with positive reinforcement is the mainstay of treatment. Children are taught to recognize the need to urinate and promptly go to the bathroom. Once in the bathroom, they are encouraged to postpone urination briefly and, thereby, exercise both the muscles that confer continence and also their tolerance of the sensation of fullness. Intentionally stopping and starting the flow of urine has a similar effect. Putative approaches to behavior modification, such as making the child wash bed linens or putting wet sheets out "to dry" in public, should be discouraged.

Nocturnal enuresis can be treated by restructuring fluid intake (e.g., none after 7 p.m.), routinely waking the child a few hours after falling asleep for bladder voidance, and, perhaps most effectively, using an enuresis alarm. As many as 60% to 80% of children initially respond to an **enuresis alarm system**, although relapses may require multiple trials. Cases of enuresis that prove refractory to behavioral approaches may benefit from either desmopressin or a TCA such as imipramine.

Encopresis

The etiology of encopresis includes temperamental type, genetic predisposition to constipation, and environmental factors such as diet and temperamental "fit" with caregivers. Children with encopresis tend to have a "difficult" temperament (i.e., frequent negative mood, low adaptability, and high intensity). Affected children are also more likely to be delayed in motor, communication, and social development. Mothers of children with encopresis may be anxious or depressed. Constipation, which may be chronic or the result of an acute illness, change in diet, or dehydration, usually precedes encopresis. The constipated child often experiences significant pain with defecation and begins to avoid bowel movements, inadvertently worsening the gastrointestinal condition.

Successful treatment is team based and addresses physiological, behavioral, and psychological aspects of the condition. Promoting in the child an internal, as opposed to external, sense of control for toileting is an overarching goal. When constipation is present, a pediatrician or pediatric gastroenterologist can assist with bowel evacuation. Recognition and discussion of the social difficulties inherent with fecal soiling foster the working alliance. In developmentally appropriate language, educating the child about the gastrointestinal system, assessing and encouraging the child's interest in change, and reframing the child's perception of the potential for success all promote cooperation. Parent–child dyadic work may also be useful.

Bowel retraining should include routine, often postprandial, time on the toilet, as well as ample **positive reinforcement**. Bowel retraining can take up to 6 months for an effect, because chronic constipation results in bowel distention. Alternating remissions and stress-induced recurrences may persist for several years, but encopresis usually **resolves by early puberty**.

EXTERNALIZING DISORDERS

ATTENTION-DEFICIT HYPERACTIVITY DISORDER (ADHD)

Diagnostic and Clinical Features

Attention-deficit hyperactivity disorder (ADHD) is a neurobiological condition that results in significant impairment (see DSM-5). The diagnosis has aroused controversy among clinicians, teachers, parents, policymakers, and the media, with variations in opinion about its diagnosis, treatment, and causes.

Children and adolescents with ADHD experience **hyperactivity** (generalized behavioral overreactivity), **impulsivity** (inability to inhibit behaviors driven by impulses), and **inattention** (inability to maintain focused attention). Key diagnostic features include onset of symptoms and related impairment **before 12 years** of age, and symptoms of at least **6 months duration**. The symptoms must cause impairment in at least **two different settings** (e.g., at home and in school) and be maladaptive and inappropriate for the child's developmental age. Previously, ADHD was referred to as "hyperactivity," "hyperkinetic syndrome," and "attention deficit disorder." DSM-5 specifies three subtypes: combined type (criteria are met for both inattention and hyperactivity-impulsivity), predominantly inattentive type, and predominantly hyperactive-impulsive type (see DSM-5). The predominantly inattentive type is similar to the entity the DSM-III described in 1980 as "attention deficit disorder" (ADD). Children with predominantly inattentive type ADHD, sometimes described as "daydreamers" or "spacey," tend to have fewer conduct and behavior problems and, therefore, are less likely to be seen in treatment. The DSM-5 modifies the (B) criterion from symptoms present prior to age 7 years to symptoms present prior to age 12 years. Additionally, DSM-5 requires that symptoms are not solely a manifestation of oppositional behavior, defiance, hostility, or failure to understand tasks or instructions. The DSM-5 allows older adolescents and adults (age 17 and older) to have only five (rather than six) symptoms of either inattention or hyperactivity and impulsivity for the diagnosis of ADHD.

Making the diagnosis requires **collateral** information from adults (i.e., parents and teachers), as well as careful clinical examination. In disruptive behavior disorders, self-reports are often discrepant with (and suggest less severity than) caregiver reports. Unlike the diagnosis of internalizing disorders, the diagnosis of disruptive behavior disorders is more valid when based on adult reports. Reports of parents and teachers are often concordant, but symptoms and impairment can vary with the structure and requirements of the environment. Symptoms are more likely to be noted in settings where specific tasks are required of the child.

Structured rating scales have been used to identify cases of ADHD on the basis of cutoff points that deviate from normality. Scales such as the Conners' Teacher Rating Scale and the Vanderbilt ADHD Teacher Rating Scale have been shown to be highly correlated with more definitive structured diagnostic interviews. The use of standardized scales from caregivers and teachers coupled with clinical evaluation is the best diagnostic approach. Neuropsychological tests (such as the Continuous Performance Test) are useful in research and, sometimes, diagnostic corroboration. They are, however, neither necessary nor sufficient diagnostically.

In July of 2013, The U.S. Food and Drug Administration (FDA) approved the Neuropsychiatric EEG-Based Assessment Aid (NEBA) System to help diagnose ADHD in children and adolescents aged 6 to 17 years. Children and adolescents with ADHD have been shown to have a higher theta wave–to–beta wave ratio than those who do not have the disorder. The NEBA can be used to calculate that ratio and, together with medical and psychological assessment, results can confirm a diagnosis of ADHD or indicate further testing.

ADHD is frequently comorbid with other psychiatric disorders. Language and learning problems are present in 25% to 35% of patients with ADHD. The impairment in interpersonal, academic, and occupational functioning associated with ADHD can result in low self-esteem, and up to one-third of children with ADHD have a depressive disorder.

Etiology

ADHD is a heterogeneous syndrome, and its precise etiology remains unknown. A family history of ADHD, learning disorders, conduct disorder, antisocial personality disorder, and substance use disorders are often present in individuals with ADHD. Twin studies have shown the **heritability** of ADHD to be 76%, and at least seven genes are associated with ADHD.

Environmental risks include **low birth weight, perinatal complications** (e.g., prolonged maternal labor, low Apgar scores at 1 minute, antepartum hemorrhage), **traumatic brain injury, maternal smoking during pregnancy, and early deprivation**. Studies of association between dietary factors (e.g., sugars, preservatives, additives, dyes) and ADHD have been inconclusive. Children exposed to lead are at increased risk of hyperactivity and inattention.

Ultimately, dysfunction in the **prefrontal cortex** is thought to impair "executive functioning" such as planning, organizing, and controlling impulses. Imaging studies have demonstrated anatomical differences (e.g., in frontal lobe volume, symmetry of the caudate nucleus, and volume of the cerebellar vermis) in areas of the brain associated with executive functioning, and these differences tend to be more prominent in subjects who have not received treatment than in those who have received long-term medication treatment. Multiple neurotransmitter systems are involved in ADHD, including most notably those mediated by norepinephrine and dopamine.

Treatment and Prognosis

Long-term studies demonstrate that a majority (60%-85%) of children with ADHD continue to suffer with the disorder during their teenage years, although hyperactivity tends to lessen. Most individuals have fewer symptoms as they enter adulthood, but 40% of 18- to 20-year-olds who grew up with ADHD still meet full diagnostic criteria, and 90% have at least five symptoms of ADHD. While many individuals with ADHD learn coping strategies that decrease impairment over time, adults with a childhood history of ADHD have higher rates of injuries, accidents, employment and marital difficulties, and antisocial and criminal behavior. The National Comorbidity Survey Replication estimated the adult rate of ADHD to be 4.4%.

Psychostimulants are the first-line treatment of ADHD (see Pharmacotherapy). Atomoxetine is a nonstimulant, noradrenergic reuptake inhibitor that has been shown to be superior to placebo in the treatment of ADHD and has FDA approval for the treatment of ADHD in children, adolescents, and adults. Additionally, two long-acting alpha-2-adrenergic agonists, guanfacine XR (Intuniv) and clonidine XR (Kapvay), have been FDA approved for the treatment of ADHD and for augmentation of a stimulant in the treatment of ADHD. Other nonstimulant medications that are used when first-line approaches are unsuccessful, though not FDA approved for this indication, include bupropion, tricyclic antidepressants, and short-acting alpha-2-adrenergic agonists (i.e., clonidine, guanfacine).

Effective psychosocial interventions for ADHD include individual psychotherapy, educational interventions, and family interventions. **Behavior therapies** that reinforce positive behaviors and extinguish negative behaviors can alleviate some symptoms of ADHD. Educational approaches must take into consideration the possibility of a comorbid learning disorder and facilitate an environment that fosters unique learning styles. Parent management training can assist otherwise effective parents in the sometimes challenging parenting of children with ADHD. A National Institute of Mental Health (NIMH)-funded study found, however, that subjects randomized to medication treatment only had better outcomes than those randomized to psychosocial or community treatment only, and that the combination of medication and psychosocial treatment fared no better than medication only (MTA Cooperative Group 1999).

OPPOSITIONAL DEFIANT DISORDER (ODD)

Diagnostic and Clinical Features

Children with oppositional defiant disorder (ODD) have a recurrent pattern of **disobedient, defiant, negativistic, and argumentative behaviors toward authority figures** that is more intense and frequent than would be expected for a child of similar chronological or developmental age (see DSM-5). Unlike patients with conduct disorder, there is no serious violation of others' rights. Children with ODD can be stubborn, aggressive, and challenging, particularly with parents, but also with teachers. Children with ODD may prefer forfeiting a toy or privilege over losing a battle or argument. They can frustrate and exhaust parents, who may then relinquish all efforts at discipline or resort to excessively punitive discipline.

Etiology

Brain imaging studies have found abnormalities in regions that mediate reason, judgment, and impulse control. Psychosocial factors likely include inconsistent methods of discipline, lack of structure and limit setting, limited time with parents, and exposure to abuse or community violence.

Treatment and Prognosis

In the majority of children with ODD, symptoms improve over time, especially with appropriate interventions. About one-third of children with ODD go on to develop conduct disorder, and as many as 10% will ultimately develop antisocial personality disorder. Early-onset ODD in particular is associated with later conduct disorder, ADHD, mood disorders, and anxiety disorders.

Psychosocial interventions, including **problem-solving skills training** and **parent management training**, are first-line treatments and should be consistent, enduring, and coordinated between home and school. Psychotropic medication is generally reserved for the treatment of comorbid and exacerbating disorders such as ADHD or a mood disorder.

CONDUCT DISORDER (CD)

Diagnostic and Clinical Features

Children with conduct disorder demonstrate a persistent pattern of behavior that violates the rights of others as well as social norms or rules. Diagnostically, there are four main categories: (1) aggression toward people and animals, including bullying, fighting, and cruelty; (2) destruction of property, including fire setting; (3) deceitfulness or theft, including lying, "conning," stealing, and breaking into homes; and (4) serious violation of rules, which includes failure to adhere to social norms and expectations (see DSM-5). Children and adolescents with CD are at increased risk of school dropout and failure, adult unemployment, injury due to physical altercations, sexually transmitted disease, and substance use disorders.

Childhood-onset CD is diagnosed if at least one criterion for CD is present before age 10 years. It is often preceded by a diagnosis of ODD and is frequently comorbid with ADHD. More closely associated with physical aggression, impaired peer relationships, and later antisocial personality disorder, childhood-onset CD has a **poorer prognosis**. Low IQ and family history of antisocial personality disorder also negatively affect the long-term prognosis.

"Limited prosocial emotions" is specified when an individual persistently displays over at least 12 months in multiple settings and relationships at least two of the following characteristics: (1) lack of remorse or guilt; (2) callousness or lack of empathy; (3) absence of concern about performance; and (4) shallow or deficient affect.

Posttraumatic stress disorder and a history of abuse are often comorbid with CD, especially in youth in the juvenile justice system. Learning disorders are often comorbid. Mood disorders may be comorbid, and episodes can exacerbate CD. Anxiety disorders are common, especially in postpubertal females. Substance use disorders can exacerbate impulsivity and aggression and impair judgment.

Etiology

CD likely results from an interaction of genetic and neurobiological predisposition (e.g., temperamental type, psychiatric morbidity, resilience) and environmental exposure (e.g., abuse, parental rejection, loss of primary caregiver).

Differential Diagnosis of Externalizing Disorders

There is significant comorbidity among the externalizing, or disruptive behavior, disorders. Over half to three-quarters of children and adolescents with ADHD have comorbid ODD, and up to 50% of children with CD also suffer from ADHD. The hyperactive/impulsive subtype of ADHD can be difficult to differentiate from ODD, particularly because ODD is more likely to occur in families with a history of ADHD, as well as substance use disorders and mood disorders.

The hyperactive/impulsive subtype of ADHD can be difficult to differentiate from ODD, but children with ADHD fail to conform to requests of others, specifically in situations that require sustained attention or sitting still. Depressive and bipolar disorders can generate irritability and defiant behavior and, when explanatory, preclude the diagnosis of ODD. DMDD is characterized by more frequent, severe, and chronic temper outbursts than ODD and, like other mood disorders, trumps the diagnosis of ODD. Children and adolescents with both CD and ODD conflict with authority figures, but behaviors of ODD are less severe than those of CD and exclude aggression toward people and animals, destruction of property, and patterned theft or deceit. Furthermore, ODD is characterized by emotional dysregulation, but CD is not. Anxiety disorders (e.g., social anxiety disorder, separation anxiety disorder) should be considered because youngsters' attempts to avoid anxiogenic situations not infrequently take the form of oppositional and defiant behavior. What differentiates CD from ODD, ADHD, mood disorders, and intermittent explosive disorder (IED) are, respectively, (1) aggression toward individuals or animals (ODD), (2) violation of societal norms or the rights of others (ADHD),

(3) conduct problems without concurrent emotional disturbance (mood disorders), and (4) premeditated, as opposed to only impulsive, aggression (IED).

The differentiation of ADHD from bipolar disorder can be complex. A late and abrupt onset of ADHD symptoms is more suggestive of substance use disorders and mood disorders (see Figure 15.2). Consideration of schizophrenia or other psychotic disorder is necessary.

Treatment and Prognosis

Although adolescent-onset CD is more often associated with gang activity, it is more likely to respond to therapeutic interventions. Even with psychiatric comorbidity and involvement in the juvenile justice system, many adolescents with CD adjust to adulthood successfully. In addition to onset in adolescence, better premorbid social skills and positive peer relationships are favorable prognostic indicators.

Treatment is multidisciplinary and multimodal. Because children and adolescents with CD may underestimate or underreport symptoms and only reluctantly cooperate with both assessment and treatment, the involvement of caregivers, school personnel, and other relevant parties (e.g., the juvenile justice system) is critical.

Psychosocial treatments develop communication and problem-solving skills and enhance impulse control and anger management. Family-focused treatments, such as parent management training, positively reinforce acceptable social behavior and decrease power struggles between parents and their affected child. Based on systems theory, multisystemic therapy involves extensive contact between the therapist and the youth's various environments, including home and school.

Pharmacotherapy should target comorbid disorders and aggression. Assessment resulting in appropriate identification and treatment can be critical. For example, individuals with CD and ADHD have been shown to be less aggressive when the comorbid ADHD is treated with stimulant medications. Absent another disorder, aggression that is refractory to psychosocial interventions can be symptomatically targeted with mood stabilizers and antipsychotic medications.

ADDITIONAL DISORDERS

SCHIZOPHRENIA

While psychotic disorders only rarely begin in childhood, parental worries about psychosis are more common. A parent may bring a child with worrisome behaviors, thoughts, or perceptions to clinical attention with the question, "Could this mean that my child is becoming psychotic?"

Diagnostic and Clinical Features

Children and adolescents with schizophrenia present with a range of "**positive**" **symptoms**, including hallucinations, delusions, and disorganization in thought and behavior, as well as "**negative**" **symptoms**, including affective flattening, alogia, and avolition (see DSM-5). Presenting problems that raise the specter of schizophrenia must be differentiated from imaginary friends and fantasy figures. Establishing the presence of positive psychotic symptoms in children can be relatively challenging, and the developmental context must be considered. For example, preschool and early school-age children, who are in a prelogical stage of cognitive development, are given to egocentrism, magical thinking, and an active fantasy life often populated with imaginary friends. Even once children have progressed cognitively, fantasy remains a characteristic defense, especially in stressful settings (e.g., during transitions in school, in the midst of family discord, or, for some children, in a darkened room at bedtime). Organization of thought and behavior, functioning across domains, and the range and appropriateness of affect are a few features by which these normative and prognostically benign phenomena can be distinguished from psychotic disorders.

Diagnostic criteria for schizophrenia in children and adolescents are largely the same as for adults (see Chapter 4, Schizophrenia and Other Psychotic Disorders), with one notable exception: failure to realize an expected level of interpersonal, academic, or occupational functioning can suffice to meet the diagnostic criterion of dysfunction in children and adolescents, rather than deterioration in social or occupational function. However, it is not unusual that childhood schizophrenia is, in fact, characterized by significant **deterioration in functioning** at school and with family and friends.

The onset of schizophrenia in children or adolescents is most often pubertal or peripubertal and tends to be insidious, with prominent negative symptoms. Acute onset before 9 years of age is exceedingly rare. Among children who develop schizophrenia, about half have early abnormalities in social, cognitive, language, or motor development and low-average to borderline IQ. In fact, approximately one-third of children who develop schizophrenia also have an autism spectrum disorder. Features that may reflect a **prodromal** phase of schizophrenia include attenuated positive symptoms (e.g., unusual thought content, suspiciousness, paranoia, grandiosity, perceptual abnormalities, or disorganized communication), brief intermittent psychotic symptoms, and significant decline in functioning along with heightened genetic risk (i.e., having either a first-degree relative with a psychotic disorder, or a diagnosis of schizotypal personality disorder). Usually the phase is declared "prodromal" in retrospect, only after the diagnostic criteria for schizophrenia have been met. The prodromal phase of schizophrenia may last anywhere from days to months or even years.

Differential Diagnosis

Autistic spectrum disorder (ASD) should be considered in the differential diagnosis of childhood-onset schizophrenia (see Figure 15.3). Differentiation of schizophrenia and ASD is complicated by similarities in phenomenology (e.g., social impairment, inappropriate affect, unusual or impoverished thought content, illogical thinking) and observed comorbidity (as many as one-third of children with schizophrenia also meet criteria for ASD). In the context of ASD, prominent delusions or hallucinations must be present for at least a month to make the additional diagnosis of schizophrenia. Helpful in their differentiation are age of onset (ASD typically begins before 5 years of age, whereas early-onset schizophrenia tends to be peripubertal or pubertal) and early development (deficits in infancy are the rule in ASD, whereas about half of children with schizophrenia have normal early development).

Assessment of mood symptoms during the initial evaluation of a child or adolescent with psychotic disturbance can be challenging. Up to one-half of children with **major depressive disorder** present with hallucinations, and adolescent-onset **bipolar disorder** often presents with mania complicated by psychotic features. It can, therefore, be difficult to ascertain the relative durations of affective and active-phase psychotic disturbances.

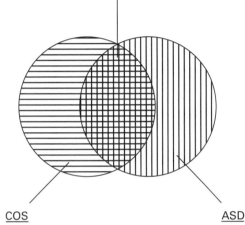

Shared Features of
COS and ASD

Social impairment (e.g., lack of reciprocity or
motivation to share experience)
Decreased spontaneity of speech or alogia
Inappropriate affect
Impoverished or unusual thought content
Illogical thinking
+/– Cognitive impairment

COS

Positive symptoms
(e.g., hallucinations & delusions)
Age of onset typically peripubertal
Half of children have normal early
development

ASD

Age of onset & developmental
delays in first few years of life
Repetitious & stereotyped
behavior
Strong preference for sameness

FIGURE 15.3 Childhood-Onset Schizophrenia (COS) & Autism Spectrum Disorder (ASD)

Evaluation over time may be most useful in their differentiation from schizophrenia as well as **schizoaffective disorder**.

Posttraumatic stress disorder and **obsessive-compulsive disorder** should also be considered. Children with posttraumatic stress disorder can act or feel as if traumatic events are recurring with psychotic intensity. Furthermore, they may have dissociative experiences (depersonalization, derealization) and a constricted range of affect, both suggestive of psychotic disorders. In childhood obsessive-compulsive disorder, intrusive thoughts and images, as well as ritualistic behaviors, can be challenging to differentiate from psychotically disturbed cognition, perception, and behavior, particularly because insight into the symptomatic nature of the obsessions and compulsions is less common in children.

Although not commonly diagnosed before 18 years of age, certain **personality disorders**, or at least their precursors, should be considered in the differential diagnosis of childhood-onset schizophrenia. Schizotypal, schizoid, paranoid, and borderline personality disorders in adulthood may have antecedent psychotic-like symptoms in childhood.

Visual hallucinations, which are more common in childhood-onset schizophrenia, necessitate ruling out **disturbances in sleep** (e.g., narcolepsy, medication-induced sleep disturbances) that are associated with relatively benign hypnagogic or hypnopompic hallucinations (i.e., those occurring immediately before falling asleep, or just after wakening, respectively).

Finally, a range of neurological, endocrinological, metabolic, autoimmune, infectious, and toxic causes should be ruled out with a **neurological examination** and other tests as clinically indicated. These causes include but are not limited to seizure disorders; congenital, mass, and vascular abnormalities of the central nervous system; delirium; hypothyroidism; Wilson's disease; Huntington's disease; lipid storage disorders; systemic lupus erythematosus; HIV, encephalitis, and meningitis; and encephalopathies due to illicit drugs, prescription drugs (especially corticosteroids, anticholinergics, amphetamines, and methylphenidate), solvents, heavy metals, and other environmental toxins.

Etiology

Recent studies of childhood-onset schizophrenia have found genetic abnormalities, including 22q11 deletion (velocardiofacial syndrome), X-chromosome abnormalities (trisomy, atypical Turner's syndrome), and translocations. Some children with schizophrenia have rare copy-number variants on genotyping.

Treatment and Prognosis

Both psychosocial and pharmacological interventions are generally indicated in the treatment of schizophrenia in children and adolescents, as they are in adults. Useful adjuncts might include psychoeducation for the child or adolescent and family, parent support, family therapy, neuropsychological assessment, and appropriate special educational services. The course of illness is phasic, as it is with adults. In general, childhood-onset schizophrenia has a poorer prognosis than adult-onset illness.

The treatment of a presumptive prodrome to psychosis is controversial. An association has been observed between longer duration of untreated psychosis and worse prognosis, but causality is unclear. In other words, untreated psychosis could lead to worse prognosis, or other factors associated with worse prognosis—for example, an insidious onset—could be associated with delays in treatment. At this time, there is inadequate evidence to support the treatment of individuals with attenuated psychotic features with antipsychotic medications. Children and adolescents at heightened risk for or presumed to be prodromal to schizophrenia are best treated supportively, not preemptively.

PERSONALITY DISORDERS

Diagnostic and Clinical Features

The diagnosis of personality disorders (see Chapter 8, Personality Disorders) in the pediatric population is controversial. Because children and adolescents are developing both psychologically and neurologically, personality is rarely as consolidated or as fixed as it is in adults. The diagnostic criteria in the pediatric and adult populations are the same, with two exceptions: a **1-year duration** is required to make the diagnosis of a personality disorder in children and adolescents, and antisocial personality disorder cannot be diagnosed before 18 years of age; children and adolescents with traits of antisocial personality disorder are diagnosed with conduct disorder. Personality disorders in adolescents may overlap more broadly than in adulthood. For example, adolescents with a cluster B borderline personality disorder may also have schizotypal personality disorder, which is classified in cluster A.

Differential Diagnosis

Mood disorders, anxiety disorders (especially OCD and PTSD), and psychotic disorders should be considered. Additionally, any concern about abuse or neglect should be thoroughly evaluated.

Etiology, Treatment, and Prognosis

Given the significant role of the social group in adolescence, contagion by and social reinforcement of problem behaviors (e.g., nonsuicidal self-injury) can play a role in the etiology of adolescent-onset personality disorders. Psychotherapies that are effective in adults may be effective in adolescents. Dialectical behavior therapy (DBT) has been adapted for adolescents with chronic suicidal ideation, self-harming behaviors, or borderline personality disorder. It is difficult to predict the persistence of personality disorder features into adulthood.

PSYCHOSOCIAL TREATMENTS

Working with Parents

Working effectively with the parents of children and adolescents in psychiatric treatment is of the utmost importance. In order to engage parents as collaborators in treatment, the physician must provide **psychoeducation** about the diagnosis, therapeutic options, and prognosis. The physician may discuss genetic risk posed by the family psychiatric history, explore changes in family structure (e.g., a divorce) as important psychosocial stressors, or address aspects of parenting that exacerbate or perpetuate presenting problems. During these discussions, great care must be taken to **avoid blaming parents** for their child's difficulties. Frequently, parents are already struggling with feelings of incompetence, frustration, self-blame, and guilt. If inadvertently exacerbated, these feelings can compromise the effectiveness and viability of their child's treatment. The surest way the physician can circumvent this risk is to engage parents proactively in the treatment.

Such engagement begins with the psychiatric assessment, in which parents are crucial informants, and continues throughout treatment, in which parents are essential collaborators. The extent of parental involvement in treatment varies. For example, parent management training, an effective treatment for children and preadolescents with disruptive behavior disorders, involves conducting the therapeutic work exclusively with parents. In parent–child interaction therapy, an effective treatment for children with a variety of behavioral and emotional problems, most of the therapeutic work occurs with the parent and child simultaneously, and none occurs with the child alone. Treatments such as cognitive-behavioral therapy and interpersonal therapy for adolescents principally work individually with the child or adolescent, yet both incorporate parents to varying degrees.

Even psychoanalytically oriented treatment of children and adolescents, perhaps the quintessentially individual therapeutic modality, must involve parents. Incorporating parents into therapeutic play with children offers important benefits: the physician gains an invaluable window into the world of the child, in which the quality of parent–child interaction factors prominently; and the parents gain an appreciation for the mind of their child, an improved capacity to play with their child, and an expanded ability to promote their child's development and recovery. In the psychoanalytically oriented treatment of adolescents, parents may not be included in many (or any) sessions with the adolescent, but the physician will still communicate with the parents about the goals and progress of treatment while respecting the adolescent's confidentiality.

Parents' ambivalence about their children's treatment can make working with the parents challenging. While parents desperately want help for their child, they often have a number of concerns: they do not want their child labeled or stigmatized with a psychiatric disorder; they do not want to feel supplanted in their capacity to help; and they do not want to be found at fault.

Not infrequently, parents of children and adolescents in psychiatric treatment struggle themselves with mental illness. In such cases, parents may need to be referred for their own treatment. Research has clearly shown that the effective treatment of maternal depression significantly reduces the burden of mental illness in children (Weissman et al. 2006). Particularly when parents lack insight into their own difficulties, making such a referral can be a delicate task.

Cognitive-behavioral therapy, interpersonal therapy, and psychodynamic psychotherapy are the most common and effective psychotherapies currently recommended for children and adolescents.

Cognitive-Behavioral Therapy (CBT)

CBT has been found to be an efficacious treatment in children and adolescents for separation anxiety disorder, social anxiety disorder, generalized anxiety disorder, specific phobias, panic disorder, obsessive-compulsive disorder, posttraumatic stress disorder, major depressive disorder, and dysthymic disorder (Verdeli et al. 2006). In more severe cases, the combination of CBT and medication should be considered. To engage meaningfully in CBT, patients should be verbal and of at least average intelligence, given that many therapeutic interventions are made in the cognitive sphere. It is also useful if the child or adolescent has some insight into the problems (e.g., depressed mood, anxious avoidance) and motivation to change. Patients with significant learning or language disabilities or with a borderline or lower IQ may be more amenable to behavioral interventions. Behavior therapy has been employed in the treatment of children and adolescents with intellectual disability, autism spectrum disorder, attention-deficit hyperactivity disorder, tic disorders, feeding disorders, elimination disorders, oppositional defiant disorder, and conduct disorder.

The process of CBT with children and adolescents parallels that with adults: psychoeducation about the working diagnosis is provided in a medical model; the triad of thoughts, behaviors, and feelings is introduced and reinforced; the effectiveness of CBT is explained, instilling hope of change and enhancing motivation for the therapeutic work; and adaptive coping skills are developed collaboratively. Those skills include recognizing and rating feelings (i.e., "mood monitoring") and somatic symptoms (e.g., fatigue, stomachache, tachypnea, nausea, headache); gaining awareness of thoughts (e.g., "automatic thoughts," "core beliefs"); recognizing behaviors and behavioral inclinations (e.g., avoidance); learning diaphragmatic breathing and other methods of affect regulation; evaluating the evidence for and effects of negative (distorted, maladaptive) thoughts; entertaining alternative thoughts; effective problem solving; and considering and choosing behavioral alternatives (e.g., "behavioral activation," progressive exposure, and response prevention). Therapeutic work is pursued actively and transparently, both during and between sessions (with modeling, role-play, and homework). Treatment is usually relatively time-limited (e.g., 16–20 weekly sessions), with follow-up or "booster" sessions periodically as needed.

In several ways, however, the process of CBT with children and adolescents differs from that with adults. First, **parents are frequently involved**, actively and collaboratively. They may play a role in the completion of intersession homework and are often "managers" of rewards and punishments. Second, therapeutic techniques and foci must be **geared to the developmental age** of the patient. For example, one efficacious manualized CBT for anxiety in children ages 8–13, the *Coping Cat* (Kendall 1992), was subsequently modified for patients ages 14–17, in the *C.A.T. Project* (Kendall et al. 2002). Whereas the *Coping Cat* engages children and, perhaps less successfully, young adolescents in the transformation of a "scaredy cat" into a "coping cat," particularly around fears of separation and animals, the *C.A.T. Project* takes leave of the feline character, affords the adolescent autonomy in both naming and directing the treatment, and locates adolescent anxiety more fittingly in the academic and social domains.

Interpersonal Therapy

Interpersonal therapy has been developed for the treatment of **depressed adolescents** (IPT-A) and has been shown to be effective. Treatment is time-limited (e.g., 12 weekly sessions), usually involves telephone contact between sessions, and frequently includes parents. IPT-A comprises three phases of treatment: initial, middle, and termination.

In the initial phase, the physician confirms the diagnosis of a depressive disorder, provides **psychoeducation** about the diagnosis and treatment options for both the adolescent and his or her parents, conducts an **inventory** of significant **interpersonal relationships**, and identifies the problem areas that will focus the treatment. IPT-A is designed to address the same **four problem areas** that IPT addresses with adults: grief, interpersonal role disputes, role transitions, and interpersonal deficits. In adolescence, disputes are sometimes pronounced in the process of separating and individuating from parents (i.e., transitioning between developmental stages), peer conflicts can take on particular significance given the normal adolescent task of developing identity in the peer group setting, and role transitions may prove particularly challenging with changes in family structure (e.g., separation, divorce, remarriage) that are associated with depression.

In the middle phase of IPT-A, the physician helps the depressed adolescent to **develop strategies for negotiating interpersonal difficulties** more successfully. Effective therapeutic techniques include expressing feelings, clarifying expectations in relationships, interpersonal problem solving, and role-playing with the therapist various options for interpersonal interaction. Sometimes parents participate in the middle phase of treatment (e.g., by discussing a dispute in session). Given the developmental thrust in adolescence toward autonomy, the transparency with which these therapeutic techniques advance the overarching treatment goal of developing a skill set for negotiating relationships more effectively is enormously helpful in engaging adolescents in treatment.

In the final, or termination, phase of IPT-A, the physician helps the adolescent to consolidate the skills learned and applied in the middle phase, to assess depressive symptoms and consider the need for ongoing treatment, and to appreciate a greater sense of interpersonal mastery.

Psychodynamic Psychotherapy

In psychodynamic psychotherapy the mode of communication varies with developmental age. Younger children have relatively undeveloped verbal skills and tend to reveal and explore the reality of their lives and the workings of their minds more through action than through words. As such, **play and drawing** are useful and appropriate therapeutic media with young children. Play and drawing also permit "displacement" of anxiety, as the expression of fear, worry, or conflict in a dollhouse or a drawing can be far less threatening. The physician will often clarify, confront, and interpret entirely within the play or drawing. Attempts to link the material of play or drawing explicitly and verbally to the life or mind of the child are undertaken selectively, as time and cognitive development permit. Therapeutic change occurs by working with unconscious material in play. With school-age and preadolescent children, games are often incorporated into the increasingly verbal therapeutic process as a useful medium for exploring themes of competition and the pursuit of mastery. Adolescent patients are usually able to work verbally, with progressively less "displacement" of anxiety-provoking material.

Psychodynamic therapists of children and adolescents will offer reassurance and guidance, thus functioning not only as transference objects but also as developmental objects. The therapist engenders change not only by interpreting transference and, thereby, opening up a new way of relating, but also by serving as a new object who facilitates the patient's active developmental course.

PHARMACOTHERAPY

Recommending psychiatric medication for a child or adolescent is a serious clinical decision, and the physician should be clear about indications and therapeutic goals. It is important to assess the patient's and family's attitudes, beliefs, and fears about psychopharmacological treatment. It is also important to educate the child or adolescent and family about how the medication works, as well as about potential therapeutic and adverse effects. When starting psychopharmacological treatment with an adolescent, possible teratogenic effects and the use of contraception should be discussed.

Until recently, most of the information about prescribing psychiatric medications for children and adolescents was based on information derived from clinical trials and experience with adults. Fortunately, much more is known about the effectiveness and safety of these medications in the pediatric population as a result of recent advances in research.

Selective Serotonin Reuptake Inhibitors (SSRIs)

SSRIs are the primary agents used for pediatric **depressive** and **anxiety** disorders. **Fluoxetine** is FDA approved for depression in children 8–17 years of age, and **escitalopram** is FDA approved for adolescents 12–17 years of age. No other SSRIs currently have an FDA indication for pediatric depression. Fluoxetine, sertraline, fluvoxamine, and clomipramine have FDA indications for the treatment of pediatric obsessive-compulsive disorder. Despite their smaller average body size, children and adolescents have considerable hepatic capacity to metabolize these compounds. Therefore, therapeutic doses are often similar to those used in adults.

The evidence available from various studies of SSRIs in depressed or anxious children and adolescents has suggested a small increased risk of suicidal thinking. Although the data do not clearly support or refute this concern, the FDA has placed a warning on antidepressant product labels. The warning highlights the need for careful monitoring of worsening depression and the **emergence of suicidality** in children treated with these medications. For children and adolescents started on antidepressant medications, the FDA has recommended weekly visits for 4 weeks, then visits every other week for 4 weeks and, subsequently, monthly visits. Once symptoms of depression and anxiety are in remission, treatment should be maintained for 1 year, after which a medication-free trial, at a low-stress time, can be considered.

Serotonin-Norepineprhine Reuptake Inhibitors (SNRIs)

Several studies have demonstrated efficacy of extended-release venlafaxine in the treatment of pediatric **anxiety** disorders. Venlafaxine has shown efficacy in adolescents with **depressive** disorders, but mixed results in children. Changes in vital signs and the emergence of suicidal ideation and behaviors must be carefully monitored.

Bupropion

A study of bupropion in adolescents with **comorbid major depressive disorder** and **attention-deficit hyperactivity disorder** has shown efficacy in treating the symptoms of both disorders. Bupropion's profile of adverse effects, including an increased risk of seizure at total daily doses exceeding 300 mg, is the same in children and adolescents as it is in adults.

Tricyclic Antidepressants (TCAs)

TCAs have demonstrated efficacy in the treatment of pediatric **anxiety disorders**, but they are used only when first-line options (e.g., SSRIs) have been ineffective. They are not efficacious in the treatment of pediatric depression. Dosing is based on body weight, and serum concentrations must be monitored. Cases reports have described sudden unexplained death in children prescribed desipramine for attention-deficit hyperactivity disorder. Consequently, **serial ECGs** are recommended for children treated with TCAs.

Stimulants

Methylphenidate and amphetamine preparations are equally efficacious, **first-line** treatment for children with attention deficit hyperactivity disorder. Immediate-release preparations require multiple administrations during the day. A variety of longer-acting preparations can be administered once daily and improve adherence to treatment. Dosing schedules are based on age and weight. Dose response is, however, highly individual. Once treatment has been initiated, the dose should be increased every 1 to 3 weeks until target symptoms have subsided or the maximum recommended has been reached. At each dose adjustment, symptoms should be rated by parents, teachers, and the patient.

Common adverse effects include **decreased appetite, weight loss, insomnia, and headache**. Less common adverse effects include tics, irritability, and affective lability. Low doses of clonidine, guanfacine, bupropion, trazodone, or an antihistamine can be used alternatively or adjunctively. Because the risk of sudden death posed by stimulant medications remains unclear, the Pediatric Advisory Committee of the FDA has considered adding a warning label to stimulant medications. Prior to initiating treatment with any stimulant medication, the physician should complete a thorough **cardiac history** of the child or adolescent and family. If symptoms or history reveal possible or known cardiac disease, nonstimulant treatment options should be considered, or the cardiac risks posed by a stimulant should be further characterized in collaboration with a pediatric cardiologist.

Antipsychotics

Antipsychotics are used for the treatment of schizophrenia, bipolar disorder, severe tic disorders, and aggression (particularly in autism spectrum disorder) in children and adolescents. Second-generation (atypical) antipsychotics have largely supplanted the first-generation (typical) compounds as treatment for children and adolescents. Aripiprazole is FDA approved for the treatment of schizophrenia and manic or mixed affective episodes in adolescents; risperidone, for the treatment of schizophrenia, irritability in autism spectrum disorder, and manic or mixed affective episodes in adolescents. Depending on the target symptoms, doses vary but are, in general, higher for acute psychosis and lower for tics. Side effects are similar across age groups. Those of greatest concern include **extrapyramidal effects** (i.e., acute or tardive dystonia, dyskinesia, and akathisia), **sedation, cognitive slowing, hyperprolactinemia** (resulting in gynecomastia in boys, galactorrhea or amenorrhea in girls), **QTc prolongation** (particularly with ziprasidone), and **metabolic syndrome** (obesity, hypertension, glucose intolerance, and dyslipidemia). The following parameters should be assayed at baseline, at 3 months, and then annually: body mass index, waist circumference, fasting lipid panel, and fasting glucose.

Mood Stabilizers

First-line agents include traditional mood stabilizers such as **lithium** and **valproate**. Lithium is FDA approved for both acute treatment of mania and maintenance treatment of bipolar disorder in patients 12 years of age and older. The combination of a traditional mood stabilizer and an atypical antipsychotic, or two traditional mood stabilizers, may be necessary in treatment-refractory cases.

Use of these medications requires careful monitoring, as in an adult population. Before initiation of treatment, baseline laboratory assessments that are tailored to specific adverse event concerns should be obtained, and they should be repeated over time during the course of treatment. Prior to the initiation of lithium, a complete blood count; urinalysis; thyroid function tests; blood urea nitrogen, creatinine, and serum calcium levels; ECG; and, in girls, a pregnancy test should be obtained. Subsequently, serum lithium level, thyroid function, and kidney function should be monitored every 3 to 6 months. For valproate, a baseline complete blood count, liver function tests, and, in girls, a pregnancy test should be obtained and then monitored every 3 to 6 months. Because of the risk of polycystic ovarian disease, girls receiving valproate should be carefully monitored for weight gain and disturbances in the menstrual cycle.

In open-label studies, **lamotrigine** has been efficacious in the treatment of adolescent bipolar disorder but carries a significant risk of Stevens-Johnson syndrome (it occurred in approximately 0.8 % in patients less than 16 years of age who received lamotrigine as adjunctive treatment of epilepsy).

Benzodiazepines

The efficacy and safety of benzodiazepines in the treatment of pediatric anxiety disorders and in the adjunctive treatment of pediatric major depressive disorder are unclear. Benzodiazepines are sometimes used to relieve somatic symptoms while another medication (e.g., SSRI) is titrated to therapeutic effect. The initial dose should be low, and close monitoring of tolerability is appropriate. Generally, side effects are similar to those in adults, but children may be more vulnerable to behavioral disinhibition when treated with these compounds.

REFERENCES CITED

Kendall, P. C. *Coping Cat Workbook*. Ardmore, PA: Workbook Publishing, 1992.

Kendall, P. C., M. Choudhury, J. Hudson, and A. Webb. *The C.A.T. Project Manual for the Cognitive Behavioral Treatment of Anxious Adolescents*. Ardmore, PA: Workbook Publishing, 2002.

March, J., S. Silva, S. Petrycki, J. Curry, K. Wells, J. Fairbank, B. Burns, M. Domino, S. McNulty, B. Vitiello, and J. Severe; Treatment for Adolescents with Depression Study (TADS) Team. Fluoxetine, cognitive-behavioral therapy, and their combination for adolescents with depression: Treatment for Adolescents with Depression Study (TADS) randomized controlled trial. *JAMA: Journal of the American Medical Association* 292:807–820, 2004.

MTA Cooperative Group. A 14-month randomized clinical trial of treatment strategies for attention-deficit/hyperactivity disorder. *Archives of General Psychiatry* 56:1073–1086, 1999.

Pediatric OCD Treatment Study (POTS) Team. Cognitive-behavior therapy, sertraline, and their combination for children and adolescents with obsessive-compulsive disorder. *JAMA: Journal of the American Medical Association* 292:1969–1976, 2004.

Verdeli, H., L. Mufson, L. Lee, and J. A. Keith. Review of evidence-based psychotherapies for pediatric mood and anxiety disorders. *Current Psychiatry Reviews* 2:395–421, 2006.

Walkup, J., A. M. Albano, J. Piacentini, B. Birmaher, S. N. Compton, J. T. Sherrill, G. S. Ginsburg, M. A. Rynn, J. McCracken, B. Waslick, S. Lyengar, J. S. March, and P. C. Kendall. Cognitive behavioral therapy, sertraline, or a combination in childhood anxiety. *New England Journal of Medicine* 359:2753–2766, 2008.

Weissman, M. M., D. J. Pilowsky, P. J. Wickramaratne, A. Talati, S. R. Wisniewski, M. Fava, C. W. Hughes, J. Garber, E. Malloy, C. A. King, G. Cerda, A. B. Sood, J. E. Alpert, M. H. Tivedi, and A. J. Rush; STAR*D-Child Team. Remissions in maternal depression and child psychopathology: a STAR*D-child report. *JAMA: Journal of the American Medical Association* 295:1389–1398, 2006.

Winnicott D. W. The squiggle technique. In McDermott, J. F., and S. I. Harrison, eds., *Psychiatric Treatment of the Child*. Lanham, MD: Jason Aronson Publisher, 1977.

SELECTED READINGS

Birmaher, B., and D. Brent. Practice parameter for the assessment and treatment of children and adolescents with depressive disorders. *Journal of the American Academy of Child and Adolescent Psychiatry* 46:1503–1526, 2007.

Cannon T. D., K. Cadenhead, B. Cornblass, S. W. Woods, J. Addington, E. Walder, L. J. Seidman, D. Perkinds, M. Tsuang, T. McGlashan, and R. Heinssen. Prediction of psychosis in youth at high clinical risk. *Archives of General Psychiatry* 65:28–37, 2008.

Connolly, S. D., and G. A. Bernstein. Practice parameter for the assessment and treatment of children and adolescents with anxiety disorders. *Journal of the American Academy of Child & Adolescent Psychiatry*, 46:267–283, 2007.

Corcoran, C., D. Malaspina, and L. Hercher. Prodromal interventions for schizophrenia vulnerability: the risks of being 'at risk'. *Schizophrenia Research* 73:173–184, 2005.

Correll, C. U., and H. Carlson. Endocrine and metabolic adverse effects of psychotropic medications in children and adolescents. *Journal of the American Academy of Child & Adolescent Psychiatry* 45:771–791, 2006.

Dawson, G. Early behavioral intervention, brain plasticity, and the prevention of autism spectrum disorder. *Development and Psychopathology* 20:775–803, 2008.

Greenhill, L., S. Pliszka, and M. Dulcan. Practice parameter for the use of stimulant medications in the treatment of children, adolescents, and adults. *Journal of the American Academy of Child & Adolescent Psychiatry* 41:526–623, 2002.

McCracken, J. T., J. T. McGough, B. Shah, et al. Research Units on Pediatric Psychopharmacology Autism Network. Risperidone in children with autism and serious behavioral problems. *New England Journal of Medicine* 347:314–321, 2002.

MTA Cooperative Group. Moderators and mediators of treatment response for children with attention-deficit/hyperactivity disorder: the multimodal treatment study of children with attention-deficit hyperactivity disorder. *Archives of General Psychiatry* 56:1088–1096, 1999.

Mufson, L, D. Moreau, and M. M. Weissman. *Interpersonal Psychotherapy for Depressed Adolescents*, 2nd ed. New York: Guilford Press, 2004.

Novick, K., and J. Novick. *Working with Parents Makes Therapy Work*. New York: Jason Aronson, 2005.

Peterson, B. S., and D. J. Cohen. The treatment of Tourette's syndrome: multimodal, developmental intervention. *Journal of Clinical Psychiatry* 59(Suppl 1):62–72, 1998.

Pliszka, S. Practice parameter for the assessment and treatment of children and adolescents with attention-deficit/hyperactivity disorder. *Journal of the American Academy of Child & Adolescent Psychiatry* 46:894–921, 2007.

Rapin, I., and R. Tuchman. What is new in autism? *Current Opinion in Neurology* 21:143–149, 2008.

Rapoport, J, A. Chavez, D. Greenstein, A. Addington, and N. Gogtay. Autism spectrum disorders and childhood-onset schizophrenia: clinical and biological contributions to a relation revisited. *Journal of the American Academy of Child and Adolescent Psychiatry* 48:10–18, 2009.

Rogers, S., and L. Vismara. Evidence-based comprehensive treatments for early autism. *Journal of Clinical Child and Adolescent Psychology* 37:8–38, 2008.

Shaywitz, B. A., K. R. Pugh, J. M. Fletcher, and S. S. Shaywitz. What cognitive and neurobiological studies have taught us about dyslexia. In Greenhill, L., ed. *Learning Disabilities: Implications for Psychiatric Treatment (Review of Psychiatry Series*, Oldham, J. M., and M. B. Riba, eds.) Washington, DC: American Psychiatric Publishing, 2000.

Wiener, J. M., and M. K. Dulcan, eds. *The American Psychiatric Publishing Textbook of Child and Adolescent Psychiatry*, 3rd ed. Washington, DC: American Psychiatric Press, 2004.

/// 16 /// Pharmacotherapy, ECT, and TMS

JESSICA ANN STEWART, L. MARK RUSSAKOFF, AND JONATHAN W. STEWART

Psychoactive medications have played a prominent role in psychiatric treatment for over 50 years, and there has been a virtual explosion of drugs available for treating psychiatric patients in the past 20 years (see Box 16.1). Pharmacotherapy is currently part of the recommended treatment for nearly all psychiatrically hospitalized patients. There is not always "better living through chemistry," however. As these agents do not directly address the psychosocial problems that cause, exacerbate, and result from psychiatric disturbances, psychopharmacology is only one component of an integrated treatment approach. At the same time, these new agents have broadened the range of problems for which psychiatrists have effective interventions and reduced the psychosocial costs of psychiatric disorders.

Before modern psychopharmacological agents became available, most patients with psychotic disorders were managed in long-term asylums, while nonpsychotic problems were either not treated or addressed with psychotherapy. As the timeline in Box 16.1 indicates, insulin coma was the first somatic treatment; its complexity and dangers limited its availability. Electroconvulsive therapy (ECT) was introduced next. While often effective, ECT was also problematic before the advent of modern anesthesia techniques. The first psychotropic medications were administered to psychotic inpatients who recovered sufficiently to be discharged, sometimes following decades of hospitalization. As physicians became experienced with these new medications, they began administering them to outpatients, sometimes preventing the need for hospitalization. These changes in psychiatric practice contributed to the emptying of state psychiatric hospitals in the 1960s and 1970s. They also enabled a shift from chronic, long-term hospitalization for the most severely ill to community and outpatient maintenance treatment that included psychotropic agents.

GENERAL PRINCIPLES

The first step in psychopharmacological intervention is to obtain a history in order to establish a firm diagnosis. While the diagnosis does not necessarily indicate a specific treatment, it does suggest a range of likely and unlikely candidate medications.

Once the diagnosis is established, the next step is for the physician to explain to the patient what the diagnosis entails and what treatment is recommended. This explanation

---

BOX 16.1

HISTORY OF SOMATIC TREATMENTS: TIMELINE OF "FIRSTS"

1927—Insulin coma

1937—Dextroamphetamine

1938—Electroconvulsive therapy (ECT)

1949—Lithium identified as antimanic

1952—First antipsychotic (chlorpromazine)

1954—Reserpine and meprobamate introduced in the United States

1956—First monoamine oxidase inhibitor (MAOI) (iproniazid)

1958—First tricyclic antidepressant (TCA) (imipramine)

1960—First benzodiazepine (chlordiazepoxide)

1967—Thioxanthenes and haloperidol introduced in the United States

1970—Lithium, carbamazepine, and valproic acid marketed in the United States

1982—First alternative to TCA and MAOI (trazodone)

1988—First selective serotonin reuptake inhibitor (SSRI) (fluoxetine) marketed in the United States

1989—First alternative to tardive dyskinesia-producing antipsychotic (clozapine)

1994—First serotonin/norepinephrine reuptake inhibitor (SNRI) (venlafaxine)

   —First non-benzodiazepine marketed for anxiety (buspirone)

1996—Mirtazapine introduced

2006—First transdermal antidepressant medication (selegiline)

---

begins the process of **informed consent** and should include the following elements: a description of what the patient can and cannot expect to occur with medication treatment, including any likely negative consequences; the likelihood of the treatment being helpful; the likely results if no medication is taken; the time frame in which improvement can be expected; anticipated changes in dosing; alternatives to the recommended treatment; the criteria for determining that the treatment is not effective; and what the next step would be.

The bottom line in treating patients with medications is **adherence**. Thus, it is an axiom of psychopharmacology that an unused treatment will not help. A corollary is that suboptimal treatment lessens the odds of benefit. Therefore, it is imperative to address adherence at the beginning of treatment, including the consequences of poor adherence on likelihood of benefit. Part of this education should be the time frame during which observable change can be expected. Many psychotropic agents are not effective immediately, often requiring weeks to months before maximal effects occur. Educating the patient about side effects and timing of improvement will help build a trusting relationship that, in turn, will contribute to adherence and allow an adequate test of the drug's ability to help during acute treatment and to maintain its effectiveness during later continuation and maintenance treatment. For example, benzodiazepines and stimulants are effective 30–60 minutes after ingestion and remain effective for some number of hours thereafter, and then the effects dissipate unless another dose is taken. So, the patient should know soon after the first use whether that dose of that medication will help. With antidepressant medications, by contrast, improvement is typically not seen for several weeks after initiation of treatment, although side effects usually result from initial doses.

Patients are often ambivalent about taking medications, especially for mental and emotional problems. They may worry, "if I take medication, there is something wrong with me" (implying that if they do not take the medication they do *not* have something wrong with them). While logically the patient has the disorder regardless of whether medication is prescribed, exploration of such **emotional resistance** to accepting the need for treatment is often an important part of the initial treatment planning process. Absent this discussion, some patients will find taking a pill to relieve their symptoms a "bitter pill to swallow," and may either not take the medication or only take it too sporadically for it to provide benefit. Such patients may then inappropriately conclude that "medications do not work." Attention to the patient's concepts, concerns, attitudes, and hesitancies about taking the medication will engender adherence and better allow both patient and physician to discover which treatment will be most helpful.

Another important psychoeducational issue is to help patients understand that psychiatric medications most often do not cure illness but rather ameliorate symptoms. Because this amelioration occurs through compensatory mechanisms involving biochemical and neurophysiological processes, stopping the medication will likely allow the aberrant pathophysiological process to recur, with return of the original emotional and behavioral symptoms. Thus, the physician must clearly delineate how to take the medication and for how long, as well as what to do should symptoms recur or side effects develop.

All medications have **side effects** and other risks. The side effects of most psychoactive drugs are relatively benign and remit when the medication is stopped. But, since the beneficial effects are often delayed, while side effects tend to occur during the first few days or weeks of treatment, patients may be tempted to discontinue medication prior to discovering its potential benefits. Close monitoring of potentially disconcerting side effects in the context of a strong relationship with the physician may help prevent unilateral discontinuation of treatment.

The patient's specific concerns about serious and dangerous adverse effects and drug–drug interactions should be addressed in making a final treatment decision. For example, a patient especially concerned with weight gain might better be started on a weight-neutral agent than on one more likely to produce weight gain. If a weight-neutral medication is not available, then it is best to discuss this risk proactively as a potential obstacle to the patient's willingness to take the medication.

One of the most important aspects of ensuring adherence is the management of side effects. Before prescribing the first dose, the physician should explain what the expected side effects are, noting that not everyone gets side effects and certainly no one experiences all those listed. Patients should be encouraged to call between appointments if they are experience troublesome side effects that tempt them to stop their medication. In judging whether a symptom is likely to be a side effect, it is useful to know whether the patient had had a similar experience before beginning the medication. For example, sleep disturbance or nausea that is similar to the patient's premedication experience seems less likely to have been caused by the medication than does a skin rash or vivid dreams that are unlike the patient's prior experience.

With regard to the **time frame**, many psychotropic medications should be begun at a low dose and then increased iteratively if they are ineffective and tolerated. This process is continued until the patient improves sufficiently, develops intolerable side effects, or the maximal dose approved by the U.S. Food and Drug Administration (FDA) is reached.

If the maximal or maximally tolerated dose does not achieve remission (i.e., cessation of symptoms), a decision should be made to either add another treatment (**augmentation strategy**) or switch to a different therapy (**switch strategy**). From a practical standpoint, if the patient is somewhat improved but still symptomatic, the current treatment is generally continued, adding an "augmenter," whereas if no symptomatic change has occurred, the initial treatment is usually discarded and a second one substituted. Unfortunately, there are almost no controlled studies demonstrating the wisdom of switching treatment for complete nonresponders and augmenting treatment for partial responders. The goal of treatment should be complete remission of symptoms. Changes in dose, medication, or other aspects of treatment are indicated as long as symptoms of illness remain. A general rule of treatment should be to minimize the number of medications and the dosage without sacrificing the ultimate goal of remission.

Knowledge of the patient's illness course and past treatment history is helpful in making **causal inferences** as treatment proceeds. If the course of illness changes after initiation of therapy, the treatment is a likely candidate for having produced the change. Conversely, if the course of illness continues as previously, there is no reason to assume the treatment is effective even if symptoms temporarily remit. For instance, a patient whose depression spontaneously remits every March who begins an antidepressant in February should not be considered a medication responder when remission occurs a month later. In contrast, a chronically anxious patient who is much less anxious when taking a benzodiazepine but becomes very anxious again during periods off medication is likely to be having a true medication response.

ANTIPSYCHOTIC AGENTS

Antipsychotics are derived from several classes of chemicals (Table 16.1). The first class of commonly used antipsychotics was the phenothiazines, which are divided into aliphatics, piperidines, and piperazines, depending on the substitution that occurs on the nitrogen of the central ring. Chlorpromazine was the first phenothiazine introduced. Several other classes of antipsychotics were produced by making other substitutions. These original, or **first-generation, antipsychotics** (FGAs) are associated with significant side effects, particularly Parkinsonism-like symptoms, and tardive dyskinesia (TD), an involuntary movement disorder of the limbs, trunk, neck, and mouth that may remit if treatment is discontinued but is often permanent.

Clozapine, a dibenzodiazepine, was synthesized in 1958 and introduced in Europe in the 1970s. Because of its high association with agranulocytosis, it was not approved for use in the United States until 1989, and then with required frequent blood monitoring. Clozapine offers three advantages over the FGAs: it is more effective than any other antipsychotic, it is particularly effective against schizophrenia's negative symptoms (paucity of thought and apathy), and it does not cause TD. Because of these major differences between clozapine and previous antipsychotics, the differences between clozapine and the FGAs were the focus of tremendous interest. It was hypothesized that clozapine's ability to block the D_2 and the 5-HT_{2A} receptors might account for its unique properties. Therefore, pharmaceutical companies sought compounds that block both receptors. This property is common to many antipsychotic agents introduced since 1989 and is associated with their designation as "atypical" antipsychotics. The term **second-generation antipsychotic** (SGA) is preferable, as each SGA has unique actions. The SGAs have more varied pharmacological effects than the FGAs. Thus far, studies have not demonstrated the clear superiority of the SGAs over FGAs on the reduction of symptoms of psychosis

TABLE 16.1 Antipsychotics

Generic Name	Brand Name	Usual Starting Dose (total per day)	Usual Dose Range (total per day)	Maximal Dose (total per day)	Sedative Effects	Extrapyramidal Effects	Orthostatic Hypotension	Anticholinergic Effects	Prodiabetes Effects
Phenothiazines									
chlorpromazine	Thorazine	150–450 mg*	50 mg–1 g	1 g	Severe	Mild	Severe	Moderate	Moderate
fluphenazine	Prolixin	1 mg	1–10 mg	10 mg	Minimal	Severe	Minimal	Minimal	Minimal?
thioridazine	Mellaril	50 mg	50 mg–800 mg	800 mg	Severe	Minimal	Severe	Severe	Moderate
trifluoperazine	Stelazine	2.5 mg	2.5–30 mg	30 mg	Mild	Moderate	Minimal	Minimal	Minimal?
perphenazine	Trilafon	16 mg	24–48 mg	64 mg	Moderate	Moderate	Minimal	Minimal	Moderate
Diphenylbutylpiperidine									
pimozide	Orap	.4 mg	4–10 mg	10 mg	Minimal	Severe	Minimal	Minimal	Unknown
Thioxanthenes									
thiothixene	Navane	4 mg	4–24 mg	24 mg	Mild	Moderate	Mild	Mild	Minimal?
Butyrophenones									
haloperidol	Haldol	1–2 mg	1–20 mg	20 mg	Minimal	Severe	Minimal	Minimal	Minimal?
Other First-Generation Antipsychotics									
loxapine	Loxitane	15 mg	15–225 mg	225 mg	Mild	Mild–moderate	Mild	Mild	Unknown
molindone	Moban	10 mg	10–100 mg	100 mg	Mild	Mild–moderate	Mild	None	Unknown

(continued)

TABLE 16.1 Continued

Generic Name	Brand Name	Usual Starting Dose (total per day)	Usual Dose Range (total per day)	Maximal Dose (total per day)	Sedative Effects	Extrapyramidal Effects	Orthostatic Hypotension	Anticholinergic Effects	Prodiabetes Effects
Second-Generation Antipsychotics									
aripiprazole	Abilify	2 mg	2–30 mg	30 mg	Minimal	Mild (moderate akathisia)	Minimal	Minimal	Minimal?
clozapine	Clozaril	50 mg	50–600 mg	900 mg	Severe	Minimal	Severe	Severe	Severe
olanzapine	Zyprexa	5 mg	2–20 mg	20 mg	Moderate	Minimal	Mild	Mild	Moderate–severe
paliperidone	Invega	3 mg	3–12 mg	12 mg	Mild	Moderate	Mild	Minimal	Moderate
quetiapine	Seroquel	50 mg	75–800 mg	800 mg	Moderate	Minimal	Moderate	Mild	Moderate
risperidone	Risperdol	1 mg	1–10 mg	16 mg	Minimal	≤6 mg: minimal >6 mg: moderate	Mild	None	Moderate
ziprasidone	Geodon	40 mg	40–200 mg	200 mg	Minimal	Mild (moderate akathisia)	Minimal	Minimal	Minimal?
lurasidone	Latuda	40 mg	40–160 mg	160 mg	Minimal	Moderate akathisia	Minimal	Minimal	Minimal
iloperidone	Fanapt	1 mg bid	6–12 mg bid	24 mg	Moderate	Minimal	Moderate at initiation	Minimal	Unknown
asenapine	Saphris	5 mg SL bid	10 mg SL bid	20 mg	Mild	Minimal	Minimal	Minimal	Unknown

*In divided doses.

at the level demonstrated by clozapine. Evidence is mixed as to whether the incidence of TD is lower for SGAs than for FGAs. Certain side effects, such as akinesia and dystonias (see Extrapyramidal Symptoms, later in the chapter), are much less common with SGAs than with FGAs, causing those treated with FGAs to be identified by their Parkinsonian appearance, posture, and gait. Patients observe that this ease of identification is less prominent with SGAs, perhaps contributing to less stigma.

The Clinical Antipsychotic Trials of Intervention Effectiveness (CATIE) was sponsored by the National Institute of Mental Health (NIMH) to be an unbiased assessment comparing SGAs to FGAs. This trial did not substantiate the superiority of the SGAs over the FGA perphenazine, dampening physician's earlier enthusiasm for SGAs. However, SGAs remain preferable because of their lower incidence of TD and other side effects.

Figure 16.1 provides a schematic of the neuronal synapse, and Figure 16.2 provides a schematic for the hypothesized mechanism of action of antipsychotics.

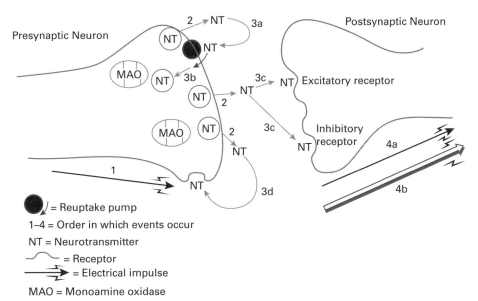

FIGURE 16.1 The Synapse: How Neurons Work. When a neuron is stimulated, an electrical impulse travels along the axon (1, arrow). When the impulse reaches the end of the axon, it releases neurotransmitter (2, NT) into the gap (synaptic cleft) between the presynaptic neuron and the postsynaptic neuron. Released NT has four possible outcomes: **A.** Most of it is taken back into the originating neuron by an energy-dependent mechanism, called a "reuptake pump" (3a, circle). NT that is pumped back into the neuron may be repackaged into vesicles ready to be re-released. Monoamine NTs such as dopamine, norepinephrine, and serotonin may be deactivated presynaptically by the mitochondrial enzyme, monoamine oxidase (3b, MAO). **B.** Some NT diffuses across the synapse and attaches to a postsynaptic receptor (3c), which can either stimulate the neuron to discharge (4a) or inhibit discharge (4b). **C.** Some NT contacts presynaptic autoreceptors (3d), which can be stimulatory but typically inhibit the presynaptic neuron. **D.** The remaining NT diffuses away from the synaptic cleft. Receptors may stimulate the neuron, making it more likely to discharge or inhibit the neuron, thus decreasing likelihood of discharge. The balance between activation and inhibition determines whether the neuron will produce an electrical impulse.

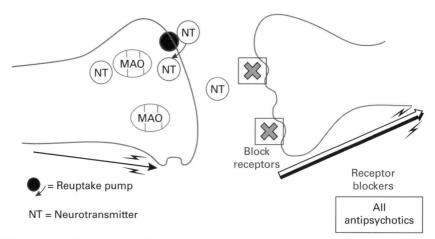

= Reuptake pump

NT = Neurotransmitter

FIGURE 16.2 How Antipsychotics Work. All drugs marketed to treat psychosis block the postsynaptic D_2 dopamine receptors. Second-generation antipsychotic medications also block other receptors; most notably, they block the postsynaptic 5-HT2A receptor.

Indications and Contraindications

The primary indications for antipsychotic medications are for the treatment of **psychotic disorders** (see Chapter 4, Schizophrenia and Other Psychotic Disorders) and **mania**, even in the absence of psychosis. Other indications include **nonpsychotic major depression that is refractory or associated with bipolar disorder** (see Chapter 3, Mood Disorders), and **obsessive-compulsive disorder**. The dosing and side effects of antipsychotic medications for nonpsychotic disorders are similar to those when they are used for psychosis, but lower doses are sometimes highly effective. This observation suggests that the antidepressant and anxiolytic effects of these agents may result from a mechanism other than D_2 receptor blockade, a common effect of all drugs effective for psychosis.

Although not FDA-approved indications, antipsychotic medications are sometimes helpful for patients with schizotypal personality disorder who have severe oddities of thinking, as well as for borderline personality disorder and other conditions characterized by **impulsivity**, excitability, or psychotic-like features. For example, a 26-year-old woman with borderline personality disorder remained emotionally labile and dysphoric despite adequate trials of several antidepressants. She denied psychotic symptoms. Trifluoperazine at 2 mg three times daily resulted in mood stabilization without her characteristic emotional overreactions to minor stresses, and she was able to discuss emotionally charged issues in her therapy without cutting or other self-injurious behavior outside the sessions. However, the adverse effects of these drugs dictate caution in their use for nonpsychotic indications.

There are few substantial medical **contraindications** for antipsychotic agents. Patients who are allergic to a class of medications should not receive other agents from that class. If a psychotic patient is intoxicated, has taken an overdose, or is obtunded for any reason, he or she should not be started on antipsychotic medications until the **intoxication** has cleared. Patients with **cardiac conduction delays** should not be given pimozide, thioridazine, or ziprasidone because they can prolong the QTc interval. Patients with or at risk for **diabetes mellitus** should first receive an SGA with a lower propensity to disrupt their metabolic state. Patients with known **liver disease** should avoid antipsychotics known to irritate the liver, such as chlorpromazine, in favor of others that minimally affect the liver, such as haloperidol. A history of agranulocytosis may constitute a relative contraindication for clozapine, although it has not been established that prior blood dyscrasias increase the risk for bone marrow suppression with clozapine. Other SGAs have cautions regarding their use in persons with histories of leukopenia.

Careful monitoring of anticonvulsant therapy in patients with a preexisting **seizure disorder** is indicated because most antipsychotics lower the seizure threshold. While routine prophylactic use of anticonvulsants is not indicated, anticonvulsant therapy may be added if seizures occur.

Pretreatment Evaluation

Before initiating treatment with an antipsychotic medication, the physician should obtain a complete psychiatric and medical history, including history of prior seizures, alcohol and substance abuse, and use of other medications, particularly medications that lower the seizure threshold or otherwise might interact adversely with an antipsychotic, such as antihypertensives. Several antipsychotic agents induce orthostatic hypotension, which may worsen when a patient is taking antihypertensives. A thorough mental status examination should confirm the presence of psychotic symptoms and the absence of cognitive dysfunction suggestive of a toxic or metabolic etiology or dementia. Vital signs should be checked. Relevant testing includes a **complete blood count, serum electrolytes, liver function tests**, and an **electrocardiogram**. If immediate treatment is necessary and there are no medical contraindications to the chosen treatment, antipsychotic medication can be started pending test results. But in nonemergent situations institution of antipsychotic medications is best left until the workup is complete.

Initiating Treatment

Relatively slow upward **dose titration** should aim for the lowest necessary effective total dose. This practice results in lower total doses and fewer side effects. **Parenteral** forms of haloperidol, aripiprazole, olanzapine, and ziprasidone are available and have been demonstrated to be efficacious in the treatment of acutely agitated psychotic patients. An advantage of parenteral medication over oral formulations is that the physician knows whether the patient received the medication, so adherence is not part of the equation should the patient not improve. Several medications are available in orally quickly dissolving formulations when placed under the tongue.

Combination Therapy

It is common to combine antipsychotic medication with a **benzodiazepine**, such as lorazepam. This combination is especially useful if the particular antipsychotic causes minimal sedation and sedation is desired. Because the antipsychotic can take a week or two to be titrated to an effective dose, use of a benzodiazepine as a sedative can allow the antipsychotic dose to be lower, reducing side effects and perhaps the risk for TD. Once the psychosis has remitted, the benzodiazepine can often be tapered and discontinued.

Patients on clozapine sometimes require supplementation with a second antipsychotic agent because clozapine's risk for seizures limits its maximum dose to 900 mg/d. There is not usually any indication for the use of multiple SGAs.

Dosing

Table 16.1 describes starting and maximum doses of antipsychotics. Because olanzapine is particularly sedating and has a long half-life, it is usually given in a single dose at bedtime. Paliperidone is an active metabolite of risperidone and both are largely excreted in the urine; thus dosage adjustments are made in renally impaired patients. Quetiapine produces significant orthostatic hypotension, so usually the dose is started low and increased slowly in order to give the body a chance to compensate. Orthostatic hypotension is more of a problem in the elderly and in women (especially in elderly women) because muscle mass helps protect against drops in blood pressure. Risperidone is increased up to 4–6 mg/d because above 6 mg/d, extrapyramidal symptoms (EPS) occur, such as tremor, dyskinesias, and bradykinesia.

Long-Acting Injectable Antipsychotics

Fluphenazine, haloperidol, risperidone, paliperidone, olanzapine, and aripiprazole are available in long-acting injectable formulations. These are useful for patients who either forget to take their medications or who refuse oral pills. Whether antipsychotic medication is "on board" is not in question with these long-acting drugs. If psychosis continues or returns, the physician knows it is a failure of the current dose of the medication rather than poor adherence. One drawback of long-acting injectable medication is that patients may suffer for several weeks if unacceptable side effects occur. It is therefore best to begin the patient on the oral formulation, and then **switch** to the injectable form **once tolerance is established** (see Box 16.2).

Side Effects

While the specific beneficial effects of antipsychotic medications may be delayed a week or two, side effects often start with the first dose.

Weight Effects

The low-potency FGAs and most SGAs cause increased appetite, decreased satiety, and **weight gain**. Whether due to these physiological effects, other direct effects of antipsychotic agents, or to other pathophysiological pathways, patients chronically treated with antipsychotic medications suffer from increased rates of **diabetes mellitus, hypercholesterolemia, atherosclerosis**, and **cardiovascular problems**. Aripiprazole and ziprasidone are relatively weight neutral. Obtaining a **baseline weight**, measurement of **abdominal girth, blood pressure**, and a baseline **metabolic profile** (fasting blood sugar, lipid profile) is recommended practice for patients who are to be treated long term with antipsychotics. An educational and weight-controlling **diet** and **exercise program** should be initiated early in treatment. Assessments should be updated periodically and adverse results addressed as part of the comprehensive treatment plan.

Extrapyramidal Symptoms (EPS)

Extrapyramidal side effects consist of tremor, akinesia, rigidity, dystonias, dyskinesias, and akathisia. The first five symptoms are sometimes called pseudoparkinsonian because they mimic Parkinson's disease.

The **tremor** of EPS is usually coarse and can be so severe as to interfere with eating and other daily activities. **Akinesia** is a paucity of motion and can be mistaken for the psychomotor retardation of depression. However, the akinesia due to EPS may remit

---

BOX 16.2

CONVERSION FROM ORAL TO LONG-ACTING INJECTABLE ANTIPSYCHOTICS

Fluphenazine enanthate is administered every 2 weeks, fluphenazine decanoate and haloperidol decanoate are administered every 3 to 4 weeks. Rough dosage equivalents are as follows: fluphenazine hydrochloride (the oral formulation) 12.5 mg/d = 0.5 mL fluphenazine enanthate/decanoate, and haloperidol hydrochloride dose multiplied by 10 = haloperidol decanoate dose. Risperdal Consta, its long-acting injectable form, is administered in doses of 25–50 mg biweekly. Invega Sustenna is a monthly long-acting injectable form of paliperidone and dose range is 39–234 mg. Zyprexa Relprevv is long-acting injectable olanzapine and is dosed every 2–4 weeks. There are recent cautions in the use of long-acting injectable olanzepine, as there have been reports of patients becoming delirious and comatose following injections. In order to administer Zyprexa Relprevv, the provider, pharmacy, and patient must be registered. Patients must be observed for 3 hours after each injection to ensure their safety. Abilify Maintenna is administered monthly, starting at 400 mg. This dose is the usual maintenance dose, but it may be reduced to 300 mg intramuscularly monthly if there are troublesome side effects. There are no simple guidelines to help individualize the dosing, which must therefore be empirically determined for each patient.

---

within an hour of administering an anticholinergic medication, whereas the psychomotor retardation of depression does not. The **rigidity** of EPS lends a wooden quality to movement and responds readily to antiparkinsonian medication. Acute **dystonias** typically appear within hours of initiating or increasing the dose of antipsychotic medications. Patients should be warned that their muscles may become tight with these drugs, and that this stiffening quickly reverses when counteractive medication is given. Unless the dystonia affects swallowing, it is not dangerous but can frighten patients, especially if they and their family are not forewarned. In the presence of delusions of being controlled, acute dystonias seem to confirm a patient's worst fears. Muscles of the eye and neck are especially prone to develop dystonias. A forced turning of the neck, or **torticollis**, and upturning of the eyes that prevents looking downward, or **oculogyric crisis**, are not medical emergencies but can be painful and frightening. Rarely, tightening of the back muscles (opisthotonos) and posturing may occur.

EPS usually remit quickly with **anticholinergic** medications, such as benztropine 1 or 2 mg daily. For acute dystonias, diphenhydramine 25 mg injected intravenously over 1 minute (or 50 mg intramuscularly) typically provides relief within minutes. Alternatively, benztropine 1–2 mg can be injected intramuscularly, but it may take 15 minutes or more to provide relief. Once EPS or dystonias appear, benztropine 1 or 2 mg/d should be continued as long as the offending agent is prescribed. Prophylactic anticholinergic agents can be prescribed in an attempt to prevent patients from experiencing these uncomfortable effects, but because not all patients experience these symptoms, use of antiparkinsonian medications can generally be limited to those having uncomfortable symptoms. However, prophylaxis is justified for patients with a history of prior EPS, particularly dystonia. EPS are commonly associated with dysphoria, but the EPS should be treated first, only resorting to antidepressant medications if significant dysphoria remains once the EPS are minimized.

Akathisia is experienced as an inner sense of restlessness ("like a motor inside" or "ants in your pants") that is discomforting. It is difficult to treat and often takes days to improve even when pharmacological intervention will be ultimately effective.

EPS and akathisia are disliked by patients and families alike. EPS are associated with poor adherence and thus should be carefully watched for and aggressively treated. **Quetiapine** and **clozapine** are the best choices for patients who find EPS and akathisia particularly difficult to tolerate, as these drugs are virtually never associated with these side effects.

Tardive Dyskinesia (TD)

TD is defined as **involuntary choreiform, athetoid, or rhythmic movements** of the tongue, jaw, or extremities that occur in association with the use of antipsychotic medications (see DSM-5). Rhythmic rocking motions of the torso also sometimes occur. Classic TD affects the **buccolingual-masticatory muscles**, leading to "fly-catcher's tongue" (the tongue's darting in and out of the mouth), bonbon sign (repeated pushing of the tongue against the cheek, as if one had a piece of candy in one's mouth), grimacing, or chewing movements. An early sign of TD is **wormlike movements** of the resting tongue. TD is more likely to develop in patients who have EPS early in their use of antipsychotic medication, in those with diabetes mellitus, in the elderly, and in patients with affective disorders.

It is speculated that the abnormal movements of TD result from chronic dopamine receptor blockade–induced postsynaptic hypersensitivity to dopamine. Two observations are consistent with this hypothesis. First, increasing dopamine receptor blockade by increasing the dose of the antipsychotic decreases or stops the movements. This is not a useful strategy, however, since eventually the movements will re-emerge, presumably as the receptors become even more hypersensitive. Second, **dopamine agonists**, such as **methylphenidate, exacerbate TD**. Interestingly, the **anticholinergics**, which so readily counteract EPS, also **exacerbate TD**, perhaps by further disrupting the balance between dopamine and acetylcholine. **Clonidine** reduces dyskinesias in some patients, but its effect is unpredictable. The best treatment is to remove the antipsychotic, as TD sometimes remits early in its course when the offending agent is removed. However, when it is contraindicated to have a potentially psychotic individual off antipsychotic medication, the doctor and patient face a dilemma that is sometimes best solved by switching to clozapine as the antipsychotic agent.

TD occurs in 15–25% of schizophrenic patients treated with FGAs and occurs in a lower percentage of those treated with SGAs. **Clozapine** not only does not cause TD, it sometimes can reverse these abnormal movements.

The **Abnormal Involuntary Movement Scale (AIMS)** is a tool used to assess TD. It consists of 10 items measuring involuntary movements of the face, mouth, jaw, tongue, upper and lower extremities, and trunk. The systematic assessment of each area with the AIMS provides identification of the location and severity of abnormal movements and a uniform methodology for following its progression over time. All patients receiving antipsychotic medications should be assessed periodically for abnormal movements.

Sedation

Sedation is common with antipsychotic medication. A general rule is that the higher-potency drugs (i.e., those requiring fewer mg to achieve efficacy) are less sedating than those requiring higher doses. Patients generally accommodate to the sedative effects of these medications once a stable dose is reached, but during dose titration they may be too sedated to participate effectively in activities. Administering the medication at bedtime sometimes helps.

Anticholinergic Effects

Symptoms of excessive anticholinergic activity include **dry mouth**, **blurred vision**, **constipation**, and **difficulty initiating urination**. Acute glaucomic crisis can be precipitated in patients with narrow-angle glaucoma. Lemon-flavored gum (sugar-free) helps with dry mouth. Increasing dietary fiber helps constipation, but sometimes stool softeners, such as docusate sodium or psyllium, are necessary. Sometimes two or three times the recommended dosing is required (e.g., docusate sodium 100 mg tid or psyllium 1–2 tablespoons tid). Urinary retention may be relieved by bethanechol 10–25 mg bid.

High doses of highly anticholinergic drugs, such as chlorpromazine, especially when used with other anticholinergic drugs, may produce an atropine-like **delirium**, characterized by mental confusion, visual hallucinations, tachycardia, flushed facies, and dilated pupils. Mucous membranes are typically dry. Discontinuation of the anticholinergic agent is the best treatment. Administration of parenteral physostigmine is fraught with cardiac complications and should not be attempted. Additionally, physostigmine is short-acting, and the anticholinergic agents are long-acting.

Hypotension

Lightheadedness on standing can occur with most low-potency FGAs because of their interference with the mechanisms that counteract a drop in blood pressure upon standing, called **orthostasis**. Among SGAs, orthostatic hypotension is most common with clozapine and quetiapine. If the blood pressure falls sufficiently, the patient loses consciousness, and the resulting falls can cause injury. Such falls are more likely when the person has been using the toilet or gets out of bed in the middle of the night. Patients should be cautioned specifically about those circumstances and advised to arise slowly and carefully while increasing blood return by moving their legs. Because muscle mass helps sustain the blood pressure, orthostatic hypotension is more problematic in the elderly and in women than in young men. In most cases, the body accommodates to orthostasis over time, so slow upward dose titration is usually sufficient to minimize this problem. If problems with dizziness and syncope persist, increasing salt intake is usually effective. In rare cases, flurinef and compression stockings can be added.

Sexual Effects

Because dopamine is the brain's main brake on prolactin release, blockade of dopamine receptors often results in increased prolactin levels, which can result in **gynecomastia** in male patients, and milk production and **menstrual irregularities** in women. **Decreased sexual interest** and **delayed orgasm** may be related directly to dopamine effects or to increased prolactin. These changes in sexual interest and functioning can be especially troublesome for patients with sexual delusions or delusions of external control. These effects are not reported with clozapine and quetiapine. Thioridazine may cause **retrograde ejaculation**, which a male with sexual delusions may consider catastrophic.

Hepatic Effects

Idiosyncratic **cholestatic jaundice** is associated with acute increases in liver enzymes. Chlorpromazine is the antipsychotic most associated with this complication. The offending medication must be discontinued and a chemically unrelated antipsychotic substituted. This problem is to be distinguished from mild benign elevations in liver enzymes, which return to normal even while continuing the medication. The general rule is to discontinue current medications if liver enzyme values exceed three times the upper limit of normal, but to continue medication and repeat enzyme tests when liver enzyme elevations are within three times the upper limit of normal values.

Dermatological Effects

Most rashes from antipsychotic medications are benign. Mild rashes often spontaneously remit even if the medication is continued. However, more serious rashes can evolve into **Stevens-Johnson syndrome**, which in its extreme can result in death. Therefore, rashes that are more than mild (e.g., cover much of the body or are accompanied by moderate pruritis and/or involvement of other organs such as the joints) should alert the physician to discontinue current medications. Phenothiazines can produce **photosensitivity** whereby patients burn easily when exposed to the sun, because of an inability to detoxify free radicals produced in the skin by the sun. Therefore, patients taking these medications require sun protection and must be warned to avoid prolonged exposure to the sun. Long-term, high-dose chlorpromazine therapy has been associated with a slate-gray appearance of the skin of Caucasians.

Hematological Effects

Agranulocytosis is uncommon with most antipsychotic medications, occurring in 1 in 10,000 patients taking chlorpromazine. However, the incidence increases to about 1 in 100 for patients taking **clozapine**. The risk is sufficiently high that when using clozapine, the patient, provider, and pharmacy must be registered with the manufacturer, and frequent blood tests are required, so that a drop in white blood cells can be noted in time to discontinue the medication. Most often, the drop in white blood cells is sufficiently gradual (suggesting a toxic mechanism) that clozapine can be discontinued in time to avert full-blown agranulocytosis. Rarely, however, the drop is precipitous, suggesting an allergic response. In the first 6 months of clozapine treatment a complete blood count is obtained weekly. Thereafter, testing is performed every 2 weeks. After 1 year, the blood is tested monthly, since the greatest risk is in the first year of treatment. However, if the patient discontinues clozapine, weekly testing should begin with reinstitution of the drug.

With all other antipsychotics, the risk of agranulocytosis is too small to warrant frequent blood tests except in patient who have histories of leucopenia. Patients should report unusual infections, however, and blood work should then be quickly obtained.

Seizure Effects

All antipsychotic drugs lower the seizure threshold. High doses of **chlorpromazine** and **clozapine** present a particularly elevated risk. **Gradual dose increases** and **divided doses** diminish the risk. Addition of an anticonvulsant is generally indicated if seizures occur.

Ophthalmological Effects

Retinitis pigmentosa has been associated with **thioridazine**, especially if the dose exceeds 800 mg/d. Therefore, use of this drug is always limited to this maximal dose. Anticholinergic medications can induce acute **narrow-angle glaucoma.**

Neuroleptic Malignant Syndrome (NMS)

All antipsychotic agents can cause NMS, which is characterized by high fever, rigidity, autonomic instability, and delirium. In its extreme, NMS may result in death. Therefore, whenever symptoms of NMS occur, the antipsychotic must be stopped and the patient hospitalized. NMS is more likely in hot weather, presumably being exacerbated by dehydration. The most critical features are **fever** (usually >102°F) and **rigidity**. Unlike Parkinsonian rigidity, however, the stiffness of NMS does not improve with anticholinergic medication. Thus, if a patient complains of stiffness and that his or her benztropine no longer helps, the physician should consider NMS and ask about fever. Discontinuation of antipsychotic medication and reporting to an emergency room are indicated in the presence of both a significant fever and benztropine-resistant rigidity.

Treatment of NMS is mainly palliative beyond discontinuation of the causative agent. NMS in its full form is a medical emergency. Fever can quickly rise to or above 106°F and must be countered with ice packs. Fluids should be pushed or given intravenously. Infection must be ruled out. In severe cases, admission to the intensive care unit is required. There are no known effective antidotes except giving the body time to rid itself of the antipsychotic. Intravenous dantrolene sodium has been administered with variable results.

Drug Interactions

All antipsychotics are metabolized by and variously inhibit the **cytochrome P-450 system** of liver enzymes. Thus, not only is the metabolism of these drugs affected by concomitantly administered medications, but the antipsychotics also affect the metabolism of coadministered drugs. Unfortunately, each of the antipsychotic medications is metabolized by and inhibits a different P-450 enzyme, so it is best to check the specific potential interactions prior to prescribing.

Medication Choice

An antipsychotic agent should be chosen on the basis of the patient's specific needs, vulnerability to particular side effects, and history of response to and tolerance of side effects in general. The SGAs generally produce fewer and less severe EPS and may have a lower risk for TD, but many also cause patients to gain considerable weight and increase the risk for development or exacerbation of diabetes and hyperlipidemia. Most SGAs are more expensive than older agents, even when available generically. While SGAs have become much preferred over FGAs, the CATIE studies have questioned whether their increased cost is sufficiently counterbalanced by either increased efficacy or decreased problems. In particular, their increased diabetogenic effects may offset any decreased TD risk.

Once a psychotic patient has **failed to benefit from at least two different classes** of antipsychotic medications, a trial with **clozapine** should be considered. Despite its limitations, clozapine has distinct advantages over other marketed antipsychotic medications. Clozapine is often very effective, both for the positive (i.e., hallucinations and delusions) and negative (i.e., apathy, cognitive slowing, paucity of thought) symptoms of schizophrenia. In fact, it is the **most effective** antipsychotic medication available. Clozapine **does not cause TD** and can sometimes ameliorate its symptoms, so presence of TD is another indication for its use.

Antiparkinsonian Agents

More than half of patients treated with FGAs experience EPS; these symptoms occur in as many as 25% of patients treated with most of the SGAs (with the exception of clozapine, olanzapine, and quetiapine). The anti-Parkinsonian treatments include anti-cholinergics and dopamine agonists.

Benztropine mesylate is an anticholinergic agent. It is the most commonly used drug to counteract EPS. It is also long-acting. The usual dose is 1 or 2 mg daily or bid, although up to 8 mg daily may be administered. **Procyclidine** is another anticholinergic agent that is highly effective, but it has a shorter half-life, so it must be given three times a day, up to 15 mg/d. **Trihexyphenidyl** is a third effective anticholinergic. It is rarely prescribed because it has street value as an agent of abuse (hallucinogenic). **Diphenhydramine** is a fourth anticholinergic; it may be used intramuscularly for the treatment of dystonias and has been used orally for treatment of akathisia. When given with drugs that have significant anticholinergic effects themselves, such as chlorpromazine, thioridazine, and olanzapine, these side effects can become severe (see Anticholinergic Side Effects, earlier in this chapter).

Dopamine agonists, such as bromocriptine, counter EPS but also exacerbate psychotic symptoms, so they are rarely used. **Amantadine** is an indirect dopamine agonist that ameliorates EPS, sometimes when anticholinergic medications are not sufficiently counteractive, without exacerbating psychosis (perhaps because it selectively affects the striatal pathways presumed to be overactive in EPS, leaving cortical dopamine sites relatively unaffected). Amantadine is also useful for patients who cannot tolerate anticholinergic effects. It is prescribed in divided doses, 100–200 mg bid.

Propranolol, a beta-blocker, can counteract tremor and akathisia. It is usually prescribed in doses up to 20 mg bid, after gradually increasing the dose while monitoring blood pressure and pulse, titrating against therapeutic effects. Intramuscular **diazepam** relieves dystonic reactions, and oral benzodiazepines ease akathisia.

ANTIDEPRESSANT AGENTS

From time immemorial, various elixirs have been used to improve mood. Alcohol, for example, has long been thought to "lift one's spirits." While one may temporarily feel better immediately after drinking an alcoholic beverage, a depressed individual generally feels worse within a few hours of any initial euphoric effects, so its benefits appear transient, and its mood effects are biphasic.

True antidepressant medications do not provide a momentary lift but instead gradually (i.e., over several weeks) alleviate depressive states together with their accompanying debilitative symptoms. The search for an improved treatment for tuberculosis led to the observation that iproniazid, a monoamine oxidase inhibitor (MAOI), lifted the spirits of patients with tuberculosis, leading to trials in depressed patients. The initial tricyclic antidepressant (TCA), imipramine, was discovered during a search for an improved antipsychotic, and the TCAs dominated the pharmacological treatment of depression for years.

Fluoxetine, the first SSRI marketed in the United States (1988), changed psychiatric practice. By the early 1990s, the older, more problematic TCAs and MAOIs had largely been relegated to second- then third-line agents, respectively, and today are little used and probably underused. The SSRIs and other newer antidepressants do not have the anticholinergic and orthostatic effects of TCAs or the dietary restrictions and other problems associated with MAOIs. They are easier to use and just as likely to be effective. Today, most previously treated depressed patients have received one or more SSRI, which have been estimated to account for 80% of initial antidepressant prescriptions. Figure 16.3 provides a schematic for the hypothesized mechanism of action of antidepressants.

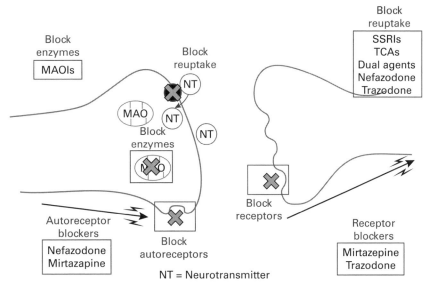

FIGURE 16.3 How Antidepressants Work. Various antidepressants have different effects. The most common mechanism is reuptake blockade, meaning the drug occupies the reuptake pump, thus preventing it from removing neurotransmitter (NT) from the synaptic cleft. Increased NT in the cleft results in increased occupancy of autoreceptors and postsynaptic receptors. Increased occupancy of stimulatory postsynaptic receptors will result in increased neurotransmission of signals from the presynaptic to the postsynaptic neuron. Increased occupancy of inhibitory postsynaptic receptors results in decreased discharge of the postsynaptic neuron. Increased occupancy of inhibitory presynaptic neurons dampens the firing rate of the presynaptic neuron. The balance between inhibitory and stimulatory inputs determines whether a neuron produces an electrical impulse.

In 2007, the FDA issued a black box warning for all antidepressants for young adults aged 18–24 years. The warning was based on pooled analysis indicating that suicidal ideation and behavior was more frequent in this age group during the initial treatment with an antidepressant (odds ratio 1.62). The frequency of suicidality was lower in adults over age 25. Nevertheless, this issue is controversial because untreated depression often leads to suicidality, too.

Indications

Despite their label as antidepressants, all of these agents can be effective for nondepressed patients with other disorders. The primary indication for all of the antidepressants is **major depression.** While most studies used by pharmaceutical companies to obtain FDA approval to market their products have required that patients meet criteria for major depression, other studies suggest that these agents may work as well for other forms of depressive illness, including persistent depressive disorder (**dysthymia**) and **premenstrual dysphoric disorder**. Antidepressants are often used effectively in the treatment of **anxiety disorders, obsessive-compulsive disorder, bulimia nervosa, and somatic symptom disorders**. In selecting a medication for patients who have prior experience with antidepressants, it is best to let that experience guide selection of previously helpful medications and avoidance of those that had been problematic.

Dosing Strategies

A general principle in using all antidepressants is to start at the lowest marketed dose, increasing every week or two up to the FDA listed maximum dose, if the patient is tolerating the drug and has not improved sufficiently. The maximal dose or highest tolerated dose should be continued for at least 4 weeks before declaring the drug ineffective.

All antidepressant medications generally produce side effects quickly, whereas their benefits are delayed. The expected time course of improvement from the medication varies with the disorder. This delay can range from days (panic disorder) to weeks (depressive disorders) to months (obsessive-compulsive disorder). Because different doses and different medications are effective for different patients, there is always a tension between continuing the same dose in the face of continuing symptoms and presuming the dose is ineffective and making a change in treatment, such as increasing the dose. If one waits sufficiently long to determine whether each dose will help, and then increasing it only to wait again, it may take several months before it is decided that the initial medication is ineffective. If it is, then it will take another several months testing an alternative treatment's effects. If benefit does not accrue until the third or fourth medication, suffering may continue for a year or more before effective treatment is found. The alternative is to raise the dose prior to fully determining that dose's ineffectiveness. In the most aggressive strategy, the dose is raised every few days up to an arbitrary amount, such as the FDA maximum, then waiting about 4 weeks at this dose level before declaring the medication ineffective. The clear advantage of this **more aggressive approach** is decreased time spent depressed and, if ineffective, a reduced wait in moving to the next medication, but the disadvantage is the likelihood of increased burden of side effects. Most patients and physicians prefer a "go slow" approach, accepting prolongation of symptoms in exchange for minimizing side effects.

Many antidepressants can produce **withdrawal** symptoms if suddenly stopped. Therefore, patients should be warned not to miss doses or discontinue their antidepressant. Instead, they should gradually taper the dose over several weeks. The withdrawal syndrome from antidepressants is not medically dangerous but may be quite uncomfortable, akin to suffering from the flu. Medications with shorter half-lives and few or no active metabolites, such as paroxetine and venlafaxine, are more likely to produce such a withdrawal syndrome.

Selective Serotonin Reuptake Inhibitors (SSRIs)

The ease of use and tolerability of SSRIs have resulted in their capture of 80% of prescriptions written for nonpsychotic drug-naive depressed patients.

Dosing

Fluoxetine's very long half-life creates differences from other SSRIs, which all have half-lives approximating 24 hours (see Table 16.2). Fluoxetine builds up in the body more slowly than other antidepressant medications, so its full effects are delayed even longer and one must wait longer than with other antidepressants, perhaps 6–8 weeks, before declaring a given dose ineffective. One advantage of fluoxetine's long half-life

TABLE 16.2 Selective Serotonin Reuptake Inhibitors

Generic Name	Brand Name	Usual Starting Dose (total per day)	Usual Dose (total per day)	Maximal Dose (total per day)	Side Effects and Comments
citalopram	Celexa	20 mg	20–40 mg	40 mg	Nausea, insomnia, somnolence, sexual dysfunction, sweating
escitalopram	Lexapro	10 mg	10–20 mg	20 mg	Nausea, insomnia, somnolence, sexual dysfunction, sweating
fluoxetine	Prozac	20 mg	20–80 mg	80 mg	Nausea, headache, akathisia, weight loss (early), weight gain (late), diarrhea, insomnia, rash, sweating, sexual dysfunction
fluvoxamine	Luvox	100 mg	100–300 mg	300 mg	Nausea, insomnia, somnolence, nervousness, sexual dysfunction, sweating; potent inhibitor of CYP 450 enzymes and thus prone to drug interactions
paroxetine	Paxil	20 mg	20–60 mg	60 mg	Sedation, nausea, headache, akathisia, diarrhea, sexual dysfunction, sweating; short half-life and no active metabolites so prone to withdrawal syndrome if doses are missed or precipitously discontinued; potent CYP 2D6 inhibitor
sertraline	Zoloft	50 mg	50–200 mg	200 mg	Nausea, headache, akathisia, diarrhea, sexual dysfunction, sweating
vilazodone	Viibryd	10 mg	10–40 mg	40 mg	Diarrhea, nausea, headache, insomnia; administer with food

is that occasional doses can be missed without losing efficacy or creating withdrawal. Adolescents, young adults, and those with chaotic schedules may be better served with such a long-acting medication that is forgiving of missed doses. Particularly sensitive individuals may experience benefit from 5 or 10 mg/d.

A conservative starting dose of **sertraline** is 25 mg, but most patients can tolerate a starting dose of 50 mg/d. **Paroxetine**'s shorter half-life (about 16 hours) means that it is associated with more frequent and problematic withdrawal symptoms so it must be tapered when discontinued, and patients need to be strongly warned about missed doses and abrupt stoppage. On the other hand, patients who suffer from sexual side effects may obtain some relief by skipping a dose. **Fluvoxamine**'s only FDA indication is for the treatment of obsessive-compulsive disorder, although in Europe it is also used for all the indications of other SSRIs. Nevertheless, in the United States this is a little-used drug. An unusual aspect of both fluvoxamine and paroxetine is that they inhibit their own metabolism, so blood levels increase disproportionately as the dose is raised. **Citalopram** and its levorotatory enantiomer, **escitalopram**, have all the usual SSRI side effects but are generally thought to be somewhat better tolerated. Nevertheless, citalopram has been associated with prolongations of the QT_c interval, thus its dose should be limited to 40 mg/d or less (20 mg/d maximum dose in patients over age 60 or with preexisting electrical abnormalities or cardiac disease). Citaloram and escitalopram also have somewhat less effect on the P450 enzyme system so may be less problematic when given with other medications. This property is most useful with patients who are prescribed multiple medications, such as many geriatric patients.

Side Effects

Nausea and overstimulation, a form of agitation, can occur within an hour of the first dose. Fortunately, these two effects do not last, as most patients accommodate quickly. **Overstimulation** is sometimes inaccurately considered to be increased anxiety. Unalerted patients may become alarmed, stop taking the SSRI, and even refuse a retrial. A second kind of agitation associated with the SSRIs is **akathisia**, or motor restlessness, similar to that produced by antipsychotics. Patients can become very uncomfortable and the akathisia may last as long as the medication is continued or an antidote is found. Anticholinergics are not helpful, whereas benzodiazepines and beta-blockers sometimes are. Usually the best strategy is to lower the dose or switch to a different medication. This form of agitation may contribute to a sense of hopelessness, helplessness, and suicidality, precipitating a catastrophic response, particularly when the agitation is unexpected. Alerting patients to the possibility of these side effects and developing a management plan in advance can avert disaster.

Nausea, occasionally accompanied by vomiting, can also occur soon after the first dose. Taking the medication with food delays absorption, thus decreasing this effect. In most cases, nausea only occurs following the first dose or diminishes over the first few days. Occasionally, however, nausea lasts as long as the medication is taken. **Headaches** usually respond to standard remedies, including aspirin or acetaminophen. Patients prone to migraine headaches may experience either exacerbation or amelioration.

Anorgasmia and **delayed orgasm** occur in both men and women. Other sexual dysfunctions, such as decreased libido, also occur but are less common and may be secondary to problems reaching orgasm. The best management strategy is to skip a dose of a short-acting SSRI until after sexual activity. Many patients are able to experience orgasm with this strategy; they take their missed dose afterward. Some use adjunctive buspirone, bupropion, yohimbine, or cyproheptadine. Unfortunately, none of these interventions is robustly effective.

Episodes of **mania** and increased cycling in bipolar patients have been attributed to all antidepressants, but it is unclear whether these represent spontaneous occurrences or drug-induced episodes that would not have happened absent the medication. Bipolar depressed patients are typically excluded from trials of antidepressants, so support for the use of antidepressants in bipolar depression is largely anecdotal, but such use is common in practice.

Initially, some of the SSRIs, particularly fluoxetine, cause **loss of appetite** and **weight loss**. Over a few weeks, normal appetite returns and, over months to years, some patients gain weight. Rarely, patients taking SSRIs develop a skin **rash**. Presence of a rash should trigger discontinuation of the medication, since in rare instances it can develop into an autoimmune vasculitis, or Steven-Johnson's syndrome, a potentially fatal condition. SSRIs are quite **safe in overdose**, a major advantage over the TCAs and MAOIs. Only when taken with other medications have SSRI overdoses been lethal.

Drug Interactions

Perhaps the most important drug–drug interaction between SSRIs and other medications is production of a **serotonin syndrome,** for example, when SSRIs are administered with a **monoamine oxidase inhibitor**. In the extreme, serotonin syndrome can be fatal. Therefore, these two classes should never be used together or in close proximity. In switching from one to the other, the patient should not have taken the discontinued medication at least 2 weeks (5 weeks with fluoxetine) prior to starting the MAOI antidepressant. Other interactions are more relative, and SSRIs can be used with virtually any other medication as long as the physician is prepared to make dosing adjustments and is aware that certain side effects may be more likely.

Drug–drug interactions may be due to pharmacokinetic or pharmacodynamic effects. **Pharmacokinetic interactions** are those in which one drug affects the absorption, metabolism, distribution, or excretion of other drugs. The most important pharmacokinetic effects of SSRIs are on the **P450 cytochrome enzyme** system, which is the major means by which the body inactivates foreign chemicals such as pharmacological agents. Drugs that induce or inhibit the main P450 enzyme that removes another drug from the system will reduce or increase blood levels of the second agent. Sometimes, as with paroxetine, a drug inhibits its own metabolizing enzyme, such that doubling the dose more than doubles steady-state blood levels. Unfortunately, each SSRI inhibits a different P450 enzyme. The most important one is 2D6, which fluoxetine and paroxetine inhibit to a substantial degree, and 3A4, which is strongly inhibited by fluvoxamine (and nefazodone, strictly speaking, not a SSRI). The 2D6 enzyme metabolizes **codeine compounds** and some **antiarrhythmics**, so caution must be exercised when using these drugs together. Blood levels of a **tricyclic** antidepressant may increase several-fold if a 2D6-inhibiting drug is added; conversely, if a TCA is added to a 2D6-inhibiting SSRI, TCA doses otherwise thought of as quite low (e.g., 50 or 75 mg/d) may yield adequate TCA blood levels. Because the 3A4 enzyme metabolizes a wide range of pharmacological agents, care must be used in prescribing 3A4-inhibiting drugs. Citalopram, escitalopram, and, to a lesser extent, sertraline have only relatively weak effects on P450 enzymes, so they are **pharmacokinetically safer** to use with most other drugs (as is mirtazapine, see Other Antidepressants).

Pharmacodynamic interactions occur when the pharmacological effects of two drugs are the same or interact with each other. Pharmacodynamic interactions are mostly **additive**, meaning that a patient taking two drugs, drug A and drug B, will experience the sum of the effects of the two drugs. Thus, a little dry mouth from A plus a little dry mouth from B might add up to a moderate degree of dry mouth from A + B. A little serotonin reuptake inhibition from A plus a little serotonin reuptake inhibition from B will produce moderate inhibition from A + B. However, occasionally, **synergism** may result, especially when drugs having different mechanisms are mixed. For example, a serotonin syndrome is difficult to produce when SSRIs or MAOIs are used alone, even in overdose, but can result if otherwise safe doses of an SSRI and MAOI are used together.

Tricyclic Antidepressants (TCAs)

TCAs were the mainstay of the pharmacotherapy of major depression until the advent of fluoxetine. Blood levels of some TCAs correlate modestly with clinical response, making them useful in monitoring both adherence and dosing. Because TCAs **delay electrical conduction** in the heart, they can be **fatal in overdose**, even with a week's supply of medication. TCAs should probably **not be used in children**, as they have been associated with sudden death (see Chapter 15, Child and Adolescent Psychiatry) and there is little evidence of efficacy.

Dosing

Most TCAs are dosed between 150 and 300 mg/d, starting with 50 mg and increasing the dose by 50 mg every few days to 2 weeks to the FDA maximum, or lower doses if remission or intolerable side effects occur (see Table 16.3). Some physicians use 25 mg as a starting and incremental dose, perhaps switching to 50 mg increments once 100 mg/d

TABLE 16.3 Tricyclic Antidepressants

Generic Name	Brand Name	Usual Starting Dose (total per day)	Usual Dose (total per day)	Maximal Dose (total per day)	Side Effects and Comments
amitriptyline	Elavil, Endep	25–50 mg	100–250 mg	250 mg	Dry mouth, sedation, urinary retention, weight gain, constipation
clomipramine	Anafranil	25–50 mg	150–250 mg	250 mg	Dry mouth, sedation, urinary retention, weight gain, constipation; blood levels may be helpful in assessing adequacy of dosing in OCD
desipramine	Pertofrane, Norpramine	25–50 mg	150–300 mg	300 mg	Dry mouth, urinary retention, weight gain, constipation, sweating; blood level 150–300 ng/mL for treatment of major depression
doxepin	Sinequan	25–50 mg	150–300 mg	300 mg	Dry mouth, sedation, urinary retention, weight gain, constipation; low bioavailability so "tolerability" may be linked to insufficient dosing
imipramine	Tofranil, Pressamine	25–50 mg	150–300 mg	300 mg	Dry mouth, sedation, urinary retention, weight gain, constipation; blood level of combined imipramine and desipramine should exceed 225 ng/mL
nortriptyline	Aventyl	25 mg	50–150 mg	150 mg	Orthostatic hypotension, constipation, dry mouth, urinary retention, weight gain; blood level should be within range of 50–150 ng/mL
protriptyline	Vivactil	10 mg	20–60 mg	60 mg	The same as amitriptyline but less severe anticholinergic effects. Very long half-life
trimipramine	Surmontil	25–50 mg	150–300 mg	300 mg	Same as amitriptyline

is reached. The upper limit for clomipramine is 250 mg/d because there is increased risk for seizures above this dose.

Blood levels may be obtained for TCAs. Levels above 500 ng/mL are rarely helpful and may be toxic. Cardiac complications, often seen in deliberate overdoses, are common when blood levels exceed 1,000 ng/mL. Nortriptyline has a "**therapeutic window**" of efficacy; that is, at least 50 ng/mL is required, but one study suggested that blood levels above 150 ng/mL interferes with benefit.

Side Effects

Anticholinergic side effects are the most common problem with TCAs, including dry mouth, difficulty initiating urination, constipation, and exacerbation of narrow-angle glaucoma. Management is the same as for the anticholinergic effects of antipsychotics (discussed earlier). An inconsequential anticholinergic effect is increased heart rate due to blockage of vagal tone.

TCAs cause **orthostatic hypotension** to varying degrees. Fortunately, increasing the dose does not seem to worsen this problem, and usually the body accommodates to it after several weeks (see Hypotension Associated with Antipsychotics, earlier in this chapter).

The **quinidine-like** effect of TCAs can exacerbate second-degree heart block, resulting in complete heart block and a ventricular rhythm. To protect against this possibility, an **ECG** should be obtained prior to initiating TCA treatment and then periodically to be sure the **QT_C interval** is not prolonged. Prolongation of the QT_C interval should alert the physician not to increase the dose of the TCA further or to lower the dose. A personal or family history of sudden unexplained loss of consciousness or sudden death indicates a vulnerability to TCA-induced arrhythmias and possible sudden death. An individual with such a history should only be given a TCA as a last resort and with frequent ECG monitoring.

Weight gain occurs over months to years in patients taking a TCA. Some patients develop a craving for sweets, while others increase their overall food intake. **Sexual dysfunction**, including delayed ejaculation and anorgasmia, occurs with TCAs, particularly those with a tertiary structure (i.e., amitriptyline, clomipramine, doxepin, imipramine, and trimipramine). TCAs **lower the seizure threshold** and may induce convulsions, especially when taken in overdose, but also occasionally at therapeutic doses. Because **sedation** is common, it is best to give these medications all in a single bedtime dose. Some patients still experience grogginess upon waking in the morning and find that taking some of the dose earlier in the evening allows sufficient time for metabolism so that they waken clear-headed by morning.

Other Antidepressants

Several antidepressants do not fall into any common group, each having its own unique structure and presumed mechanism of action (see Table 16.4). Several block serotonin reuptake so are serotonin reuptake inhibitors (SRIs), but they also have other actions so are not SSRIs. Thus, each may have actions not shared by other antidepressants, possibly providing unique relief for some patients.

Venlafaxine, **desvenlafaxine**, and **duloxetine** are dual uptake inhibitors—at high doses they block both serotonin and norepinephrine reuptake. Duloxetine is the only antidepressant that is also marketed for **pain syndromes**, such as diabetic neuropathy.

While **trazodone** is marketed as an antidepressant, its **soporific** effects are so profound that it is largely used as a nonaddicting sleep aid. Trazodone seems particularly

TABLE 16.4 Other Antidepressants

Generic Name	Brand Name	Mechanism	Usual Starting Dose (total per day)	Usual Dose (total per day)	Maximal Dose (total per day)	Side Effects and Comments
bupropion	Wellbutrin, Wellbutrin SR Wellbutrin XL, Zyban[1]	NRI, DRI[2]	75–150 mg	300–450 mg[3]	450 mg	Overstimulation, insomnia, seizures, dry mouth
duloxetine	Cymbalta	SRI, NRI	20–30 mg	60–120 mg	120 mg	Nausea, sexual dysfunction, hypertension at higher doses. Renally excreted so dosage must be decreased with renal insufficiency
desvenlafaxine	Pristiq	SRI, NRI	50 mg	50 mg	50 mg	Active metabolite of venlafaxine
maprotiline	Ludiomil	NRI	50 mg	100–250 mg[3]	250 mg	Dry mouth, constipation, sweating, rash, seizures
mirtazapine	Remeron	Inhibits α and several 5-HT receptors	15 mg	15–45 mg	45 mg	Sedation (especially at lowest doses), weight gain. Few interactions with other medications.
nefazodone	Serzone[4]	SRI, 5-HT$_{2A}$ inhibitor	50–100 mg	300–600 mg	600 mg	Sedation, hepatotoxicity, minimal sexual dysfunction
trazodone	Desyrel	5-HT$_{1A}$ inhibitor	50 mg	300–600 mg	600 mg	Very sedating, priapism. More often prescribed as an nonaddicting hypnotic than as an antidepressant
venlafaxine	Effexor, Effexor XR	SRI, NRI	37.5–75 mg	150–375 mg	375 mg	Nausea, dry mouth, sexual dysfunction, hypertension (at higher doses)

[1] Marketed at 300 mg/d for smoking cessation.

[2] While bupropion inhibits norepinephrine and dopamine reuptake, at doses used in humans, this effect appears to be minimal and possibly insufficient to account for its antidepressant activity, which remains unknown.

[3] Maprotiline should not be used above 250 mg/d and bupropion beyond 450 mg/d because of increased risk for seizures.

[4] Brand was removed from the market and only generic nefazodone is available.

safe and effective for patients who develop insomnia during the course of their treatment with other drugs, especially MAOIs and bupropion. **Nefazodone** is associated with rare cases of liver failure, and the brand product was removed from the market. It is not associated with sexual side effects and is particularly useful for patients who achieve remission with an SSRI but also have significant sexual dysfunction.

Mirtazapine blocks many receptors, including several serotonin receptors, the α-receptor and histamine receptors. Because one of the receptors that mirtazapine blocks is the anxiogenic 5-HT$_{2A}$ receptor, like nefazodone, it is anxiolytic. Its blockade of histamine receptors presumably accounts for its soporific and appetite-increasing effects, making it a good drug for depressed patients who sleep and eat poorly, such as the **elderly**. While technically a tetracyclic, **maprotiline** chemically looks like a tricyclic with a bridge across the middle ring, and its efficacy and side effect profile are similar to that of TCAs. Its early association with a pruritic rash, tendency to induce seizures, and lack of advantage over TCAs have made it an uncommonly prescribed medication.

Dosing and Side Effects

Seizures are a risk in the use of bupropion, clomipramine, and maprotiline, limiting the maximum safe doses of these drugs. Bupropion, venlafaxine, and duloxetine can increase the **blood pressure**, so readings should be obtained periodically, especially with each dose increase. Patients are particularly vulnerable to blood pressure effects at 450 mg/d of bupropion, above 225 mg/d of venlafaxine, and above 60 mg/d of duloxetine. One advantage of bupropion over other antidepressants is that it is **weight neutral**. Bupropion, nefazodone, and mirtazepine are also **not associated with the sexual dysfunction** of other antidepressants. **Venlafaxine** has a short half-life, causing a **withdrawal syndrome** with missed doses. It is also available in an extended-release formulation. At low doses venlafaxine acts as an SSRI, but at higher doses (above 225 mg/d) it is also a norepinephrine reuptake inhibitor. Thus, particularly at higher doses, venlafaxine produces not only the side effects of SSRIs but also the norepinephrine-related side effects seen with TCAs. **Duloxetine** is particularly likely to produce **nausea**, so it should be started at its lowest dose (20 mg) and given with food.

Trazodone is most commonly used as a sleep aid in doses ranging from 50 to 200 mg/d. Because it is so **soporific**, it should be given at bedtime when prescribed for its antidepressant properties. Antidepressant effects of trazodone are achieved at higher doses than needed for sleep aid effects. Trazodone produces **priapism** (a painful inability of the penis to detumesce) in about 1 in 800 males; men must be alerted to prolonged erections and warned to notify their doctor immediately and reduce the dose should they experience longer-lasting erections.

Because **nefazodone** blocks the 5-HT$_{2A}$ receptor, it can be anxiolytic. A soporific drug marketed as a twice-daily dosing, it was never popular because the morning dose typically caused daytime sedation. Then, rare reports of **liver failure** (estimated to occur once in 200,000 patient years of use) led to the brand product being removed from the market.

Mirtazepine should be given all at bedtime, starting with 15 mg; some physicians believe it is less sedating at higher doses and start patients on 30 mg/d.

Monoamine Oxidase Inhibitors (MAOIs)

There are two main classes of MAOIs, the hydrazines (phenelzine and isocarboxazid) and the nonhydrazines (tranylcypromine and selegiline) (see Table 16.5). The main practical

TABLE 16.5 Monoamine Oxidase Inhibitors

Generic Name	Brand Name	Usual Starting Dose (total per day)	Usual Dose (total per day)	Maximal Dose (total per day)	Side Effects and Comments
isocarboxazid	Marplan	10 mg	20–30 mg	60 mg	Same as phenelzine; never widely prescribed since introduced after the enthusiasm for MAOIs had waned
phenelzine	Nardil	15 mg	45–90 mg	90 mg	Weight gain, slowing of bowel activity, shifts in sleep timing, insomnia, hypersomnia, sexual dysfunction, orthostatic hypotension
selegiline	Emsam	6 mg/24^0	6–12 mg/24^0	12 mg/24^0	A patch, so may irritate skin where applied. At higher dosage, dietary restrictions apply.
tranylcypromine	Parnate	10 mg	30–60 mg	60 mg	Overstimulation, insomnia, biphasic effect on blood pressure (immediate hypertension, later orthostatic hypotension). The MAOI most associated with the "cheese reaction." Historically viewed as the most effective MAOI but never rigorously tested head to head.

difference is that hydrazines, but not nonhydrazines, are associated with a lupus-like syndrome requiring discontinuation of the medication should it occur. All MAOIs marketed in the United States are irreversible, meaning that they render the enzyme permanently nonfunctional. Reversible MAOIs are safer and can be used with fewer dietary restrictions. They are currently unavailable in the United States.

Because of the problems that MAOIs present, they are not used as first-line agents but rather are reserved for patients who have done poorly with at least two other antidepressants or who have had a prior good response to an MAOI.

Dosing

Phenelzine is the best studied and most widely used MAOI. Side effects can take a few days to a week to develop, so the dose should be increased in 15 mg/d increments every week or two, stopping at 60 mg/d. It can take several weeks for the effects of a given dose to manifest, and phenelzine is much better tolerated at 60 mg/d than at 90 mg/d. If remission does not occur after several weeks at 60 mg/d, the dose should be increased further to the FDA maximal dose of 90 mg/d. Because phenelzine's effect on sleep is idiosyncratic, some patients find taking it in the morning is best; others, at bedtime.

Tranylcypromine is begun at 10 mg/d and increased in weekly increments to 40 mg/d, and then biweekly to a maximum of 60 mg/d. Since tranylcypromine is an amphetamine-like compound, it can be quite activating and is best taken in the morning. **Isocarboxazid** is little used but dosed and used similarly to tranylcypromine.

Selegiline is of particular interest because it is administered as a **patch** applied daily and, at its lowest dose (6 mg/24 hours), it **does not require a tyramine-free diet**. Patients should be held at that dose for at least 2 weeks in order to identify the occasional patient who will improve on this dose. Application sites should be rotated among the shoulder, thigh, upper arm, and hip to avoid local irritation at the patch site. The maximal dose is 12 mg/24 hours. Usually, the patch is applied each morning. For patients who experience insomnia or are bothered by the local irritation, removal of the patch at bedtime can be helpful.

Side Effects

MAOIs inhibit the main enzyme that inactivates tyramine, a pressor compound. Ingestion of tyramine while significant MAO inhibition is present can quickly (within 30 minutes) raise the blood pressure. This hypertension can reach dangerous levels, creating a **hypertensive crisis**. A hemorrhagic stroke and, potentially, death can result, particularly in a vulnerable individual with an occult intracranial aneurysm. Therefore, **careful adherence to a tyramine-free diet** is a must whenever the irreversible MAOIs marketed in the United States are used.

A particularly troublesome blood pressure effect that seems to be specific to tranylcypromine is its **biphasic effect on blood pressure**. That is, immediately (30–60 minutes) after taking the dose, the blood pressure increases, but by 120 minutes later it is back to normal, or even below normal. In its extreme, this pressor effect of tranylcypromine can be of hypertensive crisis proportions. Therefore, the blood pressure should be checked 45–60 minutes following each dose increase of tranylcypromine, especially when the dose is above 30 mg, and the physician should add an antihypertensive agent if the systolic blood pressure rises more than 25 mm Hg or the diastolic increases more than 15 mm Hg. While ingestion of tyramine in the presence of an MAOI can cause a hypertensive crisis, the direct effect of MAOIs is **orthostatic hypotension**. Most patients accommodate to this effect (see Orthostatic Hypotension, earlier in this chapter).

Tranylcypromine can cause severe **insomnia**, usually treatable by low-dose (i.e., 50–200 mg hs) trazodone. Phenelzine and isocarboxazid can result in **daytime sleepiness**, sometimes manifesting as suddenly falling asleep in the late afternoon. Patients who experience this effect need to plan their schedules to avoid driving at the times when this **narcolepsy-like effect** is most likely to occur. Some patients on MAOIs experience marked shifts in their sleep schedule such that they cannot sleep at usual times but must sleep during the day, or they cannot fall asleep until the wee hours, then cannot waken until mid-afternoon. **Excessive sleeping** of 12 or 14 hours per day also occurs, especially with phenelzine.

Delayed orgasm and anorgasmia occur with the MAOIs, especially the hydrazines. Loss of libido and difficulty achieving or maintaining erections are also reported.

The hydrazines can cause **weight gain**, which is sometimes quite significant. Occasionally, the weight gain continues as long as patients remain on the medication, never reaching a plateau. At times patients have a general increase in their food intake. Others experience irresistible cravings for certain foods, particularly carbohydrates ("I just have to eat pasta"). Some say they get the "munchies." Others may eat in their sleep, as they deny remembering that they got up but find an entire pie or loaf of bread missing in the morning. When the eating and resultant weight gain cannot be curtailed, the medication must be stopped. Sometimes a switch to tranylcypromine can achieve the same benefit without this problem.

The hydrazines can cause peripheral edema, bowel slowing, and "electric shock–like" shooting sensations that tend to occur in the neck. These sensations are thought to be due vitamin B_6 deficiency induced by hydrazines and can be treated with B_6, 150–300 mg/d, in three divided doses.

Tyramine-Free Diet

Patients taking an MAOI must avoid ingesting tyramine, which is contained in many commonly eaten foods. Foods to be avoided include products containing **aged protein**, since tyramine is produced by the breakdown of the amino acid tyrosine. Examples of tyramine-containing foods include aged cheese (blue and cheddar cheeses are forbidden, while cottage cheese is safe) and aged fish and meats (such as lox, salami, and ham), but not fresh fish, chicken, or other meat. It is important to realize that the tyramine content of the same product may vary considerably, so patients who mistakenly eat a forbidden food should not be lulled into thinking that a particular forbidden food is safe, as the next salami sandwich might still give them a hypertensive crisis with the potential for an intracranial hemorrhage.

Drug–Drug Interactions

Meperidine and all **SSRIs** are **absolutely contraindicated** with MAOIs, as the combination can produce a **serotonin syndrome** (see SSRI Drug Interactions, earlier in this chapter). Some patients choose to wear a bracelet or carry a wallet card warning that they are taking an MAOI. Other drug interactions involving MAOIs generally only reflect an additive effect in the presence of another medication with a similar side effect profile.

Assessment of Treatment Response

The goal of treatment is generally remission. That is, the patient should no longer experience the targeted symptoms. A lessening of symptoms is certainly desired, but should be considered an inadequate response if residual symptoms remain. Additional **dosage increases** and **adding or switching to other medications or a focused psychotherapy** should be instituted until complete remission is achieved.

For patients who do not improve, the antidepressant should probably be stopped after 4 weeks at the FDA maximal or maximally tolerated dose. For depressed patients in whom it is assumed that the medication is responsible for their improvement, the medication should be continued for **at least 6 months**, as relapse is high if it is discontinued after shorter duration of treatment. For patients who have had more than two prior episodes of major depression or who are experiencing chronic depression, indefinite treatment might be suggested as a reasonable option. Indefinite treatment also seems indicated when several trials off medication have resulted in prompt relapse.

Placebo Effects

Placebo-controlled studies demonstrate that remissions that are early (first 2 weeks) and non-sustained (i.e., improvement is followed in a few weeks by return of symptoms) occur no more often in depressed patients taking an antidepressant than in those receiving an inactive pill. Therefore, physicians cannot attribute such early apparent benefit to the pharmacological effects of the antidepressant and should be aware that subsequent relapse is possible. A corollary is that delayed (i.e., more than 2 weeks) sustained remission identifies likely medication effect. Patients who experience delayed and sustained improvement should be told of the likelihood of relapse should they discontinue their medication prematurely.

Switch Strategies

When a patient has not benefited at all from the initial medication, it is usually best to discontinue its use and switch to another treatment. Generally, an agent having a different presumed mechanism of action is chosen, although data to support this strategy are currently lacking.

Augmentation Strategies

For patients experiencing **partial remission**, it is generally recommended that the same medication be continued and **another antidepressant be added**. As with switch strategies, it makes the most sense to add a drug having a **different mechanism of action**, although, again, there are few data to support this intuitive logic. Thus, if the initial treatment is with an SSRI, a commonly chosen next medication is bupropion, whether augmenting or switching.

Other effective augmenting agents include lithium, triiodothyronine, and antipsychotic medications, all of which have multiple studies demonstrating their utility when a first-line agent has not resulted in remission of symptoms. **Lithium** doses should be in the same range as those used to treat mania, aiming to achieve blood levels of 0.7–1.0 mEq/L. **Triiodothyronine** is started at 25 µg/d, increased to 75 µg/d, and continued for several months before concluding it is ineffective. Augmentation with several **antipsychotics** has been shown effective in large double-blind studies, especially for bipolar depression. But their significant side effects relating to glucose metabolism and their propensity to produce tardive dyskinesia dictate that antipsychotic augmentation should be reserved for patients who are psychotic or have not benefited from two or more standard antidepressants.

Discontinuing an Antidepressant

TCAs and SRIs are associated with **withdrawal** symptoms if abruptly discontinued. Therefore, save for dire circumstances, they should be **tapered over a week or two** prior to stopping them completely. A useful strategy for stopping any antidepressant is to taper the dose slowly as a hedge against relapse, since abrupt discontinuation might precipitate sudden recurrence of depressive symptoms in full force, perhaps including suicidal ideation or behavior. If the antidepressant is tapered slowly, mild symptoms may signal a continuing need for the medication, thus further taper should be stopped, before the full syndrome re-emerges. Once the medication has been completely stopped, the **first 2 months** are the highest risk for relapse, so patients should be seen frequently during this fragile period. Depressive symptoms occurring during these first 2 months are considered to be a **relapse** of the initial episode, whereas new symptoms appearing after 2 months signal a new depressive episode.

MOOD STABILIZERS

The first mood stabilizer, lithium, was reported by Cade in 1949 to control psychotic excitement—now conceptualized as mania. Since that time, a variety of medications have received FDA approval for dampening the mood swings characteristic of bipolar

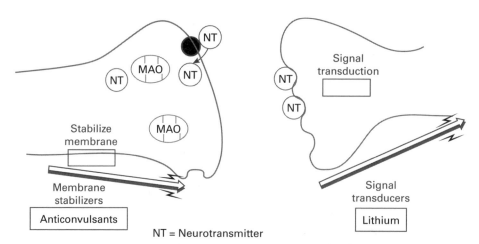

FIGURE 16.4 How Mood Stabilizers Work. Most drugs that stabilize mood stabilize the cell membrane by interfering with voltage-sensitive ion channels, particularly sodium and calcium, making spontaneous discharge less likely. They may also affect intracellular signal transduction and enhance the inhibitory effects of γ-aminobutyric acid (GABA) and glutamate. Lithium's mechanism is unknown, but it may be via effects on intracellular signaling pathways.

disorder. These include several antipsychotic medications and three anticonvulsants. Ideally, a single agent would equally lower and prevent elevated moods *and* raise and prevent depressed moods. Of currently marketed agents, lithium comes closest to this goal, yet leaves much room for improvement. Figure 16.4 provides a schematic for the hypothesized mechanism of action of the mood stabilizers.

Lithium

The main indications for use of lithium are the **acute and maintenance treatment of mania**. Lithium has also been used for other bipolar states, but its efficacy for these is less well demonstrated and less predictable. In addition, multiple studies have demonstrated lithium's utility for **aggression** and **suicidality**, as an **augmenter** of antidepressants in **treatment-refractory depression**, and to smooth out the "**hyperemotionality**" of histrionic and borderline personality disorders. These latter uses are "off-label," however (i.e., not FDA approved).

Pretreatment Evaluation

Lithium has a narrow therapeutic index and is highly **toxic** when blood levels become too high. As a chemical element, lithium is not metabolized, but excreted almost exclusively by the kidney. Therefore, prior to initiating treatment with lithium, **kidney function** (i.e., blood urea nitrogen [BUN] and creatinine) must be assessed and the patient must be carefully educated about lithium toxicity. If the BUN or creatinine is abnormal, alternative treatment should be considered. Patients' renal blood flow must be stable for lithium to be safely administered. If lithium is determined to be necessary in a patient having decreased renal function, dosage must be started very low and increased only after determining that the blood level is inadequate. Because lithium acts in the body like other salts, **electrolytes** should be checked before beginning lithium treatment to make sure that sodium and potassium levels are normal. Events that disturb electrolyte balance—persistent vomiting or diarrhea, or prolonged exposure to high heat without adequate hydration—will unpredictably alter lithium levels. Abnormal sodium and potassium levels can adversely affect lithium's efficacy and alter its excretion by the kidney. Finally, because lithium interferes with thyroid hormone synthesis, it is important to obtain thyroid function tests, particularly thyroid-stimulating hormone (**TSH**), as a pretreatment baseline for later comparison.

Dosing

Marketed in pill and capsule formulations as lithium carbonate, there is also a liquid, lithium citrate. Both salts are highly effective in the acute and maintenance treatment of mania. While the company package inserts recommend twice- or three-times daily dosing, clinical experience suggests that once-**daily dosing** is just as effective, improves patient adherence, and produces fewer side effects.

Lithium is generally started at 600 or 900 mg hs and titrated to a **blood level of 0.7–1.0 mEq/L**, at which it is maintained. Once lithium's efficacy has been demonstrated in a given patient, the effective blood level is maintained indefinitely, usually without requiring changes in dosage unless renal function changes.

Blood levels of lithium should be obtained about a week after each dosage change. Once the desired blood level is achieved, it remains stable as long as kidney function does not change. However, dehydration, diuretics, and many other medications can alter kidney function. Therefore, patients must be warned to **avoid dehydration** and to let their physician know if a diuretic, antihypertensive, or persistent dosing of a nonsteroidal anti-inflammatory medication is prescribed.

Concurrent use of **diuretics** and lithium has long been considered an absolute contraindication. Because thiazide and furosemide diuretics cause increased reabsorption of lithium by the kidney, use of these agents by patients taking lithium will result in elevation of lithium blood levels, potentially to toxic levels. Toxicity can be avoided if the lithium dose is reduced and the lithium level is monitored carefully, allowing lithium and diuretics to be used together safely. Since this combination is problematic, it is usually best to try other treatments first. Similarly, kidney disease may alter the excretion of lithium, producing toxic lithium levels. Therefore, it is important to more carefully monitor lithium levels if an acute kidney ailment develops and, in the absence of known kidney disease, to obtain **kidney function testing and a lithium level every 6 months**. Because lithium can interfere with thyroid function, a **TSH level** should be obtained **annually**. If the TSH becomes elevated, adjunctive thyroid hormone (e.g., T_3 25–75 μg/d) should be added until the TSH normalizes.

Side Effects

Common side effects of lithium treatment include **nausea, diarrhea, tremor, acne**, and **excessive urination**. The latter is due to lithium-induced diabetes insipidus and can result in dehydration and lithium toxicity if the patient fails to compensate with extra liquids. This problem is much less common if lithium is given once daily.

Lithium **toxicity** occurs at blood levels that are not much higher than those that are therapeutic, dictating that lithium blood levels, hydration, and kidney function be closely followed. Symptoms of lithium toxicity include **ataxia, myoclonus**, and **mental confusion**. These symptoms may be accompanied by **nausea, diarrhea**, and **vomiting**. The resulting loss of electrolytes may exacerbate toxicity as the kidneys strive to maintain electrolyte balance. If the afflicted individual continues to take lithium, delirium, coma, and death can ensue. Therefore, lithium-treated patients who develop incoordination or become confused should stop their lithium until further evaluation establishes that they are not lithium toxic.

For over 30 years, it has been thought that **long-term** lithium treatment damages the kidney, paralleling the experience with antipsychotics and tardive dyskinesia. Whether this is true remains unclear. It has been suggested that the renal damage stems from micro-episodes of lithium toxicity, not simply long-term treatment. Some investigators suggest that once-daily lithium dosing may minimize this risk, as lithium levels become sufficiently low in the several hours before the next lithium dose that the kidney can recover. Alternatively, others have suggested that once-daily dosing would lead to higher blood levels, through the kidney's multiplicative effect, and thus recommend divided doses so that the peaks are never too high. While both hypotheses are attractive, there is insufficient data to strongly support either one. Close collaboration between the knowledgeable and motivated patient and the physician is the best prevention against complications. Persons with a cavalier attitude about their care, who do not appreciate the modifiable risks and the benefits of lithium treatment, are poor candidates for such treatment.

Anticonvulsants

Divalproex and **carbamazepine** are indicated for **refractory mania, rapid cycling bipolar disorder, and severe mood instability**. Divalproex and probably carbamazepine are also useful to counteract **intermittent explosive disorder**, including "road rage." There is some indication that divalproex is particularly helpful for hypomania, rapid cycling, and mania that is primarily characterized by irritability, and that it is less useful for pure mania. **Lamotrigine** is indicated for bipolar depression, but it may not work well for nondepressive symptoms of bipolar disorder.

Pretreatment Evaluation
Because these agents can be toxic to the liver and bone marrow, baseline blood count and **liver function testing** must be obtained. A baseline **platelet count** is necessary when using divalproex, and a baseline **white blood cell count** when prescribing carbamazepine. A baseline **ECG** is required when using carbamazepine, which can exacerbate cardiac conduction delays.

Dosing
Divalproex sodium is better tolerated than valproic acid, which is little used. The initial dose is 250 or 500 mg/d, increasing in 250 mg/d increments, as tolerated. At 1 g/d, a blood level is drawn, seeking a level of 50–125 µg/mL. More aggressive dosing can result in more rapid achievement in therapeutic blood level and clinical response. Because of the ease and effectiveness of rapid dosing, divalproex sodium has been quickly adopted as the first-line of treatment for acute mania over lithium.

Carbamazepine used to be a problematic drug because of its short half-life requiring multiple daily dosing. A delayed-release formulation is now available, however, and its once-daily dosing is preferred. Dosing starts at 200 mg/d and increases in 200 mg/d increments to a blood level of 6–12 µg/mL, typically obtained at 1–2 g/d in dose. Blood level monitoring with carbamazepine is primarily a guide to prevent toxicity, rather than establishing a clear therapeutic level.

Because **lamotrigine** causes frequent allergic responses if too high a dose is given too quickly, dosing begins at 25 mg/d with weekly 25 mg/d dose increments until 100 mg/d is reached. Then 50 or 100 mg/d increments may be safely used without increasing the risk for drug allergy. Usual effective doses range from 100 to 400 mg/d.

Side Effects

Divalproex interferes with **platelet function**, so bruising may occur. Initial dosing may induce **nausea**, and **weight gain** can be problematic. Too high a dose can cause **incoordination** and **confusion**. Divalproex has been implicated in the production or exacerbation of polycystic ovaries, but the suggestive studies cannot be considered definitive. There have also been warnings regarding pancreatitis.

Carbamazepine routinely drops the white blood cell count into the 3,000–4,000 cells/μL range. In rare cases, however, **agranulocytosis** can occur. Therefore, white blood cell count should be monitored and the drug stopped if it drops below 1,500 cells/μL. Specifically, a **white blood cell count** should be obtained at baseline, then **biweekly** for the first month of treatment, then **every 3–6 months**. Excessive carbamazepine can cause **toxic symptoms**, such as **ataxia** and **diplopia**. Nontoxic side effects include **dry mouth** and **constipation**.

Lamotrigine causes a skin **rash** in about 10% of patients in whom the dose is started high or increased quickly, but only about 1% of the time with the recommended dosing. Occasional patients will experience **headaches, nausea, dizziness, ataxia, somnolence, diplopia, and blurred vision**. The most serious side effect associated with lamotrigine is **Stevens-Johnsons syndrome**. This **potentially fatal** side effect is associated with **too-rapid dose increases** or pharmacokinetic effects when **combined with medications such as divalproex sodium**. Therefore, it is important to monitor all of the medications taken by a patient who is prescribed lamotrigine.

ANXIOLYTIC MEDICATIONS AND HYPNOTIC AGENTS

Benzodiazepines

The first treatment marketed for nonpsychotic anxiety was meprobamate, a still available but now virtually unused medication. Since the introduction of chlordiazepoxide in 1960, the benzodiazepines have largely replaced meprobamate, because of both efficacy and safety. While occasional patients become addicted to benzodiazepines, the likelihood is low, and these are often highly effective agents for **nonspecific anxiety** and **specific anxiety disorders**. They are also used as **sleep agents, muscle relaxants**, and anticonvulsants and to **counteract withdrawal symptoms on abrupt discontinuation of other medications**, particularly alcohol. Thus, even though generally thought of as antianxiety agents, the benzodiazepines have multiple uses. Figure 16.5 provides a schematic for the hypothesized mechanism of action of the anxiolytics.

Table 16.6 lists the benzodiazepines and their indications. These indications are mostly accidents of history, in the sense that the indication listed in the FDA was the one for which the marketing company chose to demonstrate efficacy rather than necessarily being its only or best use. The main use of chlordiazepoxide is to counteract alcohol withdrawal symptoms, and clonazepam was first marketed as an antiseizure medication. Flurazepam and temazepam were marketed as sleep aids.

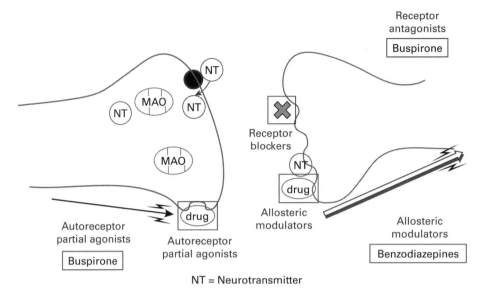

FIGURE 16.5 How Anxiolytics Work. All benzodiazepines act as positive allosteric modulators. That is, they do nothing when acting alone. However, when a benzodiazepine occupies its binding site on a γ-aminobutyric acid (GABA) receptor, GABA stimulates the receptor more strongly. Thus, benzodiazepines are helper drugs that strengthen GABA's inhibitory effect, decreasing the likelihood of affected postsynaptic neurons to discharge. Propranolol blocks the postsynaptic catecholamine β-receptor, preventing catecholamine stimulation of postsynaptic neurons via β-receptors. Buspirone is a partial agonist of the 5-HT$_{1A}$ receptor, an inhibitory presynaptic receptor.

Pretreatment Evaluation

All benzodiazepines are potentially addictive, in that occasional patients find they need to escalate the dose in order to retain benefit but have withdrawal symptoms if they do not take their medication. Therefore, dose escalation and too-frequent requests for renewal of prescriptions should alert the physician to possible dependency. The development of dependency usually means benzodiazepines cannot be used for a particular patient. **Dependency** is more common with rapidly absorbed, tightly bound, shorter half-life drugs, such as lorazepam and alprazolam, than with more slowly absorbed, less tightly bound agents, such as oxazepam, or longer half-life drugs, such as diazepam and clonazepam, although tolerance and/or withdrawal symptoms can occur with these drugs as well. If benzodiazepines are considered, it is important to take a detailed addiction history. Physicians should exercise caution in prescribing a potentially addictive drug to patients having histories of addiction. If electing to prescribe a benzodiazepine to such a patient, the physician should be particularly careful in monitoring for possible addiction.

An important issue in evaluating anxiety and insomnia is determining whether they are **primary or secondary**. That is, is another condition causing the anxiety or insomnia? Terminal insomnia, for example, is a common accompanying symptom of depression, whereas initial insomnia is frequent in anxiety disorders and can stem from going to sleep feeling angry. It is therefore important to determine whether another condition is present and whether the anxiety or insomnia may be a presenting symptom of some

TABLE 16.6 Benzodiazepines

Generic Name	Brand Name	Mechanism	Half-Life (hours)	Usual Starting Dose (total per day)	Usual Dose	Maximal Dose (total per day)	Absorption	Side Effects
Anxiolytics								
alprazolam	Xanax Xanax CR	Positive GABA-A receptor allosteric modulator*	12 ± 2	.25–.5 mg	.5 mg prn–2 mg tid	6 mg	Moderate to rapid	Sedation, incoordination, confusion, physical dependence
chlordiazepoxide	Librium	Positive GABA-A receptor allosteric modulator*	10 ± 3.4	10 mg	10 mg prn–20 mg tid	60 mg	Moderate	Sedation, incoordination, confusion, physical dependence
clonazepam	Klonopin	Positive GABA-A receptor allosteric modulator*	23 ± 5	.5 mg	.5 mg prn–2 mg tid	6 mg	Rapid	Sedation, incoordination, confusion, physical dependence
clorazepate	Tranxene	Positive GABA-A receptor allosteric modulator*	2.0 ± 0.9	30 mg	7.5–30 mg/d	90 mg	Moderate	Sedation, incoordination, confusion, physical dependence
lorazepam	Ativan	Positive GABA-A receptor allosteric modulator*	14 ± 5	.25–5 mg	.5 mg prn–2 mg tid	6 mg	Rapid	Sedation, incoordination, confusion, addiction
Hypnotics								
estazolam	Prosom	Positive GABA-A receptor allosteric modulator*	10–24	1 mg hs	1–2 mg hs	2 mg hs	Moderate to rapid	Sedation, incoordination, confusion, physical dependence
flurazepam	Dalmane	Positive GABA-A receptor allosteric modulator*	74 ± 24	30 mg hs	15–30 mg hs	30 mg hs	Rapid	Dizziness, daytime drowsiness, ataxia, headache, heartburn; may be more effective on second and third night of use
quazepam	Doral	Positive GABA-A receptor allosteric modulator*	39	15 mg hs	7.5–15 mg hs	15 mg hs	Rapid	Daytime drowsiness, headaches, fatigue, dizziness; long (72 hours) half-life active metabolite
temazepam	Restoril	Positive GABA-A receptor allosteric modulator*	11 ± 6	15 mg hs	15–30 mg hs	30 mg hs	Slow	Daytime drowsiness, headaches, fatigue, dizziness
triazolam	Halcion	Positive GABA-A receptor allosteric modulator*	2.9 ± 1.0	.25	.125–0.5 mg hs	0.5 mg hs	Rapid	Daytime drowsiness, headaches, fatigue, dizziness, anterograde amnesia

*A positive allosteric modulator has no direct action, but its presence at a receptor enhances the effect of the receptor's neurotransmitter, in this case, GABA.

other disorder. A careful course of illness history should help in this regard. For example, if each time the patient's depression recurs his or her anxiety also recurs, and whenever depressive symptoms remit anxiety also remits, it seems likely that the anxiety is a secondary symptom of the depressive illness. However, if a patient reports having significant trouble sleeping, whether depressed or not, a primary sleep disorder in addition to depression seems likely. The use of anxiolytic medications in the presence of another disorder should be approached with some caution. While their use in this circumstance may risk addiction and side effects, benzodiazepines can provide effective symptomatic relief of anxiety, whether in the context of another disorder or not. Because benzodiazepines do not usually treat depressive disorders, their use as monotherapy for anxiety in the presence of depression denies patients with symptoms of both anxiety and depression adequate treatment for their depressive disorder. Also, always treating anxiety as if separate from depression can result in overtreatment if standard treatment of the depression would have relieved the anxiety as well.

In patients with insomnia, it is important to determine the **timing** and characteristics of the sleep problem. Some patients have trouble getting to sleep but sleep well once asleep. Others easily fall asleep and sleep well for the initial portion of the night but then waken too early. Some patients experience restless, unsatisfying sleep, while others have a shift in the timing of their sleep such that they are unable to fall asleep, then sleep 8 or more hours, and others sleep more than 8 hours.

A final common source of insomnia is as a side effect of other treatments, most notably stimulants, and antidepressants such as SSRIs, bupropion, and MAOIs. The best treatment of insomnia when it is a symptom of another problem is to treat the underlying problem, although drug-induced insomnia may require counteractive treatment if the causative agent effectively treats an underlying illness and thus cannot be readily discontinued. Sleep–wake changes are common in psychosis and mania, which should be the primary focus of treatment rather than the sleep problems.

Drug Selection

The selection of a particular benzodiazepine depends on the goal of treatment. If a long-term **antianxiety** effect is desired (as when treating the chronic worry of generalized anxiety disorder or the high levels of interpanic anxiety typical of panic disorder with agoraphobia), a long half-life medication such as clonazepam or diazepam usually is best. On the other hand, for treatment of the anxiety of a social event having a short duration, a shorter half-life drug, such as alprazolam or lorazepam, may be best. Alprazolam and clonazepam may specifically relieve panic attacks, not just intercurrent anxiety.

Selection of a sleep aid depends on the **timing of the insomnia**. Generally, a short-acting drug, such as triazolam or zolpidem, is best for initial insomnia, while longer half-life agents, such as flurazepam or temazepam, are best for middle and terminal sleep difficulty.

Dosing

Dose should always be started low and increased only if insufficient relief is experienced. Dose can be increased nightly until the maximal dose is reached or sleep improves. The main danger is that a given dose may initially work well and then stop working. If the patient appears to require progressively higher doses, **tolerance** may be present. Tolerance should alert the clinician to the potential for dependence (see Chapter 7, Substance-Related and Addictive Disorders). Tolerance differs from initial ineffectiveness of a lower dose; in that case raising the dose provides important benefit.

Clonazepam is started at 0.25 or 0.5 mg with upward adjustments of 0.25 or 0.5 mg until remission of anxiety or side effects (most typically, daytime somnolence) occur. **Diazepam** is started at 2.5 or 5 mg with upward titration of 2.5 or 5 mg. Because of their long half-lives, clonazepam and diazepam are typically given once or twice daily. **Alprazolam** and **lorazepam** are started at doses similar to that of clonazepam, but these shorter half-life drugs are given as needed up to four times a day. However, if a patient is taking a short half-life medication multiple times a day, the person is probably better served by a drug having a longer half-life.

Side Effects

As noted earlier, the major problem with benzodiazepines is their potential for abuse. Withdrawal symptoms may occur if the benzodiazepines are suddenly discontinued. Also, **"rebound insomnia"** can happen the first few nights one does not take these drugs. It can take a few nights of poor sleep before a normal sleep cycle is restored once a benzodiazepine is stopped. Rebound insomnia misinterpreted as a return of the original insomnia can result in continued but unnecessary use.

Patients taking longer half-life drugs may still experience their soporific effects on wakening, thus feeling sleepy or **groggy** in the morning. This effect may be counteracted by taking some of the medication earlier in the evening or switching to a shorter half-life medication. For example, switching from flurazepam to temazepam may alleviate morning sleepiness.

Excessive benzodiazepine use can cause **incoordination** and **difficulty concentrating**. Patients must be **warned about driving** and using dangerous tools while on a benzodiazepine. Rarely, patients become **disinhibited** when they take benzodiazepines. Some agents result in **retrograde amnesia**, wherein a user seems perfectly alert and oriented but later has no recollection of the conversation, having eaten the meal, or been to the event that witnesses insist occurred.

Non-Benzodiazepine Anxiolytics and Hypnotics

Buspirone is the one non-benzodiazepine marketed only for anxiety. Its major advantage is that it is **nonaddictive**. Buspirone's disadvantage is its **delay in onset** of efficacy: it does not provide the immediate relief of symptoms afforded by the benzodiazepines. Some studies have shown that patients who are naïve to buspirone find better relief from their anxiety than those who had been previously treated with a benzodiazepine. Buspirone is begun at 5 mg, often two or three times a day, titrating with 5 mg increments to 15–30 mg bid.

Propranolol, a beta-blocker, is useful for performance anxiety, as it reduces many of the anxiety-driven symptoms that can interfere with performance, such as tremor, sweating, and tachycardia. It is prescribed at doses of 10–40 mg given 30–60 minutes before a presentation. Table 16.7 summarizes information about the non-benzodiazepine anxiolytics and hypnotics.

MEDICATIONS FOR SUBSTANCE-RELATED DISORDERS

Eight medications are marketed for the treatment of substance-related disorders: disulfiram, naltrexone, and acamprosate for alcohol use disorders; bupropion, varenicline, and nicotine for smoking cessation; and methadone and buprenorphine for opioid addiction (see also Chapter 7, Substance-Related and Addictive Disorders). Figure 16.6 provides a schematic for the hypothesized mechanism of action of these agents.

TABLE 16.7 Non-Benzodiazepine Anxiolytic and Hypnotic Medications

Generic Name	Brand Name	Mechanism	Half-Life (hours)	Usual Starting Dose (total per day)	Usual Dose	Maximal Dose (total per day)	Side Effects
Anxiolytics							
buspirone	Buspar	5-HT$_{1A}$ receptor partial agonist	2.4 ± 1.1	5 mg	15–30 mg bid	60 mg	Dizziness, headaches, nausea,
propranolol	Inderal	Beta-blocker	3.9 ± 0.4	10 mg	10–40 mg prn	120 mg	Hypotension, bradycardia
Hypnotics							
eszopiclone	Lunesta	Unknown	6	2 mg hs	1–3 mg hs	3 mg hs	Dysguisia, headache, daytime drowsiness, dry mouth, dizziness, heartburn
trazodone	Desyrel	5-HT$_{2A}$ receptor partial agonist	3–6	25–50 mg hs	25–200 mg hs	600 mg/d	Morning grogginess, priapism in males (but, probably only at higher doses)
zolpidem	Ambien	Selective binding of BZ$_1$ receptor	2.6 ± 1.2	5 mg hs	5–10 mg hs	10 mg hs	Drowsiness, dizziness, diarrhea, anterograde amnesia

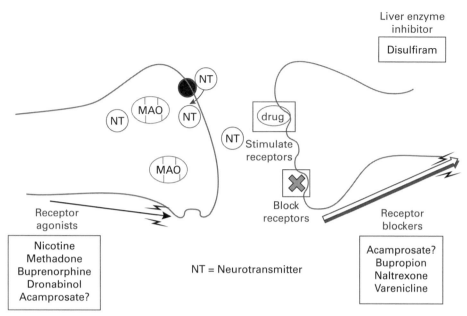

FIGURE 16.6 How Substance Abuse Drugs Work. Some drugs replace the addictive drug with a drug that stimulates the same receptors and are also addictive. Examples include nicotine at the nicotine receptor, dronabinol at the cannabinoid receptor, and methadone and buprenorphine at the opiate receptor. Other drugs confer their anti-addiction properties by blocking receptors. Examples include bupropion which may act by blocking the norepinephrine and dopamine receptors; naltrexone, which blocks opiate receptors; and varenicline, which blocks the nicotine receptor. Acamprosate may have two actions, blocking the excitatory glutamate receptor and stimulating the inhibitory γ-aminobutyric acid (GABA) receptor. Disulfiram has no effect on synapses. Rather, it blocks aldehyde dehydrogenase, the liver enzyme responsible for degrading alcohol's first metabolic product, thus allowing a buildup of the highly toxic acetaldehyde, producing noxious symptoms, including nausea and vomiting.

Bupropion is approved for the treatment of nicotine addiction. Dosing is 150 mg/d for the first 3 days, and then 300 mg/d. Patients start bupropion while still smoking and pick a stop date 1 to 2 weeks after beginning the medication. The package insert suggests stopping bupropion after 7–12 weeks, but patients often require continued bupropion in order to remain abstinent from tobacco products.

Disulfiram blocks aldehyde dehydrogenase, the enzyme that metabolizes acetaldehyde, the first metabolite of alcohol. Acetaldehyde is a toxic chemical causing nausea and vomiting. Normally, aldehyde dehydrogenase oxidizes acetaldehyde as soon as it forms, but in the presence of disulfiram, acetaldehyde accumulates, even after relatively small amounts of alcohol are consumed, and toxic gastrointestinal symptoms quickly ensue. This negative feedback is sufficient for some alcoholics to not drink. Because disulfiram has no direct effect on the urge to drink and craving for alcohol, some individuals will still drink, with dire consequences. Also, some alcoholics will stop taking it or take it only intermittently in order to return to drinking. Disulfiram is little used today but deserves consideration in the occasional appropriate patient. The best candidates for disulfiram are those who are highly motivated to stop their drinking, who fear the toxic response enough to motivate them to at least delay any drinking, and who have a significant other in their life who could oversee the daily administration of the pill. This significant other may be a family member or an employee health nurse from work.

Naltrexone was originally marketed as a treatment for opiate addiction. Because it effectively blocks the opiate receptor, heroin and other opiates are ineffective. However, patients would not take it, so it became little used. A long-duration injectable formulation has been developed, so naltrexone may yet become useful in treating this problem. Its cost, logistics for administration, and discomfort at the injection site have limited its wide adoption. The opiate addicts who did accept oral naltrexone treatment sometimes reported no longer wanting to drink alcohol, so studies were conducted that demonstrated its efficacy for treating alcohol abuse and dependence. Indeed, some alcoholics will take naltrexone and find that while it does not effectively remove their craving for alcohol, it does reduce the extent of drinking if they do drink. They seem to be unable to achieve the "high" that they had previously sought. Dosing is 25–100 mg/d. The main side effects are nausea and a "spacy" feeling, sometimes described by patients as feeling "dizzy," but without lightheadedness or vertigo. There is a risk of hepatotoxicity, which limits dosing.

Acamprosate is a GABA analog, which suggests that its mechanism may be through the NMDA receptor, although this has not been determined. Dosage is 666 mg tid. In FDA-approval studies treatment was initiated upon patients' release from an alcohol detoxification program. Such studies have demonstrated superior maintenance of abstinence relative to placebo, but efficacy of acamprosate in current alcohol users has not been demonstrated. Acamprosate is generally well tolerated; diarrhea is its main side effect. While it is difficult to comment on a medication for which outcome studies have been mixed, there is enough evidence to suggest that acamprosate may mitigate cravings.

Varenicline binds tightly to $\alpha_4\beta_2$ nicotinic acetylcholine receptors, preventing the binding of nicotine. Dosing is 0.5 mg/d, increasing to 0.5 mg bid after 3 days and gradually increasing to a maximum dose of 1 mg bid over the first 2 weeks of treatment, guided by patient tolerability. Typical side effects include nausea, vomiting, flatulence, constipation, insomnia, abnormal dreaming, and dysgeusia (abnormal tastes). There have been reports of depression with suicidal ideation emerging in patients treated with varenicline, leading to a change in labeling.

Nicotine is marketed as a gum and as a patch to be applied daily. The gum should not be vigorously chewed; rather, proper technique is to hold the gum between the cheek and teeth, called "pouching." Either formulation replaces the nicotine supplied by tobacco use but without the pulmonary problems that smoking causes. Nicotine, however, is not benign, having its own cardiovascular-stimulating properties.

Methadone is an opiate whose main use is in the treatment of opiate addiction; it also has a role in the management of chronic pain. Its primary advantages in the treatment of opiate abuse are that it can be legally obtained through licensed methadone clinics, its effects last throughout the day because of its relatively long half-life, and it can be taken orally, thus avoiding the negative consequences inherent in using injectable drugs. It is typically started at 20 mg/d, but usual maintenance doses are 50–100 mg/d. Methadone poses problems, however. First, it is an opiate, so essentially it substitutes a legal addiction for an illegal one. Second, methadone is dispensed only from federally licensed programs that require patients to come to a methadone clinic daily to receive their dose. If given a supply, some addicts will sell it rather than taking it themselves.

Buprenorphine is a mu-opioid receptor partial agonist, which means that it partially stimulates the receptor; it also is an antagonist at the kappa-opioid receptor.

Buprenorphine has a strong binding affinity and displaces other opiates from the receptor. Thus, giving buprenorphine will precipitate opiate withdrawal symptoms in a patient whose receptors are already occupied by other opiates whose binding affinity is less strong—for instance, in a patient with opiate dependence. A patient who is not opiate dependent will experience pain relief due to its partial-agonist effect. Because its half-life of about 72 hours is considerably longer than that of methadone, buprenorphine presents some advantages in treating opiate addiction. However, its propensity to induce opiate withdrawal means patients must begin experiencing withdrawal symptoms prior to beginning buprenorphine. Buprenorphine is usually given daily but may be given three times a week. It is marketed mixed with naloxone, an opiate antagonist that prevents opiate effects if injected, so it has less "street value" than methadone. It is administered sublingually in a dose of 12–16 mg/d or 24–32 mg every other day. The main side effects of buprenorphine are headache, constipation, and vasodilation.

ELECTROCONVULSIVE THERAPY

Electroconvulsive therapy (ECT) evolved from an erroneous "observation" that patients with epilepsy appeared to have a lower incidence of schizophrenia, leading to the hypothesis that epilepsy might provide protection against developing schizophrenia. For nearly two decades, ECT was the only effective treatment for severe psychosis. Its efficacy in severe states led to its use in less severe conditions. There are reports of nearly all of the psychiatric disorders "responding" to a course of ECT, although often with only anecdotal supporting evidence.

Indications and Contraindications

The primary indication for ECT is **severe major depression**, especially in acutely **suicidal** patients. Other indications are major **depression with psychotic features** and schizophrenia with **catatonic** features, as well as **treatment-resistant** mania, major depressive disorder, and obsessive-compulsive disorder.

The primary contraindication for ECT is **increased intracranial pressure**, since its use in the presence of increased intracranial pressure may result in herniation of the temporal lobe and death. Other contraindications relate to anesthesia (e.g., recent myocardial infarction, pulmonary disease, severe kyphosis of the spine). The risks associated with anesthesia must be balanced against the risks of not using ECT.

Pretreatment Evaluation

Prior to recommending ECT, a complete history and physical examination should be obtained. In particular, the eye fundi should be examined for **papilledema** (swelling of the optic nerve head indicative of increased intracranial pressure). An **ECG** should be obtained because the patient will receive atropine. **Liver function tests** should be done because hepatitis is a risk factor of anesthesia. Electroencephalography, CT scanning, or spinal radiography need not be performed routinely.

Treatment

ECT is usually administered in a recovery suite under general anesthesia. An anesthesiologist is often present, but a psychiatrist may administer it. An intravenous line is established for the administration of medications. Electrodes are strapped onto the patient's head for administering the electrical stimulus and monitoring the EEG. Atropine or glycopyrrolate is administered to prevent bradycardia or asystole during the seizure. An anesthetic or hypnotic agent (e.g., propofol, thiopental) is administered. After the patient falls asleep, the muscle relaxant succinylcholine is given to suppress the motor component of the seizure (i.e., tonic-clonic movements of the trunk and limbs); this is not necessary for efficacy but minimizes the risk of fractures. It is particularly important that patients with osteoporosis, who are at greater risk for fractures, be adequately relaxed. After the succinylcholine has taken full effect, and with the patient still unconscious, the electrical stimulus is applied.

Seizures lasting 30–90 seconds are effective. Seizures that persist after 2 minutes are terminated with diazepam given intravenously. Seizures can be assessed by EEG or by the tonic-clonic movements of the toes. The electrical stimulation should be 150% of the threshold value for inducing a seizure in order for the seizure to be effective. As the memory disturbance produced by ECT is proportional to the amount of current used, current is kept as close to the 150% level as possible.

Side Effects

The most frequent complaint that patients have after ECT is **headache.** Even though succinylcholine is given, the electrical stimulus causes tonic contraction of the jaw muscles and soreness. The headache usually responds to acetaminophen.

Bilateral administration of ECT produces both **anterograde** and **retrograde amnesia**, that is, loss of memory for events immediately prior to and after ECT. For example, patients may not remember specifically what led to their hospitalization. While this might be therapeutic for acutely suicidal patients, some find memory disturbance distressing and need reassurance that the disturbance is limited. Occasional patients complain of chronic and persistent memory troubles.

Unilateral administration of ECT to the **nondominant hemisphere** (almost always the right hemisphere) produces much **less memory loss** than bilateral administration. In some patients unilateral ECT is less effective than bilateral ECT. The risk of possible delayed efficacy and increased exposure to anesthesia must be weighed against the reduced likelihood of memory problems.

Broken teeth and fractures, especially of the vertebrae, were common in the early days of ECT, as unrestrained seizure activity can be quite violent. Now broken bones and teeth are rare, as tonic-clonic movements are markedly reduced to twitches of the eyelids by routine use of succinylcholine.

A massive surge of many different transmitters and hormones occurs during the seizure. Cardiac arrhythmias are not uncommon and require monitoring until they resolve, either spontaneously or with treatment. Transient hypertension secondary to ECT does not usually require treatment.

TRANSCRANIAL MAGNETIC STIMULATION

Repetitive transcranial magnetic stimulation (rTMS) is a noninvasive technology used to treat treatment-resistant depression. TMS passes alternating electric current through a coil placed on the scalp to generate a revolving magnetic field to then activate nerve cells. The precise mechanism of action of rTMS is unknown. TMS is superior to sham placebo treatment, but less effective than ECT for patients with acute major depressive disorder refractory to at least one antidepressant medication. The benefit of maintenance rTMS treatments is unknown.

Treatment

rTMS is typically an outpatient procedure which lasts about 30 minutes and does not use anesthesia. Treatments are 3–5 days/week for 4–6 weeks. The left dorsal lateral prefrontal cortex is generally targeted in rTMS for depression because this is an area of hypoactivity on neuroimaging. Although proconvulsant medications should be discontinued prior to rTMS, other psychotropic medications are safe to use concomitantly. TMS is contraindicated in patients with increased risk for seizures, implanted metallic hardware such as aneurysm clips, cochlear implants, implanted electrical devices such as pacemakers, and unstable medical disorders.

Side Effects

Generalized tonic-clonic seizure is the most serious adverse effect of rTMS. Headache and scalp pain may occur and are reduced with topical anesthetic. Cognitive impairment has not been shown. Switch to mania or hypomania has been described in case reports.

SELECTED READINGS

Black, D. W. Efficacy of combined pharmacotherapy and psychotherapy versus monotherapy in the treatment of anxiety disorders. *CNS Spectrums* 11(10 Suppl 12):29–33, 2006.

Davidson, J. First-line pharmacotherapy approaches for generalized anxiety disorder. *Journal of Clinical Psychiatry* 70(Suppl 2):25–31, 2009.

Galanter, M., and H. D. Kleber. *Textbook of Substance Abuse Treatment*, 4th ed. Arlington, VA: American Psychiatric Press, 2008.

Hammad, T. A., T. Laughren, and J. Racoosin. Suicidality in pediatric patients treated with antidepressant drugs. *Archives of General Psychiatry* 63:332–339, 2006.

Janicak, P. G., J. M. Davis, S. H. Preskorn, F. J. Ayd Jr., S. R. Marder, and M. N. Pavuluri. *Principles and Practice of Psychopharmacotherapy*, 4th ed. Philadelphia: Lippincott, Williams & Wilkins, 2006.

Lieberman, J. A., T. S. Stroup, J. P. McEvoy, et al. Effectiveness of antipsychotic drugs in patients with chronic schizophrenia. *New England Journal of Medicine* 353:1209–1223, 2005.

Meyer, J. M., V. G. Davis, D. C. Goff, J. P. McEvoy, H. A. Nasrallah, S. M. Davis, R. A. Rosenheck, G. L. Daumit, J. Hsiao, M. S. Swartz, T. S. Stroup, and J. A. Lieberman. Change in metabolic syndrome parameters with antipsychotic treatment in the CATIE schizophrenia trial: prospective data from phase 1. *Schizophrenia Research* 101:273–286, 2008.

Passarella, S., and M. T. Duong. Diagnosis and treatment of insomnia. *American Journal of Health-System Pharmacy* 65:927–934, 2008.

Soomro, G. M., D. Altman, S. Rajagopal, and M. Oakley-Browne. Selective serotonin re-uptake inhibitors (SSRIs) versus placebo for obsessive compulsive disorder (OCD). *Cochrane Database of Systematic Reviews* (1):CD001765, 2008.

Stahl, S. M. Stahl's *Essential Psychopharmacology: Neuroscientific Basis and Practical Applications*, 3rd ed. New York: Cambridge University Press, 2008.

Starcevic, V. Treatment of panic disorder: recent developments and current status. *Expert Review of Neurotherapeutics* 8:1219–1232, 2008.

Stein, D. J., J. C. Ipser, and A. J. Balkom. Pharmacotherapy for social phobia. *Cochrane Database of Systematic Reviews* (4):CD001206, 2004.

Stein, D. J., D. J. Kupfer, and A. F. Schatzberg. *Textbook of Mood Disorders*. Arlington, VA: American Psychiatric Press, 2006.

Swartz, M. S., T. S. Stroup, J. P. McEvoy, S. M. Davis, R. A. Rosenheck, R. S. Keefe, J. K. Hsiao, and J. A. Lieberman. What CATIE found: results from the schizophrenia trial. *Psychiatric Services* 59:500–506, 2008.

Tarsy, D. Lungu, C., and R. J. Baldessarini. Epidemiology of tardive dyskinesia before and during the era of modern antipsychotic drugs. *Handbook of Clinical Neurology* 100:601–616, 2011.

/// **17** /// Psychotherapy

DAVID D. OLDS AND FREDRIC N. BUSCH

Psychotherapy is a powerful form of treatment in which the primary instrument is talking and listening to the patient. All of the psychotherapies change the way a patient feels, thinks, and behaves, through meaningful interactions with a therapist. This chapter will describe in detail 15 of the most widely used forms of psychotherapy (see Table 17.1). These 15 therapies are sorted into four broad categories: psychoanalytic, cognitive-behavioral, multi-person, and supportive. Although the chapter describes these therapies in their relatively pure forms for the sake of clarity, in fact, each of these therapies has changed and borrowed from the others. Box 17.1 presents a brief history of the major psychotherapies.

THE THERAPEUTIC PROCESS

All therapies follow a similar progression and have beginning, middle, and ending phases (see Table 17.2).

Beginning Phase

The first therapeutic step, which takes place before therapy begins, occurs when the patient comes to the realization that he or she has been living in a precarious situation that is characterized by mental anguish, anxiety, depression, or some other symptom. This realization typically takes place after a stressor has broken through the defensive system established by the personality and has upset the patient's usual equilibrium. Patients with personality disorders often have behavioral traits that they are not aware of that nonetheless interfere with their interpersonal lives; they may begin psychotherapy at the suggestion of those around them.

At the beginning of therapy, the patient and physician enter into an explicit or implicit contract in which both parties agree to set some **basic rules** and to try to meet certain expectations. The patient is expected to come to sessions and try to communicate openly. The therapist will keep appointments, remain attentive, apply the therapeutic technique consistently, and follow the ethical code (see Box 17.2). As the beginning phase comes to a close, the patient should understand the technique being employed, the goals of the treatment, and that the rules of engagement are reasonable and beneficial.

TABLE 17.1 Overview of the Four Major Categories of Psychotherapy

	Psychoanalytic	Cognitive-Behavioral	Multiple Person	Supportive
Specific Treatments	Brief psychodynamic psychotherapy Psychoanalysis Long-term psychoanalytic psychotherapy Transference focused psychotherapy Mentalization based treatment Panic focused psychodynamic psychotherapy	Behavior therapy Cognitive-behaviorial therapy Dialectical behavior therapy	Interpersonal psychotherapy Family therapy Group therapy	Crisis intervention Medical illness Ego deficits
Underlying Theory	Disorders stem from unconscious traumatic memories or conflicts about sexual and aggressive wishes. Maladaptive or self-destructive behavior patterns learned in the past are unconsciously repeated (the repetition compulsion).	Disorders arise from maladaptive patterns of cognition and behavior. The patterns develop from learning based on behavioral conditioning.	Disorders arise from problems in relations between and among people. The self emerges from the infant caretaker dyad and forever bears the marks of early relationships.	Disorders derive from inadequate defenses and poor ego functioning, which can develop from a number of factors, including significant stressors.
Central Technical Features	Therapist's stance varies from active to expectant. Interpretation of the transference and of unconscious conflicts	Therapist is active and directive. Examination and confrontation of thought patterns and behaviors Various skills training	Therapist is active and directive. Techniques range from psychoanalytic and interpretive to supportive with behavioral and social-supportive interventions.	Therapist has an active, directive, reassuring, and encouraging stance, provides a warm supportive holding environment, and supports, rather than confronts, patients' defenses. Therapist readily provides advice and education to enhance skills and ego functions.

BOX 17.1
HISTORY OF PSYCHOTHERAPY

Various forms of psychotherapy have been present at least as far back as Neolithic times. In such primitive cultures, some of which still exist, psychotherapy is not differentiated from the medicine practiced by shamans and indigenous healers. By the time of the Greek city-states, a physiological basis for medicine had been developed. Healers understood, to some degree, that there was a difference between mental and physical illness, and that some physical diseases could be caused by psychological stress. For the most part, the healing arts of organized religion and the occult focused on a person's ailments, using prayers, nostrums, herbs, or magic, and did not clearly differentiate between mental and physical illnesses. In the nineteenth century, as medical science advanced, and the physical and infectious bases for many medical illnesses were discovered, patients with severe mental illnesses (e.g., the psychoses and severe mood disorders) began to be treated separately in asylums, which were often warehouses and prisons in which insanity was treated with barbaric methods. In France, Philippe Pinel worked to change the conditions in mental asylums, so they gradually became more humane. There was no officially recognized form of psychotherapy for patients with less severe mental illnesses, who consulted priests, family physicians, or other types of practitioners, such as soothsayers, psychics, or palmists.

In 1885, Sigmund Freud (who was by then a successful neurologist) went to Paris to study with the renowned neurologist Jean Martin Charcot and to confront the apparent physical and neurological illnesses of hysterics. Their symptoms could be brought on by psychic stresses, and they could be manipulated and sometimes cured by physicians who were skilled in hypnotic therapies. The theory and practice of psychoanalysis, which is the "parent" of most therapies practiced today, emerged from Freud's exploration of this phenomenon.

Psychotherapy has changed remarkably in the last few decades. There has been a revolution in psychiatry that is almost as profound as that which occurred in medicine when antibiotics were discovered. This transformation has taken place in two stages. The first stage was the birth and growth of psychoanalytic techniques in the first half of the twentieth century; the second stage, in the second half of the century and continuing to this day, was the blossoming of multiple kinds of therapies.

The largely supportive therapies of the nineteenth century provided the background for the first stage, which was the development of psychoanalysis and the psychoanalytic psychotherapies. The supportive therapies continue to be important and are widely used. Their purpose is to shore up the patient's temporarily or permanently inadequate defenses. But psychoanalysis provided the means to

(continued)

confront and change a person's defensive psychological structure and, therefore, to potentially cure the illness. Psychoanalysis and its "progeny" still form a major part of the theoretical basis for psychiatry.

Since the late 1950s, however, a second revolutionary phase has taken place, during which short-term, specialized techniques for individual, family, and group therapies have been developed and new psychopharmacological agents have become available. The focus of the therapies has become more specific because the diagnostic categories of psychiatric illnesses have become clearer. Many diagnostic categories have had treatments that have been tailored to fit them.

In addition, two other theoretical psychoanalytic models evolved from Freud's ego psychology and its emphasis on unconscious conflict. First, Melanie Klein moved in the direction of the earliest object relations, even in the first year of life, before the Oedipal period, which Freud considered to occur around age five. The emphasis for Klein was on early primitive, intense affects, with particular attention to rage and aggression, believed to arise from an inborn "death instinct. " Second, Heinz Kohut emphasized a developmental view in which psychopathology derives from interference with the normal progression of the individual's development of a "cohesive self" in the setting of sufficient narcissistic gratification.

Middle Phase

In the middle phase, the therapeutic model is applied as the patient and therapist work through the patient's pathological symptoms and behaviors and together set out to achieve the goals of the therapy. The goal of short-term focal therapies is to eliminate or reduce the intensity of the patient's symptom or discrete problem. Reaching this goal often produces generalized "ripple" effects, which provide more widespread benefits to the patient's personality. The more general goals for patients in longer-term therapies are to improve the personality functioning and achieve important life goals. In supportive therapy or in crisis intervention treatments, restoring and maintaining the patient's best previous level of functioning is often the goal. In most therapies the middle phase is the longest in duration. This is where the work of the therapy takes place, where the techniques defining that therapy are used to maximum advantage.

TABLE 17.2 Phases of Psychotherapy

Phase	Duration	Process
Beginning	1 or 2 sessions to several months	The patient learns the particular requirements of the technique and how the therapist and the theory work.
Middle	10 or 20 sessions—years	Work through patient's symptoms and behaviors to achieve the therapy's goals.
Ending	3–4 sessions to several months; longer in the longer treatments	Therapeutic gains are reevaluated, consolidated, and stabilized.

BOX 17.2
ETHICS IN PSYCHOTHERAPY

Although ethical considerations are important in any medical interaction, they have special significance for the practice of psychiatry and psychotherapy. In general, the ethical issues in medicine involve the beneficial and wise use of authority by the physician, specifically, the physician's commitment to do good rather than harm and to treat patients with respect and dignity. A psychiatric patient is, in many ways, as vulnerable to the therapist's power and control as an unconscious surgical patient is to the actions of the surgeon. This is because, in a sense, the therapist also has an unconscious patient. A major part of the patient's mentation is unconscious, and often provides motivations in conflict with conscious will and highly vulnerable to manipulation. Two major areas of ethical issues relevant to psychotherapy are the right to privacy and confidentiality, and the right to dignified, nonexploitative treatment.

RIGHT TO CONFIDENTIALITY

The issue of confidentiality arises every day in the practice of psychiatry. Patients impart to therapists their most intimate thoughts and memories, which range from the embarrassing or shameful to the illegal. They must feel free to speak about these things in order for certain issues that are crucial for the therapy to be addressed. They must be able to trust that the therapist will not divulge information.

RIGHT TO NONEXPLOITATIVE TREATMENT

Exploitation is the most subtle and pervasive of the ethical issues. The therapist is in a dominant position with respect to the patient; he or she is a potent transference figure in whom the patient invests much of the great power and authority that parents have over their children. The therapist must resist the temptation to take advantage of this power. The temptation is often a countertransference reaction in which the patient reminds the therapist of a disliked or seductive relative, and the therapist is tempted to react as he or she would to that person. Or the patient may behave in a seductive manner, dress provocatively, or gratify the therapist in ways that could provoke a sexual response. The results of succumbing to this temptation are always disastrous, even though the therapist may be able to rationalize that the actions are "for the patient's benefit." Much more subtle situations may also occur (e.g., when a therapist, motivated by his or her self-gratification rather than the patient's best interest, unconsciously pushes the patient into a certain career path or into a divorce). In this ethical arena, the best grounding and protection for therapists is obtained by undergoing intensive psychotherapy or analysis as part of their training. Of similar importance is consultation or supervision with a trusted colleague or a peer supervision group.

End Phase

During the end phase the therapeutic gains made by the patient are reevaluated, consolidated, stabilized, and placed in the context of the future, when the patient will no longer be seeing the therapist. The final goal of psychotherapy is for patients to be prepared to learn on their own as they did in therapy. Patients are often able to do this, having adopted the therapist's methods and ideals. Depending on the length of therapy and the patient's degree of involvement in it, the termination of the therapeutic relationship—and the consequent prospect of facing the realities of life without the therapist—can be a challenging and even wrenching experience involving a process of separation and mourning. Termination can also be the most growth-promoting part of therapy because, as with most experiences of mourning, the individual can emerge more integrated and mature. Therapies vary in the degree to which the patient's reaction to termination is employed as part of the treatment. In psychoanalytic psychotherapies, the patient's response to the end of treatment is a central focus.

BASIC CHARACTERISTICS OF PSYCHOTHERAPIES

All effective and ethical therapies share the following basic characteristics. The understanding of these characteristics originated in psychoanalytic theory, but the phenomena are found in all forms of therapy.

Transference

Transference is a ubiquitous process that occurs in a variety of relationships, for example, between student and teacher, patient and physician, client and attorney, and customer and salesperson. It is the **reactivation**, in a later stage of life, of a person's feelings, attitudes, or behavior patterns that were first **established in response to parents** or other early caretaking figures. Two commonly reactivated feelings are the awe and idealization that were felt for a beloved parent, or the rage and disappointment felt for a parent who was perceived as cruel or inadequate. Transference is usually **unconscious** and most often manifests itself as an emotional expectation that current relationships will be similar to those experienced in childhood. The **positive** transference consists of hopeful expectations and positive feelings toward the physician. These feelings and expectations arise from an attribution of power and trustworthiness to the physician as the wished-for good parent. These hopeful feelings can be associated with improvement in the patient's mood. The **negative** transference consists of feelings of mistrust and anger. Patients experiencing such negative feelings toward their therapist may sense in the therapist similarities to a hostile or cruel parent from early life.

Countertransference

Countertransference is the therapist's **response to the patient** or to the patient's transference. It is, in fact, a transference from the therapist to the patient, who may resemble, or be misperceived as resembling, a person from the therapist's early life. For instance, a patient whose constant belittling and antagonism toward the therapist resembles the behavior of the therapist's father may repeatedly be hitting a sore point and undermining the therapist's self-confidence. The therapist may respond with anger or even depression and not know why, because countertransference, like transference, is usually **unconscious**. A well-trained therapist does not act on such feelings but, instead, becomes aware of them and uses them to learn something about the way in which the patient affects other people. When properly perceived, and used as a tool for understanding the patient, countertransference can be one of the most valuable elements of a therapeutic interaction.

Corrective Emotional Experience

Corrective emotional experience refers to the new emotional experience the patient has with the therapist in which the therapist behaves differently from the patient's parents. For example, the patient may come to therapy expecting to be criticized and shamed or, perhaps, adulated and seduced. The contrast between the patient's expectation and the therapist's actual behavior is a powerful force for change. By contradicting the expectations, the therapist's responses lead the patient to new views of reality and, ultimately, to a new concept of self.

Emotional Intensity

Therapy is seldom beneficial when the patient is not engaged emotionally. Effective therapy also requires that the therapist be emotionally engaged and have an active attitude. Even in psychoanalytically based therapies, in which the therapist remains relatively quietly attentive, the therapist should be engaged emotionally and exquisitely attuned to the patient.

Resistance

Reluctance to change may emerge as gross interference, such as missing sessions, refusing to be open with the therapist, forgetting to do homework assignments, or rejecting interpretations or suggestions. At times a therapy will fail when resistance is too strong. Most therapies have ways of confronting this defensive behavior as part of the process of engaging the patient.

PSYCHOANALYTIC PSYCHOTHERAPIES

The therapies based on psychodynamics, the unconscious, and emotional conflict have their roots in the psychoanalytic theory of Sigmund Freud. The unconscious elements are either hidden traumatic memories that are kept out of the patient's awareness (e.g., episodes of physical or sexual abuse or traumatic losses in childhood) or fantasies that represent conflicts over sexual and aggressive wishes (e.g., a man was incapable of participating in any competitive activities because of the feelings of guilt and inhibition of ambition caused by the hostile, aggressive feelings he had toward a younger brother during childhood). These unconscious elements are thought to be instrumental in determining behavior and can lead to **unconscious conflicts** between incompatible wishes or ideas, which may be expressed in neurotic symptoms and pathological personality traits. Patients make use of **defense mechanisms** to prevent these unconscious elements from becoming conscious (see Box 17.3).

Psychoanalytic theory traces maladaptive patterns to their childhood origins. At the heart of the system is the basic theoretical concept of the **Oedipus complex**, which Freud and the early psychoanalysts viewed as the primary conflict at the root of all neuroses. (The reference is to Sophocles' drama *Oedipus Rex*, in which the protagonist, Oedipus, unaware that he is the son of the king of Thebes, kills his father in a chance encounter, and

BOX 17.3
DEFENSE MECHANISMS

PRIMITIVE DEFENSE MECHANISMS

Denial—the refusal to perceive or register as significant external events (e.g., the destructive consequences of one's own behavior).

Dissociation—the splitting off of thoughts and associated feelings from conscious awareness, as if to place them in a separate mental compartment. This occurs in amnesia, fugue states, multiple personality disorder, and splitting.

Splitting—seeing others in black or white terms (e.g., all good or all bad). It occurs when contradictory sets of thoughts and feelings are dissociated from each other. At any given time, the individual is under the influence of only one of the contradictory mental sets.

Idealization—seeing another person as perfect and ignoring the faults of that individual.

Devaluation—maintaining an entirely negative view of another person by ignoring the person's virtues.

Projection—attributing one's own thoughts, feelings, or impulses to another individual. Person A is sexually attracted to person B, but person A's ego blocks the desire from entering his own conscious awareness because of guilt. Person A tries to disavow the sexual desire by projecting it onto person B (i.e., by imagining that person B is attracted to Person A, rather than vice versa).

Acting out—expressing thoughts and feelings in actions rather than words (e.g., missing an appointment because one is afraid of becoming too dependent on the physician rather than keeping the appointment and discussing this fear with the physician).

Projective identification—a complex operation that involves projection and acting out and has multiple steps. Person C imagines that person D is regarding and treating person C in a particular way (e.g., contemptuously). Person C is actually feeling and behaving toward person D as he imagines person D is regarding and treating him. Person C's behavior frequently provokes person D into doing unto person C what person C already imagines is happening. In other words, person C unwittingly brings about the very reaction he or she dreads (i.e., contemptuous treatment).

MATURE DEFENSE MECHANISMS

Suppression—a partly conscious mechanism by which the individual wishes to put something unpleasant out of his or her own awareness and does so.

Repression—blocking a thought, feeling, or memory from conscious awareness (e.g., forgetting a painful experience).

Reaction formation—acting opposite to one's own desires, which one wants to disavow (e.g., a person who is conflicted over his or her own dependency yearnings who spends all of his or her time taking care of others).

(continued)

> **Intellectualization**—thinking or talking about an emotion-laden subject in an unemotional way (i.e., while experiencing and expressing no feelings).
>
> **Rationalization**—attributing one's behavior to a cause that one finds more acceptable than the actual cause, which one does not want to face or admit (e.g., a man who says that he lives with his mother because she needs him when the true reason is that he fears being separated from her).

subsequently marries the widowed queen, whom he later discovers is his mother. His discovery of the horrifying nature of his crime and his subsequent guilt and need for expiation is the focus of the play.) The complex described by Freud refers to the dynamic *process* by which a child develops sexual longings for the parent of the opposite sex and feelings of jealousy toward and fierce competition with the parent of the same sex. In Oedipal terms, successfully competing with the same-gender parent invites terrible retribution. In later life, this dynamic conflict may cause the person to have difficulties with sexual relationships, inhibitions or guilt about competition, and problems in relations with authorities.

Current psychoanalytic theory regards the Oedipal conflict as only one of many patterns that have important psychopathological effects and can be elucidated in psychoanalysis. Psychoanalytic theory no longer attempts to fit all patients into one or more basic complexes; instead, it focuses on the basic, personal, idiosyncratic, and particular unconscious psychological structures of each patient. A major issue that enters into the dynamics of any patient is the constellation around the experiences of attachment and separation. These include the outcome of the earliest childhood interactions with caretakers, leading to secure or insecure attachment, as well as the defenses activated by feelings of separation and loss (see Chapter 14, Child, Adolescent, and Adult Development).

Of increasing importance in current psychoanalytic theory is the phenomenon of the **repetition compulsion,** which refers to a person's tendency to repeat patterns. It is common, for example, for an adult who has been abused in childhood to marry an abusive spouse and **repeat** the experience of childhood (direct repetition) or to become an abusive parent in **identification** with the abusive parent. The pattern that underlies the repetition may be completely unconscious, necessitating much work for the person to see how it affects current life experience.

Insight is an improvement in the patient's understanding that may result from the therapeutic process. The gains in understanding usually relate to the causes of the patient's behavior, the particular attitudes and emotional responses that guide his or her life, the childhood events that may have influenced functioning, and the contingencies that may affect current behavior. In most patients, insight takes the form of **pattern recognition**, such as growing awareness of the repetition compulsion. A patient who always sabotages his work when he is on the verge of success and "snatches failure out of the jaws of victory" is reenacting a specific pattern. The value of the psychoanalytic phenomenon of the transference lies in its ability to induce the patient to **reenact** the pattern in his or her relationship with the therapist. For example, a patient who was in the midst of describing a recent success at work suddenly stopped and started to criticize himself because he feared that the therapist was "annoyed" with him. The analyst pointed to this sequence as an example of the patient's typical behavior pattern of needing to disavow success. To be useful, insight must have true emotional weight and the conviction born of an intense affect. Table 17.3 provides an overview of the psychoanalytic therapies.

TABLE 17.3 Overview of Psychoanalytic Therapies

	Brief Psychodynamic Psychotherapy	Psychoanalysis	Long-Term Psychodynamic Psychotherapy	Transference Focused Psychotherapy	Mentalization Based Treatment	Panic Focused Psychodynamic Psychotherapy
Patient Characteristics	Relatively healthy Highly motivated, intelligent, and psychologically minded	Relatively healthy Highly motivated, intelligent, and psychologically minded	Ego deficits Unwilling or unable to commit the resources necessary for psychoanalysis	Borderline personality disorder Severe ego deficits	Borderline personality disorder Deficits in mentalization	Panic disorder
Indications	Focal symptom disorder Discrete behavioral problem Grief reaction Adjustment disorder	Long-standing problems with work and personal relationships. Often associated with negative affects, including depression, anxiety, and anger	Long-standing problems with work and personal relationships. Often associated with negative affects including depression, anxiety, and anger.	Severe problems and unstable relationships Identity diffusion Depression and mood instability Low self-esteem Destructive behavior Emotional hyperactivity	Intense and unstable relationships Dissociation Impulsivity	Panic attacks Chronic anxiety Depression and mood instability.
Patterns	Unconscious conflicts and defenses that contribute to problems of recent origin; often triggered by life events or traumas	Unconscious conflicts and defenses that contribute to transference and repetition compulsion, and interfere with relationships, work, and overall personal development, maturation, and achievement of life goals. Maladaptive identifications and developmental fixations	Unconscious conflicts and defenses that contribute to transference and repetition compulsion, and interfere with relationships, work, and overall personal development, maturation, and achievement of life goals. Maladaptive identifications and developmental fixations. Self-destructive behaviors, including suicidality and substance abuse	Insecurity Unstable sense of self Primitive defenses of splitting, projection, and acting out Helpless dependency	Problematic expression of emotional states Difficulties identifying internal experience in self and others Insecurity leading to problematic intense relationships	Insecure attachments Anxiety in relationships and about separations Suppression of negative affects Somatization.

Frequency	Weekly	3–5 sessions per week	1–2 sessions per week	2–3 sessions per week	Weekly	2 sessions per week
Duration	15–20 sessions	Years	Months to years	Months to years	18 months	24 sessions
Therapeutic Stance	Actively interpretive	Expectant, allowing free association	Actively interpretive	Actively interpretive	Neutral	Actively interpretive
	Neutral and nondirective	Neutral and nondirective	Generally neutral and nondirective, but varying, and can include more supportive elements	Neutral when possible, but not in the face of destructive behavior.	("not-knowing"), nondirective, and collaborative	Neutral and non-directive
Techniques	Clarification of thoughts and feelings	Clarification of thoughts and feelings	Clarification of thoughts and feelings	Psychodynamic approach to unconscious and conscious conflicts	Individual and group	Phase 1 focuses on acute panic and its precipitants.
	Confrontation of defenses and resistance	Confrontation of defenses and resistance	Confrontation of defenses and resistance	Interpretations of primitive defenses and enactments	Empathize with internal state	Phase 2 focuses on vulnerability to panic, utilizing interpretation of transference and of defenses, especially somatization and defenses against anger
	Early interpretation of transference, relating it to early experience and present others (TOP)	Interpretation of the transference neurosis, linking it to childhood experiences	Early interpretation focuses on resistance	Attention to rage and aggression in the transference and the external world	Clarification of subjective state	Phase 3 focuses on separation and anxiety about termination
			Attention to childhood history		Identification of emotions	
					Mentalize the relationship between patient and therapist, as well as with group members	
Outcome	Insight into past conflicts and family issues	Insight into past conflicts and family issues	Insight into past conflicts and family issues	Integration of dissociated parts of the self, leading to a less conflict-ridden identity and more stable interpersonal relationships	Improved emotional regulation, and reduced insecurity, impulsivity and dissociation, resulting in more stable interpersonal relationships	Resolution of panic attacks.
	Resolution of conflicts leading to improved functioning in many areas	Resolution of deep conflicts and freedom to grow and mature	Resolution of conflicts, improved ego function, and freedom to grow and mature			Can lead to generalized benefit in many areas of functioning.

Brief Dynamic Psychotherapy

The theory and method of brief dynamic psychotherapy are similar to those of Freud's earliest psychoanalytic treatments, which took months rather than years. One feature of this method, which is shared by all variations of brief psychodynamic therapies, is the importance of focusing on a problem while the patient is in a state of **high emotional intensity**. The patient must enter this intense state in order to prevent intellectualization and to break through to deep emotions, and thereby gain emotionally meaningful insights into the unconscious roots and supports of his or her problems. Different means are used by the various schools of brief dynamic psychotherapy to generate this intensity, including constant attention to a central focus (Malan 1976), strict use of a time limit, and a persistently confrontational style (Davanloo 1980). This pursuit of the unconscious dynamic and conflict is the hallmark of psychoanalytic technique (see case example in Box 17.4). Other short-term nondynamic therapies do not place much importance on this pursuit.

BOX 17.4

CASE EXAMPLE OF EVALUATION FOR BRIEF DYNAMIC PSYCHOTHERAPY

A 30-year-old associate in a law firm complained of dissatisfaction with his work and difficulty in dealing with his superiors. He tended to be obsequious toward them, but was also resentful and procrastinated in doing assigned work. This behavior had not threatened his job, but he realized that he had gradually disappointed the partners with whom he worked and that, ultimately, he might not be promoted to partnership in the firm. He had a stable relationship with a girlfriend, but no definite plans for marriage. He had two good friends in whom he confided, one of whom he had known since high school. He described relations with his family as being warm and friendly, but it became clear during the interview that he felt his father was overly controlling, emotionally distant, and rather abrupt and awkward when relating to the patient and his younger sister. He was disappointed in his father and had a low-grade chronic anger toward him. He said that he felt angry with himself for his self-sabotaging style at work. He intensely wanted to succeed and become an authority in his branch of the law. He had never been seriously depressed or suicidal, did not suffer much from anxiety, and had no history of mood swings or substance abuse. He had not had the emotional crises at transition points, such as beginning school or going to college, which would suggest a major intolerance of separation. By the end of the interview, the physician surmised that the patient's issue with authorities included anger at them and an apparent need to sabotage his relations with them and, consequently, his own prospects. From a psychodynamic viewpoint, the patient's fear of authority and apparent fear of competition with older men pointed to an Oedipal focus. During the session, the psychiatrist suggested that the patient might be reacting to his senior partner with some of the feelings he had toward his father, noting that the patient, upon first entering the psychiatrist's

---

(continued)

consulting room, had asked, "Where is the head-shrinking chair?" in a somewhat belligerent tone.

The physician wondered aloud if the hostile tone the patient used in greeting him reflected his angry feelings for his father, and that he might be reacting similarly, in an unconscious way, to his senior partner. The patient at first blushed and then said, "You caught me out! But it's true, I always expect somebody above me to put me down or push me around, so 1 guess I was expecting something like that from you."

The psychiatrist made a tentative diagnosis of a personality disorder with obsessive and masochistic features and with a possible focus on the issue of anger at authority figures and fear of being punished for successfully competing with them. An appropriate treatment in this case would be brief psychodynamic therapy. According to psychoanalytic theory, this patient has both a conscious and an unconscious set of motivations. The conscious set is his desire for a family and for success in his profession. His anger at his father and his fear of competing with him is the unconscious set. The latter motivation, which is derived from his fear of being punished if he were to successfully compete with his father, leads him to unconsciously arrange for his own failure. For this patient, the focus of the treatment would be his relationships with authorities, including the passive-aggressive ways in which he expressed his anger at them, and his fear of being punished for success. The therapist would make it clear to him that even though he avoided direct confrontation by passive-aggressive means, his behavior was maladaptive enough to sabotage his prospects for success.

When unconscious motives are made conscious in a person who is otherwise relatively healthy, the contradictions become apparent and can then be resolved. The success of short-term therapy depends on the patient's ability to separate a **focal problem** from the rest of his or her personality and then, standing on the platform of a healthy personality, attack that one problem. The same kind of formula works for the patient whose pathological area is more widespread or difficult, although a longer-term therapy is required because the patient needs to have the platform of the therapeutic relationship itself.

Indications and Selection Criteria

Brief dynamic psychotherapy is generally indicated for patients who have a relatively **discrete conflict** that can become the focus of therapy. Patients should be **highly motivated, intelligent,** and reasonably **psychologically minded**. They should not be chronically isolated or untrusting, suffering from chronic substance abuse, or have a history of psychosis or severe affective disorder. A good prognostic sign is a patient's affective response to a **trial interpretation.** Brief dynamic psychotherapy would be appropriate for the patient described in Box 17.4 because he was able to feel, accept, and work with the therapist's interpretation that linked the patient's father, the senior partner in the law firm, and the therapist; and the patient did not abruptly withdraw, change the subject, or become paranoid or disorganized.

Therapeutic Process

The goal of brief dynamic psychotherapy is to resolve the patient's specific conflict through a brief treatment in which defenses are uncovered and psychodynamic interpretations that can lead to insight and change are presented. This process usually takes 15–20 sessions. Patients who have more diffuse conflicts or who tend to use more primitive defense mechanisms may require 40 or more sessions.

In the opening phase of therapy, the focus is selected, the time limits are set, and the developing transference, as well as the patient's resistance and defenses in response to the transference, is explored. In the middle phase, the patient's formerly positive transference may give way to disappointment in the therapist and in the perceived results of therapy. Negative transference issues that emerge are interpreted. The emotional dynamics that maintain the patient's pathological symptoms come under repeated scrutiny and interpretation. In the final phase, the patient's resistance to termination is an issue, and the patient's angry feelings at the perceived abandonment and defenses against those feelings are resolved. New symptoms may appear to justify the continuation of the therapy. By the end of a successful treatment, these issues will have been worked out in a rough fashion, and, in the months after therapy has ended, the patient can be expected to continue the process of working through them alone. Working through the termination is considered to be one of the most important aspects of this method.

Adherence to the **time-limited structure** is an important element of the technique because the issue of termination pervades the entire therapy, and the reality of the separation provides a tension that furthers the work on the patient's focal conflict. When a readily discernible conflict emerges, the patient and therapist agree to focus the therapy on this issue and do not attempt a broad exploration of the patient's life and personality.

An important aspect of brief dynamic psychotherapy is the **active engagement** of the therapist. (Transcripts of therapeutic sessions show some therapists to be so active that they talk as much or more than the patients, which is different from the behavior of therapists engaged in long-term analytic therapies.) The active engagement does not include making suggestions, giving advice, or offering reassurance; instead, the therapist gently, but persistently, prods the patient about his or her defenses against being aware of feelings and points out similarities that exist between, for example, the patient's reactions to loved ones and to colleagues. The most highly regarded intervention in brief dynamic psychotherapy is the "**TOP interpretation**" (e.g., the "trial interpretation" mentioned earlier), which links the transference to the *therapist*, relations with contemporary **others**, and the **parents**. Unlike other psychoanalytic therapies, the therapist does not wait expectantly for transference to develop; instead, every sign of transference is detected early on, and its relationship to the patient's history is rapidly interpreted. This method brings out transference issues quickly, although at a limited depth. For a deeper transference to develop, the more abstinent stance and frequent contact of psychoanalysis are required. A deep, regressed transference, however, is neither necessary nor desirable for patients in short-term therapy.

Psychoanalysis

Indications and Selection Criteria

Individuals with general **problems in adaptation** that are the result of **personality problems** and that do not respond to a focal treatment are good candidates for psychoanalysis (see case example in Box 17.5). Their problems usually fit the pattern

BOX 17.5

CASE EXAMPLE OF EVALUATION FOR PSYCHOANALYSIS

PART ONE. INITIAL INTERVIEWS

By the end of the first evaluation session with the lawyer described in Box 17.4, the therapist thought that the patient might be a candidate for short-term therapy, which would focus on his relationships with authorities, his problems stemming from his Oedipal conflict, and his intensely hostile relationship with his father. However, the therapist was not completely certain about this plan and thus asked the patient to return for a second interview before making a final determination.

In the second interview, the patient said that he had had a dream the night before in which he went to get a haircut, did not watch what the barber was doing, and suddenly realized that his hair had been cut much shorter than he wanted. He shouted at the barber and left in a rage. After telling the therapist about the dream, the patient seemed somewhat guarded. He steered away from discussing his work problems and instead raised issues concerning his girlfriend. It became clear that he had had serious problems relating to women since adolescence and had never really had a sexual love relationship. He had visited prostitutes several times but had been extremely anxious and unable to have an erection. He felt that he was unattractive to women, although he had reacted with arrogant aloofness when, occasionally, a woman had been interested in him. The therapist pointed out that the patient had rejected these women because he felt they would reject him. The patient agreed. He revealed more about the low level of his self-esteem, which seemed to be defended by his general supercilious arrogance that many people found irritating and distancing. He said that he was mildly depressed most of the time. Occasionally, he went on a drinking binge, which might begin at a bar and then last for several days. He normally drank one or two beers a day and did not feel that he was addicted to alcohol or impaired by drinking. He had no history of drug use, no suicidal ideation, and no evidence of psychosis.

When the physician asked the patient about the dream, the patient at first said that he did not see much in it. When the therapist pointed out that the short haircut could relate to his feelings about having short-term therapy, which had been mentioned at the end of the previous session, the patient said, "Maybe." He then said that he did not see how his problems could be solved in a few months. The interviewer agreed. They discussed the possibility of psychoanalysis, which would go to the roots of his self-esteem and his deepest defenses. Psychoanalysis would be most likely to achieve the deepest, most far-ranging changes. The hope would be that the patient would considerably improve his work style as well as his relationships, and that his fears of women and sex and traits of aloofness and arrogance would also decrease.

PART TWO. USE OF DREAMS

The patient may have recently had, or thought of having, a haircut. He had probably also had, in the past, a haircut that he did not like. These feelings seem to have become symbolically connected to the interviewer through the association with the head, especially in view of his remark about the "head-shrinking chair." The evaluator picked up the connection between short hair and short-term therapy and noted the patient's feeling about the mode of treatment. Later in analysis, when early childhood issues are closer to the surface, the analyst might connect the hair cutting with fears of the father, of being belittled or castrated, or retaliated against by the father for the patient's success. Early in therapy, these deeper connections would probably not be mentioned, because they are so far from awareness that the patient would find them silly, or a "Freudian cliché."

of a **personality disorder** that has varying degrees of **narcissistic, masochistic, obsessional, histrionic, or avoidant features.** The patients most appropriate for psychoanalysis have a **high degree of motivation, intelligence,** and **psychological mindedness.** Practical factors such as time and money are often considerations, since the cost in both is high.

Psychoanalysis is not usually recommended for patients with a history of a significant substance use disorder, psychosis, mania, or severe depression because the intense experience of analysis might aggravate such psychopathology. Other patients who are not appropriate for psychoanalysis are those who have a history of serious sociopathic behavior that would prevent them from being able to enter into a therapeutic contract or tolerate the inevitable frustrations involved; a history of paranoid features severe enough to make it impossible for the patient to establish a trusting alliance; or a history of severe narcissism, which would preclude any relationships other than superficial, exploitative ones. These criteria must be somewhat flexible because analysis may be able to help even patients with these problems. In other words, although analysis will be extremely difficult for a patient, for example, whose narcissism makes a therapeutic relationship nearly impossible, or who has a history of major self-destructive tendencies, any less inclusive techniques may not have much effect. In these cases, when analysis is chosen as the treatment, the therapist may modify the technique to fit the patient's needs.

The determining factor in choosing between brief dynamic psychotherapy and psychoanalysis is the presence or absence of focused, discrete symptoms and maladaptive behaviors. Psychoanalysis is usually indicated for patients with diffuse, **serious personality psychopathology** who have enough **ego strength** to tolerate the process. Additionally, **mental health professionals** with psychological problems of varying degrees of severity may choose to undergo psychoanalysis if they are motivated to learn more about themselves in order to become better therapists. The best way to understand how deeply therapy can probe, and how it feels to give up a defense or achieve a profound insight, is to experience it as a patient. For therapists, the best defense against potentially dangerous countertransference is to understand their own deepest motivations and areas of vulnerability.

Therapeutic Process

Psychoanalysis requires 3–5 sessions per week for an extremely variable amount of time, ranging from 3 to 7 or more years. Psychoanalysis requires the patient to **recline on a couch**, to have no visual contact with the analyst, and to free associate.

Free Association

Free association is one of the main techniques employed in psychoanalysis: the analyst tells the patient to say "**whatever comes to mind**," explaining that any thoughts or feelings that the patient experiences during the session are of interest to the analyst. The patient is not expected to interact with the analyst in the usual conversational way but to speak freely. Patients have varying abilities to do this. While some patients have no trouble pouring forth a cascade of thoughts, impressions, and feelings, others find it difficult to think, much less speak, freely and often are inhibited by their assumption that their thoughts are inappropriate or irrelevant. Most people fall within a middle category and have alternating periods of freedom and restraint. Psychoanalytic theory maintains that, as patients speak more or less openly and without constraint, they will slowly reveal a narrative life story and unconscious material. Freely associating allows a person to wander down little-used byways, sometimes encountering forgotten, surprising memories. The analyst's role is to listen to the patient's discourse while, much of the time, silently absorbing the information that is emerging and allowing it to take an understandable shape in his or her own mind. This technique fosters the emergence of the patient's story in never-ending detail and ultimately allows both the patient and analyst to understand it.

Therapeutic Neutrality

Throughout the process of psychoanalysis, the analyst stands equally between the patient's **ego** (self interest), **superego** (conscience), and **id** (drives or biological needs). In this position, the analyst remains **neutral with respect to the patient's behavior**. Remaining neutral is one of the psychoanalyst's most difficult, but nonetheless essential, tasks. For example, when a patient is endangering his or her job by constantly getting into arguments at work, the analyst might feel angry about this self-sabotage and be tempted to strongly wish for the patient to stop the behavior. The neutral approach requires that the analyst avoid siding with the patient's ego or superego and, instead, continue interpreting what the behavior means to the patient. When the analyst is successful in accomplishing this, the change in behavior made by the patient will result from self-understanding and thus be more permanent than if the change had been affected by the analyst's direct influence on the patient's behavior. (Of course, the analyst must intervene when the patient's behavior is truly life-endangering, e.g., driving extremely recklessly, or is threatening the therapeutic process itself, e.g., coming to sessions drunk.) The patient's ability to trust in the analyst's neutrality ultimately pays off in honesty and a willingness to reveal his or her deepest wishes, desires, and fears.

Clarification

Clarification is an attempt to help the patient flesh out and make clear what he or she is saying. To clarify, the therapist may **elicit more details, ask about feelings**, and **clear up apparent misunderstandings or contradictions**. For example, to a patient who said, "When I would get home from school, there was usually food or even a prepared snack in the fridge," the analyst responded by asking for more information: "You mean no one was home when you got home?" To which the patient replied, "Right. I never knew where my mother was, and I guess I felt I wasn't supposed to ask. Years later, I found out she had been having an affair." The case example in Box 17.6 provides a further illustration of clarification.

BOX 17.6

CLARIFICATION AND INTERPRETATION IN PSYCHOANALYSIS

A female patient who was obsessed with food and all aspects of eating always became depressed near the end of a meal, particularly the last meal of the day. She would look forward to it, but after a few bites, she would be unable to finish it. In the analysis of this phenomenon, its meaning became clear. Because the meal was nearly over, the patient was faced with the loss of eating in general, and eating for her meant love and caring. The last meal of the day implied an end to eating for the whole night. In tracing this issue back to childhood, it became evident that the patient's mother, who was narcissistic and unable to relate empathically to the child, used food as a substitute for normal maternal love. The patient was reenacting this conflict every time she sat down to eat. She was hungry and needed food, but eating reenacted the enraging situation in which food had to stand for love. When the patient was confronted with the repetitive nature of this scenario, she was eventually able to see the pattern. Her emotional response to food and to meals subsequently began to diminish.

Interpretation

An interpretation links together the various aspects of the patient's story. As is shown in the case examples in Boxes 17.4 and 17.6, the therapist explains **linkages and parallels** between the patient's relationships in **childhood**, relationships in the **present**, and the **transference** relationship. For example, in analytic work a patient may have been working through a tendency to provoke authority figures (including the analyst), then assume they are angry with him, and then avoid contact with the person, leading to further annoyance and disappointment. The patient might say, "The last few sessions, I've been kind of dreading coming, feeling you were somehow angry at me. Then I came late and felt that was what made you angry. I couldn't even talk about it." The analyst could reply, "This has happened before with me. And it seems similar to those times when you thought your father was mad at you, and maybe he really was, but you avoided him, and that made it worse in the end. So you have developed this pattern of avoidance, which makes your superiors angry and probably interferes with your advancement at work. You feel I will be angry, and unconsciously you are trying to make me angry, and so you react to me as though I were angry."

Defense Analysis

Throughout the treatment, the therapist will point out the ways in which the patient struggles to preserve his or her personality and its cherished defense mechanisms, for fear of being overwhelmed by anxiety, humiliation, depression, or even a loss of the sense of self. Defense analysis is one of the most important aspects of analytic technique; defenses must be interpreted and confronted repeatedly in an ongoing analysis.

Resistance

Resistance is the patient's attempt to **maintain the emotional status quo**, or "business as usual." Resistance may be manifested in defenses such as isolation of affect, intellectualization, disavowal, or acting out (see Box 17.3). The effect is to stall treatment and, when the resistance is very successful, cause the treatment to fail. The therapist must steadily, but gently, help the patient see through these defenses. **Acting out** is a particularly potent mechanism of resistance. A patient in an intense transference relationship will develop strong feelings toward the analyst. These feelings may represent unconscious feelings from childhood, and there may be strong prohibitions to becoming conscious of them. The patient may take an **action that substitutes for the unacceptable feeling** and also obscures it. For instance, if a patient has unconscious anger toward the therapist, the patient may miss sessions or frequently be late for them. Or, unconscious erotic feelings might be displaced to another person and result in an impulsive love affair. The interpretation of acting out is an important aspect of psychoanalytic therapy. As with the psychoanalytic concept of transference, resistance, in general, and acting out, in particular, occur in all types of therapy (e.g., in behavior therapy, acting out may take the form of not doing homework assignments or not "having time" to do relaxation exercises).

Dream Analysis

Freud described the dream as the "royal road to the unconscious." The current view is that dreams represent a continuation of information processing during sleep. When a person wakes up from a dream and remembers it, it carries obvious remnants of the day's experience, the "**day residue**." The narrative story of the dream, the "**manifest content**," may have deeper symbolic reference to basic themes in the patient's life, which is referred to as the "**latent content**". The analyst listens carefully to patients' retelling of their dreams, often seeing the connection of the dream to the transference and to the patient's childhood experience (see Part 2 of case example in Box 17.5). When used properly, dreams are an important source for discovering what lurks just below the surface of consciousness.

Working Through

Working through is the process by which repeated confrontations with the transference, patterns of behavior, and turmoil of feelings generated in the analytic situation lead to insight and change. The interactions with the therapist are seen as the patient's typical reactions, and they become open for revision. For example, a patient might declare, "You are looking particularly well today. I was thinking how lucky I am to have you as my analyst." The analyst responds, "Could there be more to it? I am going away for 2 weeks, and yesterday you were speaking, in what you called 'general terms,' about how offensive it is when physicians keep people waiting or suddenly cancel appointments." The patient replies, "Huh…you know it's weird. Before I was thinking how great you are, I was in this rage about how you just go away whenever you want, and I have no say in it. You know it really makes me mad." In this vignette, the analyst noticed and pointed out that the patient defended against his anger at the analyst by superimposing a more acceptable emotion, which, in this case, is idealization. The vignette also shows the value of the transference. Because of it, the patient finds the analyst's presence important enough to have strong feelings about it and to defend against these feelings in his characteristic way, which can then be examined. In this way, the transference analysis is a kind of "laboratory" in which the patient's habitual personality style can be enacted and analyzed.

Working through is probably the engine for change in all types of therapy. It is the process whereby the work of therapy leads to changes in the patient's life in the real world. This process is usually not a patient's sudden revelation of an infantile trauma, as is often portrayed in fictional accounts of psychoanalysis. The therapist must assist the patient in uncovering layers of memory and must repeatedly confront the patient's defenses against awareness and change. The **repeated confrontations and interpretations** help patients to understand their underlying motivations, enhance their ability to apply this understanding to different situations in life, and, eventually enable them to **change their self-concept and behavior** (see case example in Box 17.5).

Intersubjectivity

"Intersubjectivity" is a relatively new trend in analytic method. Analysts have increasingly appreciated that any therapeutic relationship is a dyad and that there is a constant **mutual interplay** between the therapist and patient. The analyst cannot and should not be a purely neutral figure. The patient's thoughts and feelings cannot merely be "distortions" projected onto a "mirror-like" analyst. The analyst may start late, make errors in billing, express impatience, or forget facts, and have countertransference reactions that can emerge in subtle ways. The analyst must take the patient's reactions to these events as serious information and not simply as misperceptions. In this model, the two participants are seen as more equal and reciprocally interactive.

Long-Term Psychoanalytic Psychotherapy

The goal of long-term psychoanalytic psychotherapy is to integrate the patient's personality through the combined use of supportive and interpretive techniques.

Indications and Selection Criteria

Selection criteria for long-term psychoanalytic psychotherapy include negative factors that render a patient unsuitable for a brief therapy (e.g., due to multiple diffuse problems) or psychoanalysis (e.g., due to a history of severe self-destructiveness or near psychosis), as the case example in Box 17.7 illustrates.

In patients who are significantly depressed or prone to psychotic symptoms, medication can be a useful adjunct, leading to an improvement in mood or a decrease in psychotic thinking that may strikingly enhance the alliance and therapeutic process (see discussion of integration of psychotherapy and medication treatment in Box 17.8).

Some people who might be appropriate candidates for psychoanalysis choose psychoanalytic psychotherapy because they cannot afford the time or money required for psychoanalysis. Some people who might do well in a short-term therapy for a focal symptom have more ambitious goals and therefore elect a long-term treatment. This choice is frequently made because, although analysis may be the only method that has a chance of working for some patients, many patients will receive great benefit from either treatment, and psychoanalytic psychotherapy may be the only feasible alternative.

BOX 17.7

CASE EXAMPLE OF LONG-TERM PSYCHOANALYTIC PSYCHOTHERAPY FOR A PATIENT WITH A PERSONALITY DISORDER

By the end of the first evaluation session with the lawyer described on Box 17.4, the therapist was not completely certain as to whether short-term therapy would be the best choice and so invited the patient to return.

(continued)

The second interview, instead of suggesting that psychoanalysis was the appropriate treatment, could have gone in yet a third direction, in which it became clear that he had not given an accurate or sufficiently detailed history. He had withheld the information that he had had three previous attempts at therapy. Near the beginning of each therapy, he would soon become argumentative and increasingly self-destructive and then quit in a rage. He had also failed to report that he was doing so badly at work that he was on a kind of probation, so that the next time he missed a deadline or had an argument with a partner he would be fired. In the past, these disputes at work had often involved a loss of reality testing, a feeling that colleagues were plotting against him, and the conviction that his phone was being tapped. Furthermore, the girlfriend he mentioned at first was really an acquaintance with whom he talked occasionally on the phone but rarely saw. The relationship with this woman was the closest one he had to a trusting relationship. It also turned out that he rarely saw his parents, and that the friends he mentioned were actually acquaintances. After three sessions of brief therapy, he began to show more of his true style, becoming increasingly irritable over the therapist's attempts to get further information and make tentative interpretations. It soon became clear that the patient was "faking good" in an attempt to get help and to hoodwink an authority figure. By this time, he knew what therapists expected to see in a "healthy patient." Despite this turn of events, he expressed the wish to continue in therapy because he was terrified that he would soon lose his job and had some insight that he was heading toward such a catastrophe.

The new information suggests that the patient has a severe personality disorder and poor interpersonal relations (no close friends, is suspicious and isolated). These problems cannot be adequately treated in a brief therapy. He could lose his job, which would lead to a further sense of helplessness, persecution, and chaos in his life. He does not appear to have the ego strength to tolerate the rigors of psychoanalysis. Thus, the best treatment for him is long-term psychoanalytic therapy. The therapist's tasks will be to engage him in the therapy and form a working alliance and, eventually, help him work through a very ambivalent transference to a more healthy adaptation. The therapist will probably need to direct the patient and set limits on his behavior, and should expect strong resistance to exploration and interpretation.

At the least, this therapy can help the patient achieve a stable professional life, and it may also improve his life in the interpersonal sphere by helping him to become more trusting and capable of establishing a long-term relationship. There are some positive prognostic indicators for the success of this patient's therapy. He is highly motivated, even though it is mostly out of fear of losing his job; and he is intelligent, has some ability to understand psychological issues, and can contemplate the possibility that his paranoid ideas may not be accurate. He is not currently psychotic, severely depressed, or suicidal and is not abusing alcohol or drugs.

BOX 17.8

INTEGRATION OF PSYCHOTHERAPY AND PHARMACOTHERAPY

Combining medication with psychotherapy has become standard practice. Antidepressants, for example, are used to treat chronic mood disorders even for patients who are in psychoanalysis. The results may be an improved mood and an increased ability to participate in the therapeutic process. The analysis may proceed more rapidly and with greater long-term effects. Some patients may need medication for a limited period during the analysis, and others may need it indefinitely. In acute crisis interventions, an anxiolytic or a hypnotic drug is often given temporarily to reduce the unbearable anxiety and severe insomnia that patients may experience. Medication is also frequently used in the treatment of patients with ego deficit disorders, for whom an antipsychotic drug may be prescribed to treat distorted thinking, and an antidepressant or mood-stabilizer for a mood disorder.

Some patients may refuse to consider medication as part of their treatment, for personal or philosophical reasons. The therapy may then have to proceed without it. Even for those who reject medication, the therapist's offering of it may have a positive effect, because it signifies that the therapist has heard the patient's complaint and taken it seriously. This perception alone may improve the therapeutic alliance and move the therapy forward, even though the treatment may not be optimal without the medication. On the other hand, the refusal of medication can be part of the patient's unconscious, possibly deadly, wish to defeat the therapy. When a patient is at risk for impulsive violence or suicide, the physician may have to insist upon medication and refuse to engage in treatment without it.

Another response to the physician's suggestion of medication may be an enthusiastic welcome and hope for a magical cure. This attitude has its own set of problems. A patient who thinks, "Finally, now, we're doing something real" may suffer a crashing disillusionment when his or her high hopes are not fully realized and then think, "We've played the last card. If this didn't work, nothing will." It is important for the therapist to raise the subject in a tactful manner at the right time and to avoid promising too much. The idea should be presented in a somewhat optimistic way, with the therapist pointing out that medication is an adjunctive treatment that could very well speed things up, but that it is not a last resort.

When psychotherapy is provided by nonmedical practitioners, two specialists may be involved in the patient's treatment. The therapy will be most effective when the two practitioners cooperate in a synergistic, noncompetitive manner. Conflicts between practitioners in how to manage a patient's care can lead to disruptions in treatment. For many patients, therapy conducted by a physician who can also administer medication is more effective because any problems and side effects may be detected more quickly. Also, a physician is better equipped to manage the

(continued)

behavior of patients who use the medication to act out the feelings and fantasies they are experiencing in the transference. For example, a woman who was suffering from anxiety and depression lowered the dosage of her antidepressant because she was concerned that her physician was as untrustworthy as her alcoholic father. The physician began to notice the she was becoming gradually more hostile and dysphoric, while complaining less about medication side effects. After gentle confrontation the patient was persuaded to go back on the medication before becoming unmanageably symptomatic. Certain patients with complex personality disorders, especially those who also have mood disorders, will most likely do better with one person providing therapy and medication, if this option is available. Finally, medical/psychiatric training provides physicians with an overview of biological and psychological factors that can provide a more integrated amalgam of medication and psychotherapy.

Therapeutic Process

While the duration of psychoanalytic psychotherapy is generally several years, the exact length is difficult to predict at the outset. The method of psychoanalytic psychotherapy differs from that of analysis in that the patient **sits up facing** the therapist during the sessions and there are **two or three sessions a week**. The therapist makes use of a slight positive transference to develop a therapeutic alliance. This alliance consists of a mutual feeling that the therapy can help the patient and that the therapist and patient can cooperate in the effort. The supportive alliance and the idealization of the therapist empower the patient to be more self-confident and optimistic. The patient's defenses may be interpreted gently or even ignored, with the understanding that the patient's stability is fragile and that the defenses may be necessary to prevent further disorganization. Interpretations are usually directed at the patient's negatively oriented defenses and resistances to the therapy process. The idealizing magical transference is generally not interpreted until late in treatment. Throughout treatment, the therapist will make **clarifications, correct distorted perceptions of reality**, and, at times, give advice, all of which will work to **enhance the patient's coping abilities**. The therapist's degree of activity may vary and, in general, the therapist is less talkative than he or she would be in brief therapy.

The therapeutic interaction is usually **more interactive and confrontational**. The method is similar to analysis in that the therapist tries to be nondirective, tends to listen, and intervenes infrequently with clarifications and interpretations. The style of therapy varies considerably, depending on the personal style of the therapist and the perceived needs of the patient. Some patients can talk about problems and even interpret some of their own motivations without a great deal of activity on the part of the physician. Others are more passive and need the therapist to be actively involved by frequently interjecting questions, confrontations, and clarifications.

In some ways, psychoanalytic psychotherapy is an **intermediate form of therapy** between psychoanalysis and short-term therapy. It is similar to analysis in its intensity, use of transference, long duration, and far-reaching goals. It is like short-term therapy in its use of face-to-face interactions, active dialog, and directive interventions, which may limit the depth of transference. An intense, deep transference, however, often does occur in psychoanalytic psychotherapy. With a well-motivated, self-directed patient, the results may be similar to those obtained through analysis. With a less motivated, less introspective person, the increased intensity of psychoanalysis, if it can be tolerated, might be necessary for success.

Transference Focused Psychotherapy (TFP)

Transference focused psychotherapy is based on Kernberg's conception of the central features of borderline personality disorders, including identity diffusion (contradictory or poorly defined views of self and others, with a lack of recognition of these contradictory aspects), primitive defenses such as splitting and acting out (see Box 17.3), brief disruptions in reality testing, and distorted representations of self and others (Kernberg 1975) (see Chapter 8, Personality Disorders).

Indications and Selection Criteria
TFP was developed and has been studied for the treatment of borderline personality disorder.

Therapeutic Process
The treatment begins with the development of a treatment **contract** that establishes the treatment **frame** (a minimum of 2 to 3 sessions per week) as well as limits on impulsive, self-destructive, and suicidal behaviors. In the context of an individual session, priority is given to risks of injury, when present. As the patient's split-off, primitive perceptions of self and others come alive in the transference, the therapist helps the patient identify the primitive relationship being experienced and the internalized views of self and other that are being perceived or enacted. For instance, it may emerge that the patient views the therapist as idealized in order to avoid the threat of damaging him or her with rageful feelings or impulses. Alternatively, the patient may view himself or herself as a victim of an "all bad" therapist. Efforts are made to **engage the patient's observing ego** to identify the unrealistic and defensive nature of these perceptions.

This therapeutic process includes identifying the patient's **role reversals**. For example, a patient may view himself or herself at one point as a needy child and the therapist as a rejecting mother, while at another point in the same session the patient may identify with the rejecting mother, with the therapist perceived as the needy child. These role reversals can be described to the patient, who over time gains knowledge of the shifting and split-off views and of the unconscious need to keep them separate. **Identity diffusion** is reduced as the patient develops a more complex, accurate, and integrated self-concept. The therapist is active and focuses on the "**here and now**" aspects of the transference. In addition, analysis of the transference is linked more closely to external reality than in other psychoanalytic treatments.

The background of patients with borderline personality disorder usually involves a childhood of deprivation or overt abuse, sexual or physical. In order to survive such a childhood the patient dissociated parts of the self, each of which have viewed the world from a different perspective. This unstable situation leads to wildly alternating moods, self-esteem, and identifications with others. Much of the TFP technique is devoted to bringing out these separate worldviews and helping the patient to realize that all of them belong to a single and unique self. As the patient progresses to a view of one self that can sometimes be good and sometimes bad, an improved ability to perceive the reality of relationships with other people and a more solid sense of the self as a continuous, stable entity are developed (see case example in Box 17.9).

BOX 17.9

CASE EXAMPLE OF TRANSFERENCE FOCUSED PSYCHOTHERAPY FOR BORDERLINE PERSONALITY DISORDER

A 26-year-old single woman left college in her sophomore year after being hospitalized for a suicide attempt with an overdose of the antidepressant she had been taking for several months. The attempt was apparently triggered by a violent argument with her boyfriend, leading to his threat to quit the relationship. After hospitalization, she returned home to live with her parents. Despite their constant urging, she refused to go back to school and spent most of her time in her room alone. She made a half-hearted attempt to work as a waitress, but quit after several days when she was scolded by an impatient customer. She had meals at the family table, but was usually sullen and silent. On two occasions, after arguments with her parents about her "lack of ambition," she threatened suicide. At her parents urging, she enrolled in a day hospital where there was an active TFP program. In the intake interview her mother said she had always been a "sensitive" child who would "overreact to the slightest thing, and would be inconsolable." Her mother later volunteered that the patient, as a child, had several times complained that her alcoholic uncle had on many occasions "tried to feel her up." The parents had "paid this no mind" and explained it as "just another of her exaggerations."

She began therapy with a TFP therapist, planning a schedule of three sessions a week. She and the therapist agreed on a contract to the effect that she would not make any further suicide attempts. She settled into the therapy, and after 3 weeks found a temporary clerk position at an advertising agency. After the first day on the job, the patient came to session very upset, saying, "Well you wanted me to take that job, and I lasted one day!"

The therapist asked for the story of what happened. "I had this job, the one I told you about. I got there and at first it seemed pretty good. My boss was really friendly and seemed to want to make me comfortable. I thought, "This is really nice! Maybe I'll get a permanent job here. My first assignment was to sort some bills that they had in cardboard boxes. I wanted to make a good impression, so I was working pretty fast. Well, I was about halfway through this job, when my supervisor came over and asked how much longer it would take. I said 'I'm doing it as fast as I can!' The supervisor said, 'I was just asking.' He walked off looking pissed. I could tell then that he had it in for me. I was trying to think what I would say when he came back. I couldn't concentrate. An hour later I still wasn't done with it. Then it was five o'clock, and when I left the supervisor said they wouldn't need me any more. I was so frightened of him, I ran out the door. I don't even remember where I went after that! Then I was home in my room. I have a razor blade there, and I had to cut my arm or I couldn't stand it. I made three cuts where no one would see them."

(continued)

> The therapist dealt with the cutting incident first and most urgently, and then worked through the incident at work. The therapist demanded that the patient give up the razor blades, and discussed how the patient, in her anger at the therapist, was enacting a role as the victim and cutting her skin. They spent more time discussing the contract wherein she agreed not to harm herself, and what to do in the future when she felt the need to cut or hurt herself.
>
> The therapist asked for the details of the situation at the office. The patient told her about her initial pleasant impression of the job and her supervisor, and then how things deteriorated. She said, "See how you shifted! At first you thought he was great, a kind of ideal father. Then, when he just asked a question that made you doubt yourself, you suddenly crashed into your victim self, and he became the terrible, evil father." When the patient left at the end of the session, the therapist was left with an uneasy feeling. She had barely noticed that the patient walked out rapidly and left the door open, and then slammed the outside door. "What's going on? I thought I was making a useful interpretation, but she may have seen me as criticizing her." The therapist, in examining her feelings, realized she had become impatient with the patient's behavior, and that there was an irritated tone in her voice. She had acted like the supervisor, who was himself irritated. Making use of their frequent sessions, the next day the therapist was able to point out how the experience in the session was similar to what happened in the workplace. Over many more sessions, interpretations of this sort were able to help the patient gain a more solid sense of herself.

In any psychotherapy, it is often useful to obtain advice from a colleague. TFP makes this a routine. TFP therapists usually work in a group and have scheduled meetings for peer supervision. They present their cases to the group and often benefit greatly from the feedback and suggestions. This process functions as a kind of analysis of their unconscious feelings, most often their countertransference feelings and enactments, which might otherwise undermine the treatment.

Mentalization Based Treatment (MBT)

Mentalization based treatment has been developed from Fonagy, Bateman, and colleagues' exploration of mentalization, the **awareness and identification of mental states** in self and others and their impact on behavior (Batemen and Fonagy 2004). The **capacity for mentalization**, referred to as **reflective functioning**, has been associated with a number of measures of mental health and a sense of secure attachment to others. A high level of reflective functioning provides the capacity to both better identify internal states and understand more about the motives and behaviors of others, allowing for less internal distress and greater interpersonal effectiveness. Fonagy and colleagues view borderline personality disorder as deriving from a limited capacity to mentalize or a disruption of this capacity, particularly in the context of close attachment relationships. This deficit is the source of the emotional fluctuations, impulsivity, and disrupted interpersonal relationships characteristic of the disorder. Insecure attachment, frequently found in borderline patients, interferes with the safe exploration of one's own internal states and the motives and emotions of others. An attachment strategy of hyperactivation can develop, leading to rapid and **insecure attachments**, which are typically followed by intense disappointment and rage. Poor mentalization predisposes to the development of these intense emotional states and attachments, which in turn interfere with mentalization. Loss of the capacity for mentalization leads to "pre-mentalistic" modes, including concrete thinking, dissociation, and a tendency to action, adding to interpersonal disruptions and psychic distress.

Indications and Selection Criteria

MBT has been developed and studied for the treatment of **borderline personality disorder**, but treatments focusing on enhancing mentalization capacity are being developed for a number of disorders (Bateman and Fonagy 2011).

Therapeutic Process

MBT includes an initial assessment period that identifies deficits in mentalization, attachment insecurities, and problematic strategies that the patient has developed for coping with these problems. There is an early focus on how to manage problematic behavioral expressions of internal states, which disrupt relationships. A discussion about the diagnosis of borderline personality disorder is followed by efforts at developing mentalizing capacities. The process is regarded as a collaborative investigation, with the therapist presuming that he or she does not know more than the patient about the "truth" of a given situation, referred to as a **"not-knowing" stance**. Comments about what patients "must" be feeling are avoided, as they imply knowledge about the patient that the therapist cannot be certain of and impede the development of mentalization capacities. The therapist is relatively open about his or her own thoughts regarding the patient's perspective on a given situation, presenting it as an alternative perspective to the patient's. The therapist is quick to acknowledge if he or she has misunderstood the patient's communication, furthering a collaborative, exploratory approach.

An important goal of the therapist is to help the patient avoid undue arousal in the therapeutic relationship, which disrupts mentalization, while allowing the relationship to become important enough to be experienced as a significant attachment. Types of interventions include empathizing with the internal state described by the patient, exploring and clarifying the patient's subjective state, working to identify emotions, and mentalizing the relationship between patient and therapist. The first two interventions are felt to be "safer," or less likely to cause arousal, and are therefore used more frequently early in treatment. The second two interventions are employed after the patient has developed some mentalizing capacity and can think more about intense emotional states. In contrast to TFP, MBT therapists cautiously approach transference interpretations, which they believe may invalidate the patient's experience if not handled properly. With regard to the transference, the patient is assumed to be observing some way in which the therapist is drawn into the patient's experience. Rather than a distortion, then, the patient's perception of the therapist is assumed to have some accuracy in it, and the therapist acknowledges his or her contribution. This allows for looking at different perspectives of the experience, promoting mentalizing. The patient practices mentalizing by thinking about what is going on in the mind of the therapist, and learning about how the therapist perceives the patient. After mentalizing capacities have been further developed, the patient's perceptions can be looked at as distortions that can be identified in more traditional transference interpretations.

MBT for borderline personality disorder includes weekly group therapy in addition to weekly individual therapy. The group provides additional opportunities for patients to compare their own view of self and others with the perspectives of other members of the group.

Panic Focused Psychodynamic Psychotherapy (PFPP)

Panic focused psychodynamic psychotherapy is a specialized treatment based on evidence that patients with panic disorder have neurophysiological and psychological vulnerabilities to panic that include specific psychodynamic configurations. In particular, these individuals become fearful of separation, with a belief that others are required to maintain a sense of safety or prevent helplessness. In the context of a **fearful dependency** on others, patients develop both a fear of abandonment and a sense of narcissistic injury about their inability to manage on their own. Angry feelings toward important attachment figures become particularly threatening, as patients fear that this anger will lead to disruption in the needed relationship. This **intense ambivalence** triggers the employment of particular defense mechanisms in an attempt to **deny anger** and heighten affiliative efforts, such as denial, reaction formation, and undoing (observed as patients "taking back" anger that is expressed). Another important defense is **somatization**, in which patients experience intrapsychic conflicts as bodily symptoms. However, these defenses interfere with the ability to manage conflicts with others in a more direct manner. Under conditions of specific stressors in adulthood, particularly those perceived as loss or separation, intensifying fears of loss and anger lead to panic onset.

Indications

PFPP was developed for treatment of panic disorder, but has been successfully employed in treatment of other anxiety disorders (Busch et al. 2012).

Therapeutic Process

Panic focused psychodynamic psychotherapy is a twice-weekly 24-session treatment in which the therapist is active and maintains a focus on the symptoms and conflicts surrounding panic onset and persistence. Initial efforts elucidate the context and meanings of panic to help the patient to understand that panic has not emerged "out of the blue" but has developed from particular environmental stressors and internal conflicts. Exploration of the patient's developmental history includes prior periods of severe anxiety, such as childhood separation anxiety, and any traumatic experiences. In the second phase of treatment, the therapist weaves together information about panic precipitants, meanings, and feelings with the developmental history to identify the **intrapsychic conflicts surrounding separation and anger** involved in the patient's panic episodes. For example, patients who describe a temperamental or violent parent may be particularly frightened about experiencing or expressing angry feelings. Other individuals with panic may describe a parent who is fearful and overprotective, adding to a sense of insecurity and a need to depend on others to feel safe. As with other psychoanalytic treatments, use of the transference can be a valuable tool. Anxiety about separation or expressing angry feelings and fantasies may emerge with the therapist, allowing for a direct identification of conflicts within the treatment.

Despite the brevity of the therapy, the transference is focused on when relevant, particularly as termination approaches. During termination, conflicts around separation, loss, and anger intensify as feelings about separation from and dependency on the therapist are brought to the forefront. The patient's feelings of loss and anger with the therapist typically mirror fears that occur with other important attachment figures.

Further examination of these conflicts adds to the patient's capacity to identify and reflect on feelings rather than avoid or deny them and experience them as bodily symptoms. Interpersonally, panic patients will frequently engage in submissive relationships, as they have difficulty expressing and discussing problems, fearing disruptions in attachments. As patients find their feelings less threatening, they become more willing to address tensions with significant others, rather than suppress them. Improvement in interpersonal relationships further reduces vulnerability to panic, by reducing stress and helping patients to clarify and express feelings that they previously found frightening. The goals of treatment are panic reduction, as well as increased recognition and tolerance of feelings of loss and anger, and increased ability to better manage problems in interpersonal relationships.

COGNITIVE-BEHAVIORAL THERAPIES

Cognitive-behavioral therapies lie on a continuum from those that focus on behavioral interventions to those that are primarily cognitive. Most cognitive therapies now combine cognitive and behavioral approaches. Dialectical behavior therapy consists primarily of components of cognitive behavior therapy, but it also draws from several other psychotherapeutic approaches. Table 17.4 provides an overview of the cognitive-behavioral therapies.

Behavior Therapy

Behavior therapy grew out of the work of B.F. Skinner, who conceived of the mind in generally external terms, rejecting the notion of inner subjective experience and preferring to see the mind as behavior. His model was based on the reflexive learning that occurs in all animals, in which certain stimuli are followed by certain responses. He held that the entire repertoire of human behavior could be traced back to **conditioned responses** (i.e., learned reactions) from infancy to adulthood. Language, too, was thought to be an accumulation of conditioned reflexes favoring certain phonemes, pronunciations, and syntax. In recent years, most behavior therapists have broadened their approach to accommodate the existence of internal subjective experience.

Behavior theory holds that all psychopathology arises from **inappropriate conditioning**, which mostly occurs in childhood, although it can occur later in life (e.g., a car accident might condition a person to fear driving). The conditioning model is based on the principle that one stimulus can replace another when the two stimuli occur close together in time. In Pavlov's famous experiment, food was presented to a dog at the same time that a bell was rung. Initially, only the food induced salivation in the dog. After a period of conditioning, however, the dog salivated when he heard the ringing bell. This phenomenon is known as **classical conditioning**. Another form of conditioning is **operant conditioning**, a typical example of which is the following experiment with a caged pigeon: while pecking randomly at the floor and walls of an enclosure, the pigeon occasionally happens to peck and depress a small lever at one end of the cage; this movement releases a pellet of food into the bird's cage, and, eventually, the pigeon "learns" that pecking the lever will be rewarded by food. Most behavior therapy is built upon the process of classical conditioning. When applied to patients, this theory maintains that a person cannot be anxious and relaxed at the same time. Therefore, in order to eliminate the anxiety, behavior therapists attempt to replace the patient's anxious reaction with a more relaxed one (see case example in Box 17.10).

TABLE 17.4 Overview of Cognitive-Behavioral Therapies

	Behavior Therapy	Cognitive-Behavior Therapy	Dialectical Behavior Therapy
Indications	Circumscribed anxiety disorders, including phobias Inhibitions Sexual disorders Substance use disorders Self-destructive behavior	Depression Anxiety disorders Substance use disorders Low self-esteem Inhibitions	Borderline personality disorder characterized by unstable relationships, anger, and destructive behavior
Theory of Symptom Formation	Disorders stem from inappropriate conditioning, which causes problematic learned responses.	Disorders derive from irrational beliefs and disordered thinking.	Emotional dysregulation impairs attention, increases impulsivity, and disrupts interpersonal relationships
Patterns	Anxiety triggered by situations Behaviors influenced by anxiety	Catastrophic thinking Overgeneralization Negative attribution Exaggeration Selective abstraction	Emotional hyperactivity Insecurity Unstable sense of self Primitive defenses of splitting, projection, and acting out Helpless dependency
Therapeutic Stance	Active, directive, and collaborative	Active, directive, and collaborative	Active, directive, and collaborative, including contracts and limit-setting
Techniques	Learned relaxation Exposure Systematic desensitization	Behavioral analysis Confrontation of irrational beliefs and distortions Written homework assignments	Skills training Behavioral analysis Confrontation of irrational beliefs and distortions Training in mindfulness, stress tolerance, and interpersonal skills
Outcome	Reduced anxiety decreases inhibition and allows freedom of action, assertiveness, and self-esteem.	Changes in thought patterns enhance mood and self-esteem and resolve symptoms.	Improved ego stability, interpersonal skills, self-esteem, and emotional tolerance, resulting in better functioning at work and in relationships

> ## BOX 17.10
> ## CASE EXAMPLE OF BEHAVIOR THERAPY FOR SOCIAL PHOBIA
>
> A 43-year-old architect came for a consultation because he had a fear of public speaking. For most of his career, he had been a talented assistant to senior architects. He had not been asked to make a presentation since he was a student in architecture school. At that time, he made his presentations in a state of panic, getting through them with the help of a benzodiazepine. Recently, he had been promoted to the position of senior architect on a project, which required him to make a major presentation. He was terrified.
>
> He had a stable marriage, was in good physical health, and drank moderately. He had no history of mood swings, severe depression, mania, or thought disorder. He described experiencing anxiety on other occasions, such as when first being assigned to projects and when walking into a room full of colleagues.
>
> It appeared that the architect had associated appearing in public with anxiety. He explained, "I'm afraid I'll mess up my speech. I'll forget what I plan to say. I'll be humiliated by making a fool of myself." The patient's less conscious fears might be expressed as "I'll get angry and start smashing things" or "I'll wet my pants." The skilled behaviorist tries to uncover these deeper fears as well as the conscious fears that the patient first describes.
>
> It appeared that the patient had social phobia. In beginning behavior therapy, he would be asked to rank-order his fears. A presentation to a small group of friends would be at the bottom, and a speech with no notes to an audience of a thousand would be at the top. He could also construct a list of feared outcomes, which could include any scenario, from momentarily forgetting and then remembering to going berserk and suffering complete degradation and humiliation. As the therapist and patient list these fears, they would discuss them in detail, including the likelihood of their occurrence.

Indications and Selection Criteria

Behavior therapy is appropriate for patients who suffer from a **circumscribed disorder** that includes the symptoms of **anxiety**. This therapy works best in patients who do not have long-term, chronic problems that are likely to interfere with treatment (e.g., unstable relationships, obviously self-destructive and self-sabotaging patterns, substance abuse, severe depression, or psychosis). However, when combined with cognitive therapy, these behavioral techniques are appropriate for patients with a broad range of disorders.

Therapeutic Process

The goal of behavior therapy is to diminish the anxiety associated with a particular behavior that has inhibited or blocked the patient from engaging in that behavior. The treatment is most often **short term** (4–20 once-weekly sessions). For the patient described in Box 17.10, the goal would be to weaken the association between a public appearance and his fears.

Behavior treatment is directive, informative, and focused on the patient's symptoms. The initial evaluation is particularly important and includes inquiry about the patient's symptoms, the situations associated with them, and all possible associated fantasies. The therapist explores these aspects further by asking the patient to make a list of feared situations and rank them into a **hierarchy of fears**.

The second "arm" of behavior therapy is **learned relaxation**, for which there are several methods. One method consists of the therapist leading the patient through a series of exercises designed to induce a relaxed state. In one set, for example, the patient is instructed to sit back in a recliner and, focusing on one group of muscles at a time, tense and then relax the muscles. By the end of the set, the patient usually feels more relaxed. The patient is often asked to practice this exercise two or three times each day. A variation of this method is to have the patient follow audiotaped relaxation instructions, provided by the therapist, several times a day.

Biofeedback is a relaxation technique in which electrodes placed on a muscle group (usually on the patient's forehead) are connected to electromyographic equipment that registers the tension level in the muscles by different tones or by different positions on a meter. As the patient relaxes the muscles, the tone becomes lower in pitch or the meter shows the decrease. Biofeedback is a form of operant conditioning through which the patient begins to relax almost unconsciously and is rewarded by a corresponding change in tone or reading on the meter.

Systematic desensitization is a method that combines relaxation with the patient's hierarchy of fears. In this technique, the phobic situation is disconnected from the negative affect of anxiety. After having learned how to relax, the patient is asked to imagine the items on his or her list of fears, in ascending order. As each fear is imagined, the patient is instructed to deliberately relax and thereby counter the anxiety that usually accompanies the fantasy image. The goal is for the patient to be able to relax while imagining the worst possible fear. Once the patient has made some progress in relaxing while fantasizing the phobic image, actual practice exercises are assigned. For example, the patient described in Box 17.10 might practice by first giving a presentation to the therapist, then to some friends, and then to a professional group. As a result of the "in vitro" desensitization and the "in vivo" practice, his anxiety should diminish considerably. These exercises have the supplementary effect of getting the patient to take action, which by itself counters the helplessness that patients feel about their anxiety.

Other aspects of behavior therapy that contribute to its efficacy are the patient's establishment of a positive transference to a benign authority and the patient's and therapist's collaborative investigation into the areas producing the anxiety. Separating and listing these areas exposes and objectifies them. This process is similar to the listing of thought distortions, in cognitive therapy, whereby the very act of listing the distortions helps to reduce their power. To help the patient separate an event from its associated severe anxiety, a form of classical conditioning is used in which relaxation and transference-induced confidence are substituted for the pathological fear.

As in cognitive and interpersonal treatment, a synergy exists between the effects of behavior therapy and the effects of medication. Medications that may enhance the process of dissociating the anxiety from a feared situation can be combined with behavior therapy. Benzodiazepines or beta-adrenergic blocking agents, such as propranolol, inhibit the peripheral effects of anxiety, relieving the patient of the sweaty palms, hand tremors, dry mouth, and nausea that formerly accompanied public appearances. Pharmacological intervention may also relieve the actual symptoms that plague the patient during the event. However, desensitization exercises may be more effective than medication in ameliorating the anticipatory anxiety and terrifying fantasies that are experienced before the event.

Generalized benefits, or "ripple effects," can result from this highly focused therapy. For example, as the patient described in Box 17.10 resolved his public speaking problem through behavior therapy, his self-esteem was enhanced. His ability to speak in public with much less fear increased his general sense of confidence, which, in turn, rendered him more effective at work and more likely to be promoted, further improving his self-image. This benign circle is the opposite of the vicious cycle that had been caused by his anxiety.

Cognitive-Behavioral Therapy (CBT)

Cognitive-behavioral therapy was initially designed as a short-term therapy for the treatment of depressive disorders. This treatment, which was developed by Aaron T. Beck and his colleagues (1987), focuses very closely on the patient's cognitive processes and distortions. The theory underlying the therapy is based on two principles: (1) close **correlations exist between a patient's mood and the patient's patterns of conscious thought**; and (2) certain habits of thought can **cause and maintain a patient's depressed state**. As the name suggests, the method combines a direct approach to the patient's cognitive patterns, with behavior therapy techniques, such as a directive practice and homework assignments. The theory of CBT has been subjected to research that has demonstrated a regular correlation between negative thinking and depression, although such thinking has not definitively been shown to *cause* depression. The efficacy of CBT has been demonstrated in the treatment of patients with moderate depression and compares well with other forms of psychotherapy (see Box 17.11).

Indications and Selection Criteria

CBT is well suited for patients who suffer from a mild to a moderate degree of **major depression, dysthymia**, or depressed mood due to an adjustment disorder. This method is also suitable for patients who have **anxiety disorders** or severe major depression, bipolar disorder, or psychotic symptoms and who are simultaneously receiving appropriate medications.

Patients with severe substance use disorders tend to be poor candidates for CBT. However, this therapy can be used as an adjunct to rehabilitation in patients who demonstrate their seriousness about stopping problematic substance use by regularly attending Alcoholics Anonymous or other 12-step programs or by admitting themselves to drug treatment programs. CBT is not appropriate for patients who are mired in destructive family or environmental situations. Such patients usually have far-reaching pathological syndromes that are supported by these problematic systems, against which any type of short-term therapy stands little chance of success.

Therapeutic Process

The treatment is usually **brief**, consisting of one session a week for 15–30 weeks. The goal is to help the patient achieve relief from and resolution of a **specific affective complaint**, such as depression or anxiety. The technical goal is for the patient to more objectively observe all conscious self-denigrating thoughts and then change the content of these thoughts to reflect a more positive view of the self. CBT techniques require the therapist to take an active and directive role in helping the patient uncover **pathological**

BOX 17.11

PSYCHOTHERAPY RESEARCH

An increasingly important endeavor in recent decades has been research to assess the effectiveness of various forms of psychotherapy. This research is important, because it can reassure therapists and patients that they are engaged in useful treatments, and it can be used to justify the cost of the treatments to those who pay for them, including patients, their families, and particularly insurance companies. In addition, such research will hopefully aid in determining which psychotherapies may be best suited for particular patients or disorders.

Psychotherapy research is complicated by a number of factors. Some psychotherapies (e.g., cognitive-behavioral therapies) have been studied much more extensively than others (e.g., psychoanalytic treatments) (see Thoma et al. 2012). Thus, psychotherapies that have demonstrated efficacy for specific disorders are recommended as treatment of those disorders, but the lack of study of other psychotherapies cannot be taken as evidence that they do not work. Many studies of psychotherapies examine responsiveness to short-term interventions and do not assess whether these treatments prevent or reduce recurrence of the disorder over the long term. Comparison groups can be difficult to define, as there is no "placebo" psychotherapy, and treatment as usual can vary greatly. In addition, some psychotherapy studies have not controlled for the presence of other concurrent treatments, particularly medication interventions, thus complicating assessments of the psychotherapy.

Finally, there have been problems in the quality of psychotherapy research studies, including a lack of randomized controlled trials, although evidence suggests that they have been improving over time (Thoma et al. 2012). Studies should include an adequate description of subjects and diagnostic methods, as well as clearly defined treatments and specific outcome measures. An important development in the current research environment is the use of a written manual providing explicit instructions on the technique being tested. Adherence measures can then be employed, which evaluate whether therapists are performing the specific mode of therapy being studied. Psychoanalysts in particular have been concerned that with the use of a manual some of the spontaneity and natural creativity of individual therapists may be lost, but manuals have been developed that allow for adequate flexibility for therapists to feel they are not stifled in their treatments.

Despite all the difficulties, significant findings have emerged from psychotherapy research. Cognitive-behavioral treatments (CBT) have undergone the most extensive systematic testing, with studies demonstrating efficacy for a wide variety of disorders, including major depression, panic disorder, obsessive-compulsive disorder, social phobia, posttraumatic stress disorder, generalized anxiety disorder, specific phobias, and bulimia (Hofmann et al. 2012). Although there is evidence that

(continued)

CBT is effective in the treatment of avoidant personality disorder (Emmelkamp et al. 2006), treatment of other personality disorders with CBT has been less well studied. Dialectical behavior therapy (DBT) has been found to be efficacious in the treatment of borderline personality disorder (Stoffers et al. 2012), but other adaptations of DBT have received less research attention (Rosenthal and Lynch 2009). Interpersonal psychotherapy (IPT) has demonstrated efficacy in the treatment of major depressive disorder (Cuijpers et al. 2011). Evidence suggests that maintenance IPT provides some protection against relapse in patients who have recovered from a major depressive episode. Adaptations of IPT to other diagnoses have been less well studied.

Two types of psychoanalytic treatments, mentalization based treatment (MBT) and transference focused psychotherapy (TFP), have been found to be effective in the treatment of borderline personality disorder (Bateman and Fonagy 2001; Clarkin et al. 2007). In the study of MBT, treatment gains were maintained 5 years after follow-up in comparison to the standard care group (Bateman and Fonagy 2008). One study demonstrated efficacy of panic focused psychodynamic psychotherapy (Milrod et al. 2007). Studies of psychodynamic therapies have shown promise in the treatment of depression (Leichsenring 2005). A review of studies of long-term psychodynamic psychotherapy found it to be effective in treatment of complex mental disorders and to be superior to short-term psychotherapies (Leichsenring and Rabung 2011). Studies of psychoanalysis have been less common, in part because of the complexity of studying the treatment over several years, but preliminary studies have shown promise (de Maat et al. 2013). For example, a study of children and adolescents with anxiety disorders receiving either psychoanalysis four or five times a week or once- or twice-weekly psychodynamic psychotherapy found an overall clinical improvement and a correlation between the frequency of treatment and degree of improvement (Fonagy and Target 1996).

Some studies of supportive psychotherapy involve a treatment based primarily on psychodynamic psychotherapy, whereas others involve more specific supportive interventions. Overall, supportive psychotherapies have shown a surprising degree of value for treatment of anxiety and depressive disorders, given that these are not focused treatments (Lipsitz et al. 2008).

Family therapy has been found to be effective in treatment of anorexia nervosa (Geist et al. 2000). Family interventions with schizophrenic patients, particularly surrounding psychoeducation, have been found to significantly reduce relapse rates (Pharoah et al. 2010). Various forms of group therapy have been found to be effective for treatment of bulimia nervosa (Katzman et al. 2010; Russell et al. 1987). In addition, group treatments with specific orientations, such as CBT or a group that is part of a DBT treatment, have been found to be of value for other specific disorders.

(continued)

Another area of psychotherapy research is process-outcome studies (see Busch et al. 2013). These studies focus on identifying factors that cause therapeutic change in order to develop more effective therapeutic interventions. In addition, these studies attempt to determine which types of interventions (for example, transference interpretations) are useful for specific types of patients or disorders. One significant finding from this research is that the outcome of psychotherapy, independent of the approach that is used, is related to the quality of the relationship with the therapist, referred to as the therapeutic alliance. As with outcome research, studies of process have been problematic, but increasingly sophisticated approaches and measures are being employed in this important area of study.

patterns of thought and develop ways to control them. To this end, the therapist asks the patient to complete **homework assignments** that usually involve recording in a journal conscious thoughts and feelings in reaction to certain events. Early in treatment, the therapist explains to the patient the nature of depression and the effects of pathological thoughts. In the first interview, the therapist usually elicits such thoughts from the patient and catalogues them (see case example in Box 17.12). When the cooperative efforts of the patient and therapist are successful, the patient is able to notice depressive thoughts as they occur, view them somewhat more objectively, and question their validity. The patient's belief in the correctness of such perceptions then diminishes. Throughout the therapy, although transference is not explicitly addressed, the cognitive therapist makes use of the positive transference, which gives the patient a sense of possibility, reduces the feeling of isolation, and empowers the patient to try new things and to understand that the firmly held, former convictions are reciprocally related to depression.

Dialectical Behavior Therapy (DBT)

Dialectical behavior therapy was originally developed by Marsha Linehan for treatment of borderline personality disorder (Linehan et al. 1991). Linehan conceptualizes patients with borderline personality disorder as suffering from a biologically based emotional vulnerability interacting with an "invalidating environment," interfering with the development of interpersonal skills and the capacity for emotional regulation and tolerance. Emotional dysregulation leads to **disrupted attention**, interfering with the perception of interpersonal experiences, and to **behavioral dyscontrol**, including impulsivity, aggression, and self-harm, in an attempt to manage physiological arousal.

According to the concept of dialectics, the therapist works with the patient to **resolve contradictory ideas and emotions**. The initial dialectic that burdens the patient is one between the patient's inborn emotional hyperreactivity and the environment in which expressions of feeling are invalidated, contradicted, or punished, leading to the extremes of dysregulation. These three elements lead to **recurring vicious cycles**, which can lead to self-destructive or aggressive behavior. Such behavior can allow transient escape from the painful feelings, but usually leads to deteriorating relations with all the people close to the patient, and an ever-worsening sense of self and self-esteem. The therapy makes explicit the contradictions in the patient's life through a **series of structured**

BOX 17.12

CASE EXAMPLE OF COGNITIVE BEHAVIOR THERAPY FOR DEPRESSION

A 50-year-old teacher, the married mother of two teen-aged children, had been a somewhat pessimistic person and a chronic worrier for most of her life. After her 18-year-old son left for college, she began to worry obsessively about him, telephoning him intrusively and badgering him about coming home to visit. She became impatient with her pupils at the primary school where she taught and found that she had little energy, early morning insomnia, and a general feeling of being a "bad person." Her relationship with her husband was stable but had become distant and was punctuated by frequent bickering and mutual complaining. Her relationship with her daughter, which previously had been very close and mutually dependent, had become more antagonistic and frequently erupted into screaming arguments.

The patient appeared to be suffering from a major depressive episode with a reactive component that had been triggered by her son's leaving home and her daughter's fighting for more independence, both of which signaled the end of a life phase. A likely first choice of therapy for this patient would be cognitive behavior therapy.

In the course of treatment the patient told the therapist, "My son never calls me. He has forgotten me." The therapist subsequently learned that the son called once a week. Since that could not be considered total abandonment, the patient's thought was labeled an **exaggeration,** or an example of negative thinking. The patient's next statement that "I've become totally useless to him" was an **overgeneralization**. "My husband used to be home on weekends when the kids were home. Now he plays golf all day Saturday. He obviously doesn't want to be with me." This statement could be labeled a **selective abstraction,** or a negative conclusion based on inadequate information.

When cataloguing pathological thoughts, the cognitive therapist should be careful not to label in a way that belittles the patient or suggests that the therapist thinks the patient is "just exaggerating." In order for an empathic mutual collaboration between the therapist and patient to be established, it is essential that both parties come to understand the patient's thinking. Therefore, the therapist should not automatically dismiss the patient's alleged distortions. For example, in her last statement, the patient may have touched on a potentially serious problem in her marriage. Her relationship with her husband could very well have genuine troubles and be foundering since the children left home. Another possibility is that the marriage may, in fact, be stable, but her husband prefers playing golf with his friends to being at home with his wife when she is worrying and complaining.

approaches, starting with a delineation of patient and therapist assumptions about the treatment, including a protocol to address suicidal behaviors. Using these approaches, DBT works through blocking problematic behavior intended to relieve emotional distress and teaching new, more adaptive coping strategies.

Indications and Selection Criteria

DBT has been found to be efficacious for the treatment of borderline personality disorder, particularly in reducing self-destructive behaviors. More recent efforts have involved applying DBT to a series of other disorders, such as substance abuse and antisocial behaviors, although research data on these approaches are preliminary.

Therapeutic Process

In a preliminary phase of DBT, referred to as pretreatment, the therapist discusses with the patient the expectations of the treatment, and the patient's commitment to it. In the initial stage of treatment, the goal is to develop control over behaviors that are self-destructive, interfere with treatment, and disrupt interpersonal relationships. Patients develop new emotional, cognitive, and interpersonal skills in several contexts of the treatment, with efforts then made to implement these strategies throughout the patient's life (see case example in Box 17.13).

Group Therapy

In group therapy, patients are taught new coping skills in a didactic format using a skills training manual developed by Linehan, which they then attempt to apply in homework. The results of these efforts are discussed in the following session with both the group and the individual therapist. Skill modules target the development of mindfulness, distress tolerance, emotion regulation, and interpersonal effectiveness. **Mindfulness training**, a core aspect of the treatment, focuses on acquiring nonjudgmental self-observational skills, with attention to the present moment. Patients allow thoughts and feelings to come freely into their minds, and subsequently describe and label them. Mindfulness also includes the development of effectiveness: behaving in ways consistent with values and long-term goals rather than immediate relief of distress. Improved **stress tolerance** is taught using behavioral techniques such as distraction and self-soothing. Relaxation skills, breathing, and imaginal exercises are used to help relieve distress. **Emotional regulation** is aided through increased awareness and identification of emotions, and understanding how emotions lead to problematic behaviors. Finally, the therapy helps improve interpersonal skills, challenges problematic cognitive assumptions about interpersonal situations, and teaches modulation of behavior in interpersonal contexts.

Individual Therapy

Individual sessions provide a nonjudgmental and supportive environment for the focus on developing behavioral change. Sessions are structured to avert states of high arousal that may interfere with attention required for learning. Therapists validate patients by recognizing how problematic behaviors are understandable given the patient's biological vulnerability and history. The patient maintains a **diary card** that describes emotional states, injurious behaviors, and other treatment targets. Using this list, the therapist and patient examine episodes of emotional distress and discuss the skills that were or could be implemented. **Behavioral analysis** is used to help identify antecedents and consequences of disruptive behaviors, as well as thoughts and feelings that add to distress and trigger problematic behaviors. Circumstances, thoughts and feelings, psychic distress,

BOX 17.13
CASE EXAMPLE OF DIALECTICAL BEHAVIOR THERAPY FOR BORDERLINE PERSONALITY DISORDER

The young woman described in Box 17.9 as a patient in transference focused psychotherapy would also fit the requirements for referral to dialectical behavior therapy as a recurrently suicidal patient diagnosed with borderline personality disorder. Enrolled in a course of DBT at a day hospital, the patient was seen in weekly group therapy and in individual therapy. In the group she and the other members discussed their feelings and their recent activities and problems. They were urged to express their feelings in a mindful way, nonjudgmentally, and allow the others to respond to those feelings. After she lost her second temp job, she remained in a rage for days. The group discussed how to tolerate her disappointment, humiliation, and gnawing anger. They described their own use of tactics for distress tolerance, such as distracting activities, self-soothing with hot baths or music, breathing exercises, and interruption of thought patterns. The group also discussed their individual emotions and the behavioral techniques they used for emotion regulation. They addressed the issue of interpersonal effectiveness, including ways to reduce distortions of other people's intentions and feelings, and encouraging interpersonal skills, such as how to be taken seriously and gain respect.

In the individual therapy, the therapist addressed many of the same issues. One example is their behavioral analysis of what happened when she lost her second job after being asked to sort a large number of bills by date. The therapist asked her to recall every detail that she could about the ensuing interactions and led her through the details of this scene (see description in Box 17.9). They reviewed and reiterated her commitment to the therapy and the importance of telephoning the therapist before she cut herself. She promised she would bring in all her razor blades and give them up. They went over her reaction to the supervisor's question, her distorted sense of being criticized and humiliated, as well as other possible interpretations she could have had, and ways in which she could have distracted or soothed herself. They rehearsed ways she could get the next job and how she could handle possible situations. After the session, the therapist was left with an uneasy feeling that the patient wasn't telling her everything, that something was missing.

The next day, the therapist attended a meeting of her consultation team. She vented her sense of frustration and anger at the patient; indeed, after they discussed the case, she realized she had been short-changing the effect that the patient had had on her job supervisor. He probably was angry after that interaction; it was probably not a "distortion." The patient tended to make people angry, just as she, the therapist, was angry a day later. This perspective helped her "get a grip" on her feelings and make use of them in the next session.

and behaviors are examined to determine changes that patients can make and to develop new coping strategies. Individual therapy further develops patients' skills through **rehearsal**, including role-playing of interpersonal situations with practicing of skills and rehearsing challenges to problematic emotions or cognitions. Therapists reinforce effective behavior and ignore or coolly respond to problematic behavior. In addition, therapists help patients to recognize troubling emotions in sessions, and practice thoughts and behaviors that could block urges to behave in a destructive manner.

Telephone Consultation

Telephone consultation is employed as a tool of therapy, with therapists setting clear limits around timing and length of calls to maintain appropriate boundaries and avoid reinforcing problematic behavior. The possibility of a phone call provides a supportive lifeline to the therapist. It allows for brief contacts in which adaptive behavior can be encouraged, and in which a temporarily desperate patient can get help in stopping a self-injurious behavior. At the same time, it can offer a bridge between the weekly sessions.

Consultation Team

Finally, DBT provides a consultation team to support and validate individual therapists in their work with difficult patients. The team consists of a group of like-minded DBT therapists who meet weekly. They provide emotional support for each other in dealing with difficult and often suicidal patients. They also provide an opportunity to discuss problems, and try to give nonjudgmental mutual supervision. In addition, the team can offer new perspectives and strategies when a therapist is feeling that treatment is at impasse.

THE MULTIPLE-PERSON THERAPIES

The treatment methods based on interpersonal systems have become more important in recent years and many of their concepts have been integrated into the individual therapies. Interpersonal psychotherapy (IPT) is included in this section to highlight its valuable application of the two-person model, although it uses some cognitive and psychodynamic principles and is an individual psychotherapy. The growing understanding of the development of the individual as part of a dyad, starting with the earliest relationship with the caretaker, has contributed to the foundation of IPT as well as the group and family therapies. Table 17.5 provides an overview of the multiple-person therapies.

Interpersonal Psychotherapy

Interpersonal psychotherapy emerged from Harry Stack Sullivan's interpersonal school of psychiatry and was further developed by Gerald Klerman, Myrna Weissman, and their colleagues (Klerman et al. 1984). It is a well-organized technique based on the theory that **depression is a problem in interpersonal relations**. According to interpersonal theory, depression is often correlated with events that occur in relation to other people. Depression not only contributes to the cause of interpersonal problems but also aggravates any preexisting difficulties a person is having in interpersonal relations. These difficulties then perpetuate the vicious cycle by increasing the depression. The interpersonal psychotherapist directs the patient to improve his or her communication and interpersonal skills and to develop more accurate perceptions of feelings. These changes enable the patient to engage in more fulfilling and pleasurable interpersonal interactions, which

TABLE 17.5 Overview of Multiple-Person Therapies

	Interpersonal Psychotherapy	Family Therapy	Group Therapy
Indications	Depression Grief reactions Interpersonal disputes Role transitions Interpersonal deficits	Conflicts between family members resulting in overt distress in the family Pathology in one family member	Problems with socialization due to anxiety, anger, psychosis, sociopathy, or immaturity Level of impairment can range from mild to severely disabled Particularly useful for substance use disorders.
Theory of Symptom Formation	Disorders stem from problems in interpersonal relationships.	Psychodynamic approach: pathological patterns within the family arise from the dynamics within and between individual family members. Systems approach: pathological patterns stem from the system, rather than individuals.	Varies with patient and group characteristics
Patterns	Communication problems Distrust Dependency issues Low self-esteem	Communication problems Individual pathology alters dynamics within the family. Alliances and enmities disturb dynamics within the family.	Avoidance of other people Interpersonally tends to be irrational, paranoid, and irritable Lack of social skills
Therapeutic Stance	Active, directive, and collaborative	Active, directive, and supportive	Active, directive, reassuring, and encouraging
Techniques	Examination of thought patterns Communication analysis Interpersonal inventory Guided rehearsal and practice	Weekly sessions with the entire family in which members express feelings and interact with each other. Psychodynamic approach: exploration of family history to elucidate the nature of family conflicts and contributing transferences, allowing for interpretations linking past and present. Systems approach: active manipulations of family patterns, including paradoxical instructions, relabeling, and reframing, to bring forth and address conflicts within the system.	May be in conjunction with individual treatment. Techniques range from psychoanalytic and interpretive to supportive with behavioral and social-supportive interventions.
Outcome	Improved interpersonal skills result in relief of mood symptoms and enhanced relationships and self-esteem.	Insight and habit change engendered by interpretation and manipulations of the system reduce family conflicts and allow each family member to grow.	May include insight, symptom relief, and behavior change

make the patient feel less helpless. The final ideal outcome of the therapy is the resolution of the patient's depression.

Indications and Selection Criteria

Interpersonal psychotherapy is indicated for patients with a mild to moderate degree of **major depression, dysthymia**, or depressed mood due to an adjustment disorder whose primary concerns involve relationships, especially when bereavement or a significant life change is involved.

Therapeutic Process

Interpersonal therapy consists typically of **12–20 weekly sessions**. In the initial interview, the therapist inquires about recent crises or changes involving other people in the patient's life. Such problems fall into four general categories: (1) a **grief reaction** to the loss or death of a loved one; (2) an **interpersonal dispute** (e.g., a feud with a boss or a friend or some other major disagreement); (3) a **role transition** (e.g., graduation, retirement, or, as in the case presented in Box 17.12, a change in the parental role as the "nest" begins to empty); and (4) an **interpersonal deficit,** which is often a more chronic problem of insensitivity to others, inability to get along with others, or inability to form a relationship.

After first explaining the nature and usual course of depression, its damaging effects on a person's life and relations with others, and the rationale for inquiry into the patient's social world, the therapist then encourages the patient to describe in detail relationships and interactions with other people. Together, they explore the patient's interpersonal world and develop an **interpersonal inventory**. As the patient's story unfolds, a history of many interpersonal difficulties may emerge, including difficulties in communicating feelings, problems with understanding the mutual obligations in relationships, and a poor sense of what to expect from other people. The therapist and patient examine what these interpersonal difficulties imply about the ways in which the patient affects other people.

The therapist then encourages the patient to become aware of and express his or her feelings about other people. This focus on affect is part of the process by which the patient learns how to acknowledge feelings and how to express them more clearly in relationships. The therapist conducts a **communication analysis** to remedy faulty communication skills, including failure or refusal to communicate, which often contribute to interpersonal problems. The interpersonal therapist approaches faulty communication in much the same way that a cognitive therapist approaches cognitive distortions: by pointing them out to the patient when they occur and exploring ways in which they can be changed (see the case example in Box 17.14).

Family Therapy

Family therapy includes the treatment of whole families, parts of families, and couples. The most obvious difference between this form of therapy and other therapies is that family therapy treats more than one person. Important changes in technique are required because the focus is not on an individual but a system of individuals and the communication patterns within the system.

Systems Approach

Systems theories of family therapy focus on the **current structural entities** within the family. These structures are either Oedipal triangles involving two parents and one child or

---

BOX 17.14

CASE EXAMPLE OF INTERPERSONAL PSYCHOTHERAPY FOR DEPRESSION

The depressed mother discussed in Box 17.12 as a patient in cognitive-behavioral therapy might also be an appropriate candidate for interpersonal psychotherapy. The referring doctor noted that her depression was occurring in the context of a major phase shift in her life, namely the emptying of her nest. The IPT therapist in the first interview asked about her symptoms and soon began to concentrate on her relations with her family members. In the interpersonal inventory, the therapist asked her to provide details of her interactions with her husband by asking her to describe what happened when he came home from work. The patient answered that he hung up his coat, put his briefcase in the study, and looked for her. She was usually in their darkened bedroom in bed and responded to his inquiries with complaints about her day and their daughter's behavior, reiterating that their son had not called in 3 days and declaring that he must be in some sort of trouble. "I know I shouldn't but I can't stop myself, I start berating him: why has he come home so late, and doesn't he know I worry? Yesterday he was 15 minutes later than usual; I told him I'd been worrying that he had been in an accident, mugged, or some other horrible thing. I said he must not love me any more and why should he? I'm worthless, and he must be looking for someone else."

The therapist focused on understanding these interactions and exploring possible ways to improve them. For example, the therapist asked the patient how she thought her husband felt about her tirades, and together they speculated that he might find this unchanging pattern painful and guilt-provoking, and that it might eventually make him angry. He might very well not look forward to coming home, not because she is "worthless" but because her behavior caused him pain. The therapist suggested that if the patient discussed feeling depressed and hopeless with her husband in a non-accusatory way he might become more sympathetic, and they could possibly have a more pleasant evening. The successful outcome of this work would be for the patient to understand her behavior and its underlying motivation, see beyond her set opinion that she is simply worthless, communicate better with her husband, and take action to alter this particular homecoming greeting.

---

sibling triangles involving two children and one parent. Dyads occur as structural systems within the family as well, as does, of course, the family as a whole. Using the family systems approach, the therapist attempts to understand and describe to the family the **pathological patterns** in their relationships and **manipulate** the family in order to help resolve these pathological patterns. Box 17.15 describes a case example of a systems approach in which the family structure is confronted by enactments and suggested changes.

Psychodynamic Approach

The **psychodynamic model** of family therapy incorporates the psychoanalytic principles of ego psychology and object relations and focuses on individual psychodynamics

BOX 17.15

CASE EXAMPLE OF FAMILY THERAPY—SYSTEMS APPROACH

The depressed woman referred to in Boxes 17.12 and 17.14 might experience the following family crisis. A few months after Peter, their son, left for college and the mother began therapy, their daughter, Nancy, now a junior in high school, began showing signs of disturbance. Her grades had dropped, and she had joined a group of semi-delinquent drug-abusing classmates. At home she was increasingly withdrawn and angry, occasionally erupting in a rage at her mother. Recently, while she was drunk, she wrecked the family car but miraculously escaped injury. Her parents realized that she might soon succeed in killing herself.

As a result of this family crisis, the father and daughter agreed to go with the mother to family therapy. Although brief individual psychotherapy might have helped Nancy, she did not seem to have much motivation to seek therapy for herself and probably would not show up for appointments. More importantly, even if all three members of the family were engaged in individual therapies, certain problems in the family system would not be addressed.

The family went to the first appointment with a strategic family therapist. In the office, they found a circle of five chairs. It seemed natural for the daughter to sit next to her mother and for her father to sit opposite them with an empty chair on each side of him. The therapist said nothing directly about the seating arrangement but asked the daughter if she would please sit next to her father. She looked surprised but complied, and the therapist sat between her and her mother. The therapist had initially sensed that the mother and daughter were bonded and that the father was isolated. He was not surprised to find out rapidly that the bond between mother and daughter was ambivalent and hostile, and that Nancy's separation from her father was painful to both of them. The therapist had been well briefed beforehand and knew that there was a fourth silent, but still present, member in the empty chair. He knew that there was some risk if he sat in a chair that could have been Peter's and failed to address this fact. He said, "I know that you are all missing Peter, now away at college; I hope you are not offended if I have taken his seat." This acknowledgment immediately brought Peter's absence into the foreground, and for most of the session, the initial complaint about the "designated patient," Nancy, was forgotten.

The therapist's manipulation of the seating arrangement in order to enact a family pattern that would challenge the unspoken relationship patterns was a common strategic systems maneuver that forced the family to talk about their relationships and, at the same time, to feel the forces that were at work within the family. This kind of intervention may also be used as a homework assignment in which the family would be asked to sit at different positions at their dinner table.

(continued)

Early in the treatment the therapist reframed the initial complaint about the designated patient's behavior (e.g., the daughter's semi-delinquent behavior) as part of the family system to which everyone contributes. It became clear that missing Peter was not the family's only problem. The family dynamics were such that the mother, who doted on her son, had been comparatively indifferent to Nancy, who did not feel that she could turn to her father, and felt rejected by him, because he had always been emotionally isolated and unable to relate comfortably to her. As she had developed and become somewhat provocative at puberty, he had become uneasy and withdrew further. She and her father were both isolated in the home where the mother and son were a team. Peter's absence had, among other things, upset this stable equilibrium. It had left the mother without her ally. She had wanted to turn to her husband for support, but he could not provide it and withdrew. Nancy, who had long been envious of her brother because he was her mother's favorite, felt extremely guilty about that envy. In her guilt, she felt the need to cling to her mother, partly out of spite toward her father and despite her feeling that her mother did not really love her and would have been much less unhappy if she herself had gone away instead of her brother.

The daughter's bond with her mother, indeed both parents, included a great deal of rage, which she enacted in her delinquent, self-destructive behavior. This behavior got the attention of her parents and was, therefore, being perversely rewarded. This behavior also provided a focus for her mother's worry, which, in fact, helped relieve her mother's depression. It also forced the father to become closer to the mother as they dealt jointly with the daughter. Before her brother's departure, the family situation had been a hard but stable compromise for the daughter.

By intuitively suggesting the seating arrangement, the therapist had effectively brought out the family's dynamic and countered the prevailing family structure by separating Nancy from her mother and uniting her with her father. This arrangement gratified the daughter and made her a less reluctant participant, although it angered her mother. But by placing himself next to the mother, the therapist had implicitly substituted himself for her son and the father, thus gratifying her. The father's isolation was at least confronted by having his daughter sit next to him.

During the ensuing months, the family met for 12 sessions, and the therapist became a dominant force in the family as he manipulated the family structure to make it change. One technique that he used was **paradoxical instruction**, as he observed that the father withdrew and let the mother intercept the message whenever the daughter tried to speak to her father. The next time that this happened, the therapist instructed the daughter to address her father while the father remained silent and the mother interrupted; in other words, he asked the family to act out their habitual pattern. This technique provides the family members with an immediate experience of a system that they had been participating in out of their awareness. Once seen, the pattern becomes more difficult and even embarrassing for them to continue.

within the context of a family system and on the conflicts that have emerged. The family context includes the family's history, the interactions within the family, the process by which family members internalize one another, and the established patterns, based on these internalizations, of relating to each other. When a family does not provide for the needs of its members, it is "dysfunctional." The inner psychic struggles of family members result in pathological behavior patterns, which usually lead to conflict within the family.

The primary technique in the psychodynamic model of family therapy involves defining existing relationships within the **history of the family** and the **transferences** between its members. Transference is a very important concept in this form of therapy: a parent may see a child as being "just like" one of his or her parents or may feel and act like one of his or her own parents in dealing with the child. The therapist, whose role is analytic and inquisitive rather than active or manipulative, focuses more on understanding the family's history and interpreting that history than on examining current interactions (see case example in Box 17.16).

Couple therapy is a variant of family therapy in which the focus is on adults in their romantic, marital, and sexual relations. Some couple therapists sub-specialize in sex therapy, which may use behavioral, cognitive, and psychodynamic methods in dealing with sexual dysfunctions.

Group Therapy

Both group therapy and family therapy examine the interactions within a group of people, instead of focusing on the individual. Many of the same principles underlie both techniques, although in group therapy the group is composed of unrelated people whose history as a particular group is short, unlike the long shared history of a family. The important feature in group therapy is the current interrelationships of the members. The goal of **psychoanalytically oriented group therapy** is to induce in the patient a greater understanding of how he or she perceives others and is perceived by others, by challenging defenses and producing insights. Some groups focus on current interaction between group members, while the more psychoanalytic groups use the transferences

---

BOX 17.16

CASE EXAMPLE OF FAMILY THERAPY—PSYCHODYNAMIC APPROACH

In contrast to the systems style that was used by the family therapist in Box 17.15, a therapist taking a psychodynamic approach might have entered the session and sat in the customary chair. Sooner or later, the therapist would ask the family members to explain why they are sitting where they are, how they feel about it, and what they might like to change about it. A discussion of the family members' feelings toward each other and the ways in which they reflect certain transferences toward each other might then ensue. For example, the mother might say that she had felt very dependent on, and at the same time rejected by, her own mother and, fearing that she would do something similar to her daughter, she clung to her in an overwhelmingly intrusive way. The psychodynamic approach concentrates more on interpretation than enactment and is less dramatic, but it is often equally effective.

within the group to help recall childhood experiences. In either case, an important result is to induce in the patient a greater understanding of how he or she functions in a social environment (see case example in Box 17.17).

The most variable element in group therapy is the explicit purpose of each group. There are probably more different functional types of therapy in the group mode than in any other therapeutic modality. Groups serve many different purposes; for example, there are medical support groups, daily management groups for psychotic inpatients, and interactional outpatient groups that promote personality growth and change. In addition to psychodynamically oriented groups, there are groups that employ primarily cognitive

---

BOX 17.17

CASE EXAMPLE OF GROUP THERAPY FOR AN ADOLESCENT

The daughter, Nancy, whose course of family therapy is described in Box 17.15, participated in the family therapy for 6 months. During that time, the interactions within her family improved considerably, and at the end of 6 months, the family made a decision, with which the therapist agreed, to end therapy. The therapist was well aware that the daughter still had problems, but sensed that her motivation to work them out in the presence of the family was coming to an end. She had found a way to live with her family. Next, she would need to learn how to separate from them as she approached young adulthood. She would clearly do better in another kind of therapy, without her family. In referring this patient for further treatment, the therapist considered two forms of therapy, individual psychoanalytically oriented therapy and group therapy, each of which had advantages and both of which were available in the community. Individual therapy would have the patient work through an intense transference in which she would react to the therapist in the same angry way she had reacted to her parents. The therapist would repeatedly interpret this pattern so that the patient would learn about her distorted expectations and then be able to change them. However, if the patient proved to be relatively unmotivated and antagonistic toward the parental figure/therapist, the interpretations might go unheeded. The therapist decided to send the patient to group therapy, having concluded that therapy in a group of peers with similar experiences would better serve her.

The group therapist was an experienced woman who had a reputation for working well with adolescents who are acting out their feelings. There were eight people in the group ranging in age from 16 to 22 years. Because of their similarity in age, the members tended to band together as siblings and developed a strong transference to the middle-aged therapist. This group experience was beneficial for the patient in a number of ways. She quickly realized that her age-mates had similar problems with their families. Some things that she had regarded as her own unique secrets were, in fact, universal issues that the members in the group talked about openly. Learning

(continued)

that some of the older members had worked through problems like hers and were becoming college students helped to reduce her feeling of hopelessness. She also acquired valuable information, including answers to many questions that she had "always wanted to ask but was afraid to." In particular, she learned important information about birth control and about the hazards of drug abuse, which was imparted in ways that she could not have accepted from a parent.

She began to be genuinely concerned about other group members and realized that they were interested and concerned about her. This newly developed altruism led her out of her self-pitying self-preoccupation, so that she looked forward to the group meetings. The group was very helpful in teaching her new techniques for socialization and letting her know that her sullen, pouting style was not the best way to win friends. She learned how to meet people, how to make small talk, and how to be less awkward in groups. Imitative behavior was important in helping her with socialization. She found herself imitating one of the more socially graceful women in the group and realized that this approach worked much better than her former mode of relating to people.

As she became more comfortable in the group, she experienced an important realization: she was able to express her feelings with less expectation of ridicule or criticism. She again told the story of her family, but this time, she felt a warm, empathic response, which became another step in her long mourning process. It is helpful to relive an experience in different contexts because each re-experience adds something unique and provides new relief. Telling her story in the group and revealing her thoughts, feelings, and weaknesses generated a strong bond with the group. The patient gradually became more open to feedback from the group. At the same time, she brought her problems into an arena outside herself, which encouraged her to gain perspective on herself and a new objectivity. Through this interpersonal learning, she began to see her problems as less unspeakable than before. At the same time, she was able to take some personal responsibility for her problems and began to feel that her difficulties were not completely the fault of her parents. This realization, in turn, gave her a sense of empowerment to do something about her problems.

or interpersonal approaches. **Specialized groups** are made up of people with particular problems, such as eating disorders, phobias, sexual dysfunctions, drug and alcohol addictions, and obsessive-compulsive disorder. The leaders and members of these groups are expert in dealing with a specific problem, such as drug abuse, in which all members of the group have had the same experiences and used similar rationalizations and defenses to perpetuate their addictions. They can often see through self-justifications that might fool a sympathetic individual therapist. The message "I have been there, too" that is expressed by the other members is a powerful, engaging device that can get through to the most resistant patient.

Supportive groups for medical disorders include groups for diabetic, hypertensive, and cancer patients and for the relatives of such patients. **Supportive groups for psychiatric disorders** include daily groups for hospitalized patients, monthly groups for chronic patients who are taking psychotropic medications, and groups for other patients in need of supportive therapy. For these groups, the model is similar to that of supportive individual therapy, and the purpose is to maintain patients at their best possible level of functioning. In addition to receiving reassurance and advice and having a stable object to whom they can relate, patients gain the benefits derived from companionship and the feeling that a number of people are interested in their welfare.

SUPPORTIVE PSYCHOTHERAPIES

Supportive psychotherapy is the oldest type of therapy. The shamans of primitive cultures, the priests of the Middle Ages, the general practitioners who talk to their patients, and the coaches who say, "You can do it!" all provided a form of supportive psychotherapy, the purpose of which is to support the personality at its best level of functioning. Because this functioning is largely accomplished by aiding the patient's personality defenses, supportive therapy has been given second-class status when compared with therapies that promote improvement and psychological change. The importance of supportive psychotherapy should not be underestimated, however, because it may still be the most widely practiced form of psychotherapy.

The therapies of the twentieth century developed from and made systematic use of specific techniques from the repertoire of supportive therapy. For instance, pioneers in hypnosis and psychoanalysis distilled the magical power and omnipotence attributed to the therapist into a positive transference, which became the keystone of therapy. The inevitable disappointment in the idealized therapist became the equally important negative transference. The therapist's hortatory statement, "You can do it. Maybe you could just start a conversation in the hall" (with the woman to whom you are attracted but by whom you are intimidated), has been appropriated by the behaviorist as the basic form of "in vivo" desensitization. The encouraging statement, "You are thinking very negatively. You have no evidence that she hates you," is a pre-systematic form of cognitive therapy. Interpersonal psychotherapy uses many supportive techniques in helping to improve interpersonal relationships.

Crisis Intervention

The normal response to trauma or loss is a period of grief followed by a natural healing process, which may take months or years. In some cases, the trauma is so great and the patient so vulnerable that this process is prolonged. The goal of supportive psychotherapy is to speed up the process and ensure a better outcome for the patient. In the same way that a physician supports a patient with a physical trauma or a severe viral illness by maintaining vital physical functions until the body can heal itself, the therapist's support of the patient's temporarily weakened psychological defenses allows normal functioning to be regained more quickly. Although restoration of normal function is the goal, patients frequently achieve more than that. By opening up their defenses, and then confronting and emerging from a severe existential crisis, patients often experience psychological maturation and growth. Through interpretations and reassurance, the therapist may take advantage of the opportunity to help the patient become even stronger than before. The goal of supportive psychotherapy in this situation is to **restore the patient's normal defenses** and resolve his or her grief, insofar as this is possible.

Indications and Selection Criteria

Patients best suited for this type of supportive psychotherapy are those who are in **crisis situations**, which may involve a **loss**, an **acute medical illness**, or a **major trauma**. These patients may have previously been in good psychological health or have had varying degrees of pathological symptoms. The goal is to return them to their former level of adaptation.

Therapeutic Process

The duration of supportive psychotherapy ranges from just a few sessions to many months. Individuals tend to regress during a crisis, and the supportive psychotherapist may have to accept, without interpretation, the patient's need to believe and unrealistically expect that the therapist's magical power can undo the tragedy. During the acute phase, instead of confronting the patient's intellectualization, rationalization, or denial, the therapist may encourage and support the patient's habitual defenses or, at least, let them be. The therapist's most important task is to maintain a warm, confident, supportive stance and provide a **holding environment** (i.e., a positive therapeutic alliance that offers a solid, reliable source of help). The therapist responds empathically to the patient's feelings and demonstrates acceptance of the way the patient is reacting to the crisis. Although the therapist may counter exaggerated fears or excessive pessimism with encouraging doses of reality, this alternative perspective must be carefully presented. Patients usually experience tactless or unrealistic reassurances as evidence that the therapist does not understand their situation. The supportive therapist does not employ the usual methods of increasing intensity and tension (e.g., through silence or confrontation) and should not set strict time limits on the therapy or adhere firmly to a specific focus. As time goes by and the patient emerges from the acute phase, the therapist may bring up painful issues and interpretation becomes more useful. The therapist may then interpret the transference and ultimately confront the termination of the therapy.

Medical Illness

A variant of crisis intervention is helpful to many patients with problems of indefinite duration, the most common of which is severe **medical illness** (see Chapter 11, Psychological Factors Affecting Medical Conditions). Patients who poorly manage their severe diabetes, for example, or suffer from cancer can benefit from the close support of an empathic, reliable physician who is skilled in knowing when to support and when to gently challenge a patient's defenses. The techniques and other aspects of this therapy are similar to those used in crisis intervention. Since therapy may continue for years, an intense, dependent transference can develop, which may remain uninterpreted if it does not interfere with the patient's functioning outside of the treatment. Supportive psychotherapists understand their patients' emotional dynamics and defenses and use this understanding to guide their support.

The psychodynamic life narrative developed by Viederman (1983) is one technique that has been effective in consultation-liaison work with medical patients and, in certain aspects, is similar to nonconfrontative forms of brief dynamic psychotherapy. The goal of this brief intervention, which attempts, in only a few sessions, to place the patient's illness into the context of his or her life and psychodynamics, is to bring the patient to an even better than usual level of adaptation.

Ego Deficits

The goal of supportive psychotherapy for patients with chronic ego deficits is to help them maintain the highest possible level of functioning and emotional well-being. The therapist supports the patient's defenses, not only to sustain his or her psychological status quo but also to enable the patient to make striking gains and later be able to engage in a much more intensive, confrontative therapy. Like a surgeon's decision not to operate, the decision not to challenge the patient's defenses is a very important option in the therapist's repertoire of approaches.

Indications and Selection Criteria

While the goal of supportive psychotherapy for chronic ego deficits is the same as the goals of other forms of supportive therapy, the type of patient is different. Instead of a patient with a relatively healthy ego who has been afflicted by trauma or illness, the patient is poorly functioning and in need of support to survive, even in normal circumstances. Therefore, therapy usually continues for a long time, often for life.

Supportive psychotherapy helps patients with severe problems and ego deficits who cannot make use of the other forms of therapy. Patients with psychotic illnesses may be made worse in intensive psychotherapy. Patients with poor impulse control, an inability to tolerate negative affects, or uncontrollable swings of affect cannot tolerate the negative feelings encountered in an intense, change-oriented therapy. They may become suicidally depressed or may quit therapy in a rage. A patient who has severe problems with relationships, is suspicious and withdrawn, and has no friends will probably be suspicious and withdrawn and have severe problems in a therapeutic relationship that challenges his or her defenses or has any degree of intensity. A patient with a chronically flat affect will be frightened of anything more than a superficial, nonthreatening therapeutic relationship. Some patients with cognitive deficits, who may have limited intelligence, low introspective ability, poverty of abstraction, and inability to communicate, will not be able to make use of more challenging therapies.

Therapeutic Process

All of the techniques described in this section are useful in supportive therapy for chronic ego deficits, and, as in the other two forms of supportive therapy, the key factor is the "auxiliary ego" role played by the therapist, who thinks out loud with and for the patient and makes up for the patient's temporary or chronic deficiencies in ego function. Some additions and modifications are often made, such as providing a high degree of involvement, empathy, and reassurance for a needy, self-hating, insecure patient, or keeping a distance and maintaining a stance of benign interest for a schizoid, isolated person. **Suggestions** from and **education** by the therapist, which may include giving advice on how to dress better or role-playing in preparation for a job interview, are often very important for these patients, who have not learned to cope adequately with life.

At times, confrontation and interpretation may be helpful and even necessary, especially when the therapist must deal with a negative transference or the loss of the therapeutic alliance. In some ways, supportive psychotherapy requires that the therapist have a richer repertoire of methods than is required by other treatments.

REFERENCES CITED

Bateman, A., and P. Fonagy. 8-year follow-up of patients treated for borderline personality disorder: mentalization-based treatment versus treatment as usual. *American Journal of Psychiatry* 165:631–638, 2008.

Bateman, A., and Fonagy, P. *Handbook of Mentalizing in Mental Health Practice*. Washington, DC: American Psychiatric Publishing, 2011.

Bateman, A., and Fonagy, P. *Psychotherapy for Borderline Personality Disorder: Mentalisation Based Treatment*. Oxford, UK: Oxford University Press, 2004.

Bateman, A., and P. Fonagy. Treatment of borderline personality disorder with psychoanalytically oriented partial hospitalization: an 18-month follow-up. *American Journal of Psychiatry* 158:36–42, 2001.

Beck, A. T., A. J. Rush, B. F. Shaw, and G. Emery. *Cognitive Therapy of Depression*. New York: Guilford Press, 1987.

Busch, F. N., B. L. Milrod, M. Singer, and A. Aronson. *Panic-Focused Psychodynamic Psychotherapy, Extended Range*. New York: Routledge, 2012.

Busch, F. N., B. L. Milrod, and N. C. Thoma. Teaching clinical research on psychodynamic psychotherapy to psychiatric residents. *Psychodynamic Psychiatry* 41:141–162, 2013.

Clarkin, J. F., K. N. Levy, M. F. Lenzenweger, and O. F. Kernberg. Evaluating three treatments for borderline personality disorder: A multiwave study. *American Journal of Psychiatry* 164:922–928, 2007.

Cuijpers, P., A. S. Geraedts, P. van Oppen, G. Andersson, J. C. Markowitz, and A. van Straten. Interpersonal psychotherapy of depression: a meta-analysis. *American Journal of Psychiatry* 168:581–592, 2011.

Davanloo, H., ed. *Short-Term Dynamic Psychotherapy*. New York: Jason Aronson, 1980.

de Maat, S., F. de Jonghe, R. de Kraker, F. Leichsenring, A. Abbass, P. Luyten, J. P. Barber, Van Rien, and J. Dekker. The current state of the empirical evidence for psychoanalysis: a meta-analytic approach. *Harvard Review of Psychiatry* 21:107–137, 2013.

Emmelkamp, P. M., A. Benner, A. Kuipers, G. A. Feiertag, H. C. Koster, and F. J. van Apeldoorn. Comparison of brief dynamic and cognitive–behavioural therapies in avoidant personality disorder. *British Journal of Psychiatry* 189:60–64, 2006.

Fonagy, P., and M. Target. Predictors of outcome in child psychoanalysis: a retrospective study of 763 cases at the Anna Freud Centre. *Journal of the American Psychoanalytic Association* 44:27–77, 1996.

Geist, R., M. Heinmaa, D. Stephens, R. Davis, and D. K. Katzman. Comparison of family therapy and family group psychoeducation in adolescents with anorexia nervosa. *Canadian Journal of Psychiatry* 45:173–178, 2000.

Hofmann, S. G., A. Asnaani, I. J. Vonk, A. T. Sawyer, and A. Fang. The efficacy of cognitive behavioral therapy: a review of meta-analyses. *Cognitive Therapy and Research* 36:427–440, 2012.

Katzman, M. A., N. Bara-Carril, S. Rabe-Hesketh, U. Schmidt, N. Troop, and J. Treasure. A randomized controlled two-stage trial in the treatment of bulimia nervosa, comparing CBT versus motivational enhancement in phase 1 followed by group versus individual CBT in phase 2. *Psychosomatic Medicine* 72:656–663, 2010.

Kernberg, O. F. *Borderline Conditions and Pathological Narcissism*. New York: Jason Aronson, 1975.

Klerman, G. L., M. M. Weissman, B. J. Rounsaville, and E. S. Chevron. *Interpersonal Psychotherapy of Depression*. New York: Basic Books, 1984.

Leichsenring, F. Are psychodynamic and psychoanalytic therapies effective? A review of empirical data. *International Journal of Psychoanalysis* 86:841–868, 2005.

Leichsenring, F., and S. Rabung. Long-term psychodynamic psychotherapy in complex mental disorders: update of a meta-analysis. *British Journal of Psychiatry* 199:15–22, 2011.

Linehan, M. M., H. E. Armstrong, A. Suarez, D. Allmon, and H. L. Heard. Cognitive-behavioral treatment of chronically parasuicidal borderline patients. *Archives of General Psychiatry* 48:1060–1064, 1991.

Lipsitz, J. D., M. Gur, D. Vermes, E. Petkova, J. Cheng, N. Miller, J. Laino, M. R. Liebowitz, and A. J. Fyer. A randomized trial of interpersonal therapy versus supportive therapy for social anxiety disorder. *Depression and Anxiety* 25:542–553, 2008.

Malan, D. H. *The Frontier of Brief Psychotherapy*. New York: Plenum Press, 1976.

Milrod, B., A. C. Leon, F. N. Busch, M. Rudden, M. Schwalberg, J. Clarkin, A. Aronson, M. Singer, W. Turchin, E. T. Klass, E. Graf, J. J. Teres, and M. K. Shear. A randomised controlled clinical trial of psychoanalytic psychotherapy for panic disorder. *American Journal of Psychiatry* 164:265–272, 2007.

Pharoah, F., J. Mari, J. Rathbone, and W. Wong. Family intervention for schizophrenia. *Cochrane Database of Systematic Reviews* 4:CD000088, 2010.

Rosenthal, M. Z., and T. L. Lynch. Dialectical behavior therapy. In Sadock, B. J., V. J. Sadock, and P. Ruiz, eds. *Comprehensive Textbook of Psychiatry*, 9th ed. Philadelphia: Lippincott Williams & Wilkins, 2009.

Russell, G. F., G. I. Szmukler, C. Dare, and I. Eisler. An evaluation of family therapy in anorexia nervosa and bulimia nervosa. *Archives of General Psychiatry* 44:1047–1056, 1987.

Stoffers, J. M., B. A. Völlm, G. Rücker, A. Timmer, N. Huband, and K. Lieb. Psychological therapies for people with borderline personality disorder. *Cochrane Database of Systematic Reviews* 8:CD005652, 2012.

Thoma, N. C., D. McKay, A. J. Gerber, B. L. Milrod, A. R. Edwards, and J. H. Kocsis. A quality-based review of randomized controlled trials of cognitive-behavioral therapy for depression: an assessment and metaregression. *American Journal of Psychiatry* 169:22–30, 2012.

Viederman, M. The psychodynamic life narrative: a psychotherapeutic intervention useful in crisis situations. *Psychiatry* 46:236–246, 1983.

SELECTED READINGS

Basch, M. F. *Understanding Psychotherapy: The Science Behind the Art*. New York: Basic Books, 1988.

Caligor, E., O. F. Kernberg, and J. F. Clarkin. *Handbook of Dynamic Psychotherapy for Higher Level Personality Pathology*. Washington, DC: American Psychiatric Publishing, 2007.

Cutler J. L., A. Goldyne, J. C. Markowitz, M. J. Devlin, and R. A. Glick. Comparing cognitive behavior therapy, interpersonal psychotherapy and psychodynamic psychotherapy. *American Journal of Psychiatry* 161:1567–1573, 2004.

Gabbard, G., B. Litowitz, and P. Williams, eds. *The American Psychiatric Publishing Textbook of Psychoanalysis*. Washington, DC: American Psychiatric Publishing, 2011.

Grant, P., P. R. Young, and R. J. DeRubeis. Cognitive and behavioral therapies. In Gabbard G. O., J. Beck, and J. Holmes, eds. *Oxford Textbook of Psychotherapy*. New York: Oxford University Press, 2005.

Gunderson, J. G. *Borderline Personality Disorder: A Clinical Guide*. Washington, DC: American Psychiatric Publishing, 2000.

Linehan, M. M. *Cognitive Behavioral Treatment of Borderline Personality Disorder*. New York: Guilford Press, 1993.

Linehan, M. M., and L. Dimeff. Dialectical behavior therapy in a nutshell. *California Psychologist* 34:10–13, 2001.

Markowitz, J. C., and G. L. Klerman. *Manual for Interpersonal Psychotherapy of Dysthymia*. New York: Department of Psychiatry, Cornell University Medical College, 1993.

Milrod, B., F. N. Busch, T. Shapiro, and A. M. Cooper. *Manual of Panic-Focused Psychodynamic Psychotherapy*. Washington, DC: American Psychiatric Publishing, 1997.

Robbins, M. S., T. L. Sexton, and G. R. Weeks. *Handbook of Family Therapy: The Science and Practice of Working with Families and Couples*. New York: Brunner-Routledge, 2003.

Sullivan, H. S. *The Interpersonal Theory of Psychiatry*. New York: Norton, 1953.

Yalom, I. D. *The Theory and Practice of Group Psychotherapy*. New York: Basic Books, 1985.

INDEX

Abnormal Involuntary Movement Scale (AIMS), 524

Abstinence model, 241–243

Abstraction, selective, 593b

Abstract thought, adolescent, 443

Acamprosate, for alcohol use disorder, 249, 551f, 552

Acting out, 575

Action stage, 242b

Activity, goal-directed, in mania, 55

Acute stress disorder
  diagnostic and clinical features of, 180–181
  differential diagnosis of, 185, 187
  etiological issues in, 188–194
  interview for, 181–183, 181b
  medical evaluation in, 187–188
  treatment of, 194–197
    cognitive-behavioral therapy in, 195–197
    pharmacotherapy principles in, 194–195
    psychodynamic psychotherapy in, 197

Adaptive regression, 352

Addiction, 208–209
  to benzodiazepines, 546
  pharmacogenetics of, 239
  relative, of specific substances, 223, 223t
  treatment of, 241–254 (See also under Substance-related and addictive disorders)

Adherence
  to pharmacotherapy, 514–515
  psychosocial aspects of, 383–385
    clinical features of, 383–384
    interview in, 384
    management of, 384–385

Adjustment disorders
  in elderly, 453, 454b
  in preschoolers, 435
  in school-age child, 440–441

Adjustment disorder with depressed mood, *vs.* mood disorder, 75

Adolescent development, 441–447, 443t
  progression of, 441–445
    abstract thought in, 443
    case example of, 444b
    gender-related issues in, 443–444
    identity consolidation and emotional maturity in, 442
    independence through groups in, 441
    risk-taking in, 444–445
    sexuality in, 444
   vulnerabilities in, 445

Adolescents, mood disorder in, 78–79

Adult development, 445–451
  progression of, 445–450
    cognitive awareness in, 449
    emotional maturity in, 449
    love gratification in, 448–449
    parenthood in, 448–449
    sexual function and dysfunction in, 449–450
    work gratification and failure in, 445–448, 448b
  psychopathology in, 451
  vulnerabilities in, 450

Adversarial relationships, in bipolar disorder, 72

Advocacy, for schizophrenia, 126

Affect, 47. *See also* specific disorders and types
  blunted, 11t, 101–102, 102t
  constricted, 11t
  flat, 11t, 101–102, 102t
  inappropriate, 11t
  labile, 11t
  regulation of, infant, 420–422, 421t

Aggression
  from head trauma, 159
  in violent patients
    physical, 406–407, 407b
    verbal, 405–406, 406b
Agitation. *See also* Psychomotor agitation
  medical causes of, 361t–362t
Agoraphobia
  diagnostic and clinical features of, 171
  differential diagnosis of, 183t
  etiology of, 197–198
  pheochromocytoma in, 136, 137b, 158
  screening questions for, 37b
  treatment of
    cognitive-behavioral therapy in, 197–198
    pharmacotherapy in, 197
Agranulocytosis, from antipsychotic agents, 5, 21,
    118, 526
  carbamazepine, 545
  chlorpromazine, 526
  clozapine, 118, 516, 521, 526
Ainsworth, 419t, 422
Akathisia
  from antidepressant agents, 53
  from antipsychotic agents, 479, 510, 517t, 522,
    524
  in depression, 53
  from SSRIs, 53, 531t, 532
  treatment of
    diphenhydramine in, 528
    propranolol in, 528
Akinesia, from antipsychotic agents, 522–523
Alanine aminotransferase (ALT), in alcohol use
    disorder, 236
Alarm reaction, 356
Alcohol-induced psychotic disorder with halluci-
    nations or delusions, 210
Alcohol use disorder
  anxiety disorder from, 202
  case example of, older adult, 222b
  course of illness in, 221
  with depression, 202
  diagnostic and clinical features of, 209–210,
    209t–213t
  epidemiology of, 205b
  kindling in, 202
  medical evaluation of, 137t, 233–238,
    234t–235t
    general approach in, 233–236, 234t–235t
    laboratory tests in, 236
  vs. mood disorder, 77

safe drinking guidelines and, 228b
  screening questions for, 38b
  suicide risk in, 396
  treatment of (*See also under* Substance-related
    and addictive disorders)
    detoxification in, 249–250
    pharmacotherapy in, 249–250
Alcohol Use Disorders Identification Test
    (AUDIT), 225
Alcohol withdrawal
  anxiety disorder from, 176–177
  vs. bipolar disorder, 142
  classic, 176–177
  Clinical Institute Withdrawal of Alcohol Scale
    for, 210, 211t–213t
  mental disorders due to, 142
  nocturnal withdrawal syndrome in, 177
  symptoms of, 210, 210t
Alcoholics Anonymous, 245, 245t
Alertness
  fluctuating, in delirium, 106
  heightened
    from amphetamines, 231b
    from hallucinogens, 218
    in hypomania, 57
Alexithymia, 51
Alliance, therapeutic. *See* Therapeutic alliance
Aloof personality traits, 367
Alprazolam, 545–549, 547t. *See also*
    Benzodiazepines
Alzheimer's disease
  neurocognitive disorder from, 131t, 133b, 134,
    154
  preventative measures for, 166
  treatment of
    anticholinesterase inhibitors in, 164
    memantine in, 164
    operant-behavior treatment in, 160, 160b
    Vitamin E and B complexes in, 164
Amantadine, for Parkinson's, 528
Ambivalence
  in anorexia nervosa, to gaining weight, 307, 318
  in anxiety, 584
  to manic patients, 72
  in preschoolers, 437
  in schizophrenia, 99b
  to substance use treatment, 242, 242b, 247
  in toddler development, 428, 429, 430t, 431b
Amitriptyline, 534t. *See also* Tricyclic antide-
    pressants (TCAs)
Amphetamine preparations, pediatric, 509

Amphetamine use disorder
    anxiety disorder from, 176, 176b
    diagnostic and clinical features of, 214–216, 215t
    epidemiology of, 206b
    life-threatening effects of, 216
    withdrawal from, 215–216, 215t
Amygdala, 80–81, 159, 190–192, 191f, 194,
        197–198, 240, 285, 303–304b
Anabolic-androgenic steroid use, 219, 220t
Anesthetic use disorder, 220, 220t
Anger. See also Violence
    about pharmacotherapy, 515
    in adolescents, 450
    in bipolar disorder, 72
    in countertransference, 562
    denial of, 584
    in depressive disorders, 71, 72, 74b
    in dialectical behavior therapy, 586t, 595b
    family therapy for, 162
    Freud on, 84
    group therapy for, 597t
    in major depression, 71–72, 71b
    in mania, 55, 56
    in negative transference, 562, 582b
    in panic focused psychodynamic psychother-
        apy, 584
    parental, about child's treatment, 450, 505
    in psychotherapy, 566t–567t, 568b–569b, 575,
        584
    in reaction to medical illness, 360–362,
        361t–362t
    in reaction to physical illness, 352, 356,
        360–362
    from substance withdrawal, 214t
    in suicide risk, 392–394
Anger intrapsychic conflicts surrounding, 584
Anhedonia, 51, 51b, 53
    in major depression, 58
    from stimulant withdrawal, 215
Anorexia nervosa. See also Feeding and eating
        disorders
    with bulimia nervosa, 299, 301b
    case example of, 293b–294b
    diagnostic and clinical features of, 292–294
    differential diagnosis of, 309
        vs. body dysmorphic disorder, 341
    epidemiology and course of, 298–304
        age of onset in, 298–299
        incidence and prevalence in, 298
        long-term course in, 301–304, 305
    etiology of, 316

amplifying or maintaining factors in, 311, 311f
    biological theories in, 311–314
    cultural factors in, 314–316
    precipitating factors in, 310–311, 311f
    predisposing factors in, 310, 311f
    psychosocial theories in, 314
interview in, 306–308
perfectionism in, biology of, 301, 304b
screening questions for, 38b
signs and symptoms of, 300t
subtypes of, 292–293
treatment of, 317–319
    behavior, 317–318
    pharmacotherapy in, 318–319
    psychotherapy in, 318
Anorgasmia
    in female orgasmic disorder, 450
    from SSRIs, 532
    from tricyclic antidepressants, 535
Anticholinergic agents. See specific types
Anticholinergic effects
    of antipsychotic agents, 88, 525
    of tricyclic antidepressants, 535
Anticholinesterase inhibitors, for dementia, 164
Anticipatory anxiety
    in panic disorder, 170
    in specific phobias, 173
Anticonvulsant agents. See also specific agents and
        disorders
    for bipolar disorder, 88
    for chronic pain, 382
    dosing of, 544–545
    indications for, 544
    as mood stabilizers, 544–545
        for suicide risk, 400
    for neurocognitive disorders, 165–166
    pretreatment evaluation for, 544
    side effects of, 545
Antidepressant agents, 528–541. See also specific
        agents and disorders
    for bulimia nervosa, 321
    for children and adolescents, 509
    for chronic pain, 382
    for depression, 85–87
        in neurocognitive disorders, 164–165
    dosing strategies with, 530
    history of, 528–529
    indications for, 529–530
    mechanism of action of, 80–81, 528, 529f
    for somatic symptom disorder, 347
    for suicide risk, 399–400

Antiparkinsonian agents, 527–528

Antipsychotic agents, 516–528. *See also specific agents and disorders*

  antiparkinsonian agents in, 527–528

  for bipolar disorder, 89

  for children and adolescents, 510

  choice of, 527

  classes of, 516, 517t–518t

  combination therapy with, 521

  dosing of, 517t–518t, 522

  drug interactions of, 527

  first-generation, 516, 517t–518t

  history of, 516–519

  indications and contraindications for, 520–521

  initiating treatment with, 521

  long-acting injectable, 522, 523b

    conversion from oral form to, 523b

  long-term use of, 119–120

  mechanism of action of, 519, 519f, 520f

  for obsessive-compulsive disorder, 199

  pretreatment evaluation for, 521

  for psychosis, in neurocognitive disorders, 165

  for schizophrenia

    acute episodes of, 118–119

    adherence to, 120

    general use of, 118

    history of, 117–118

  second-generation, 516–519, 517t–518t

  side effects of, 517t–518t, 522–526

    anticholinergic, 525

    dermatological, 526

    extrapyramidal symptoms, 522–524

    hematological, 526

    hepatic, 525–526

    hypotension, 525

    neuroleptic malignant syndrome, 526–527

    ophthalmological, 526

    sedation, 524–525

    seizure, 526

    sexual, 525

    tardive dyskinesia, 524

    weight, 522

Antisocial personality disorder

  course of illness in, 272–273

  diagnostic and clinical features in, 266–267, 267b

  interview in, 273–282, 279t

Anxiety

  anticipatory

    in panic disorder, 170

    in specific phobias, 173

  benzodiazepine receptors in, 190

  from cannabis use, 214

  from chronic illness, 371–377 (*See also* Chronic illness, psychosocial aspects of)

  definition of, 168

  due to another medical condition, 158–159

  forms of, 168, 169b

  with major depression, 61

  in mood disorders, 51

  normal *vs.* maladaptive, 168

  range of, 168

  in reaction to medical illness, 356–358

  separation

    in children and adolescents, 485–487

    in toddlers, 428

  stranger, in infant development, 422–423

Anxiety disorders, adult, 168–202

  diagnostic and clinical features of, 169–181

    acute stress disorder, 180–181

    agoraphobia, 171

    anxiety disorder due to another medical condition, 173–174, 175b, 175t

    classification in, 169

    generalized anxiety disorder, 173, 174b

    panic disorder, 170, 171b

    social anxiety disorder, 172–173, 172b

    specific phobia, 172–173

    substance/medication-induced, 174–178, 175t, 176b

    substance/medication-induced, alcohol withdrawal, 176–177

    substance/medication-induced, benzodiazepine and barbiturate withdrawal, 177

    substance/medication-induced, caffeinism, 176, 176b

    substance/medication-induced, opioid withdrawal, 177

    substance/medication-induced, paradoxical reactions, 178

    substance/medication-induced, stimulant intoxication, 176, 176b

  differential diagnosis of, 183–187

    acute stress disorder, 185, 187

    agoraphobia, 183t

    anabolic-androgenic steroid withdrawal, 219

    anxiety disorder due to another medical condition, 187

    generalized anxiety disorder, 183, 183t

    hallucinogen use, 218

panic disorder, 183t, 184
social anxiety disorder, 183t, 184
specific phobia, 184
substance/medication-induced anxiety
disorder, 187
due to another medical condition, 136,
137b
differential diagnosis of, 187
eating disorders with, 299
etiology of, 188–194
generalized anxiety disorder, 201
neurobiological, genetics and environmental
interactions, 189–190
neurobiological, hypothalamic–pituitary–
adrenal axis, 191
neurobiological, neurocircuitry, attention,
and learning, 191–193
neurobiological, neurotransmitters,
190–191, 191f
panic disorder and agoraphobia, 197–198
psychosocial, cognitive-behavioral, 193
psychosocial, psychodynamic, 193–194
social anxiety disorder, 198
specific phobias, 201
substance/medication-induced, 202
interview for, 181–183, 181b
medical evaluation in, 187–188, 187b,
188b
overview of, 168
in preschoolers, 435
in school-age child, 440
screening questions for, 37b
symptoms in, 169b
threshold for, 168–169
treatment of, 194–197
generalized anxiety disorder, 201
panic disorder and agoraphobia, 197–198
pharmacotherapy principles in, 194–195
posttraumatic stress disorder, 200–201
psychotherapy principles in,
cognitive-behavioral therapy, 195–197,
587, 589
psychotherapy principles in, psychodynamic, 197
social anxiety disorder, 198–199
specific phobias, 201–202
Anxiety disorders, child and adolescent,
485–489
diagnostic and clinical features of,
485–488
fundamentals of, 485

generalized anxiety disorder, 487
panic disorder, 488
separation anxiety disorder, 485–487
social phobia, 488
specific phobia, 488
differential diagnosis of, 488–489
epidemiology of, 486t–487t
treatment and prognosis in, 489
Anxiolytics, 165, 545–550. *See also specific agents
and types*
benzodiazepines, 545–549, 547t (*See also
Benzodiazepines)*
mechanism of action of, 545, 546f
non-benzodiazepine, 549, 550t
Anxious distress, 61
Apathy
from brain lesions or tumors, 159
in dementia, 75
in depression, 52
in major neurocognitive disorder,
134
in mental disorders due to another medical
condition, 136–137
in neurocognitive disorders, 137
with psychomotor retardation, 52
in schizophrenia, 75, 102
in vascular depression, 64
Appetite
decreased
in depression, 58
from SSRIs, 532
increased, in depression, 59
Aripiprazole, 517t. *See also* Antipsychotic agents
for children and adolescents, 510
Arithmetic, in school-age children, 437–438
Aspartate aminotransferase (AST), in alcohol use
disorder, 236
Assertive community treatment (ACT),
125
Assessment, 1–20. *See also specific disorders*
case write-up in, 1–2, 2f, 3t, 12, 13b–18b
chief complaint in, 2–4, 3b, 4b, 13b
history in, 4–9
family, 9, 15b
past medical, 6–7, 14b
past psychiatric, 5, 7b, 14b
of present illness, 4–5, 6b, 13b
psychosocial, 7–9, 8b, 9b, 14b–15b
review of systems in, 7, 14b
impressions in, 18–20
case summary in, 16b, 19

Assessment (*Cont.*)
 differential diagnosis in, 16b, 19–20
 predisposing and precipitating factors in, 16b–17b, 20
 laboratory tests in, 16b, 18
 mental status examination in
  in adults, 9–12, 10t–12t, 15b–16b
  in children and adolescents, 463, 464b–465b
 physical examination in, 12, 15b
Associations, loosening of, 11t
 in mania, 56
 in schizophrenia, 102–103
Ataxia
 from carbamazepine, 545
 in delirium, 132t
 from lamotrigine, 545
 from lithium, 543
 from phencyclidine, 218t
Atomoxetine, for attention-deficit hyperactivity disorder, 498
Attachment
 avoidant, 421
 disorganized, 427, 427b
 in infant development, 421–422, 422b
 resistant, 421
 secure, 421
Attention
 deficits of, in delirium, 130
 disrupted, 592
Attention-deficit hyperactivity disorder (ADHD), 483f, 496–499
 diagnostic and clinical features of, 496–497
 vs. disruptive mood dysregulation disorder, 482, 483f
 DSM-5 classification of, 468
 etiology of, 498
 in preschoolers, 435
 in school-age child, 440
 treatment and prognosis in, 498–499
"Attenuated psychosis syndrome," 121
Auditory hallucinations, in schizophrenia, 100t, 101
Augmentation strategies, 516, 541
Autism spectrum disorder, 473–475, 503f
 attachment in, 420–421
 in children and adolescents, 473–475
 diagnostic and clinical features of, 473–474
 differential diagnosis of, 474
  vs. schizophrenia, 111, 474, 502, 503f

 etiology of, 474–475
 in infants, 425
 treatment and prognosis in, 475
Automatic thoughts, 90
 negative, in anxiety disorders, 193
Autonomous self, in preschoolers, 432–433
Autonomy
 in adolescents, 441, 442, 443, 446b, 463
 in elderly, 452
 fear of, in cluster C personality disorders, 260t, 268
 in latency-age child, 440b
 in preschoolers, 432–433
 in relationships, adult, 448
 in toddlers, 421t, 425b, 427, 430t, 431b
 involuntary commitment *vs.*, 126
Avoidance behavior, 11t
 in agoraphobia, 171, 283
 in anorexia nervosa, 294, 301, 304b
 in anxiety disorders, 168, 169, 169b
 in binge-eating disorder, 321
 in cluster C personality disorders, 259, 260t
 in illness anxiety disorder, 328
 in panic disorder, 170
 in phobia, 11t, 170
 in posttraumatic stress disorder, 179
 in social anxiety disorder, 172, 184
 in specific phobia, 172, 173
Avoidant attachment, 421
Avoidant personality disorder
 course of illness in, 273
 diagnostic and clinical features in, 268, 268b
 interview in, 273–282, 279t
Avoidant/restrictive food intake disorder
 diagnostic and clinical features of, 492
 differential diagnosis of, 493
 etiology, treatment and prognosis in, 493–494
Avolition, in schizophrenia, 102, 102t
Awareness, cognitive, 449
 in adults, 449

Barbiturates
 for alcohol and sedative detoxification, 249–250
 anxiety disorder from withdrawal from, 177
 paradoxical reactions from, 178
Basal ganglia, 154, 199, 304b, 479
Basic rules, 557
Basic trust, 420, 421t, 425b
Beck, Aaron T., 589

Behavioral analysis, in dialectical behavior therapy, 594
Behavioral contract, for regression, 354–355
Behavioral dyscontrol, 592
Behavior therapy, 585–589, 586t. *See also* Cognitive-behavioral therapies (CBT)
    for anorexia nervosa, 317–318
    case example of, 587b
    dialectical (*See* Dialectical behavior therapy (DBT))
    for enuresis, 496
    indications and selection criteria for, 587
    for intellectual disability, 470
    origins and theory of, 585
    for sexual disorders, 450
    for substance-related disorders, 248
    therapeutic process in, 587–589
Benzodiazepine receptors, anxiety and, 190
Benzodiazepines, 545–549, 547t. *See also specific types*
    addiction and dependency with, 546
    for alcohol and sedative detoxification, 249–250
    for anxiety
        as in reaction to medical conditions, 356–357
        in neurocognitive disorders, 165
    for anxiety disorders, 194–195
        generalized anxiety disorder, 201
        panic disorder, 197
    for bipolar disorder, 89
    for children and adolescents, 511
    for conversion disorder, 347
    for depression, 87
    dosing of, 547t, 548–549
    history of, 545
    mechanism of action of, 545, 546f
    paradoxical reactions from, 178
    pretreatment evaluation for, 546–548
    selection of, 548
    side effects of, 547t, 549
    for suicide risk, 400
    tolerance to, 548
    withdrawal from, anxiety disorder from, 177
Benztropine mesylate, for Parkinson's, 528
Bereavement, normal, 74–75
β-carbolines, in anxiety, 190–191
Binge-eating disorder. *See also* Feeding and eating disorders
    biology of reward in, 299–300, 302b–303b
    differential diagnosis of, 309–310

    epidemiology and course of, 298–304, 305
        age of onset in, 298–299
        incidence and prevalence in, 298
        long-term course in, 305
        morbidity and mortality in, 299–301
    etiology of, 316
        amplifying or maintaining factors in, 311, 311f
        biological theories in, 311–314
        cultural factors in, 314–316
        precipitating factors in, 310–311, 311f
        predisposing factors in, 310, 311f
        psychosocial theories in, 314
    interview in, 308–309
    treatment of, 321
Binge eating, in bulimia nervosa, 294. *See also* Bulimia nervosa
Biofeedback, 588
Biological factors, in treatment plan, 20
Biopsychosocial approach, 20
Biopsychosocial model, for mood disorders, 79–85. *See also* Mood disorders, etiology of
Bipolar disorder, 47
    bipolar I, 47, 54–55, 55f
    bipolar II, 55, 55f
    catatonic features in, 62–63
    in children and adolescents, 480–481, 483f
    classification of, 47, 48f
    course of illness in, 67f, 68–69, 68b
    cycle length and episode number in, 66, 66f
    cycling in, 67, 67f, 68–69, 68b
        rapid, 61–62, 66–67, 68, 68b
    diagnostic and clinical features of, 54–55, 55f, 68–69, 68b
    differential diagnosis of
        alcohol withdrawal, 142
        schizophrenia, 111
    due to another medical condition, 136
    in elderly, 64
    epidemiology of, 64–66, 65t
    interview in, 72–74, 73b, 74b
    mixed features in, 62
    recurrence of, 68
        natural history of, 67, 67f
    seasonal pattern of, 61, 61b
    substance use disorder with, 233
    symptoms of, 47
    treatment of, 93–94
        depression in, 87–88
        mood-stabilizing medication in, 88–89
        objection to, 72

Bizarre behavior, in schizophrenia, 103
Blackouts, from alcohol use, 210
Bleuler, Eugene, 99b
Blocking, 11t
Blood pressure
    antipsychotic agents on, 525
    MAOIs on, 539
Blunted affect, 11t
    in schizophrenia, 101–102, 102t
Body dysmorphic disorder
    vs. anorexia nervosa, 341
    case example of, 330b
    course of illness in, 334–336, 335t
    diagnostic and clinical features of, 325t,
        329–330
    differential diagnosis of, 340–341, 340t
    etiology of, 345
    medical evaluation of, 342
    treatment of, 348
Body integrity identity disorder, 341
Borderline personality disorder
    course of illness in, 272
    diagnostic and clinical features in, 264–265,
        265b
    with factitious disorder, 345–346
    interview in, 273–282, 279t
    treatment of
        dialectical behavior therapy in, 594, 595b
        mentalization based treatment in, 287,
            566t–567t, 582–585
        transference focused psychotherapy in,
            581b–582b
Bowel retraining, 496
Bowlby, 419t, 424t, 430t, 432t
Brain-derived neurotrophic factor, in depression,
    81
Brain infarctions, neurocognitive disorders from,
    154
Brain injury, anoxic, personality change from,
    136–137, 137b
Brain tumor, 36, 101, 105, 142, 153, 159, 283,
    340t, 412
Brief psychodynamic psychotherapy, 566t–567t,
    568–570
    case example of, 568b–569b
    indications and selection criteria in, 569
    vs. psychoanalysis, 572
    theory and method in, 568–569
    therapeutic process in, 570
Brief psychotic disorder. See also Psychotic
    disorders

case example of, 105b
diagnostic and clinical features of, 97, 105
epidemiology of, 98t
vs. mood disorder, 77
pharmacotherapy for acute episodes of,
    118–119
Bright lights, 61
Broadband rating scales, 466b
Bromocriptine, for Parkinson's, 528
Bulimia nervosa. See also Feeding and eating
    disorders
    with anorexia nervosa, 299, 301b
    case example of, 295b–296b
    diagnostic and clinical features of, 294–297
    differential diagnosis of, 309–310
    epidemiology and course of, 298–304
        age of onset in, 298–299
        incidence and prevalence in, 298
        long-term course in, 305
        morbidity and mortality in, 299–301
    etiology of, 316
        amplifying or maintaining factors in, 311,
            311f
        biological theories in, 311–314
        cultural factors in, 314–316
        precipitating factors in, 310–311, 311f
        predisposing factors in, 310, 311f
        psychosocial theories in, 314
    interview in, 308–309
    screening questions for, 38b
    signs and symptoms of, 300t
    treatment of, 319–321
        cognitive-behavior therapy in, 320
        overview of, 319
        pharmacotherapy in, 320–321
        psychotherapy in, 319–320
Buprenorphine
    for opioid use disorder, 252, 551f, 552–553
    for opioid detoxification, 252
Bupropion, 536t. See also Antidepressant agents
    for adolescents, 509
    for bipolar depression, 87
    for depression in reaction to medical illness,
        360
    side effects of, 537
    for smoking cessation, 253
    for substance-related disorders, 551, 551f
Buspirone, 549, 550t
    for anxiety, 165
Butyrophenones, 517t. See also Antipsychotic
    agents

Caffeinism, 176
  anxiety disorder from, 176, 176b
  case example of, 176b
CAGE screening instrument, 225, 225t
Calcium channel blockers, 158
Candidate gene, 83, 114
  association studies, 189
Cannabis use disorder
  diagnostic and clinical features of, 213–214,
    214t
  treatment of, pharmacologic, 253
  withdrawal from, 214, 214t
Carbamazepine, 544–545
  for bipolar disorder, as prevention, 89
  for chronic pain, 382
Carbohydrate-deficient transferrin (CDT), in
    alcohol use disorder, 236
Cardiovascular disease, depression from, 158
Caretaking relationships, in infant development,
    423, 426b
Case summary, 16b, 19
Case write-up, 1–2, 2f, 3t, 12, 13b–18b
Cataplexy, in bipolar disorder and major depres-
    sive disorder, 62
Catatonia
  in bipolar disorder and major depressive disor-
    der, 50t, 62–63
  in neuroleptic malignant syndrome, 63
  in schizophrenia, 99b, 103
Cerebrovascular disease, 64, 105
Charcot, Jean Martin, 559b
Chief complaint, 2–4
  for identical problems, different, 2–4, 4b
  misleading, 2, 3b
  write-up of, 13b
Child abuse, in Munchausen's syndrome by
    proxy, 333–334
Child and adolescent disorders, 468–511. See also
    specific disorders
  DSM-5 classification of, 468–469
  epidemiology of, 486t–487t
  externalizing disorders, 496–501
    attention-deficit hyperactivity disorder,
      483f, 496–499
    conduct disorder, 499–501
    differential diagnosis of, 500–501
    oppositional defiant disorder, 499
  internalizing disorders, 480–496
    anxiety, obsessive-compulsive, and stress
      disorders, 485–489
    bipolar disorder, 480–481, 483f

disruptive mood dysregulation disorder,
    481–483, 483f
  elimination disorders, 494–496
  feeding and eating disorders of childhood,
    491–494
  major depressive disorder, 483–485
  mood disorder, 78–79
motor disorders, 478
neurodevelopmental disorders, 469–477
  autism spectrum disorder, 473–475, 502,
    503f
  communication disorders, 471–472
  intellectual disability, 469–471
  specific learning disorders, 475–477
personality disorders, 504–505
schizophrenia, 501–504
somatic symptom and related disorders,
    489–491
tic disorders, 478–480
treatment of, pharmacotherapy, 508–511
  antipsychotics in, 510
  benzodiazepines in, 511
  bupropion in, 509
  fundamentals of, 508
  mood stabilizers in, 510
  selective serotonin reuptake inhibitors in,
    508–509
  serotonin-norepinephrine reuptake inhibi-
    tors in, 509
  stimulants in, 509–510
  tricyclic antidepressants in, 509
treatment of, psychosocial, 505–508
  cognitive-behavioral therapy in, 506–507
  interpersonal therapy in, 507–508
  psychodynamic psychotherapy in, 508
  working with parents in, 505–506
unwanted, 448–449
Child and adolescent psychiatry, 456–468
  assessment in
    psychiatric, 456
    psychological, 468
  case examples of
    collateral information in, 458, 458b
    drawing and storytelling in, 462, 462b
    observing child-parent interactions in, 460,
      461b
    rating scales in, 465, 466b, 467b
  interview in, 457–465
    of adolescent, 463
    of child, 460–462, 461b, 462b
    collateral information in, 458, 458b

Child and adolescent psychiatry (*Cont.*)
    components of, 457, 457t
    fundamentals of, 457–458
    mental status examination in, 463,
      464b–465b
    multiple evaluation sessions in, 458, 459f
    with parents, 458–460, 459f
    with parents and child, 462
    rating scales in, 463–465, 466b, 467b
    medical evaluation in, 465–468
      fundamentals of, 465–466
      laboratory testing in, baseline, 466–467
      laboratory testing in, special, 467–468
      psychological assessment in, 468
Child Behavior Checklist, 466b
Child development, 420–447. *See also specific stages*
    in adolescence, 441–447, 443t
    infancy, 420–427, 424t
    preschool, 432–435, 432t
    school-age, 435–441, 436t
    toddler, 427–432, 430t
Childhood-onset fluency disorder, 472
Child's response to physical illness
    in adolescents, 446b–447b
    in latency-age child, 440b
    parents of infants in, 426b
    in preschooler, 436b
    in toddler, 431b
Chlordiazepoxide, 547t. *See also* Benzodiazepines
Chlorpromazine, 516, 517t. *See also* Antipsychotic
    agents
Cholecystokinin, in eating disorders, 314
Cholestatic jaundice, from antipsychotic agents,
    525–526
Chronic depressive disorder, 53–54
Chronic illness, psychosocial aspects of, 371–377
    case example of, 372b–373b
    clinical features of, 371–374
    interview in, 374–377
    management of, 377
    primary and secondary gain in, 375b–376b
Chronic mental illness. *See also specific types*
    public mental health system and, 124b
Chronic pain. *See* Pain, chronic
Chronobiological theories, for mood disorders, 82
Circumstantial thought process, 11t
Citalopram, 531t. *See also* Selective serotonin
    reuptake inhibitors (SSRIs)
Clang associations
    in mania, 56
    in schizophrenia, 103

Clarification
    in psychoanalysis, 573, 574b
    in personality disorders interview, 275–276,
      275b–276b
Classical conditioning, 585
    in anxiety disorders, 193
Clinical Institute Withdrawal of Alcohol Scale,
    210, 211t–213t
Clinical Opiate Withdrawal Scale, 216–217,
    217t–218t
Clock test, 151b
Clomipramine, 534t, 535. *See also* Tricyclic anti-
    depressants (TCAs)
    for obsessive-compulsive disorder, 199, 489,
      508
Clonazepam, 545–549, 547t. *See also*
    Benzodiazepines
Clonidine
    for attention-deficit hyperactivity disorder, 498
    for opioid detoxification, 252
Clorazepate, 547t. *See also* Benzodiazepines
Closed-ended questions, 29b
Clozapine, 516, 517t. *See also* Antipsychotic
    agents
    agranulocytosis from, 526
    for schizophrenia, 118
    for suicide risk, 400
Clubhouse programs, 125
Cluster A personality disorders. *See also*
    Personality disorders
    course of illness in, 271
    diagnostic and clinical features in, 260t,
      261–263
      paranoid, 262, 262b
      schizoid, 262, 263b
      schizotypal, 263, 263b
      shared features in, 261–262
    interview in, 273–282, 279t
Cluster B personality disorders. *See also*
    Personality disorders
    course of illness in, 271–273
      antisocial, 272–273
      borderline, 272
      histrionic, 271–272
      key features in, 271
      narcissistic, 272
    diagnostic and clinical features in, 260t,
      263–267
      antisocial, 266–267, 267b
      borderline, 264–265, 265b
      histrionic, 265, 266b

narcissistic, 265–266, 267b
   shared features in, 263–264
   interview in, 273–282, 279t
Cluster C personality disorders. *See also*
      Personality disorders
   course of illness in, 273
   diagnostic and clinical features in, 260t,
      268–270
      avoidant, 268, 268b
      dependent, 268–269, 269b
      key features in, 268
      obsessive-compulsive, 269, 270b
   interview in, 273–282, 279t
Cocaine use disorder
   anxiety disorder from, 176
   course of illness in, 221–223
   diagnostic and clinical features of, 214–216,
      215t
   epidemiology of, 205b–206b
   life-threatening effects of, 216
   pharmacotherapy for, 252
   psychosis from, 155
   withdrawal from, 215–216, 215t
Cognition
   in mental status testing, 150b
   mood and, 47
Cognitive development, 433–434
   stages of, 430t, 432t, 436t, 443t
Cognitive-behavioral therapies (CBT), 585–596.
      See also specific types and disorders
   for anxiety disorders, 589
      acute stress disorder, 195–197
      agoraphobia, 197–198
      in children and adolescents, 489
      cognitive-behavioral psychotherapy in,
         195–197
      panic disorder, 197–198
      principles of, 195–197
      social anxiety disorder, 198–199
      specific phobias, 202
      stress disorders, 195–197
   behavior therapy in, 585–589, 586t
   for body dysmorphic disorder, 348
   for bulimia nervosa, 320
   case example of, 593b
   for children and adolescents, 506–507
   dialectical behavior therapy in, 586t, 592–596
   for dysthymia, 589
   for illness anxiety disorder, 347–348
   indications and selection criteria in, 589
   for major depressive disorder

   in adults, 589
   in children and adolescents, 484–485
   for neurocognitive disorders, 160–161, 160b,
      161b
   for obsessive-compulsive disorder, 199–200
   origins and theory of, 589
   for personality disorders, 287–288
   for posttraumatic stress disorder, 200–201
   research on, 589, 590b–591b
   for schizophrenia, 122
   for somatic symptom disorder, 347
   for substance-related disorders, 247–248
   therapeutic process in, 589, 592
Cognitive deficits
   alcohol-induced, 210
   in major depression, 52
   in major neurocognitive disorder, 130
Cognitive development, Piaget's stages of, 419t,
      422, 423t
Cognitive distortions, in anxiety disorders, 193
Cognitive enhancers, for dementia, 164
Cognitive remediation (CR), for schizophrenia,
      123
Cognitive restructuring techniques, for anxiety
      disorders, 196–197
Cognitive theory, of mood disorders, 84
Cognitive therapy, for mood disorders, 90, 91b
Columbia Suicide Severity Rating Scale
      (C-SSRS), 389b, 391
Commitment, involuntary
   for schizophrenia, 126
   for suicide risk, 401
   for violence, 416
Communication. *See also* Interview, psychiatric;
      Language
   in mania, 72
   patient
      nonverbal, 26
      verbal, 26
Communication analysis, in interpersonal
      therapy, 598
Communication disorders
   childhood-onset fluency disorder, 472
   differential diagnosis of
      vs. autism spectrum disorder, 474
      vs. schizophrenia, 111
   in infants, 425
   language disorder, 471
   in preschoolers, 435
   in school-age child, 440
   social (pragmatic) communication disorder, 472

Community reinforcement and family training (CRAFT), 248
Competence in school-age children, acquiring, 435–437
Complaint, chief, 2–4, 3b, 4b
    for identical problems, different, 2–4, 4b
    misleading, 2, 3b
    write-up of, 13b
Compulsion
    definition of, 178
    repetition, 565
Concentration deficits, in delirium, 130
Conditioned responses, 585
Conditioning
    classical, 585
        in anxiety disorders, 193
    operant, 585
    for substance-related disorders, 248
Conduct disorder, 499–501
Confidentiality
    right to, 561b
    in suicide risk, 401
    with violent patients, 416–417
Conflict, unconscious, 563
Confrontation
    in bipolar disorder, 73, 74b
    in brief dynamic psychotherapy, 568
    in crisis intervention, 606
    of denial, 356
    for factitious disorder, 339, 339b
    in mania, 73, 74b
    in psychoanalysis, 559t, 567t, 575, 576, 579, 579b
    in schizophrenia, 108
    in substance use disorder, 223, 247
    in supportive psychotherapy, 607
Confusion
    in delirium, 130
    in major depression, 52
Congregate supportive housing, 125
Conscience, in preschoolers, 433
Consciousness levels
    fluctuating, in delirium, 130
    mental status testing for, 148b (See also Mental status examination)
Constipation, childhood, 496
Constricted affect, 11t
Constricted emotional range, 47
Consultation team, in dialectical behavior therapy, 596
Controlled personality traits, 363–364, 364b

Conversion disorder
    case examples of
        with inconsistent sensory nerve distribution, 327, 327b
        with underlying emotional conflict, 326, 327b
    in children and adolescents, 489–491
    course of illness in, 334–336, 335t
    diagnostic and clinical features of, 325t, 326–328
    differential diagnosis of, 340–341, 340t
    etiology of, 344–345
    interview in, 337–338, 337b, 338b
    treatment of, 347
Co-occurring disorders, 232
Coping skills, for anxiety disorders, 196
Coping styles, in school-age children, 437
Coprolalia, 479
Copropraxia, 479
Corrective emotional experience, 563
Corticostriatal circuit, in obsessive-compulsive disorder, 199
Cortisol, 81, 191, 200, 300t
Corticotropin-releasing hormone, in eating disorders, 313
Cotard's syndrome, 59
Countertransference, 562–563
Coup-contra-coup lesions, 156
Couple therapy, 602
Crack cocaine, psychosis from, 156
Creutzfeldt-Jakob disease, neurocognitive disorder from, 131t, 135, 155
Crisis intervention, 605–606
    for schizophrenia, 126
    for suicide risk, 398
    for violence, 413
Cultural formulation, 20
Culture, 8, 41b–42b, 240–241, 316, 344, 397, 413, 444
    definition of, 41b
    in interview, 40, 42b–43b
Cycling
    in bipolar disorder, 67, 67f, 68–69, 68b
    length of, and episode number, in mood disorders, 66, 66f
    rapid, 61
        in bipolar disorder, 61–62, 66–67, 68, 68b
    ultrafast, 62
Cyclothymia, 55, 58. See also Bipolar disorder
Cytokines, proinflammatory, in major depression, 80

Day residue, 575
Decentering, in toddler development, 428
Defectiveness, 50
Defense analysis, 574
Defense mechanisms, 563, 564b–565b
Deinstitutionalization, for schizophrenia, 124b
Delayed discounting, 240
Delirium, 110
    case example of, 113, 113b, 132b
    course of, 130, 132t, 134–135
    diagnostic and clinical features of, 130
    epidemiology of, 132t
    etiology of, 152–153
    iatrogenic, 144
    life-threatening
        case example of, 133b
        symptoms of, 132t
    manic, 56–57
    medication-induced, 153
    vs. neurocognitive disorder, 142
    reticular activating system in, 152–153
Delirium tremens (DTs), 210
Delusional disorder. See also Psychotic
        disorders
    diagnostic and clinical features of, 97, 105
    epidemiology of, 98t
    vs. mood disorder, 77
    pharmacotherapy for acute episodes of,
        118–119
Delusions
    in alcohol-induced psychotic disorder, 210
    case examples of, 99, 100b
    definition of, 11t, 98
    in depressive episodes, 59
    grandiose (See Grandiosity)
    in major depression, 70, 70b
        nihilistic, 59
    persecutory, 59
    in psychotic disorders, 97
    in schizophrenia, 97, 98–101, 100t
        case examples of, 99, 100b
    screening questions for, 36b–37b
    from stimulant use, 215
    from substance use, 156
Dementia, 75. See also Alzheimer's dis-
        ease; Neurocognitive disorders;
        Pseudodementia
    alcohol-induced, 210
    cognitive enhancers for, 164
    from inhalant use, 220
    underlying, 360

Dementia praecox, 99b
Demoralization, 54
    in bipolar disorder, 69
Denial, 564b
    acting out in, 564b
    of anger, 584
    case example of, 355b
    in reaction to medical illness, 355–356,
        355b
Dependence. See also Substance-related and
        addictive disorders; specific substances
    with benzodiazepines, 546
    fearful, 584
    physical, 207–209, 208b
Dependent personality disorder
    course of illness in, 273
    diagnostic and clinical features in, 268–269,
        269b
    interview in, 273–282, 279t
Dependent personality traits, 363
Depersonalization, 12t
    in hallucinogen use, 218
Depressed mood, 48
Depression. See also Major depression
    in bipolar disorder, 54–55
    chronic, 53–54
    from chronic illness, 371–377 (See also Chronic
        illness, psychosocial aspects of)
    in cyclothymia, 55
    double, 54
    due to another medical condition, 136, 136b
        alcohol withdrawal, 210
        anabolic-androgenic steroid withdrawal,
            219
        herbs, 158
        Huntington's disease, 157
        hyperthyroidism, 157
        hypothyroidism, 157
        Parkinson's disease, 157
        prescription drugs, 158
        stroke, 157
        substance use, 210
    in major neurocognitive disorder, 134
    masked, 51
    mild, 54
    psychotic features in, 59
    in reaction to medical illness, 358–360,
        359b
    screening questions for, 36b
    unipolar, 54
    vascular, 64

Depression with atypical features, 59

Depressive disorders, 47

  classification of, 47, 48f

  differential diagnosis of

    vs. alcohol withdrawal, 210

    in bipolar disorder, 54–55

    vs. pseudodementia, 75, 142–144, 144b

    Wilson's disease in, 142, 143b

  from obstructive sleep apnea, 147, 148b

  substance use disorder with, 233

  suicide risk in, 396

Depressive personality, 54

Derealization, 12t

  in hallucinogen use, 218

Desensitization, systematic, 588

Desipramine, 534t. *See also* Tricyclic antidepressants (TCAs)

Desvenlafaxine, 536t. *See also* Antidepressant agents

  for depression, 535, 536t

Detoxification units, 245

Devaluation, 564b

Development, 418–454. *See also specific stages*

  in adolescents, 441–445, 443t

  in adulthood, 445–451

  approach to study of, 418

  in infancy, 420–427, 424t

  in old age, 451–454

  patterns of, 418–419

  in preschool child, 432–435, 432t

  in school-age child, 435–441, 436t

  stress and trauma on, 420

  temperament in, 419

  theories of, 419t

  toddler, 427–432, 430t

Developmental coordination disorder, 478

Developmental delay, 469

Developmental delay, global, 469

Dexamethasone suppression test (DST), 81

Dialectical behavior therapy (DBT), 288, 586t, 592–596

  for borderline personality disorder, 594, 595b

  for bulimia nervosa, 320

  case example of, 595b

  indications and selection criteria in, 593b

  origins and theory of, 592–594

  research on, 591b

  therapeutic process in

    consultation team in, 596

    fundamentals of, 594

    group therapy in, 594

    individual therapy in, 594–596

    telephone consultation in, 596

Diary card, 594

Diazepam, 545–549, 547t. *See also* Benzodiazepines

Diet pills, anxiety disorder from, 176

Differential diagnosis, 16b, 19–20

Difficult-to-engage patient, interview of, 33, 33b–35b

DiGeorge's syndrome, schizophrenia with, 114

Dimethyl-tryptamine (DMT) use

  diagnostic and clinical features of, 217–219, 218t, 219t

  epidemiology of, 207b

Diphenhydramine

  delirium from, 144

  for dystonia, acute, 523

  for Parkinson's, 528

Diphenylbutylpiperidine, 517t. *See also* Antipsychotic agents

Disinhibition

  from brain lesion or trauma, 159

  in major neurocognitive disorder, 134

  in mental disorders due to another medical condition, 136

Disorganized attachment, 427, 427b

Disorganized patient, interview of, 32–33

Disorganized thought, in mania, 56

Disorientation, 149b

  in delirium, 56, 130

  in neurocognitive disorder, 135

Disrupted attention, 592

Disruptive mood dysregulation disorder, 481–483, 483f

Dissociation, 564b

Disulfiram, for alcohol use disorder, 248, 249, 551, 551f

Diurnal variation, in major depression, 53

Divalproex sodium, 544–545

Dopamine

  in antipsychotic mechanism of action, 520f

  in eating disorders, 313

  in fear conditioning, 191

  in schizophrenia, 115–116, 115f

  in substance use, 239

Dopamine agonists, for Parkinson's, 528

Double depression, 54

Doxepine, 534t. *See also* Tricyclic antidepressants (TCAs)

Drawing, in child interview, 461

Dream analysis, 575

Drug Abuse Screening Test (DAST), 225
Dual uptake inhibitors, 535–537, 536t
Duloxetine, 536t. *See also* Antidepressant agents
   for chronic pain, 382
   for depression, 535–537, 536t
   for pain syndromes, 535
Duty to protect, 416–417
Duty to warn, 416–417
Dyslexia, 475–477
Dysphoric mania, 62
Dysthymic disorder
   in children and adolescents, 484
   diagnostic and clinical features of, 53–54
   treatment of
      cognitive-behavioral therapy in, 589
      interpersonal psychotherapy in, 598
Dystonia
   from antipsychotic agents, 510, 519, 522–524
   diphenhydramine for, 528
   propranolol for, 528
   from stimulants, 215t

Early-morning awakening, in major depression, 52, 58
Eating disorders. *See* Feeding and eating disorders
Echolalia
   in bipolar disorder and major depressive disorder, 62
   definition of, 62
   in schizophrenia, 103
Echopraxia
   in bipolar disorder and major depressive disorder, 62
   definition of, 62
   in schizophrenia, 103
Ecstasy use, 217–219, 219t
Ego, 573
Ego deficits, supportive psychotherapy for, 607
Egodystonic, 5, 11t
Egosyntonic, 5, 11t, 281b, 306
Ejaculation
   delay in, from tricyclic antidepressants, 535, 544
   premature, 450
Elderly
   response to physical illness in, 451b
   substance use in, 232
Elderly development, 451–454
   case examples of
      poor adjustment, 454b
      response to aging, 453b

progression of, 451–453
   changing relationships in, 451–452
   gradual decline in, 452
   sexuality in, 452–453
   psychopathology in, 454
   vulnerabilities in, 453
Electrocardiogram (ECG), 187, 188b, 300t, 310, 317, 468, 509, 535, 553
Electroconvulsive therapy (ECT), 553–554
   for depression, 89
   for mania, 89
   for suicide risk, 400
Electroencephalogram (EEG), 113, 144–147, 468, 497, 554
Elimination disorders, child and adolescent, 494–496
   diagnostic and clinical features of
      encopresis, 495
      enuresis, 494–495
   differential diagnosis of
      encopresis, 495
      enuresis, 495
   etiology, treatment, and prognosis in
      encopresis, 496
      enuresis, 495–496
Emergency services, for schizophrenia, 126
Emotional experience, corrective, 563
Emotional history, interview for, 40
Emotional intensity, 563
   high, 568
Emotional maturity
   in adolescents, 442
   in adults, 449
Emotional range, constricted, 47
Emotional regulation, in dialectical behavior therapy, 594
Emotional resistance, 515
Emotional responses, physician, 26, 27b
Emotional status quo, 574
Emotions, 47
Empathic listening, 23, 26
Encephalopathy, alcohol-induced, 210
Encopresis
   diagnostic and clinical features of, 495
   differential diagnosis of, 495
   etiology, treatment, and prognosis in, 496
Energy
   goal-directed
      in hypomania, 57
      in mania, 55
      increased, in mania, 56

Enuresis
diagnostic and clinical features of, 494–495
differential diagnosis of, 495
etiology, treatment, and prognosis in, 495–496
Enuresis alarm system, 496
Environment
holding, 606
in personality disorders, 284–286
in schizophrenia, 116–117
Erikson's stages of psychosocial development, 419t, 420, 421t
Escitalopram, 531t. *See also* Selective serotonin reuptake inhibitors (SSRIs)
for children and adolescents, 508
Estazolam, 547t. *See also* Benzodiazepines
Eszopiclone, 550t
Ethics, in psychotherapy, 561b
Euphoria, abnormal
in mania, 55, 59–60
from steroid use, 219
Euphoric mood, 11t
Euthymia, 48
Exaggeration, in cognitive-behavioral therapy, 593b
Expansive mood, 11t
Exposure therapy, for anxiety disorders, 196
Exposure with response prevention, for bulimia nervosa, 320
Externalizing disorders, child and adolescent, 496–501
attention-deficit hyperactivity disorder, 483f, 496–499
conduct disorder, 499–501
differential diagnosis of, 500–501
oppositional defiant disorder, 499
Extrapyramidal symptoms, of antipsychotic agents, 522–524

Factitious disorder
with borderline personality disorder, 345–346
course of illness in, 335t, 336
diagnostic and clinical features of, 330–333, 331t
ambiguous physical symptoms in, 324–325
classification of, 323–324, 324f, 324t
differential diagnosis of, 339b, 341
etiology of, 345–346
fundamentals of, 323
interview in, 39b, 338–339, 341, 341b
medical evaluation of, 342–343

with predominantly physical signs and symptoms, 331–332, 332b
with predominantly psychological signs and symptoms, 332–333
multiple symptoms in, 333b
preexisting psychiatric disorders in, 334b
treatment of, 348–349
virtual, 334
Factitious disorder imposed on another
diagnostic and clinical features of, 333–334
government agency notification in, 348
Family history, 9, 15b. *See also specific disorders*
interview for, 40, 43
Family therapy, 597t, 598–602, 600b–602b
case example of
psychodynamic approach, 602b
systems approach, 599, 600b–601b
for conduct disorder, 501
couple therapy in, 602
for neurocognitive disorders, 161–163, 162b, 163b
psychodynamic approach in, 599–602
research on, 591b
for schizophrenia, 122
structural, 162–163, 162b
for suicide risk, 400
systems approach in, 598–599
Fatigue, in depression, 60
Fear. *See also* Anxiety disorders
conditioned responses to, in anxiety disorders, 192
hierarchy of, 588
in toddlers, 429–430
Fear and avoidance hierarchy, 196
Fear conditioning, dopamine in, 191
Fear learning, 192
Feeding and eating disorders, 291–321
addiction model of, 321
comorbidities of
anorexia nervosa and bulimia nervosa, 299, 301b
anxiety disorders, 299
depression, 299
obsessive-compulsive disorder, 299
personality disorders, 300–301
substance use disorders, 299–300
diagnostic and clinical features of, 291–298
anorexia nervosa, 292–294, 293b–294b
binge-eating disorder, 297
bulimia nervosa, 294–297, 295b–296b
core shared features in, 291–292

night eating syndrome, 297–298
other specified feeding or eating disorders, 297
purging disorder, 297
differential diagnosis of
anorexia nervosa, 309
bulimia nervosa and binge-eating disorder, 309–310
epidemiology and course of, 298–304
age of onset in, 298–299
incidence and prevalence in, 298
long-term course, anorexia nervosa, 301–304
long-term course, bulimia nervosa, 305
morbidity and mortality in, 299–301
etiology of, 310–317
amplifying or maintaining factors in, 311, 311f
in anorexia nervosa, 301, 304b, 316
in binge-eating disorder, 299–300, 302b–303b
biological theories in, 311–314
biological theories in, gastrointestinal, 313–314
biological theories in, genetic, 312
biological theories in, neuroendocrine, 313
biological theories in, neurotransmitters and neuropeptides, 312–313
in bulimia nervosa and binge-eating disorder, 316
cultural factors in, 314–316
precipitating factors in, 310–311, 311f
predisposing factors in, 310, 311f
psychosocial theories in, 314
historical perspective on, 315b
interview in, 305–309
in anorexia nervosa, 306–308
in bulimia nervosa and binge-eating disorder, 308–309
fundamentals of, 305–306
guidelines for, 307b
medical evaluation in, 310
presenting complaints in, 306b
screening questions for, 38b
signs and symptoms of, 300t
sleep-related, 298
treatment of, 317–321
anorexia nervosa, 317–319
binge-eating disorder, 321
bulimia nervosa, 319–321
types of, 291

Feeding and eating disorders of childhood, 491–494
diagnostic and clinical features of
avoidant/restrictive food intake disorder, 492
pica, 491–492
rumination disorder, 492
differential diagnosis of
avoidant/restrictive food intake disorder, 493
pica, 492
rumination disorder, 493
etiology, treatment and prognosis in
avoidant/restrictive food intake disorder, 493–494
pica, 493
rumination disorder, 493
Female orgasmic disorder, 450
Fight-or-flight response, 170
First-generation antipsychotic agents (FGAs), 516, 517t
Flashbacks
from hallucinogen use, 219
in posttraumatic stress disorder, 179
Flat affect, 11t
in depression, 51
in factitious disorder, 341
in mental status examination, 10t
in schizophrenia, 101–102, 102t
Flight of ideas, 11t
in mania, 56
Fluency disorder, childhood-onset, 472
Flumazenil, for alcohol and sedative detoxification, 250
Fluoxetine, 531t. See also Selective serotonin reuptake inhibitors (SSRIs)
for children and adolescents, 508
major depressive disorder in, 485
Flurazepam, 547t. See also Benzodiazepines
Fluvoxamine, 531t. See also Selective serotonin reuptake inhibitors (SSRIs)
Fortune telling, in anxiety disorders, 193
Frame, setting, 28–30
Free association, 573
Freud, Sigmund, 419t, 424t, 428, 430t, 432t, 436t, 443t, 559b, 563
Frontal assessment battery, 152, 152b
Frontal lobe lesions, on personality, 159
Frontotemporal lobar degeneration, 131t, 134, 155
Frustration, physician
with bipolar patients, 72–73, 73b
with hypomanic patients, 73–74

Functional neurological symptom disorder, 326
  in children and adolescents, 489–491

GABA, in anxiety disorders, 190
Gabapentin, for chronic pain, 382
Gain
  primary, 375b
  secondary, 375b–376b
γ-glutamyl transpeptidase (GGT/GGTP), in
    alcohol use disorder, 236
Gender
  in adolescents, 443–444
  in preschoolers, 435
  in school-age children, 438
  in toddlers, 429
Gender identity, 429
Generalized anxiety disorder. *See also* Anxiety
    disorders
  case example of, 174b
  diagnostic and clinical features of, 173
    in children and adolescents, 487
  differential diagnosis of, 77, 183, 183t
  etiology of, 201
  screening questions for, 37b
  treatment of, 201
Genetic factors. *See also specific disorders*
  in addiction, 239
  in anxiety disorders, 189–190
  in eating disorders, 312
  in mood disorders, 83–84
  in personality disorders, 285
  in schizophrenia, 114–115, 114t
  in substance-related disorders, 238–239
Geriatric issues, in mood disorders, 64, 88, 165
Gessell, 419t, 424t, 430t, 432t, 436t
Glaucoma, from antipsychotic agents, 526
Global developmental delay, 469
Glutamate
  in anxiety disorders, 191
  in mood disorders, 81
Goal-directed activity
  in hypomania, 57
  in mania, 55
Goals. *See also specific disorders and therapies*
  Patient's, 20
Good psychiatric management (GPM), for
    borderline personality disorder, 288
Grandiosity
  in hypomania, 57
  in mania, 55, 60
  in schizophrenia, 100–101

Gratification, adult
  in love, 448–449
  in work, 445–448, 448b
Grief reaction, 598
Group therapy, 597t, 602–605
  case example of, adolescent, 603b–604b
  in dialectical behavior therapy, 594
  for personality disorders, 288
  purpose of, specific group in, 603–604
  for schizophrenia, 122
  specialized groups in, 604
  supportive groups in, 605
  theory and goal of, 602–603
Guanfacine, for attention-deficit hyperactivity
    disorder, 498
Guilt, 50
  in depressive episodes, 59
  in major depression, 70–71
Gustatory hallucinations, in schizophrenia, 101
Gynecomastia, from antipsychotic agents, 525

Habit reversal training, 480
Hallucinations, 12t
  in alcohol-induced psychotic disorder with hal-
    lucinations or delusions, 210
  in delirium, 130
  in depressive episodes, 59
  in hallucinogen use, 218
  in psychotic disorders, 97
  in schizophrenia
    adult, 97, 100t, 101
    child and adolescent, 503
  sensory-deprivation, 156
  in stimulant use, 215
  substance-induced, 156
Hallucinogen use
  course of illness in, 221–223
  diagnostic and clinical features of, 217–219,
    218t, 219t
  epidemiology of, 207b
  withdrawal from, 219
Haloperidol, 517t. *See also* Antipsychotic agents
  for Tourette's disorder, 480
Harm reduction model, 241–242
Head trauma
  aggression from, 159
  disinhibition from, 159
  major neurocognitive disorder from, 155
  neurocognitive disorder from, 135b
Hearing impairment, 472
Heart block, from tricyclic antidepressants, 535

Helplessness
    in depressive disorders, 51, 70, 71
    in factitious disorder, 338
    in neurocognitive disorders, 138
    in suicide, 396
Hepatic effects, of antipsychotic agents, 525–526
Here and now, 580
Heroin use. *See also* Opioid use disorder
    epidemiology of, 207b
    withdrawal from, anxiety disorder in, 177
Hierarchy of fears, 588
Hippocampus, 80–81, 114, 155, 190–192, 191f,
        200, 240
History, 4–9. *See also specific disorders and treatments*
    family, 9, 15b
    past medical, 6–7, 14b
    past psychiatric, 5, 7b, 14b
    of present illness, 4–5, 6b, 13b
    psychosocial, 7–9, 8b, 9b, 14b–15b
    review of systems in, 7, 14b
History of present illness, 4–5, 6b, 13b
History-taking phase, interview, 32–44
    challenges in, 32–35
        with difficult-to-engage patient, 33, 33b–35b
        with disorganized patient, 32–33
    culture in, 40, 41b–43b
    family history in, 40, 43
    fundamentals of, 32
    mental status examination in, 43–44
    past psychiatric and medical history in, 35–36
    psychosocial history in, 30b, 39–40, 44b
    review of systems in, 36, 36b–39b
Histrionic personality disorder
    course of illness in, 271–272
    diagnostic and clinical features in, 265, 266b
    interview in, 273–282, 279t
Holding environment, 606
Homework assignments, 592
Hopelessness, 50–51
    in depression, 50, 51, 57, 70, 71
    in neurocognitive disorders, 138
    in personality disorders, 77
    in schizophrenia, 396
    in suicide, 63, 390, 394, 395, 399b
Human immunodeficiency virus (HIV) infection
    neurocognitive disorder from, 131t, 155
    psychosocial aspects of, 371–377 (*See also*
        Chronic illness, psychosocial aspects of)
Huntington's disease
    mood disorders from, 156–158
    neurocognitive disorder from, 155

Hydrocephalus, normal-pressure, neurocognitive
        disorder from, 156
5-Hydroxytryptamine transporter-linked
        polymorphic promoter region
        (5-HTTLPR), in mood disorders, 83
Hyperactivity
    in alcohol and sedative withdrawal, 210, 210t
    in attention-deficit hyperactivity disorder, 483f,
        496–499, 497 (*See also* Attention-deficit
        hyperactivity disorder (ADHD))
    in autism spectrum disorders, 473
    in personality disorders, 77
    in psychomotor agitation phase of violence, 404
    in toddlers, 432
Hypersomnia
    in depression, 49t, 52, 59, 60
    from MAOIs, 539
    in pica, 492
    in stimulant withdrawal, 215t
Hypertension
    from MAOIs, 539
    in schizophrenics, 119–120, 127
Hypertensive crisis, from MAOIs, 539
Hyperthyroidism
    anxiety disorder from, 174, 175b
    mood disorders from, 157
Hypnotic agents, 545–550. *See also* Anxiolytics;
        specific agents
Hypochondriasis. *See* Illness anxiety disorder
Hypomania
    anxiety in, 61, 62
    in bipolar disorder, 54–55, 55f, 94 (*See also*
        Bipolar disorder)
    in cyclothymia, 55, 58
    diagnostic and clinical features of, 55f, 57–58
    mild, productive, 73–74
    in mood disorders, 48f, 67f
    in substance use, 77
Hypomanic alert, 58
Hypotension
    in anorexia nervosa, 300t
    from antipsychotic agents, 525
    from beta-receptor antagonists, 415
    from MAOIs, 539
    orthostatic
        from antipsychotic agents, 517t–518t, 521,
            522, 525
        from MAOIs, 538t, 539
        from propranolol, 550t
        from tricyclic antidepressants, 534t, 535
    from prazosin, 200

Hypothalamic–pituitary–adrenal axis (HPA)
in anxiety disorders, 191
dexamethasone suppression test for, 81
in major depression, 80, 82
in substance use disorders, 239
Hypothalamic–pituitary–gonadal axis, in eating
disorders, 313
Hypothyroidism, mood disorders from,
157–158
Hysteria. *See* Conversion disorder
Hysteria, mass, 327

Iatrogenic delirium, 144
Id, 573
Idealization, 564b
of caretakers, 352
Ideas of reference, 11t
Identification, 565
projective, 564b
Identity
in adolescents, consolidation of, 442
gender, 429
Identity diffusion, 580
Idiosyncratic cholestatic jaundice, from
antipsychotic agents, 525–526
Illness anxiety disorder, 328, 329b
case example of, 329b
in children and adolescents, 489–491
course of illness in, 334–336, 335t
diagnostic and clinical features of, 325t, 328
differential diagnosis of, 340–341, 340t
etiology of, 345
interview in, 337–338, 337b, 338b
medical evaluation of, 342
treatment of, 347–348
Illusions, 12t
in alcohol and sedative withdrawal, 210t
in "attenuated psychosis syndrome", 121
in hallucinogen use, 218
in mental status examination, 10t, 464b
in neurocognitive disorders, 130
Imaginative play, in preschoolers, 433
Imipramine, 534t. *See also* Tricyclic
antidepressants (TCAs)
Imminent risk, meaning of, 401
Impressions, 18–20
case summary in, 16b, 19
differential diagnosis in, 16b, 19–20
predisposing and precipitating factors in,
16b–17b, 20
Impulsivity

in attention-deficit hyperactivity disorder, 497
in mania, 57, 57b
in suicide risk, 397
in violence, 412
Inadequacy, 50
Inappropriate affect, 11t
Independence, through groups, in adolescents,
441
Individual psychotherapy
in dialectical behavior therapy, 594–596
for schizophrenia, 122
Infant development, 420–427, 424t
case example of, 425b
progression of, 420–423
affect regulation in, 420–422, 421t
attachment in, 421–422, 422b
object permanence in, 422, 423t
stranger anxiety in, 422–423
vulnerabilities in, 423–427
physical illness and caretaking relationships
in, 423, 426b
psychopathology in, developmental
disorders, 425
psychopathology in, disorganized
attachment, 427, 427b
psychopathology in, parental, 426–427
Infantile sexuality, 429
Inhalant use
diagnostic and clinical features of, 220, 220t
epidemiology of, 207b
Inpatient rehabilitation, for substance-related
disorders and addictions, 245–246
Insight, 565
definition, 10t
impaired, in mania, 56
Insomnia
in alcohol withdrawal, 177, 210t
in anxiety, 169, 183t (*See also* Anxiety
disorders)
in benzodiazepine and barbiturate withdrawal,
177
in depressive disorders, 49t, 52, 58, 69, 358
in dysthymia, 53
in hyperthyroidism, 157
in mania, 56
in mania, dysphoric, 52
from MAOIs, 538t, 539
in nicotine withdrawal, 214t
in night eating syndrome, 297
in opioid withdrawal, 216t
rebound, with benzodiazepines, 549

from SSRIs, 531t
from stimulants, 509–510
in stimulant withdrawal, 215t
in substance use disorder, 234t–235t
in suicide risk, 396
terminal, 546
from tranylcypromine, 539
treatment of
benzodiazepines in, 545–549 (*See also*
Benzodiazepines)
trazodone in, 87
Intellectual disabilities, 469–471
vs. schizophrenia, 111
Intellectualization, 565b
Interleukin -6, in major depression, 80
Internalizing disorders, child and adolescent,
480–496
anxiety, obsessive-compulsive, and stress
disorders, 485–489
bipolar disorder, 480–481, 483f
disruptive mood dysregulation disorder,
481–483, 483f
elimination disorders, 494–496
feeding and eating disorders of childhood,
491–494
major depressive disorder, 483–485
Internal representations, in toddlers, 428–429
Interpersonal and social rhythm therapy
(IPSRT), for bipolar disorder, 93–94
Interpersonal deficit, 598
Interpersonal dispute, 598
Interpersonal inventory, 598
Interpersonal psychotherapy (IPT)
for bulimia nervosa, 320
case example of, 599b
for children and adolescents, 507
indications and selection criteria in, 598
for major depression, 598, 599b
for mood disorders, 90–92
origins and theory of, 596–598
research on, 591b
therapeutic process in, 598
Interpersonal sensitivity, in depression, 59
Interpretation, 574, 574b
repeated, in psychoanalysis, 576
Intersubjectivity, 576
Interviewing, motivational, for substance-related
disorders, 242b, 247
Interview, psychiatric, 22–45. *See also specific
disorders*
conducting, 28–45 (*See also specific phases*)

concluding phase in, 44–45
history-taking phase in, 32–44
preparatory phase in, 28–31
general principles of, 22–28
attention to process in, 26–28, 27b, 29b–30b
empathic listening in, 23, 26
guidelines in, 23b
vs. medical interviews, 22–23
physician emotional responses in, 26, 27b
psychological perspective in, 23, 24b–25b
with personality disorders, 5, 6b
Intoxication, 209. *See also specific substances*
vs. medical condition, 360
Intrapersonal theory, of mood disorders, 84
Involuntary commitment
for schizophrenia, 126
for suicide risk, 401
for violence, 416
Irritability, in mania, 55
Isocarboxazid, 538t. *See also* Monoamine oxidase
inhibitors (MAOIs)
dosing of, 538t, 539
side effects of, 539–540

Jails, schizophrenia patients in, 127
Jaundice, idiosyncratic cholestatic, from antipsy-
chotic agents, 525–526
Joint attention, 420
Judgment, definition, 10t

Kernberg, 282, 580
Ketamine, 106, 237t, 347
for depression, 81
Kindling
in alcohol use, 202
in mood disorders, 82
Kleine Levin, 492
Klein, Melanie, 560b
Klerman, Gerald, 596
Kluver-Bucy syndrome, 492
Kohut, Heinz, 560b
Korsakoff's syndrome, 156
Kraepelin, Emil, 99b

La belle indifference, 327b
Labile affect, 11t
in borderline personality disorder, 279t
from brain lesions, 159
in major neurocognitive disorder, 134
in mental disorders due to another medical
condition, 136

Laboratory tests, 16b, 18. *See also specific disorders*
Lamotrigine, 544–545
  for bipolar depression, 87
  for children and adolescents, 510
Language
  difficulties with, in delirium, 130
  in interview, 31
  symbolic, in toddlers, 428
Language disorder, 471
Latency-age child, 438, 439b, 440b
Latent content, 575
Leaden paralysis, in depression, 59
Learned relaxation, 588
Learning disorders
  in school-age child, 440
  specific, 475–477
Learning, fear, 192
Leptin, in eating disorders, 313
Lethargy
  in anorexia nervosa, 293
  in depression, 60, 360
  in inhalant use, 220t
Leukopenia, 300t, 466, 521
Level of consciousness
  fluctuating, in delirium, 130
  mental status testing for, 148b (*See also* Mental
    status examination)
Lewy body disease
  anticholinesterase inhibitors for, 164
  neurocognitive disorder from, 131t, 134, 154
Libido, 77, 93,145, 532, 539
Light deprivation, in depression, 60–61, 61b
Light therapy, for depression, 61, 61b
Limbic system, 115f, 154, 159, 190, 444
Linkages, in psychoanalysis, 574
Listening, empathic, 23, 26
Lithium (carbonate), 542–544
  for bipolar disorder
    as prevention, 89
    as treatment, 88–89
  for children and adolescents, 510
  for depression, 86
  dosing of, 543
  indications for, 542
  for mania, in neurocognitive disorders, 165
  monitoring of, 89
  pretreatment evaluation for, 542–543
  side effects of, 543–544
  for suicide risk, 400
Liver function tests, 113, 146, 300t, 466, 510, 521,
  553

Locus coeruleus, 190, 191f
Long-suffering personality traits, 365
Long-term psychoanalytic psychotherapy,
  566t–567t, 576–580
  case example of, with personality disorder,
    576b–577b
  indications and selection criteria in, 576
  research on, 591b
  therapeutic process in, 579–580
Loosening of associations, 11t
  in mania, 56
  in schizophrenia, 102–103
Lorazepam, 545–549, 547t. *See also*
    Benzodiazepines
  for anxiety reaction to medical conditions,
    356–357
Love, gratification in, adult, 448–449
Lupus, psychotic disorders from, 135–136, 135b
Lurasidone, 518t. *See also* Antipsychotic agents
  for bipolar depression, 88
Luteinizing hormone, in eating disorders, 313
Lying, pathological, 332
Lysergic acid diethylamide (LSD) use, 217–219,
  219t

Magical thinking, in preschoolers, 433–434
Mahler, Margaret, 427
Major depression. *See also* Depression; Depressive
  disorders
  anger in, 71–72, 71b
  anxiety with, 61
  with atypical features, 59
  catatonic features in, 62–63
  in children and adolescents, 483–485
  course of illness in, 67–68, 67f
  cycle length and episode number in, 66, 66f
  diagnostic and clinical features of, 48–53,
    49b–50b, 67–68
    anhedonia in, 51, 51b
    behavioral signs and symptoms in, 50–53
    DSM-5 criteria in, 49t–50t, 51
    psychological signs and symptoms in,
      48–50, 50b
  diurnal variation in, 53
  eating disorders with, 299
  epidemiology of, 64–66, 65t
  interview in, 69–72, 70b, 71b
  mood reactivity in, 53
  peripartum, 61
  with peripartum onset, 61
  physician responses in, 71–72, 71b

psychotic features in, 59
rating scales for, 53
in reaction to medical conditions, 358–360, 359b
recurrence of, 67, 67f
vs. schizophrenia, 111
seasonal pattern in, 60–61, 61b
specifiers for, melancholic features in, 58
suicidal thoughts in, 63–64, 63b, 71–72, 71f
suicide risk in, 396
treatment of
    cognitive-behavioral therapy in, 589, 593b
    interpersonal psychotherapy in, 598, 599b
    transcranial magnetic stimulation in, 554–555
Major neurocognitive disorder. *See also* Neurocognitive disorders
course of, 132t, 134–135
diagnostic and clinical features of, 130, 133
epidemiology of, 132t
etiology of, 153–156
    Alzheimer's disease in, 154
    frontotemporal lobar degeneration in, 155
    HIV infection in, 155
    Huntington's disease in, 155
    Lewy body disease in, 154
    normal-pressure hydrocephalus in, 156
    Parkinson's disease in, 154
    prion disease in, 155
    thiamine deficiency in, 156
    traumatic brain injury in, 155–156
    vascular disease in, 154
Malingering
diagnostic and clinical features of
    ambiguous physical symptoms in, 324–325
    classification of, 323–324, 324f, 324t
fundamentals of, 323
interview in, 341, 341b
Mania
anxiety in, 61, 62
in bipolar disorder, 54–55, 55t (*See also* Bipolar disorder)
communication in, 72
diagnostic and clinical features of, 55–57, 55f, 57b
dysphoric, 62
manipulation in, 72
mixed features in, 62

in mood disorders, 67f
peripartum, 61
psychotic features in, 59
recurrence of, 67, 67f
vs. schizophrenia, 111
screening questions for, 36b
from SSRIs, 532
from substance use, 156
treatment of, objection to, 72
Manic delirium, 56–57
Manic-depressive illness. *See* Bipolar disorder
Manifest content, 575
Manipulation, in mania, 72
Maprotiline, 536t. *See also* Antidepressant agents
    for depression, 536t, 537
Marijuana use
course of illness in, 221–223
epidemiology of, 205b
panic attack from, 176
Masked depression, 51
Mass hysteria, 327
Mass psychogenic illness, 327
Math skills
impairment in, 475–477
in school-age children, 437–438
Maturity, emotional
in adolescents, 442
in adults, 449
MDMA use, 217–219, 219t
Medical history, past, 6–7, 14b. *See also specific disorders*
interviewing for, 35–36
Medical illness, supportive psychotherapy for, 606–607
Melancholia, 58
Memantine, for Alzheimer's disease, 164
Memory deficits
in neurocognitive disorders, 130, 131t, 133b
in pseudodementia, 142
Memory loss, after ECT, 554
Memory, in major depression, 70
Memory testing
immediate recall, 149b
intermediate, 150b
long-term, 150b
short-term, 149b–150b
Menstrual irregularities
from antipsychotic agents, 525
from eating disorder, 300t
from valproate, 510

Mental disorders due to another medical
    condition, 129–166
  definition of, 129
  diagnostic and clinical features of, 135–137
    anxiety disorders, 136, 137b
    course in, 137
    depressive and bipolar disorders, 136, 136b
    general, 129
    personality change, 136–137, 137b
    psychotic disorders, 135–136, 135b
  differential diagnosis of, 141–145
    alcohol withdrawal, 142
    iatrogenic delirium, 142
    medical history in, 141
    partial complex seizures, 144–145, 145b
    pseudodementia, 142–144, 144b
    specific syndrome and etiology in, 141b, 142
    steps in, 141
    substance-induced disorders, 144
    timeline in, 142
  etiology of, 156–159, 157f
    in anxiety and OCD-related disorders,
      158–159
    in mood disorders, 156–158
    in personality changes, 159
    in psychotic disorders, 156
  interview in, 137–140
    family, 140
    guidelines for, 137–138, 138b
    questions in, 139
    setting in, 139
    therapeutic interventions in, 139–140
  medical evaluation in, 145–152 (See also under
    Neurocognitive disorders)
  preventative measures for, 166
  treatment of, 159–166
    behavior therapy in, 159–161, 160b, 161b
    family therapy in, 161–163, 162b, 163b
    pharmacotherapy in, 163–166
    psychotherapy in, 159
Mental illness. See also specific types
  chronic, public mental health system and, 124b
  stigma of, 46
Mentalization based treatment (MBT), 287,
    566t–567t, 582–585
  indications and selection criteria in, 583
  research on, 591b
  theory and principles of, 582–583
  therapeutic process in, 583–584
Mentalization, capacity for, 582
Mental status examination, 9–12, 10t

  in children and adolescents, 463, 464b–465b
  definitions of findings in, 11t–12t
  in interview, 43–44
  Mini Mental Status Exam, 152, 153b
  recording of, 9, 12, 12t, 15b–16b
Mental status testing, 147–152
  clock test, 151b
  cognitive ability in, 150b
  frontal assessment battery, 152, 152b
  level of consciousness in, 148b
  memory in
    immediate recall, 149b
    intermediate-term, 150b
    long-term, 150b
    short-term, 149b–150b
  Mini Mental Status Exam, 152, 153b
  orientation to time, place, and person in,
    148b–149b
  set word test with word intrusion, 151b
  standardized outcome measures, 152b
Meperidine
  MAOIs and, 540
  withdrawal from, anxiety disorder from, 177
Mescaline use, 217–219, 219t
Methadone
  for opioid use disorder, 250–252
  for opioid detoxification, 252
  for substance-related disorders, 551f, 552
  withdrawal from, anxiety disorder from, 177
Methamphetamine use
  anxiety disorder from, 176
  case study on, evolution of dependence, 208b
  diagnostic and clinical features of, 214–216,
    215t
  epidemiology of, 206b–207b
  life-threatening effects of, 216
  psychosis from, 155
  withdrawal from, 215–216, 215t
Methylphenidate
  for children and adolescents, 509
  for depression in reaction to medical illness, 360
  epidemiology of, 206b
Michigan Alcoholism Screening Test (MAST),
    225
Middle-of-the-night awakening, in major
    depression, 52
Midlife crisis, 450
Mild neurocognitive disorder. See also
    Neurocognitive disorders
  diagnostic and clinical features of, 133–134
  etiology of, 153–156

Milieu response, 85
Mindfulness
    for anxiety disorders, 195
    in group therapy, 594
Mini Mental Status Exam, 152, 153b
Mirtazapine, 536t. *See also* Antidepressant agents
    for depression, 360, 536t, 537
Mitral valve prolapse, in panic disorder, 188
Mixed features, mood episodes with, 62
Modesty, in school-age children, 438, 439b
Monoamine oxidase inhibitors (MAOIs),
        537–539, 538t
    augmentation strategies for, 540
    for bulimia nervosa, 320
    classes of, 537–538, 538t
    for depression, 85–86
    discontinuation of, 540
    dosing of, 538–540, 538t
    drug–drug interactions of, 540
    meperidine and SSRIs with, 540
    placebo effects of, 540–541
    response to, assessment of, 540
    side effects of, 539–540
    for social anxiety disorder, 198
    switch strategies for, 541
    tyramine-free diet for, 540
Mood
    affect and, 47
    constricted emotional range in, 47
    definition of, 46
    vs. emotions, 47
    euphoric, 11t
    expansive, 11t
    features of, 46–48
Mood-congruent psychotic features, 59–60, 60b
Mood disorder due to another medical condition,
        75, 76t
    obstructive sleep apnea, 147, 148b
    substance use, 156–158
Mood disorders, 46–85. *See also specific types*
    affect in, 47
    classification of, 47, 48f
    cognition in, 47
    constricted emotional range in, 47
    course of illness in, 66–69, 66f, 67f
        in bipolar disorder, 67f, 68–69, 68b
        cycling and episode number in, 66–67, 66f,
            67f
        in major depression, 67–68, 67f
    diagnostic and clinical features of, 46–64
        bipolar disorder, 54–55, 55f, 68–69, 68b
    cyclothymia, 55, 58
    fundamentals of, 46–48, 48f
    geriatric issues in, 64
    hypomania, 55f, 57–58
    major depression, 48–53, 49b–50b, 67–68
    mania, 55–57, 55f, 57b
    persistent depressive disorder (dysthymia),
        53–54
    premenstrual dysphoric disorder, 54
    specifiers in, 58–64, 60b, 61b, 63b (*See also
        specific types and disorders*)
    differential diagnosis of, 74–79, 76t
        adjustment disorder with depressed mood,
            75
        bereavement, normal, 74–75
        brief psychotic disorder, 77
        in children and adolescents, 78–79
        delusional disorder, 77
        dementia, 75
        generalized anxiety disorder, 77
        mood disorder due to another medical
            condition, 75, 76t
        panic disorder, 77
        Parkinson's disease, 75
        personality disorders, 77–78
        pseudodementia, 75, 142–144, 144b
        schizoaffective disorder, 76
        schizophrenia, 75–76
        schizophreniform disorder, 77
        sleep apnea, 78
        substance use, 77
    due to another medical condition, 136, 156–158
    emotions in, 47
    epidemiology of, 64–66, 65t
    etiology of, 79–85
        biopsychosocial model in, 79
        neurobiological theories in, 79–84
        neurobiological theories in, chronobiologi-
            cal theories, 82
        neurobiological theories in, genetic factors,
            83–84
        neurobiological theories in, neuroendocrine
            hypotheses, 81
        neurobiological theories in, neurotransmit-
            ter hypotheses, 80–81
        neurobiological theories in, sensitization
            and kindling theory, 82–83
        psychosocial theories in, 84–85
    interview for, 69–74
        in bipolar disorder, 72–74, 73b, 74b
        in depressive disorders, 69–72, 70b, 71b

Mood disorders (*Cont.*)
  medical evaluation of, 79
  postpartum, 61
  predominant symptom of, 47
  recurrence of
    cycles of, 47–48, 66–67, 66f
    natural history of, 67, 67f
  in school-age child, 440
  screening questions for, 36b
  self-worth in, 47
  stigma of, 46
  suicidal thoughts in, 63–64, 63b
  suicide risk in, 396
Mood disorders treatment, 85–94
  for bipolar disorder, 93–94
  electroconvulsive therapy in, 89–90
  hospitalization in, 85
  pharmacotherapy in, 85–90
    adjunctive, benzodiazepines, 87
    adjunctive, trazodone, 87
    antidepressant agents, 85–87
    for bipolar depression, 87–88
    mood stabilizers for bipolar disorder,
      88–89
    preventive, 89
  principles of, 85
  psychotherapy in, 90–94
    cognitive therapy, 90, 91b
    interpersonal psychotherapy, 90–92
    long-term, 92
    with pharmacotherapy, 92–93
    preventive, 92
    principles, 90
    psychodynamic psychotherapy, 90, 91b
Mood episodes with mixed features, 62
Mood-incongruent psychotic features, 59, 60
Mood reactivity
  in depression, 59
  in major depression, 53
Mood stabilizers, 541–545. *See also*
    Anticonvulsant agents; Lithium; *specific*
    agents
  anticonvulsants as, for suicide risk, 400
  for bipolar disorder, 88–89
  for children and adolescents, 510
  history of, 541–542
  mechanism of action of, 542, 542f
Morality
  in preschoolers, 432–433
  in school-age children, 437
Motivational enhancement therapy, 242b, 247

Motivational interviewing, for substance-related
    and addictive disorders, 242b, 247
Motor activity, increased, in mania, 56
Motor disorders. *See also specific types*
  in children and adolescents, 478
  in infants, 425
Mourning, in parents of adolescents, 442
MRI, 18, 64, 79, 113, 145–146, 154, 284
Multiple-person therapies, 596–605. *See also*
    specific therapies
  concepts of, 596
  family therapy in, 597t, 598–602, 600b–602b
  group therapy in, 597t, 602–605
  interpersonal psychotherapy in, 596–598, 597t,
    599b
Munchausen's syndrome. *See* Factitious disorder
Munchausen's syndrome by Internet, 334
Munchausen's syndrome by proxy, 333–334, 348
Mutism
  in bipolar disorder and major depressive
    disorder, 62
  selective, 435, 474

Nadolol, for aggressive behavior, 415
Naloxone challenge, 250
Naloxone, for opioid use disorder, 250
Naltrexone
  for alcohol use disorder, 249
  for opioid use disorder, 250
  for substance-related disorders, 551f, 552
Narcissistic personality disorder
  course of illness in, 272
  diagnostic and clinical features in, 265–266, 267b
  interview in, 273–282, 279t
Narrow-angle glaucoma, from antipsychotic
    agents, 526
Narrow-band rating scales, 466b
Nefazodone. *See also* Antidepressant agents
Nefazodone, for depression, 536t, 537
Negative automatic thoughts, 90, 193
Negative reinforcement, in substance use, 240
Negatives, pertinent, 5, 12
Neologism, 10t, 11t, 102t, 103
Neuritic plaques, in Alzheimer's disease, 154
Neurocognitive disorders, 129–166. *See also*
    Delirium; Major neurocognitive disorder;
    Mild neurocognitive disorder
  case examples of
    Alzheimer's, 130, 133b
    head trauma, 135b
    life-threatening delirium, 133b

defining feature of, 129
diagnostic and clinical features of, 129–135,
    133b, 135b
  delirium, 130, 133b
  general, 129
  major neurocognitive disorder, 130,
    133–135
  major neurocognitive disorder, Alzheimer's,
    133b
  major neurocognitive disorder, traumatic
    brain injury, 134, 135b
  mild neurocognitive disorder, 133–134
differential diagnosis of, 141–145
  delirium, 142
  delirium, iatrogenic, 142
  medical history in, 141
  mood disorder, 75
  partial complex seizures, 144–145, 145b
  pseudodementia, 142–144, 144b
  specific syndrome and etiology in, 141b, 142
  steps in, 141
  substance-induced disorders, 144
  timeline in, 142
  Wilson's disease, 142, 143b
epidemiology of, 132t
etiology of, 152–156
  delirium, 152–153
  major and mild neurocognitive disorders,
    153–156
interview in, 137–140
  family, 140
  guidelines for, 137–138, 138b
  questions in, 139
  setting in, 139
  therapeutic interventions in, 139–140
medical evaluation in, 145–152
  electroencephalogram in, 146–147, 148b
  laboratory tests in, 146
  mental status testing and neurobehavioral
    assessment in, 147–152, 148b–153b
    (See also Mental status testing)
  neuroimaging in, 146, 147b
  neurological examination in, 146
  physical examination in, 145
  review of systems in, neurological, 145
  sleep studies in, 147
preventative measures for, 166
screening questions for, 37b
treatment of, 159–166
  behavior therapy in, 159–161, 160b, 161b
  family therapy in, 161–163, 162b, 163b

  pharmacotherapy in, 163–166
  psychotherapy in, 159
Neurodevelopmental disorders, child and
    adolescent, 469–477
  autism spectrum disorder, 473–475, 502, 503f
  communication disorders, 471–472
  intellectual disability, 469–471
  vs. schizophrenia, 111
  specific learning disorders, 475–477
Neuroendocrine hypotheses, for mood disorders,
    81
Neurofibrillary tangles, in Alzheimer's disease, 154
Neuroleptic malignant syndrome, 526–527
Neuron functioning, 519, 519f
Neurotransmitter
  hypotheses, for mood disorders, 80–81
  role in mechanism of action, medication, 519f,
    520f, 529f, 542f, 546f, 551f
Nicotine
  replacement, 552
  withdrawal from, 213, 214t
Nicotine use disorder
  diagnostic and clinical features of, 213, 214t
  epidemiology of, 205b
  pharmacotherapy for, 253, 254b
  with schizophrenia, 232–233
Night eating syndrome, 297–298
Nihilistic delusions, in severe depression, 59
NMDA antagonists
  for Alzheimer's disease, 164
  for depression, 81
Nocturnal withdrawal syndrome, alcohol, 177
Nonexploitative treatment, right to, 561b
Nonverbal communication, patient's, 26
Noradrenergic neurons, in locus coeruleus, 190, 191f
Norepinephrine
  in anxiety disorders, 190
  in attention-deficit hyperactivity disorder, 498
  in eating disorders, 312
  in feeding and eating disorders, 312
  in mood disorders, 80, 83
  in neurons, 519f
  in pain, 343
Normal-pressure hydrocephalus, neurocognitive
    disorder from, 156
Nortriptyline, 534t. See also Tricyclic
    antidepressants (TCAs)
Nucleus accumbens, in substance use disorder, 239

Object constancy, 429
Objection to treatment, in mania, 72

Object permanence, in infant development, 422, 423t

Obsession, 11t, 178

Obsessive-compulsive disorder (OCD)
 case example of, 179b
 in children and adolescents, 485–489
  diagnostic and clinical features of, 487–488
  epidemiology of, 486t
  vs. schizophrenia, 503
  school-age child, 440
  tic disorder and, 480
 diagnostic and clinical features of, 178
 differential diagnosis of, 183t, 184–185
 due to another medical condition, 158–159
 eating disorders with, 299
 etiology of, 188–194, 199
  neurobiological, 188–193
  psychosocial, 193–194
 interview for, 181–183, 181b
 medical evaluation in, 187–188
 screening questions for, 37b–38b
 treatment of, 194–197
  cognitive-behavioral therapy in, 199–200
  pharmacotherapy in, 199
  pharmacotherapy principles in, 194–195
  psychotherapy principles in,
   cognitive-behavioral therapy, 195–197
  psychotherapy principles in, psychodynamic, 197

Obsessive-compulsive personality disorder
 course of illness in, 273
 diagnostic and clinical features in, 269, 270b
 interview in, 273–282, 279t

Obstructive sleep apnea
 depressive disorder due to, 147, 148b
 vs. mood disorder, 78

Oculogyric crisis, from antipsychotic agents, 523

Oedipal stage, 432, 432t

Oedipus conflict, 563–565

Olanzapine, 518t. See also Antipsychotic agents
 for bipolar depression, 87

Olanzapine-fluoxetine, for bipolar depression, 87

Old age. See Elderly

Older patients. See Elderly

Olfactory hallucinations, in schizophrenia, 101

Open-ended question, 23b, 27b, 29-30b, 32, 108,
  138b, 139, 460

Operant-behavioral treatment, for neurocognitive
  disorders, 160, 160b

Operant conditioning, 585
 for substance-related disorders, 248

Opioid, 216
 overdoses of, 216, 216t

Opioid use disorder
 diagnostic and clinical features of, 216–217,
  216t–218t
 epidemiology of, 206b
 treatment of
  pharmacotherapy in, 250–252
  in physician, 251b
 withdrawal from, 216–217, 216t–218t
 anxiety disorder in, 177

Opportunistic illnesses, HIV, neurocognitive
  disorders from, 155

Oppositional defiant disorder, 499

OPRM1 gene, 239

Orgasm
 delayed
  from antipsychotic agents, 525
  from MAOIs, 539
  from SSRIs, 532
 in elderly, 452–453
 in female orgasmic disorder, 450

Orientation to time, place, and person,
  148b–149b

Orthostatic hypotension
 from antipsychotic agents, 517t–518t, 521, 522,
  525
 from MAOIs, 538t, 539
 from propranolol, 550t
 from tricyclic antidepressants, 534t, 535

Outreach services, for schizophrenia,
  125–126

Overdose. See also specific agents
 assessment for, 391, 393b

Overeating. See also Feeding and eating
  disorders
 in depression, 60

Overgeneralization, in cognitive-behavioral
  therapy, 593b

Overvalued idea, 11t

Pain, chronic
 classification of, 378
 clinical features of, 378–379
 definition and examples of, 377–378
 psychological aspects of, 377–383
  case example of, 380b–381b
  clinical features of, 378–379
  definition and examples of, 377–378
  interview in, 379–382
  management of, 382–383

Pain disorder. *See* Somatic symptom disorders
Pancreatic carcinoma, depressive disorder from, 136, 136b
Panic attack, 170
Panic disorder
  case examples of, 171b
  diagnostic and clinical features of
    in adults, 170, 171b
    in children and adolescents, 488
  differential diagnosis of, 183t, 184, 341
    hallucinogen use, 218
    mood disorder, 77
  etiology of, 197–198
  medical evaluation in, 187, 188b
  mitral valve prolapse in, 188
  pheochromocytoma in, 136, 137b, 158
  screening questions for, 37b
  from stimulant use, 215
  treatment of
    cognitive-behavioral therapy in, 197–198
    pharmacotherapy in, 197
Panic focused psychodynamic psychotherapy (PFPP), 566t–567t, 584–585
Panicogen, 197
Paradoxical instruction, 601b
Paradoxical reactions, anxiety disorder from, 178
Parallel psychosocial history, 9, 9b
  with medical condition, 370
  for somatic symptom disorders, 338, 338b
Paralysis, leaden, in depression, 59
Paranoia, alcohol-induced, 210
Paranoid ideation, 11t
  from cannabis use, 214
  in mental disorders due to another medical condition, 137
  in schizophrenia, 100
  from stimulant use, 215
Paranoid personality disorder
  course of illness in, 271
  diagnostic and clinical features in, 262, 262b
  interview in, 273–282, 279t
Parenthood, 448–449
Parents
  anger of, about child's treatment, 450, 505–506
  of infants
    in child's response to illness, 426b
    on development, 426–427
  interview with, 458–460, 459f
    child in, 462
  working with, 505–506

Parkinson's disease
  mild depression in, 136
  vs. mood disorder, 75
  mood disorders from, 156–158
  neurocognitive disorder from, 154
Paroxetine, 531t. *See also* Selective serotonin reuptake inhibitors (SSRIs)
Partial complex seizures, *vs.* mental disorders, 144–145, 145b
Past medical history, 6–7, 14b. *See also specific disorders*
  in interview, 35–36
Past psychiatric history, 5, 7b, 14b
  in interview, 35–36
Pathological lying, 332
Patient expectations, 1
Patient perspective, 1
Patient's goals, 20
Pediatric autoimmune neuropsychiatric disorders associated with streptococcus (PANDAS), 199, 480
Pediatric bipolar disorder, 78, 481–482, 483f
Peer support, for schizophrenia, 122–123
Peptide YY, in eating disorders, 313
Perceptual disturbances, 12t. *See also* Hallucinations; Schizophrenia
  in delirium, 130
  in hallucinogen use, 218
Perfectionism, in anorexia nervosa, 301, 304b
Performance specifier, of social anxiety disorder, 172
Persecutory delusions, 59
Perseveration of speech, in major neurocognitive disorder, 130, 133
Persistent depressive disorder. *See* Dysthymic disorder
Personality, 258
Personality change
  due to another medical condition, 136–137, 137b, 158
  from frontal lobe lesions, 159
  from partial complex seizures, 144–145, 145b
Personality disorders, 257–289
  case examples of, 257
  in children and adolescents, 504–505
  common features of, 258–259
  course of illness in, 270–273
    cluster A, 271
    cluster B, 271–273

Personality disorders (*Cont.*)
    cluster C, 273
        general principles of, 270–271
    diagnostic and clinical features in,
        259–269, 260t
        cluster A, 261–263
        cluster B, 263–267
        cluster C, 268–270
        general features and classification of,
        259–261, 260t
    differential diagnosis of, 282–284
        another medical condition, 283
        another psychiatric disorder, 282–283
        comorbid personality disorders, 284
        mood disorder, 77–78
    eating disorders with, 300–301
    etiology of, 284–286
        environment in, 285–286
        neurobiology in, 285
        temperament and environment in,
        284–285
    history taking in, 5, 6b
    interview in, 273–282
        challenges in, 279–280, 280b–282b
        current symptoms in, 274
        disorder-specific key features in, 279t
        interpersonal interaction in, 279–280, 279t
        leisure time in, 278
        open-ended inquiry in, 274
        personality and level of functioning in, 274
        present complaints and history in, 273–274
        psychiatric and medical history in, 274
        relationship evaluation and clarification in,
        274–276, 275b–276b
        self-concept in, 278–280
        use of, 273
        vocational functioning in, 276–278
    medical evaluation of, 284
    prevalence of, 257
    suicide risk in, 396
    treatment of, 286–289
        cognitive-behavioral therapy in, 287–288
        fundamentals of, 286
        group psychotherapy in, 288
        pharmacotherapy in, 288–289
        psychodynamic psychotherapy in, 286–287
        supportive psychotherapy in, 288
Personality style, 258
Personality traits, 258, 362
    medical illness and, 362–367
        aloof, 367

        controlled, 363–364, 364b
        dependent, 363
        fundamentals of, 362–363
        long-suffering, 365
        self-dramatizing, 364–365
        superior, 366–367, 366b
        suspicious, 365–366
Pessimism, 50–51
    in depressive episodes, 59
Pharmacotherapy, 513–553. *See also specific agents
    and disorders*
    adherence in, 514–515
    antidepressant agents in, 528–541
    antipsychotic agents in, 516–528
    anxiolytic medications and hypnotic agents in,
        545–550
    augmentation strategy in, 516
    causal inferences in, 516
    general principles of, 513–516
    history of, 513, 514t
    mood stabilizers in, 541–545
    with psychotherapy, 578b–579b
    for substance-related disorders, 549–553
    switch strategy in, 516
    time frame for, 515–516
Phencyclidine (PCP) use, 217–219, 218t, 219t
Phenelzine. *See also* Monoamine oxidase
    inhibitors (MAOIs)
    dosing of, 538, 538t
    side effects of, 539–540
Phenothiazines, 517t. *See also* Antipsychotic agents
Pheochromocytoma, anxiety disorders in, 136,
    137b, 158
Phobia, 11t
Phobias, specific. *See also* Agoraphobia
    diagnostic and clinical features of
        in adults, 172–173
        in children and adolescents, 488
    differential diagnosis of, 184
    etiology of, 201
    in preschoolers, 435
    social (*See* Social anxiety disorder)
    in toddlers, 430
    treatment of
        cognitive-behavioral therapy in, 202
        pharmacotherapy in, 201
Phobic avoidance, 170
Phobic companion, 171
Photosensitivity, from antipsychotic agents, 526
Physical aggressive phase, 406–407, 407b
Physical dependence, 207–209, 208b

Physical examination, 12, 15b
Physician emotional responses, 26, 27b
Physician reactions, 396, 410,
Physician responses, 71
Physostigmine, 525
Piaget's stages of cognitive development, 419t,
    422, 423t, 424t, 430t, 432t, 436t
Pica
    diagnostic and clinical features of,
        491–492
    differential diagnosis of, 492
    etiology, treatment and prognosis in, 493
Pick's disease, 131t, 134, 155
Pimozide, 517t. *See also* Antipsychotic agents
    for Tourette's disorder, 480
Pinel, Philippe, 559b
Play
    in child interview, 461–462
    imaginative, in preschoolers, 433
    symbolic, 428
Polythetic system, 260
"Poppers," 220, 220t
Positive reinforcement
    for encopresis, 496
    for enuresis, 496
    in substance use, 240
Postpartum mood disorders, 61
Posttraumatic stress disorder (PTSD)
    case example of, 180b
    in children and adolescents, 488
        preschoolers, 435
        vs. schizophrenia, 503
        school-age child, 440
    course of, 180
    diagnostic and clinical features of
        in adults, 178–180
        in children and adolescents, 488
    differential diagnosis of, 185, 503
    etiological issues in, 188–194
    etiology of, 200
    interview for, 181–183, 181b
    medical evaluation in, 187–188
    prevalence of, 179–180
    treatment of, 194–197
        cognitive-behavioral therapy in, 200–201
        pharmacotherapy in, 200
        pharmacotherapy principles in, 194–195
        psychotherapy principles in,
            cognitive-behavioral therapy, 195–197
        psychotherapy principles in,
            psychodynamic, 197

Pragmatic communication disorder, 472
Precipitating factors, 16b–17b, 20
Predisposing factors, 16b–17b, 20
Prefrontal cortex, 80–81, 114, 115f, 116, 159,
    191-192, 191f, 303b, 343, 397, 445, 498,
    555
Pregnancy, unplanned, 448–449
Premature ejaculation, 450
Premenstrual dysphoric disorder, 48f, 54, 529
Preparatory phase, interview, 28–31
    interview setting in, 31
    language in, 31
    safety in, 31
    setting the frame in, 28–30
Preschool child development, 432–435, 432t
    case example of, 434b
    progression of, 432–435
        autonomous self and morality in, 432–433
        imaginative play in, 433
        magical thinking in, 433–434
        sexuality in, 434–435
        vulnerabilities in, 435
Priapism, 536t, 537, 550t
Primary gain, 375b
Prion, 155
Prion disease, 131t, 135, 155
Prison, schizophrenics in, 127
Problem solving, for anxiety disorders, 197
Process, interview
    attention to, 26–28, 27b, 29b–30b
    before content, example of, 33, 33b–35b
    definition of, 27
Process-outcome studies, 592b
Procyclidine, for Parkinson's, 528
Prodromal symptoms, in schizophrenia, 75, 104,
    106, 107f, 121
    in children and adolescents, 502
Prognosis, 18b, 21
Proinflammatory cytokines, in major depression,
    80
Projection, 564b
Projective identification, 564b
Propellant use, 220, 220t
Propranolol
    for aggressive behavior, 415
    for Parkinson's, 528
    for performance anxiety, 549, 550t, 588
    mechanism of action of, 546f
Protect, duty to, 416–417
Protriptyline, 534t. *See also* Tricyclic
    antidepressants (TCAs)

Pseudocyesis, 328
Pseudodementia
    differential diagnosis of, 142–144, 144b
        vs. mood disorder, 75, 142–144, 144b
    in major depression, 52
Pseudoseizures, 490
Psilocybin use
    diagnostic and clinical features of, 217–219,
        218t, 219t
    epidemiology of, 207b
Psychiatric history, past, 5, 7b, 14b
    interviewing for, 35–36
Psychoanalysis, 566t–567t, 570–576
    vs. brief psychodynamic psychotherapy,
        572
    case example of, 571b–572b
    indications and selection criteria in, 570–572
    research on, 591b
    therapeutic process in, 573–576
        clarification in, 573, 574b
        defense analysis in, 563, 564b–565b, 574
        dream analysis in, 575
        free association in, 573
        interpretation in, 574, 574b
        intersubjectivity in, 576
        resistance in, 574–575
        therapeutic neutrality in, 573
        working through in, 575–576
Psychoanalytically oriented group therapy,
    602–605. *See also* Group therapy
Psychoanalytic psychotherapies, 563–585.
    See also specific therapies
    brief psychodynamic psychotherapy,
        566t–567t, 568–570
    defense mechanisms in, 563, 564b–565b, 574
    Freud in, 563
    identification in, 565
    insight in, 565
    long-term, 566t–567t, 576–580
        case example of, with personality disorder,
            576b–577b
        indications and selection criteria in, 576
        therapeutic process in, 579–580
    mentalization based treatment, 287,
        566t–567t, 582–584
    Oedipus conflict in, 563–565
    panic focused psychodynamic psychotherapy,
        566t–567t, 584–585
    with pharmacotherapy, 578b–579b
    psychoanalysis, 566t–567t, 570–576
    repetition compulsion in, 565

transference focused psychotherapy, 287,
    566t–567t, 580–582
    unconscious in, 563
Psychodynamic model, 23
Psychodynamic psychotherapies. *See also specific*
    types and disorders
    for anxiety disorders, 197
    brief, 566t–567t, 568–570
        case example of, 568b–569b
        indications and selection criteria in, 569
        vs. psychoanalysis, 572
        theory and method in, 568–569
        therapeutic process in, 570
    for bulimia nervosa, 320
    for children and adolescents, 507–508
    for mood disorders, 90, 91b
    for obsessive-compulsive disorder, 197
    panic focused, 566t–567t, 584–585
    for personality disorders, 286–287
    for stress disorders, 197
    for suicide risk, 400
Psychodynamic theory, of mood disorders,
    84–85
Psychoeducation. *See also specific disorders*
    for illness anxiety disorder, 348
    for neurocognitive disorders, 161–162,
        162b
    on pharmacotherapy, 514–515
    for schizophrenia, 122
Psychological factors, in medical conditions,
    351–385. *See also specific factors*
    diagnostic features of, 351–352
    psychological aspects of chronic pain in,
        377–383
    psychological reactions to physical illness in,
        352–367
    psychosocial aspects in
        adherence, 383–385
        chronic illness, 371–377
        on medical condition, 367–371
Psychological perspective, 23, 24b–25b
Psychological reactions to physical illness,
    352–367
    anger and agitation in, 360–362, 361t–362t
    anxiety in, 356–358
    denial in, 355–356, 355b
    depression in, 358–360, 359b
    importance of, in healing, 352
    personality traits and medical illness in,
        362–367
        aloof, 367

controlled, 363–364, 364b
dependent, 363
fundamentals of, 362–363
long-suffering, 365
self-dramatizing, 364–365
superior, 366–367, 366b
suspicious, 365–366
regression in, 352–355
clinical features of, 352–354, 353b
interview in, 354, 354b
management of, 354–355, 354b
Psychomotor agitation, 11t
in alcohol and sedative withdrawal, 210t
in children and adolescents, 483t
in delirium, 130
in major depression, 49t, 53, 58
in mania, 56
in phencyclidine use, 218t
in schizophrenia, 103
in stimulant withdrawal, 215t
Psychomotor agitation phase, 404–405, 405b
Psychomotor retardation, 11t
vs. extrapyramidal symptoms, 522–523
in inhalant use, 220t
in major depression, 52–53, 58, 63, 70
in mental disorders due to another medical
condition, 137
in schizophrenia, 103
in stimulant withdrawal, 215t
Psychosis, 19
electroconvulsive therapy for, 553–554
in mood episodes with mixed features, 62
from partial complex seizures, 144
in schizophrenia and other psychotic disorders,
97 (*See also* Schizophrenia)
Psychosocial aspects
of adherence, 383–385
clinical features of, 383–384
interview in, 384
management of, 384–385
of chronic illness, 371–377
case example of, 372b–373b
clinical features of, 371–374
interview in, 374–377
management of, 377
primary and secondary gain in, 375b–376b
Psychosocial development, Erikson's stages of,
419t, 420, 421t
Psychosocial factors affecting medical condition,
367–371
case examples of, 369b, 370b

clinical features of, 367–368
interview in, 368–370, 369b, 370b
management in, 371
Psychosocial history. *See also specific disorders*
in assessment, 7–9
parallel, 9, 9b
sample, 8b
write-up of, 14b–15b
in interview, 30b, 39–40, 44b
parallel, for somatic symptom disorders, 338,
338b
Psychosocial interventions, for children and adolescents, 505–508. *See also specific disorders and therapies*
for attention-deficit hyperactivity disorder,
498–499
for autism spectrum disorders, 475
cognitive-behavioral therapy in, 506–507
for conduct disorder, 501
interpersonal therapy in, 507–508
parents in, working with, 505–506
psychodynamic psychotherapy in, 508
Psychosocial stress, in mood disorders, 67
Psychostimulants. *See also specific types*
for attention-deficit hyperactivity disorder, 498
Psychotherapy, 557–608. *See also specific types and
disorders*
for anorexia nervosa, 318
for bulimia nervosa, 319–320
characteristics of, basic
corrective emotional experience in, 563
countertransference in, 562–563
emotional intensity in, 563
resistance in, 563
transference in, 562
cognitive-behavioral, 558t, 585–596
for conversion disorder, 347
ethics in, 561b
history of, 559b–560b
for mood disorders, 90–94 (*See also under*
Mood disorders)
multiple-person therapies, 558t, 596–605
for neurocognitive disorders, 159
with pharmacotherapy, 578b–579b
psychoanalytic, 558t, 563–585
long-term, 566t–567t, 576–580
psychodynamic (*See* Psychodynamic
psychotherapies)
research on, 590b–592b (*See also* Research,
psychotherapy)
for schizophrenia, 122

Psychotherapy (*Cont.*)
   for substance-related disorders, 247–248
   for suicide risk, 400–401
   supportive, 558t, 605–607
   therapeutic process in, 557–562
     beginning phase of, 557, 560t
     end phase of, 560t, 562
     middle phase in, 560, 560t
Psychosis, 97
Psychotic disorder due to another medical condition
   diagnosis of, 105–106
   differential diagnosis of, 110
Psychotic disorders. *See also* Schizophrenia;
     specific disorders
   alcohol-induced, with hallucinations or
     delusions, 210
   brief psychotic disorder, 105
   in children, 474, 481–482, 501–504
   delusional disorder, 105
   differential diagnosis of, 110–113
     depression, mania, and bipolar disorder, 111
     intellectual disabilities and communication
       disorders, 111
     medical condition, 110, 111b
     neurodevelopmental disorders, 111
     observation in, long-term, 112–113
     substance-induced psychosis, 112, 112b
   due to another medical condition, 105,
     135–136, 135b, 156
   epidemiology of, 98t
   interview in, 108–110, 108b–110b
   medical evaluation of, 113, 113b
   schizoaffective disorder, 104
   schizophreniform disorder, 104
   substance/medication-induced, 106
   suicide risk in, 394
   treatment of, 513
   violent risk in, 403, 415–416
Psychotic features
   in bipolar disorder, 59
   in mania, 59–60
   mood-congruent, 59–60, 60b
   mood-incongruent, 59, 60
   peripartum, 61
Puberty, 107f, 441–442, 443t, 444b
Public mental health system, chronic mental
     illness and, 124b
Purging disorder, 297

Quazepam, 547t. *See also* Benzodiazepines
Quetiapine, 518t. *See also* Antipsychotic agents

for bipolar depression, 88

Racing thoughts, in mania, 63
Rapid cycling, 61
   in bipolar disorder, 61–62, 66–67, 68, 68b
   ultrafast, 62
Rapid eye movement (REM) sleep latency, in
     major depression, 52
Rapprochement crisis, 428
Rashes, from antipsychotic agents, 526
Rating scales. *See also specific types*
   for attention-deficit hyperactivity disorder, 497
   broadband, 466b
   for children and adolescents, 463–465, 466b,
     467b
   for major depression, 53
   narrow-band, 466b
Rationalization, 565b
Rational Recovery, 246–247
Reaction formation, 564b
Reactive attachment disorder, 426, 432
Reading
   impairment in, 475–477
   in school-age children, 437–438
Reality testing, 11t, 19, 33, 44, 97, 108–109, 137,
     159, 456, 468, 577b, 580
Rebound insomnia, with benzodiazepines, 549
Recovery oriented psychosocial treatment for
     schizophrenia, 121–123, 125–126
Reenactment, 565
Reexperiencing, in posttraumatic stress disorder, 179
Reference
   delusions of, 100t, 100b
   ideas of, 11t
Reflective functioning, 582
Regression, 420
   adaptive, 352
   case example of, 353, 353b
   in reaction to medical illness, 352–355
     clinical features of, 352–354, 353b
     interview in, 354, 354b
     management of, 354–355, 354b
Rehearsal, in dialectical behavior therapy, 596
Reinforcement
   positive
     for encopresis, 496
     for enuresis, 496
   in substance use, 240
Relationships. *See also specific disorders*
   in adults, 448–449
   in elderly, 451–452

in interview
    interpersonal, 5, 23
    peer, 8
Relaxation
  learned, 588
  for somatic symptom disorder, 347
Repetition compulsion, 565
Repetitive transcranial magnetic stimulation
    (rTMS), 554–555
Representations, internal, in toddlers, 428–429
Repression, 564b
Research, psychotherapy, 590b–592b
  on cognitive-behavioral therapies, 589,
    590b–591b
  on dialectical behavior therapy, 591b
  on family therapy, 591b
  on interpersonal psychotherapy, 591b
  on long-term psychoanalytic psychotherapy, 591b
  on mentalization based treatment, 591b
  process-outcome studies in, 592b
  on supportive psychotherapy, 591b
  on transference focused psychotherapy, 591b
Residential therapeutic communities, 246–247
Residual symptoms, in schizophrenia, 106, 107f
Resistance
  acting out in, 575
  emotional, 515
  in psychoanalysis, 574–575
  in psychotherapy, 563
Resistant attachment, 421
Respondent conditioning, for substance-related
    and addictive disorders, 248
Responses, conditioned, 585
Retardation, psychomotor, 11t
Reticular activating system, in delirium, 152–153
Retinitis pigmentosa, from thioridazine, 526
Retirement, 451–452
Review of systems, 7, 14b. *See also specific disorders*
  in interview, 36, 36b–39b
  screening questions for, 36, 36b–39b
Reward
  in binge-eating disorder, 299–300, 302b–303b
  in biofeedback, 588
  in cognitive-behavioral therapy in children, 506
  in community reinforcement approach, 247, 248
  dopamine in, 239, 313
  in operant-behavioral treatment, 160
  in operant conditioning, 193, 248, 585
Rigidity
  in anorexia nervosa, 294, 294b
  from antipsychotic agents, 523

in autism spectrum disorders, 489
in depression, 136
in neuroleptic malignant syndrome, 526–527
in Parkinson's disease, 134
personality, 258, 259 (*See also* Personality
    disorders)
from phencyclidine, 218t
in schizophrenia, 103
Risk-taking, in adolescents, 444–445
Risperidone, 475, 480, 510, 518t, 522
Role reversals, 580
Role transition, 598
Rumination disorder
  diagnostic and clinical features of, 492
  differential diagnosis of, 493
  etiology, treatment and prognosis in, 493

Sad feelings, 48, 50–51
Safe drinking guidelines, 228b
Safety
  in interview, 31
  suicide risk and, 388–391
  in violent patient interview, 404–407
    calm phase, 404
    physical aggressive phase, 406–407, 407b
    plan for, 414, 414b
    psychomotor agitation phase, 404–405,
      405b
    verbal aggressive phase, 405–406, 406b
Scatter-site housing, 125
Schema-based therapy, 288
Schizoaffective disorder. *See also* Psychotic
    disorders
  case example of, 111, 112b
  diagnostic and clinical features of, 97, 104
  epidemiology of, 98t
  vs. mood disorder, 76
Schizoid personality disorder
  course of illness in, 262, 263b
  diagnostic and clinical features in, 262, 263b
  interview in, 273–282, 279t
Schizophrenia, adult, 97–117
  case examples of, delusions in, 99, 100b
  definition of, 97
  diagnostic and clinical features of, 97–108
    course in, 106–108, 107f
    diagnosis of, DSM-5, 104
    severity in, 104
    symptoms in, disorganized, 102–103, 102t
    symptoms in, negative, 101–102, 102t
    symptoms in, positive, 98–101, 100t

Schizophrenia, adult (*Cont.*)
    differential diagnosis of, 110–113
        vs. depression, mania, and bipolar disorder,
            111
        vs. hallucinogen use, 219
        vs. intellectual disabilities and
            communication disorders, 111
        vs. medical condition, 110, 111b
        vs. mood disorder, 75–76
        vs. neurodevelopmental disorders, 111
        observation in, long-term, 112–113
        vs. substance-induced psychosis, 112, 112b
    epidemiology of, 98t
    etiology of, 114–117
        neurobiology in, 114–117
        neurobiology in, environmental factors,
            116–117
        neurobiology in, genetic and neurodevelop-
            mental factors, 114–115, 114t
        neurobiology in, neurochemical factors,
            115–116, 115f
        psychosocial factors in, 117
    historical perspectives on, 99b
    interview in, 108–110, 108b–110b
    medical evaluation of, 113, 113b
    ocular smooth pursuit movements in, 115
    psychosis in, 97
    Schneider's first-rank symptoms of, 100
    screening questions for, 36b–37b
    substance use disorder with, 232–233
    suicide risk in, 396
Schizophrenia, child and adolescent, 501–504
    diagnostic and clinical features of, 501–502
    differential diagnosis of, 502–503, 503f
        autism spectrum disorders, 474, 502, 503f
        obsessive-compulsive disorder, 503
        posttraumatic stress disorder, 503
    etiology of, 504
    treatment and prognosis in, 504
Schizophrenia prodrome, 75, 104, 106, 107f, 121
    in children and adolescents, 502
Schizophrenia treatment, 117–127
    electroconvulsive therapy in, 553
    overcoming barriers to, 126–127
        advocacy in, 126
        inpatient and outpatient commitment in,
            126
        jails and prisons in, 127
        physical health comorbidity in, 127
        stigma in, 126
        substance use comorbidity in, 126

pharmacotherapy in, 117–120
    for acute episodes, 118–119
    adherence in, 120
    antipsychotics in, 118
    history of, 117–118
    long-term use of, 119–120
for prodromal and first-episode schizophrenia,
    120–121
psychosocial, 121–123
    cognitive remediation in, 123
    family therapy in, 122
    group therapy in, 122
    individual psychotherapy in, 122
    peer support and self-help groups in,
        122–123
    principles and goals in, 121
    psychoeducation in, 122
    self-management techniques in, 123
    vocational programs in, 123
therapeutic settings in, 123–126
    community-based psychosocial rehabilita-
        tive programs in, 125
    crisis intervention and emergency services
        in, 126
    deinstitutionalization in, 124b
    institutional and residential, hospital,
        123–124
    institutional and residential, housing,
        124–125
    outreach services and case management in,
        125–126
Schizophreniform disorder. *See also* Psychotic
    disorders
    diagnostic and clinical features of, 97, 104
    epidemiology of, 98t
    vs. mood disorder, 77
    pharmacotherapy for acute episodes of,
        118–119
Schizotypal personality disorder. *See also*
    Psychotic disorders
    course of illness in, 263, 263b
    diagnostic and clinical features of, 97, 263,
        263b
    epidemiology of, 98t
    interview in, 273–282, 279t
Schneider's first-rank symptoms of schizophrenia,
    100
School-age child development, 435–441, 436t
    progression of, 435–439
        competence in, acquiring, 435–437
        coping styles and morality in, 437

gender differentiation in, 438
  latency-age child in, 438, 439b, 440b
  reading, writing, and arithmetic in, 437–438
  sexual curiosity and modesty in, 438, 439b
Screening questions, for review of systems, 36, 36b–39b
Seasonal patterns
  of mood disorders, 58, 60–61, 61b, 82
  of schizophrenia birth rates, 116
Secondary gain, 337b, 375b–376b
Second-generation antipsychotic agents (SGAs), 516–519, 517t–518t
Secure attachment, 421
Sedative use disorder
  diagnostic and clinical features of, 209–210, 209t, 210t
  epidemiology of, 206b
  pharmacotherapy for detoxification in, 249–250
  withdrawal symptoms in, 210, 210t
Seizures
  from antipsychotic agents, 526
  partial complex, *vs.* mental disorders, 144–145, 145b
  tricyclic antidepressants on, 535
Selective mutism, 435, 474
Selective serotonin reuptake inhibitors (SSRIs), 530–533, 531t. *See also specific agents*
  for anxiety disorders, 194
    in children and adolescents, 489
    generalized anxiety disorder, 201
    social anxiety disorder, 198
  for anxiety reaction to medical conditions, 356
  for body dysmorphic disorder, 348
  for bulimia nervosa, 320
  for children and adolescents, 508
  for chronic pain, 382
  for depression, 85–86
    in reaction to medical conditions, 359
  dosing of, 530–532, 531t
  drug interactions of, 533
  for illness anxiety disorder, 347–348
  MAOIs and, 540
  for obsessive-compulsive disorder, 199
  for personality disorders, 288–289
  for posttraumatic stress disorder, 200
  side effects of, 531t, 532
  for suicide risk, 399–400
Selegiline. *See also* Monoamine oxidase inhibitors (MAOIs)
  dosing of, 538t, 539
  side effects of, 539–540

Self, autonomous, in preschoolers, 432–433
Self-concept, in personality disorder, 277–279
Self-dramatizing personality traits, 364–365
Self-harm, deliberate nonsuicidal, 387
Self-help groups, for schizophrenia, 122–123
Self-Management and Recovery Training (SMART), 246
Self-management techniques, for schizophrenia, 123
Self-medication hypothesis, of substance use, 240
Self-neglect
  in depression, 52
  in mania, 57
Self-reflection, 449
Sensitization
  in mood disorders, 82–83
  in somatic symptom disorder, 344
Sensory-deprivation hallucinations, 156
Separation anxiety
  in children and adolescents, 485–487
  in toddlers, 428
Separation-individuation
  in adolescents, 442
  in toddlers, 427
Separation, intrapsychic conflicts surrounding, 584
Serotonin
  in anxiety disorders, 190
  in eating disorders, 312–313
  in mood disorders, 80
  on suicide risk, 397
Serotonin-norepinephrine reuptake inhibitors (SNRIs)
  for anxiety disorders, 194
    generalized anxiety disorder, 201
    social anxiety disorder, 198
  for children and adolescents, 508
  for chronic pain, 382
  for depression in reaction to medical illness, 359
Serotonin syndrome, 533, 540
Sertraline, 531t. *See also* Selective serotonin reuptake inhibitors (SSRIs)
  for anxiety disorders, in children and adolescents, 489
  for depression in reaction to medical illness, 360
Setting
  interview, 31
  therapeutic (*See specific disorders and treatments*)

Setting the frame, 28–30
Set word test with word intrusion, 151b
Sexual drive, increased
    in hypomania, 57
    in mania, 56
Sexual dysfunction, 449–450
Sexual function, 449
Sexual interest, decreased
    from antipsychotic agents, 525
    in major depression, 52
Sexuality
    in adolescents, 444
    curiosity and modesty about, in school-age
        children, 438, 439b
    in elderly, 452–453
    infantile, 429
    in preschoolers, 434–435
Sexual trauma, 450
Shame, 70, 70b
Short Michigan Alcoholism Screening Test
    (MSAST), 225
Skills training. See also Cognitive-behavioral
    therapies (CBT)
    for personality disorders, 288
    for substance-related disorders, 248
Skinner, B.F., 585
Sleep abnormalities
    in bipolar disorder, 68
    in depression, 52, 59, 60
    in mania, 56
    from MAOIs, 539
    in mood disorders, 82
    in persistent depressive disorder, 53
Sleep apnea
    vs. mood disorder, 78
    obstructive, depressive disorder due to, 147,
        148b
Sleepiness
    daytime, from MAOIs, 539
    in delirium, 130
Sleep maintenance insomnia, 52
Sleep-onset insomnia, 52
Sleep-related eating disorders, 298
Smoking cessation, 253, 254b
Social anxiety disorder
    behavior therapy for, 587b
    case example of, 172b
    diagnostic and clinical features of
        in adults, 172–173
        in children and adolescents, 488
    differential diagnosis of, 183t, 184

etiology of, 198
screening questions for, 37b
treatment of
    cognitive-behavioral therapy in, 198–199
    pharmacotherapy in, 198
Social communication disorder, 472
Social factors, in treatment plan, 20–21
Social learning, for neurocognitive disorders,
    160–161
Social phobia. See Social anxiety disorder
Social referencing, 420–421
Social smile, 421
Solvent use, volatile, 220, 220t
Somatic management, for anxiety disorders, 195
Somatic symptom disorders, 323–349
    in children and adolescents, 489–491
    course of illness in, 334–336, 335t
        factitious disorders, 335t, 336
        somatic symptom and related disorders,
            334–336, 335t
    diagnostic and clinical features of, 323–334,
        324f, 324t, 325t
        ambiguous physical symptoms, 324–325
        body dysmorphic disorder, 325t, 329–330,
            330b
        classification of, 323–324, 324f, 324t
        dissociative subtype, 325t, 326–328, 327b
        factitious disorder, 330–333, 331t, 332b,
            333b, 334b
        factitious disorder imposed on another,
            333–334
        factitious disorder, virtual, 334
        obsessional cognitive subtype, 325t,
            328, 329b
        somatic/sensory subtype, 325–326, 325t
    differential diagnosis of
        conversion disorder, 340
        factitious disorder, 341, 341b
        unrecognized illness, 340, 340t
    etiology of, 343–346, 344f
        body dysmorphic disorder, 345
        conversion disorder, 344–345
        factitious disorder, 345–346
        illness anxiety disorder, 345
    fundamentals of, 323
    interview in, 337–339
        factitious disorder, 39b, 338–339
        guidelines for, 337b
        parallel psychosocial history in, 338, 338b
        somatic symptom and related disorders,
            337–338

medical evaluation in, 342–343
treatment of, 346–349
    body dysmorphic disorder, 348
    conversion disorder, 347
    factitious disorder, 348–349
    general guidelines for, 346
    illness anxiety disorder, 347–348
    somatic symptom disorder, 346–347
Somatic symptom disorder with predominant
        pain, in children and adolescents,
        489–491
Somatization, 584
Somatization disorder. *See* Somatic symptom
        disorders
Somatoform disorders. *See* Somatic symptom
        disorders
Somatosensory amplification, 491
Specific learning disorders, 475–477
Specific phobias. *See also* Agoraphobia
    diagnostic and clinical features of
        in adults, 172–173
        in children and adolescents, 488
    differential diagnosis of, 184
    etiology of, 201
    in preschoolers, 435
    social (*See* Social anxiety disorder)
    in toddlers, 430
    treatment of
        cognitive-behavioral therapy in, 202
        pharmacotherapy in, 201
Speech. *See also* Communication disorders;
        specific disorders
    in alcohol and sedative use disorders, 209t, 235t
    in bipolar disorder, 68, 72
    in brief psychotic disorder, 105
    in depression, 52
    in histrionic personality disorder, 265
    in infants, 424t, 425, 425b
    in inhalant use, 220t
    interview, 26
    in mania, 56
    in mental status examination, 9, 10t, 11t, 15b,
        464b
    in neurocognitive disorders, 138, 139, 143b
    in opioid use, 216t
    perseveration of, 130–131
    in schizophrenia, 102t
        childhood-onset, 503f
    in schizotypal personality disorder, 263
    in stimulant use, 215
    in tic disorders, 478–479

Speech sound disorder, 471–472
Splitting, 564b
Standardized outcome measures, for cognitive
        assessment, 152b
Statins, 158
Starvation, in anorexia nervosa, 299
Status quo, emotional, 574
Stereotypic movement disorder, 478
Steroid use disorder, 219, 220t
Stevens-Johnson syndrome
    from antipsychotic agents, 526
    from lamotrigine, 545
Stigma
    of mood disorders, 46
    of schizophrenia, 126
Stimulants. *See also specific types*
    for children and adolescents, 509
Stimulant use disorder
    anxiety disorder from, 176, 176b
    diagnostic and clinical features of, 214–216, 215t
    epidemiology of, 206b
    life-threatening effects of, 216
    withdrawal from, 215–216, 215t
Story-telling, in child interview, 461
Stranger anxiety, 422–423
Strange situation paradigm, 421–422, 422b
Strategic family therapy, 163
Strengths, 20
Stress disorders
    in children and adolescents, 485–489, 487t
    diagnostic and clinical features of, 180–181
    etiological issues in, 188–194
    interview for, 181–183, 181b
    medical evaluation in, 187–188
    screening questions for, 38b
    treatment of, 194–197
        pharmacotherapy principles in, 194–195
        psychotherapy principles in,
            cognitive-behavioral therapy, 195–197
        psychotherapy principles in,
            psychodynamic, 197
Stress, on development, 420
Stress, psychological, in hospitalized patients,
        352–353
Stress, psychosocial
    on medical conditions, 367–371
        case examples of, 369b, 370, 370b
        clinical features of, 367–368
        interview in, 368–370, 369b, 370b
        management in, 371
    in mood disorders, 67

Stress response system, HPA axis in, 191
Stress tolerance, 594
Stroke, mood disorders from, 156–158
Structural family therapy, 162–163, 162b
Structured approaches, series of, 592–594
Stupor
    in alcohol and sedative use, 209t
    in bipolar disorder and major depressive
        disorders, 62
    in dissociative fugue, 186b
    in inhalant use, 220t
    in schizophrenia, 99b, 102t
Stuttering, 472
Subjective Units of Distress (SUDS) scale, 196
Substance-induced psychosis
    case example of, 112b
    vs. schizophrenia, 112, 112b
Substance/medication-induced anxiety disorder
    diagnostic and clinical features of, 174–178,
        175t
        alcohol withdrawal, 176–177
        benzodiazepine and barbiturate withdrawal,
            177
        caffeinism, 176, 176b
        opioid withdrawal, 177
        paradoxical reactions, 178
        stimulant intoxication, 176, 176b
    differential diagnosis of, 187
    etiology of, 202
Substance/medication-induced psychotic
    disorder, 106
Substance-related and addictive disorders,
    204–241
    aggression and violence with, 412
    course of illness in, 220–223
        addiction in, 223, 223t
        with alcohol, 221
        general features of, 220–221
        with recreational drugs, 221–223
    diagnostic and clinical features of, 204–220
        alcohol and other sedatives, 209–210,
            209t–213t
        anabolic-androgenic steroids, 219, 220t
        cannabis, 213–214, 214t
        DMS-5, 204
        hallucinogens, 217–219, 218t, 219t
        inhalants, 220, 220t
        intoxication, 209
        methamphetamine, 208b
        nicotine, 213, 214t
        opioids, 216–217, 216t–218t

psychiatric symptoms, 209
        stimulants, 214–216, 215t
        substance-induced disorders, 209–220
            (See also Substance-induced disorders)
        substance use disorders, 207–209
    differential diagnosis of, 144, 232–233
        vs. mood disorder, 77
    epidemiology of, 205b–207b
        alcohol, 205b
        cocaine, 205b–206b
        hallucinogens, 207b
        heroin, 207b
        inhalants, 207b
        marijuana, 205b
        methamphetamine, 206b–207b
        opioid pain relievers, 206b
        sedatives, 206b
        stimulants, 206b
        tobacco, 205b
    etiology of, 238–241
        neurobiological, genetic, 238–239
        neurobiological, neuroendocrine, 239
        neurobiological, neurotransmitters, 239
        psychological, 239–240
        social, 240–241
    interview in, 223–232
        CAGE screening instrument in, 225, 225t
        in children and adolescents, 230, 230t, 231b
        in elderly, 232
        evaluation guidelines in, 223, 224b
        family, social, and legal histories in, 225–226
        history timeline in, 226, 227f
        patient engagement in, 228–230, 290b
        patient reliability assessment in, 226–228
        screening tests in, 225
        substance use history in, 223, 224b
    vs. medical condition, 360
    medical evaluation of, 137t, 233–238,
        234t–235t
        general approach in, 233–236, 234t–235t
        laboratory tests in, alcohol-related disorders,
            236
        laboratory tests in, drug-related disorders,
            236–238, 237t
    pharmacotherapy for, 549–553 (See also specific
        agents)
        acamprosate, 249, 551f, 552
        buprenorphine, 252, 551f, 552–553
        bupropion, 253, 551, 551f
        disulfiram, 249, 551, 551f
        mechanism of action of, 551

methadone, 250, 551f, 552
naltrexone, 249–250, 251b, 551f, 552
nicotine, 253, 552
varenicline, 253, 551f, 552
prevalence of, 204
with psychiatric co-morbidities, 232–233
bipolar disorder, 233
depression, 233
schizophrenia, 232–233
suicide risk in, 396
Substance-related and addictive disorder
treatment, 241–254
12-step treatment in, 245, 245t, 246
harm reduction model in, 241–242
for opioid-addicted physician, 251b
pharmacotherapy in, 248–253, 549–553
for alcohol, 249
for cannabis, 253
for cocaine, 252
detoxification from alcohol and sedatives in,
249–250
for nicotine, 253, 254b
for opioids, 250–252
principles of, 248–249
psychotherapy in, 247–248
recovery in, 241–243, 242b
smoking cessation in, 254b
therapeutic settings in, 243–247
general points on, 243–245
inpatient and residential chemical
dependence programs in, 245–246
outpatient, 246
residential therapeutic communities in,
246–247
transtheoretical model of, 242, 242b
Substance use disorders, 207–209
addiction in, 208–209, 223, 223t
definition of, 207
eating disorders with, 299–300
physical dependence in, 207–209, 208b
with schizophrenia, 126
screening questions for, 38b
tolerance in, 207
withdrawal in, 207
Suffocation alarm mechanism, 197
Suicidal behavior, risk assessment for, 394
Suicidal ideation, 387
risk assessment for, 391–394
Suicidal intent, 387
Suicidality, chronic, 401
Suicidal thoughts, in major depression, 71–72, 71f

Suicide (risk), 387–401
in case summary, 19
characteristics of high-risk individuals, 390b
clinical features of, 387–388
differential diagnosis of, 396
epidemiology of, 387, 388b
etiology of, 397
interview for, 388–396
collateral information in, 391, 393b
history taking in, 391, 392b, 393b
overdose assessment in, 391, 393b
physician reactions in, 396
risk assessment in, 389b, 391–395
risk assessment in, family history in, 395
risk assessment in, psychiatric psychosocial
history in, 394–395, 395b
risk assessment in, psychiatric symptoms
and diagnoses in, 394
risk assessment in, suicidal behavior in, 394
risk assessment in, suicidal ideation in, 391–394
safety in, 388–391
sample questions and tips in, 391, 392b
screening in, 388, 389b, 390b
legal issues in
confidentiality in, 401
involuntary commitment in, 401
lethality, 387, 391, 392b
in mood episodes, 63–64, 63b
screening questions for, 38b–39b
treatment of, 397–401
electroconvulsive therapy in, 400
motivation for, 397
pharmacotherapy in, 399–400
psychotherapy in, 400–401
therapeutic settings in, hospital, 398, 399b
therapeutic settings in, outpatient, 398
Suicide attempt, 387
Sullivan, Harry Stack, 596
Sundowning, 148b
Superego, 573
Superior personality traits, 366–367, 366b
Supportive groups, 605
Supportive housing, 125
Supportive psychotherapies, 605–607
crisis intervention in, 605–606
for ego deficits, 607
for medical illness, 606–607
origins and theory of, 605
for personality disorders, 288
research on, 591b
Suppression, 564b–565b

Suspicious personality traits, 365–366
Switch strategies, 516
  for antidepressants, 541
  for antipsychotics, 516
  for monoamine oxidase inhibitors, 541
Symbolic thought, in toddlers, 428
Sympathetic nervous system overactivity, in
    anxiety disorder, 174
Synaptic pruning, 445
Synesthesia, from hallucinogens, 218
Systematic desensitization, 588

Tactile hallucinations, in schizophrenia, 101
Tangential thought process, 11t
Tarasoff decisions, 416–417
Tardive dyskinesia, from antipsychotic agents, 87,
    516, 524, 541
Tardive dystonia, from antipsychotic agents, 360
Telephone consultation, 596
Temazepam, 547t. *See also* Benzodiazepines
Temperament, 419
Temper tantrums
  in major depressive disorder, 483
  in toddlers, 428
Terminal insomnia, 546
  in major depression, 52, 58
Testosterone, 219
Testosterone use disorder, 219, 220t
Tests, laboratory, 16b, 18. *See also specific disorders*
Tetrahydrocannibinol (THC), 213–214, 214t
Therapeutic alliance, 26. *See also specific disorders*
    and treatments
  for adherence, 385
  with bipolar patients, 73, 73b
  in eating disorders, 306
  interview in, first, 30, 30b
  with personality disorders, 287
  in suicide risk, 400
Therapeutic neutrality, 573
Therapeutic process, psychoanalytic, 573–576
  clarification in, 573, 574b
  defense analysis in, 563, 564b–565b, 574
  dream analysis in, 575
  free association in, 573
  interpretation in, 574, 574b
  intersubjectivity in, 576
  resistance in, 574–575
  therapeutic neutrality in, 573
  working through in, 575–576
Thiamine deficiency, neurocognitive disorder
    from, 156

Thioxanthenes, 517t. *See also* Antipsychotic
    agents
Thought
  abstract, in adolescents, 443
  automatic, 90
    negative, in anxiety disorders, 193
  circumstantial process of, 11t
  disorganized, in mania, 56
  disturbances of, in schizophrenia, 102–103,
    102t
  magical, in preschoolers, 433–434
  pathological patterns of, 592
  racing, in mania, 63
  symbolic, in toddlers, 428
  tangential process of, 11t
Thought blocking, in schizophrenia, 102t,
    103
Thought broadcasting, 100
Thought content, 11t
Thought insertion, 100
Thought process, 11t
Thought withdrawal, 100
Three-item verbal recall, 149b
Thyroid hormone, for depression, 86
Tic disorders
  in children and adolescents, 478–480
  in school-age child, 441
Tics, 478–479
Time-limited structure, 570
Tobacco use. *See* Nicotine use disorder
Toddler development, 427–432, 430t
  case example of, 431b
  progression of
    ambivalence in, 428
    autonomy in, 427
    decentering and symbolic thought in, 428
    gender identity in, 429
    internal representations in, 428–429
  vulnerabilities in
    psychopathology in, 430–432, 431b
    transient symptoms in, 429–430
Tolerance. *See also* Substance-related and
    addictive disorders; *specific drugs*
  to benzodiazepines, 548
  stress, 594
  in substance use disorders, 207
TOP interpretation, 570
Topirimate, 249
Torticollis, from antipsychotic agents, 523
Tourette's disorder, 479
Traits, personality. *See* Personality traits

Transcranial magnetic stimulation (TMS), 554–555

Transference, 562
  in family therapy, 602
  in psychoanalysis, 574

Transference focused psychotherapy (TFP), 287, 566t–567t, 580–582
  case example of, 581b–582b
  indications and selection criteria in, 580
  research on, 591b
  therapeutic process in, 580, 582

Trans-institutionalization, 127

Transitional object, 429

Translator, for interview, 31

Transtheoretical model, 242, 242b

Tranylcypromine. *See also* Monoamine oxidase inhibitors (MAOIs)
  dosing of, 538t, 539
  side effects of, 539–540

Trauma
  on development, 420
  head
    aggression from, 159
    disinhibition from, 159
    major neurocognitive disorder from, 155–156
    neurocognitive disorder from, 135b
  posttraumatic stress disorder from (*See* Posttraumatic stress disorder (PTSD))
  sexual, 450

Traumatic brain injury (TBI)
  on development, 420
  neurocognitive disorder from, 131t, 134, 135, 155–156

Trazodone, 550t
  for depression, 87, 535–537, 536t (*See also* Antidepressant agents)

Treatment. *See also specific disorders and treatments*
  objection to, in mania, 72

Treatment plan, 17b–18b, 20–21

Tremor. *See also* Parkinson's disease
  in alcohol withdrawal, 176, 210, 210t, 211t, 360
  from antipsychotic agents, 102, 522
  in anxiety disorders, 169b, 174
  from hyperthyroidism, 157
  in inhalant use, 220t
  from lithium, 543
  in opioid withdrawal, 177, 217t
  propranolol for, 528, 549

Triadic relationships, in preschoolers, 432

Trial interpretation, 569

Triazolam, 547t. *See also* Benzodiazepines

Tricyclic antidepressants (TCAs), 533–535
  for bulimia nervosa, 320
  for children and adolescents, 509
  for chronic pain, 382
  for depression, 80, 85–86
  dosing of, 534–535, 534t
  history of, 533–534
  side effects of, 534t, 535

Trihexyphenidyl, for Parkinson's, 528

Trimipramine, 534t. *See also* Tricyclic antidepressants (TCAs)

Trust, basic, 420

Tryptophan depletion, 80

Tumor necrosis factor alpha (TNFα), in major depression, 80

12-step program
  for binge-eating disorder, 321
  for substance use disorders, 245, 245t, 246

Tyramine-free diet, 540

Ultrafast rapid cycling, 62

Unconscious, 563

Unconscious conflicts, 563

Unipolar depression, 54

Valproate, 544–545
  for bipolar disorder, 89
  for children and adolescents, 510

Varenicline
  for smoking cessation, 253, 552
  for substance-related disorders, 551f, 552

Vascular depression, 64

Vascular disease, neurocognitive disorder from, 131t, 154

Vegetative signs and symptoms, in major depression, 51–52

Velocardiofacial syndrome, schizophrenia with, 114

Venlafaxine
  for children and adolescents, 508
  for depression, 535–537, 536t (*See also* Antidepressant agents)
  for social anxiety disorder, 198

Ventral tegmental area, in substance use, 239

Verbal aggressive phase, 405–406, 406b

Verbal communication, patient, 26

Vilazodone, 531t. *See also* Selective serotonin reuptake inhibitors (SSRIs)

Violence, 403–417
  clinical features of, 403–404
  etiology in, 412–413
  interview in, 404–410
    history in, 407–410
    history in, guidelines for, 407, 408b
    history in, interview questions in, 407, 409b
    history in, past, 409–410
    history in, psychosocial, 410
    history in, recent, 408–409
    physician reactions in, 410
    safety in, 404–407
    safety in, calm phase, 404
    safety in, physical aggressive phase,
      406–407, 407b
    safety in, psychomotor agitation phase,
      404–405, 405b
    safety in, verbal aggressive phase, 405–406,
      406b
  prevalence of, 403
  risk assessment in, 410–412
  treatment of, 413–417, 414b
    crisis formulation in, 413
    legal issues in, confidentiality, 416–417
    legal issues in, duty to warn and duty to
      protect, 416–417
    legal issues in, involuntary commitment,
      416
    pharmacotherapy in, 415–416
    psychotherapy in, 416
    therapeutic settings in, choice, 413
    therapeutic settings in, hospital, 413–414,
      414b
    therapeutic settings in, outpatient, 414–415
    therapeutic settings in, postdischarge pre-
      vention safety plan in, 414, 414b
Visual and tactile recall, 149b–150b
Visual hallucinations, in schizophrenia, 100t, 101

Vitamin B complexes, for Alzheimer's disease,
  164
Vitamin E, for Alzheimer's disease, 164
Vocational programs, for schizophrenia, 123
Volatile solvent use, 220, 220t
Volition, loss of, in schizophrenia, 102, 102t
Vorbeireden, 339
Vulnerabilities, 20

Warn, duty to, 416–417
Waxy flexibility, in schizophrenia, 103
Weight gain
  from antipsychotic agents, 522
  from hydrazines, 539–540
  from tricyclic antidepressants, 535
Weight loss
  in anorexia nervosa, 292
  in major depression, 58
  from SSRIs, 532
Weissman, Myrna, 596
Wilson's disease, 142, 143b
Winicott's squiggles, 461–462
Withdrawal. See also specific types
  vs. medical condition, 360
  in substance use disorders, 207, 209
Word intrusion, 151b
Word salad, 11t, 103
Work
  failure in, 447–448, 448b
  gratification in, 445–447
Working through, 575–576
Write-up, case, 1–2, 2f, 3t, 12, 13b–18b
Writing, in school-age children, 437–438
Written expression, impairment in, 475–477

Ziprasidone, 518t. See also Antipsychotic agents
  for Tourette's disorder, 480
Zolpidem, 550t